Master Techniques in Orthopaedic Surgery

Knee Arthroplasty

Third Edition

Master Techniques in Orthopaedic Surgery

Editor-in-Chief
Bernard F. Morrey, MD

Founding Editor
Roby C. Thompson, Jr., MD

Relevant Surgical Exposures
Bernard F. Morrey, MD
Matthew C. Morrey, MD

Peripheral Nerve Surgery
Robert J. Spinner, MD

Reconstructive Knee Surgery
Douglas W. Jackson, MD

The Hand
James Strickland, MD
Thomas Graham, MD

Soft Tissue Surgery
Steven L. Moran, MD
William P. Cooney III, MD

Pediatrics
Vernon T. Tolo, MD
David L. Skaggs, MD

The Foot and Ankle
Harold B. Kitaoka, MD

The Hip
Robert L. Barrack, MD

The Spine
David S. Bradford, MD
Thomas A. Zdeblick, MD

The Shoulder
Edward V. Craig, MD

The Elbow
Bernard F. Morrey, MD

The Wrist
Richard H. Gelberman, MD

Fractures
Donald A. Wiss, MD

Master Techniques in Orthopaedic Surgery

Knee Arthroplasty

Third Edition

Editors

Paul A. Lotke MD
Professor Emeritus, Orthopaedic Surgery
University of Pennsylvania School of Medicine
Philadelphia, PA

Jess H. Lonner, MD
Director, Knee Replacement Surgery
Booth, Bartolozzi, Balderston Orthopaedics
Pennsylvania Hospital
Director, Philadelphia Center for Minimally Invasive Knee Surgery
Philadelphia, PA

Illustrator

Caspar Henselmann
New York, New York

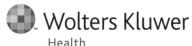
Wolters Kluwer
Health

Lippincott
Williams & Wilkins

Acquisitions Editor: Robert A. Hurley
Managing Editor: David Murphy
Marketing Manager: Sharon Zinner
Production Editor: John Larkin
Designer: Teresa Mallon
Compositor: Maryland Composition/ASI

Third Edition

Copyright © 2009 Lippincott Williams & Wilkins, a Wolters Kluwer business

351 West Camden Street   530 Walnut Street
Baltimore, MD 21201   Philadelphia, PA 19106

Printed in China

9 8 7 6 5 4 3 2

Library of Congress Cataloging-in-Publication Data

Knee arthroplasty / [edited by] Paul A. Lotke. -- 3rd ed.
     p. ; cm. -- (Master techniques in orthopaedic surgery)
  Includes bibliographical references and index.
  ISBN 978-0-7817-7922-7
  1. Knee--Surgery. 2. Total knee replacement. 3. Total knee replacement--Reoperation. I. Lotke, Paul A. II. Series.
  [DNLM: 1. Arthroplasty, Replacement, Knee--methods--Atlases. 2. Knee--surgery--Atlases. 3. Postoperative Complications--prevention & control--Atlases. 4. Reoperation--methods--Atlases. WE 17 K68 2009]
  RD561.K573 2009
  617.5'82059--dc22

                                2008043857

DISCLAIMER

Care has been taken to confirm the accuracy of the information present and to describe generally accepted practices. However, the authors, editors, and publisher are not responsible for errors or omissions or for any consequences from application of the information in this book and make no warranty, expressed or implied, with respect to the currency, completeness, or accuracy of the contents of the publication. Application of this information in a particular situation remains the professional responsibility of the practitioner; the clinical treatments described and recommended may not be considered absolute and universal recommendations.

The authors, editors, and publisher have exerted every effort to ensure that drug selection and dosage set forth in this text are in accordance with the current recommendations and practice at the time of publication. However, in view of ongoing research, changes in government regulations, and the constant flow of information relating to drug therapy and drug reactions, the reader is urged to check the package insert for each drug for any change in indications and dosage and for added warnings and precautions. This is particularly important when the recommended agent is a new or infrequently employed drug.

Some drugs and medical devices presented in this publication have Food and Drug Administration (FDA) clearance for limited use in restricted research settings. It is the responsibility of the health care provider to ascertain the FDA status of each drug or device planned for use in their clinical practice.

To purchase additional copies of this book, call our customer service department at **(800) 638-3030** or fax orders to **(301) 223-2320**. International customers should call **(301) 223-2300**.

Visit Lippincott Williams & Wilkins on the Internet: **http://www.lww.com.** Lippincott Williams & Wilkins customer service representatives are available from 8:30 am to 6:00 pm, EST.

To my wife, Ami, and our children, Carson and Jared.
To my mentors and peers, past and present, that have taught me
to appreciate the science and nuance of knee surgery and
encouraged and challenged me to teach the same.

Jess H. Lonner, MD

To my wife, Dorothy-Sue, and my children, Michael, Eric, and
Pam, who have accepted and supported the time consuming
lifestyle of an orthopaedic surgeon.

Paul A. Lotke, MD

Contents

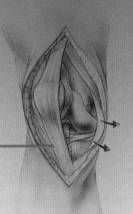

PART VI   Alternatives to Total Knee Arthroplasty   311

Series Preface

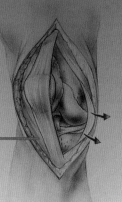

Since its inception in 1994, the *Master Techniques in Orthopaedic Surgery* series has become the gold standard for both physicians in training and experienced surgeons. Its exceptional success may be traced to the leadership of the original series editor, Roby Thompson, whose clarity of thought and focused vision sought "to provide direct, detailed access to techniques preferred by orthopaedic surgeons who are recognized by their colleagues as 'masters' in their specialty," as he stated in his series preface. It is personally very rewarding to hear testimonials from both residents and practicing orthopaedic surgeons on the value of these volumes to their training and practice.

A key element of the success of the series is its format. The effectiveness of the format is reflected by the fact that it is now being replicated by others. An essential feature is the standardized presentation of information replete with tips and pearls shared by experts with years of experience. Abundant color photographs and drawings guide the reader through the procedures step-by-step.

The second key to the success of the *Master Techniques* series rests in the reputation and experience of our volume editors. The editors are truly dedicated "masters" with a commitment to share their rich experience through these texts. We feel a great debt of gratitude to them and a real responsibility to maintain and enhance the reputation of the *Master Techniques* series that has developed over the years. We are proud of the progress made in formulating the third edition volumes and are particularly pleased with the expanded content of this series. Six new volumes will soon be available covering topics that are exciting and relevant to a broad cross-section of our profession. While we are in the process of carefully expanding *Master Techniques* topics and editors, we are committed to the now-classic format.

The first of the new volumes is *Relevant Surgical Exposures*, which I have had the honor of editing. The second new volume is *Essential Procedures in Pediatrics*. Subsequent new topics to be introduced are *Soft Tissue Reconstruction*, *Management of Peripheral Nerve Dysfunction*, *Advanced Reconstructive Techniques in the Joint*, and finally *Essential Procedures in Sports Medicine*. The full library thus will consist of 16 useful and relevant titles.

I am pleased to have accepted the position of series editor, feeling so strongly about the value of this series to educate the orthopaedic surgeon in the full array of expert surgical procedures. The true worth of this endeavor will continue to be measured by the ever-increasing success and critical acceptance of the series. I remain indebted to Dr. Thompson for his inaugural vision and leadership, as well as to the *Master Techniques* volume editors and numerous contributors who have been true to the series style and vision. As I indicated in the preface to the second edition of *The Hip* volume, the words of William Mayo are especially relevant to characterize the ultimate goal of this endeavor: "The best interest of the patient is the only interest to be considered." We are confident that the information in the expanded *Master Techniques* offers the surgeon an opportunity to realize the patient-centric view of our surgical practice.

Bernard F. Morrey, MD

Preface

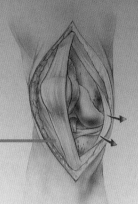

We've learned a great deal over the past three decades with regards to techniques and technologies related to knee arthroplasty. Innovative approaches to total and partial knee arthroplasty continue to evolve, even though many critical principles remain the same. Providing the optimal care for our patients requires a balance between an understanding of the basic principles and scientific basis of knee replacement surgery and a proficiency in the skills needed to master the performance of the surgery and deal with its complications. The intent of this textbook is to expose the reader to the preferred techniques and procedures of a number of highly skilled knee surgeons of our time and to convey some of the nuances of clinical decision making and surgery that make primary and revision knee replacement surgery part science, part art.

This textbook provides a "how to" approach to both basic and complex issues that we commonly deal with either routinely or infrequently in the surgical management of knee arthritis. It is not a comprehensive text that delves into theory and the scientific basis of treatment. In essence, it cuts to the point. The chapters have been written by a number of leading authorities in knee arthroplasty—recognized as "Masters" in the field. These authors were asked to contribute to this textbook, not only because of their acknowledged reputations in the field but also because they continue to better themselves and advance the care of their patients by learning from their own and others experiences. These master surgeons present their preferred solutions to a variety of clinical situations or problems that we encounter in the care of patients with arthritis of the knee or complications related to knee arthroplasty. Several of these authors have contributed to the first two editions of this text. Since 2003, when the 2nd edition of *Master Techniques in Orthopaedic Surgery: Knee Arthroplasty* was published, many principles have stayed the same, but numerous approaches, techniques, technologies, and management strategies have evolved. It is clear in this book that the contributors have not stagnated; the chapters are a clear endorsement of the changes that we've seen in the early part of the millennium. Surgical techniques presented in this edition may be different than those presented in earlier editions. We have asked the contributors not to exhaust the breadth and variety of treatment options that might be applied for a particular condition, but rather to focus on their preferred techniques. That has helped sharpen the focus of the chapters and avoid extraneous material. In essence this textbook is a "traveling fellowship" that gives us a glimpse into the operating rooms of a number of masterful surgeons who have honed their skills over a period of time to optimize the care of patients with knee arthritis.

The textbook is organized into sections which have been reformatted from earlier editions. The first part deals with surgical approaches to the knee, including traditional extensile approaches and newer minimally invasive approaches to knee arthroplasty. Clearly the latter has gained momentum since the last iteration, although minimally invasive surgery has not been adopted by all surgeons for all procedures. The details of those surgical approaches to the knee are invaluable for surgeons at all levels of experience. Regardless of what particular approach is selected, the tenets of exposure are the same—namely gaining access to the knee safely without compromising the soft tissues, bone preparation, or visualization of the joint and to allow accurate implantation of the knee arthroplasty without compromising the outcome.

The second part is devoted to basic but essential principles of primary total knee arthroplasty, whether using posterior stabilized or posterior cruciate retaining designs and measured resection or a balanced gap technique for bone preparation. This section reviews the most fundamental tenets of knee replacement surgery including bone preparation, ligament balancing, component alignment, and sizing, among others.

Part three addresses the role of computer navigation for total knee arthroplasty. This topic has gained some momentum since the last edition of this textbook, although while it has been tried by many, it has not yet been embraced by all users as a routine part of knee arthroplasty in its current form. Further evolution in computer assisted knee arthroplasty surgery will likely lead to greater utility and relevance.

Part four deals with complex issues with which we are frequently confronted in primary total knee arthroplasty such as severe fixed coronal deformity, recurvatum, extra- articular deformity, pre-operative stiffness, collateral ligament insufficiency, and patellar problems such as baja, deficiency and malalignment. These difficult scenarios require more than a cook book approach to knee arthroplasty; and "muscle memory" alone is not enough to get through these difficult cases. The chapters will provide effective strategies for dealing with these conditions effectively so that outcomes can be optimized.

The fifth part deals with revision of the failed total knee arthroplasty, which challenge us even as techniques improve and methods for dealing with bone and ligament loss become more sophisticated. It is our hope that the explicit details provided in these chapters will make even the most complicated revisions manageable for those willing to take them on. Critical elements of revision knee arthroplasty, including removing well-fixed implants, prosthesis selection (based on necessary degree of constraint), dealing with bone and ligament deficiencies with a variety of techniques, and implanting the revision knee prosthesis are presented.

The sixth part is an affirmation that we continue to strive for less invasive and more conservative approaches for patients with arthritis localized to one compartment of the knee. Techniques and technologies continue to evolve in the area of limited resurfacing, and this section will address conventional and robotic-arm assisted unicompartmental arthroplasty and patellofemoral arthroplasty. Additionally, while distal femoral and proximal tibial osteotomies have been losing their luster amongst arthroplasty surgeons over the past few years, they remain valuable and viable options for younger patients with unicompartmental arthritis, particularly as biological resurfacing evolves over time.

The final part deals with the management of complications, which unfortunately continue to plague a relatively small percentage of knees after arthroplasty. It deals with management of periprosthetic fractures, extensor mechanism disruption, stiff total knees, wound problems, and infection. Ultimately fewer tertiary centers may be willing to accept complications from external sites, making it critical that surgeons feel comfortable managing their own complications.

The intricate step-wise details presented by the authors who have contributed to this text will enlighten and inform both the casual knee arthroplasty surgeon as well as the high volume subspecialist. As editors, we have learned a great deal from the Masters who have shared their expertise with us. We have no doubt that you will find their contributions equally valuable to you as you manage your patients with problem knees.

Jess H. Lonner, MD
Paul A. Lotke, MD

Acknowledgments

The "Masters" who have contributed their insight and expertise for this textbook are no doubt stretched thin. Each has a busy clinical practice and is typically called on for numerous academic endeavors. We are therefore profoundly indebted to them for taking their time to "bring us into their operating rooms" so that we may benefit from their years of experience. These authors will admit that they have become better surgeons over the years not only by learning from their mentors and peers but also by personally experiencing successes and failures in the operating room. Those lessons, which are so clearly shared throughout this text, will enable each of us to become better knee arthroplasty surgeons.

We would like to thank the publishers and their staff at Wolters-Kluwer, Lippincott Williams and Wilkins, but particularly David Murphy, Eileen Wolfberg, and Robert Hurley, who enthusiastically and diligently worked with us towards completion of this textbook.

Finally, once again we would like to thank our spouses and families for their patience and support while we took "time away" to complete this book.

Contributors

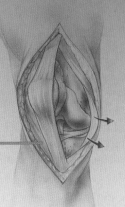

Rodney K. Alan, MD
Fellow in Orthopaedic Surgery
Palmetto Orthopaedic and Sports Medicine Center
Sumter, SC

Annunziato Amendola, MD
Professor, Department of Orthopaedics and Rehabilitation
Director, University of Iowa Sports Medicine
University of Iowa
Iowa City, IA

Martin Bedard, MD FRCS (C)
Arthroplasty Fellow
University of Southern California
Los Angeles, CA

Bryce Bederka, MD
Sports Medicine and Pediatric Trauma
The Bone and Joint Clinic
Portland, OR

Michael E. Berend, MD
Clinical Assistant Professor
Department of Medicine
Indiana University School of Medicine
Indianapolis, IN

Keith R. Berend, M.D.
Clinical Assistant Professor
Department of Orthopaedics
The Ohio State University
Mount Carmel Health System
New Albany, OH

Daniel J. Berry, MD
Department of Orthopaedic Surgery
Mayo Clinic
Rochester, MN

Hari P. Bezwada, MD
Assistant Clinical Professor
Department of Orthopaedic Surgery
University of Pennsylvania School of Medicine
Pennsylvania Hospital
Philadelphia, PA

Robert E. Booth, Jr, MD
Clinical Professor
Department of Orthopaedic Surgery
University of Pennsylvania School of Medicine
Chief, Orthopaedic Surgery
Pennsylvania Hospital
Philadelphia, PA

Robert B. Bourne, MD, FRCSC
Professor, Department of Surgery (Orthopaedics)
University of Western Ontario
London, Ontario, Canada

Henry D. Clarke MD
Assistant Professor of Orthopedics
Mayo Clinic College of Medicine
Mayo Clinic Arizona
Phoenix, AZ

Michael R. Dayton, MD
Assistant Professor
Adult Reconstruction, Department of Orthopaedics
University Colorado at Denver and Health Science Center
Aurora, CO

Craig J. Della Valle, MD
Associate Professor of Orthopaedic Surgery
Rush University Medical Center
Chicago, IL

Douglas A. Dennis, M.D
Adjunct Professor
Department of Biomedical Engineering
University of Tennessee
Knoxville, TN
Assistant Clinical Professor
University of Colorado Health Sciences Center
Colorado Joint Replacement
Rocky Mountain Musculoskeletal Research Laboratory
Denver, CO

Bradley S. Ellison, MS, MD
Senior Orthopedic Resident
Department of Orthopedic Surgery
The Ohio State University Medical Center
Columbus, OH

Gerard A. Engh, MD
President
Director, Knee Research
Anderson Orthopaedic Research Institute
Alexandria, VA

Thomas Keith Fehring, MD
Ortho Carolina Hip and Knee Center
Charlotte, NC

William F. Flynn, Jr, MD
Adult Reconstructive Surgery
Hospital for Special Surgery
New York, NY

Steven Haas, MD, MPH
Associate Professor Weil Cornell Medical School
Chief of Knee Service
Hospital for Special Surgery
New York, NY

Arlen D. Hanssen, MD
Professor
Department of Orthopaedics
Mayo School of Medicine
Rochester, MN

William L. Healy, MD
Lahey Clinic
Burlington, MA
Boston University Medical Center
Boston, MA

Richard A Hocking, FRACS
Attending Orthopaedic Surgeon
Capital Orthopaedics
Canberra, ACT
Australia

Stephen J. Incavo, MD
Professor
Department of Orthopaedic Surgery
Adult Reconstructive Surgery
The Methodist Hospital for Orthopaedics
Houston, TX

Richard Iorio, MD
Senior Attending Orthopaedic Surgeon
Lahey Clinic
Burlington, MA
Boston University Medical Center
Boston, MA

Richard E. Jones, MD
Orthopedic Specialists
Dallas, TX

E. Michael Keating, MD
Center for Hip and Knee Surgery
St. Francis Hospital
Mooresville, IN

Raymond H. Kim, MD
Colorado Joint Replacement
Rocky Mountain Musculoskeletal Research Laboratory
Denver, CO

Kenneth A. Krackow, MD
Professor, Full Time Faculty
Department of Orthopaedics
State University of New York at Buffalo
Clinical Director of Orthopaedics
Kaleida Health System
Buffalo, NY

Paul F. Lachiewicz, MD
Professor
Department of Orthopaedic Surgery
University of North Carolina
Chapel Hill, NC

Adolph V. Lombardi, Jr., M.D., F.A.C.S.
Clinical Assistant Professor
Departments of Orthopaedics and Biomedical Engineering
The Ohio State University
Mount Carmel Health System
New Albany, OH

William J. Long, MD FRCSC
Attending Orthopaedic Surgeon
Insall Scott Kelly Institute
New York, NY

Jess H. Lonner, MD
Director, Knee Replacement Surgery
Booth, Bartolozzi, Balderston Orthopaedics
Pennsylvania Hospital
Director, Philadelphia Center for Minimally Invasive
Knee Surgery
Philadelphia, PA

Paul A. Lotke, MD
Professor Emeritus, Orthopaedic Surgery
University of Pennsylvania School of Medicine
Philadelphia, PA

Steven J. MacDonald MD, FRCS(C)
Division of Orthopaedic Surgery
University of Western Ontario & London Health
Sciences Centre
London, Ontario, Canada

John B. Meding, MD
Center for Hip and Knee Surgery
St. Francis Hospital
Mooresville, IN

Douglas D.R. Naudie, MD, FRCSC
Assistant Professor
Department of Surgery–Orthopaedics
University of Western Ontario
London, Ontario, Canada

Charles L. Nelson, MD
Associate Professor
Department of Orthopaedic Surgery
University of Pennsylvania
Philadelphia, PA

Javad Parvizi, MD
Associate Professor
Department of Orthopedic Surgery
Rothman Institute at Thomas Jefferson University,
Philadelphia, PA

Trevor R. Pickering, MD
Fellowship Director
Center for Hip and Knee Surgery
St. Francis Hospital
Mooresville, IN

Chitranjan S. Ranawat, MD
Professor of Clinical Orthopaedic Surgery
Weill Medical College of Cornell University
Chairman
Department of Orthopaedic Surgery
Lenox Hill Hospital
New York, NY

Michael D. Ries, MD
Professor of Orthopaedic Surgery
University of California, San Francisco
San Francisco, CA

Aaron G. Rosenberg, MD
Professor
Department of Orthopaedic Surgery
Rush University Medical Center
Chicago, IL

Alexander P. Sah, MD
Department of Orthopaedic Surgery
Massachusetts General Hospital
Boston, MA

Eugenio Savarese
Department of Orthopaedic Surgery
University Hospital of Rome "Tor Vergata"
Rome, Italy

Richard D. Scott
Professor of Orthopaedic Surgery
Harvard Medical School
Senior Attending Surgeon
Brigham and Womens Hospital
New England Baptist Hospital
Boston, MA

Giles R. Scuderi, MD
Director, Attending Orthopaedic Surgeon
Insall Scott Kelly Institute
New York, NY

John M. Siliski, MD
Harvard Medical School and Department of Orthopaedic
Surgery
Massachusetts General Hospital
New England Baptist Hospital, Tufts Medical School
Boston, MA

James B. Stiehl, MD
Associate Clinical Professor
Department of Orthopaedic Surgery
Medical College of Wisconsin
Milwaukee, WI

Michael J. Stuart, MD
Professor and Vice-Chairman
Department of Orthopedics
Co-Director
Sports Medicine Center
Mayo Clinic
Rochester, MN

Alfred J. Tria, Jr, MD
Clinical Professor of Orthopaedic Surgery
Robert Wood Johnson Medical School
New Brunswick, NJ

Robert T. Trousdale
Professor of Orthopaedics
Department of Orthopaedic
Surgery
Mayo Clinic
Rochester, MN

Kelly G. Vince, MD FRCS (C)
Orthopedic Surgeon
Auckland City Hospital
Auckland, New Zealand

David Watson, MD, FRCS(C)
Trauma and Adult Reconstruction
Florida Orthopedic Institute
Tampa, FL

PART ONE
SURGICAL APPROACHES

1 Traditional Medial Approaches to the Knee

Douglas D.R. Naudie and Robert B. Bourne

INTRODUCTION

The intent of this chapter is to provide an illustrative description of the traditional medial approaches to the knee for total knee arthroplasty (TKA). Since its inception, TKA has most commonly been performed using some variation of a medial parapatellar approach. Von Langenbeck originally described the dissection of the vastus medialis from the quadriceps tendon extending distally through the medial patella retinaculum and along the patellar ligament leaving a small cuff of tissue for closure (1). Insall described a modification of this approach whereby the quadriceps mechanism was opened with an incision in the quadriceps tendon dividing its medial one-third from the lateral two-thirds (2). Rather than skirting the medial border of the patella and leaving a cuff of tissue, he brought the incision straight distally, directly over the medial aspect of the patella. Insall believed that modification improved quadriceps healing (tendon to tendon) and was less disruptive to the extensor mechanism. Hofmann and associates advocated a subvastus approach to the knee, which divides the vastus medialis at the intermuscular septum leaving the muscle largely untouched (3). Other than some advocates of the mini-subvastus approach (see Chapter 3), the standard subvastus approach is not commonly used because of difficulties gaining exposure, risk of bleeding, and unclear benefits. Engh popularized the midvastus approach, which spares the quadriceps tendon but requires splitting of the muscle fibers of the vastus medialis obliquus muscles (4). This approach is utilitarian, has reduced the need for lateral release in some series, and has been embraced by enthusiasts of the minimally invasive techniques for knee replacement surgery (see Chapter 3).

INDICATIONS AND CONTRAINDICATIONS

We prefer a traditional medial parapatellar arthrotomy for the vast majority of primary total knee arthroplasties at our institution, although the other referenced approaches to the knee are also appropriate and effective in select patients. For instance, the lateral parapatellar arthrotomy is particularly utilitarian in severe, fixed valgus deformities; and the extensile subvastus aproach is effective in cases of retained medial hardware on the distal femur (for example, from a previous distal femoral valgus osteotomy). However, some of these approaches have potential disadvantages. It has been our experience that the subvastus and midvastus approaches can be difficult in short, obese, and muscular individuals. These two approaches are also not conducive to the placement of a navigation array on the distal femur in cases in which we employ computer navigation. We have found that a lateral approach for severe valgus knees can compromise the ability to seal the arthrotomy from the subcutaneous space just beneath the skin incision.

The medial parapatellar approach can be used in virtually every case regardless of the preoperative deformity and range of motion. It is safe, extensile, and gives excellent access to the intra-articular and periarticular structures around the knee. This approach can be shortened to allow for a minimally invasive unicompartmental or TKA. If necessary, it can be extended both proximally and distally to allow for a quadriceps snip or tibial tubercle osteotomy, respectively. In fact, there are relatively few contraindications to its use. It does not, for instance, allow direct exposure to the popliteal fossa. It can even be used, if a very extensile approach is selected, for antero-lateral procedures such as lateral closing wedge high tibial osteotomies or other isolated procedures to the lateral side of the knee, although alternative laterally based incisions can also be selected for these procedures.

PREOPERATIVE PREPARATION

One of the important aspects of the preoperative planning for TKA is an understanding of the patient's anatomy. The blood supply to the skin should be respected at all times, especially when prior incisions are present or multiple incisions are planned. Most of the blood supply to the skin arises from the saphenous artery and the descending geniculate artery on the medial side of the knee (6). The vessels perforate the deep fascia, form an anastomosis superficial to the deep fascia, and continue through the subcutaneous fat to supply the epidermis (Fig. 1-1A). There is little communication in the superficial layer; therefore, dissection should be deep to the fascia to maintain the blood supply to the skin.

The skin incision must be selected carefully. Because the fascial perforators arise from the medial side, the most lateral incision giving appropriate exposure should be used. Transverse scars can be crossed with a longitudinal perpendicular incision, as these do not appear to affect the healing of the vertical anterior medial approach. When possible, the anterior incision should incorporate other previous longitudinal incisions about the knee.

The blood supply to the skin should not be confused with the blood supply to the patella (5). The patella is separated from the skin by the prepatellar bursa, through which few blood vessels pass. The patella has a rich plexus of arteries surrounding it, arising from various sources (Fig. 1-1B). These branches include the four genicular arteries (superior medial, inferior medial, superior lateral, and inferior lateral) and the anterior tibial recurrent artery. Medial retinacular incisions will disrupt the three medial blood vessels contributing to the anastomosis around the patella. A recent study using laser Doppler flowmetry of 10 patients undergoing TKA did not demonstrate a significant change in patellar blood flow with a standard medial parapatellar approach (6). If a lateral retinacular release is added, however, one or both of the lateral vessels will be disrupted, potentially compromising patellar blood flow.

The nerve supply to the skin is similar in distribution to the blood supply. Branches of the saphenous nerve traverse laterally to the anterior aspect of the joint to provide cutaneous sensation. The infrapatellar branch of the saphenous nerve is typically transected with vertical skin incisions (particularly anterior and anteromedial incisions), resulting in an area of transient or permanent cutaneous hypoesthesia on the skin over the anterolateral knee. Patients should be made aware of this possibility. The terminal branches of the saphenous nerve innervate the vastus medialis. Electromyographic and nerve conduction studies have been performed and show no evidence of permanent vastus medialis muscle denervation with the midvastus approach to the knee (7,8).

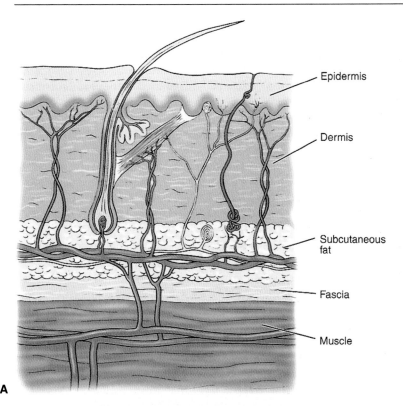

A

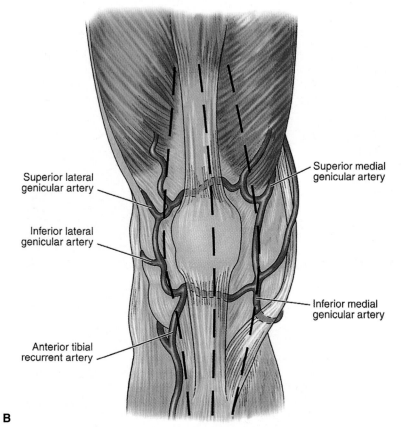

B

FIGURE 1-1

(A,B) Diagram outling the blood supply to the skin and patella. (Reprinted with permission from Scuderi GR. *Surgical Approaches to the Knee: Surgery of the Knee*, vol. 1. New York: Churchill Livingston; 2001.)

TECHNIQUE

TKA is always performed with the patient in the supine position. The operating table should be level. A protective belt is applied across the upper body to allow tilting of the table as needed. A tourniquet is applied to the upper thigh after the correct patient and extremity have been identified and marked (Fig. 1-2A). The tourniquet should be applied snugly and as far proximally as practical. In the very obese patient, the fat may be pulled distally from beneath the tourniquet, causing it to bulge from the distal edge of the tourniquet. This prevents it from migrating and ensures that the tourniquet is placed as far proximal as practical. We use a commercially available footrest placed at the bulkiest part of the calf to suport the knee in flexion during the procedure. Alternatively, a sandbag can be used, provided it is taped securely to the bed. We also use a lateral bolster placed at the proximal third of the patient's thigh to prevent external hip rotation (Fig. 1-2B). This step is particularly helpful in obese patients. The contralateral leg is well padded, especially under the heel, to reduce the risk of pressure sores.

There are many ways to prepare and drape a patient for TKA, but we have found that suspending the heel in a leg holder gives excellent access to the knee and allows surgical personnel to be available for other purposes (Fig. 1-2C). We shave the hair around the area of the planned incision just prior to sterile preparation of the leg. The nurses first scrub the leg with an iodine solution as the surgical team scrubs their hands. The entire leg is then prepared with an iodine solution. In patients with an iodine allergy, we use a chlorhexidine scrub and preparation solution. Additionally, alternative preparation solutions are emerging and being used with greater frequency.

The calf is supported with a sterile towel, the foot is removed from the footrest, and the remainder of the leg (including the foot) is prepared. A sterile drape is placed on the operating table. An impermeable, waterproof stockinette is placed over the prepped foot, after which a cloth stockinette is placed over the entire leg and over the tourniquet. A sterile U-shaped drape is placed proximally

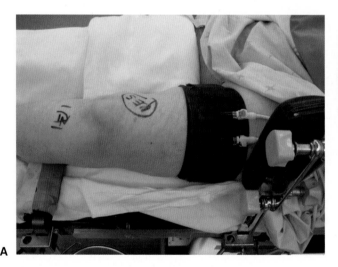

A

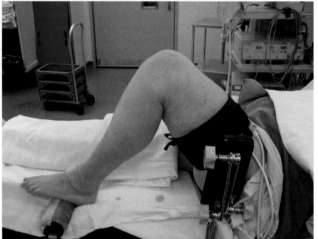

B

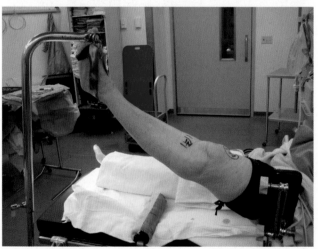

C

FIGURE 1-2

(A) The leg is marked and initialed, and a tourniquet is placed on the thigh as proximal as possible. **(B)** A footrest and lateral bolster are secured into proper position to allow the leg to be supported with minimal assistance. **(C)** The leg is suspended and ready for scrubbing and prepping.

around the stockinettte at the level of the tourniquet. A limb extremity sheet with a rubberized central portion with a hole in it is then placed over the stockinette and pulled proximally to the tourniquet level (Fig. 1-3A). The foot and ankle are wrapped to prevent the stockinette from sliding during manipulation of the limb during the procedure. As an alternative to an impermeable stockinette, a cloth stockinette can be placed over the entire leg, and a sterile surgical glove can be placed over the foot. A window is cut in front of the stockinette on the anterior aspect of the knee, and the appropriate landmarks about the knee are palpated and marked with a sterile pen. The incision is then drawn, and transverse lines are made to assist with skin edge alignment at the time of closure. A betadine-impregnated sterile adhesive surgical drape is then applied to encricle the limb around the surgical site (Fig. 1-3B).

A tourniquet is used for all total knee arthroplasties, except in patients with known peripheral vascular disease and absent pulses confirmed by Doppler examination. These patients have a consultation with a vascular surgeon preoperatively. Relative contraindications to tourniquet use include obese patients with a short thigh (in which a tourniquet is potentially ineffective) or patients with known peripheral neuropathy. Patients with neuropathy should be warned that exacerbation of the neuropathy can occur with tourniquet use. The tourniquet is usually inflated to 300 mm Hg, to have the tourniquet at least 100 mm Hg above the systolic blood pressure. The pressure can be elevated as high as 350 mm Hg in hypertensive or obese patients. The leg is usually elevated for 30 seconds before inflating the tourniquet, or exsanguinations of the limb can be performed with an elastic bandage (e.g., Esmarch bandage). Prophylactic antibiotics are given within 30 minutes before tourniquet inflation.

Skin incisions must be modifed in the presence of prior incisions around the knee, as discussed previously, to avoid regions of potential skin necrosis. It is important to check that enough skin area is exposed for the entire incision. The initial exposure is done with the knee in flexion. Generally, we use a standard straight, vertical skin incision, measuring approximately 15 cm long. It is centered over the shaft of the femur, in its midportion over the patella, and distally just medial to the tibial tubercle. Using a new blade, the dissection is taken to the anterior border of the quadriceps tendon, patella, and medial border of the patellar tendon. It is important to avoid elevating large skin flaps and creating dead space. The subcutaneous dissection is concentrated on the medial side to allow for a medial parapatellar arthrotomy. Elevation laterally over the dorsal surface of the patella is kept to a minimum. In the severely obese patient, however, lateral dissection may be more extensive and necessary to create a subcutaneous pocket in which the patella may sit, allowing it to evert (Fig. 1-4A,B).

The quadriceps tendon is then identified. We have found that a Cobb elevator is useful to remove any tissue adherent to the quadriceps tendon. The medial and lateral edges of the arthrotomy at the level of the superior pole of the patella are marked with a sterile marking pen to facilitate an

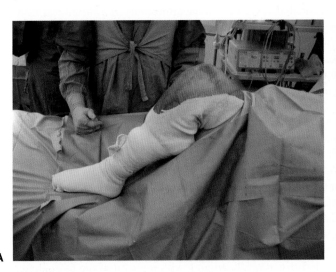
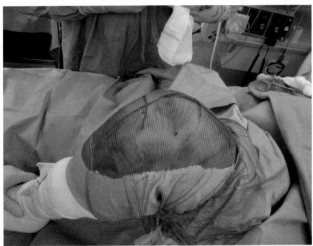

A   B

FIGURE 1-3

(A) The foot and ankle are wrapped with an elastocrepe bandage, and a limb extremity sheet with a rubberized central portion with a hole in it is then placed over the stockinette and pulled proximally to the tourniquet level. **(B)** A window is cut in front of the stockinette on the anterior aspect of the knee, and the incision is drawn; a betadine-impregnated sterile adhesive plastic surgical drape is then applied to encircle the leg around the surgical site.

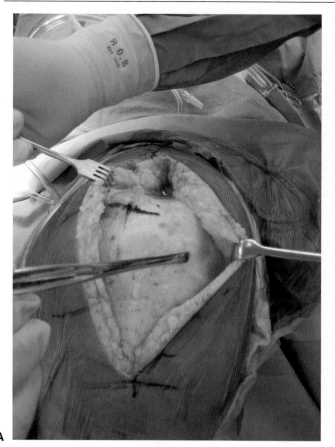

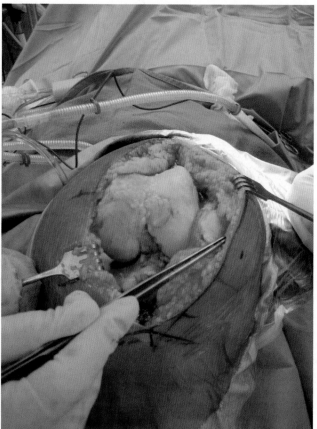

A

B

FIGURE 1-4

(A,B) In this severely obese patient with a body mass index of over 45, lateral dissection is extended to create a subcutanous pocket in which the patella may sit during eversion.

anatomic closure at the end of the procedure. As discussed, there are many variations to the traditional medial parapatellar arthrotomy (Fig. 1-5A). We incise the quadriceps tendon in line with its fibers, about 0.5 to 1 cm from the vastus medialis. We extend the arthrotomy in a curvilinear fashion distally along the medial edge of the patella and gently back along the medial border of the patellar tendon (Fig. 1-5B). A soft tissue cuff is preserved at the superior pole of the patella and at the tibial tubercle to facilitate closure. The arthrotomy incision is made with a large scalpel blade through the medial retinaculum, capsule, and synovium.

At the joint line, it is important to cut the anterior horn of the medial meniscus. The exception is when a patellofemoral arthroplasty is performed, when it is critical to leave the medial meniscus intact. The remainder of the exposure can be done in flexion or extension based on surgeon preference. Our preference is to extend the leg for further exposure at this juncture. A sharp rake is usually placed on the cut edge of the medial segment of the meniscus and gently retracted, while the foot is externally rotated (Fig. 1-6A). This aids in exposing the medial side of the joint by subperiosteal dissection of the medial collateral ligament. The medial collateral ligament is dissected in a continuous flap using electrocautery with vertical strokes, for a variable distance depending on the type and degree of preoperative deformity. We have found a small Cobb elevator or osteotome useful in this stage of the exposure. It is imperative not to over-release medially in more severe valgus deformities in which the medial collateral may already be stretched or attenuated. We prefer a stepwise release of the medial structures, beginning with removal of the osteophytes on the medial tibial plateau and medial femoral condyle with a rongeur (Fig. 1-6B). In most cases, it is necessary to expose the posterior medial corner to allow for proper external rotation, anterior translation, and tibial exposure.

After exposing the medial side, we work in a systematic fashion (clockwise for left knees and counterclockwise for right knees) to release extra-articular adhesions from the medial gutter, suprapatellar pouch, and lateral side of the knee. We routinely reflect the anterior synovium on the femur to expose the supracondylar region of the femur to ensure proper and precise sizing of the femoral

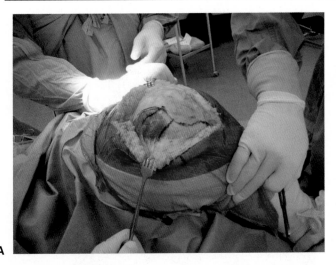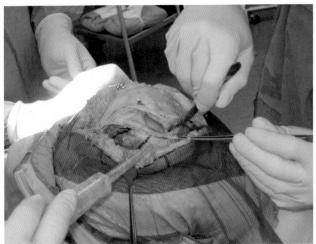

A   B

FIGURE 1-5

(A) The subvastus, midvastus, Von Langenbeck, and traditional medial parapatellar arthrotomy are marked with a sterile marking pen. **(B)** The quadriceps tendon is incised in line with its fibers, about 0.5 to 1 cm from the vastus medialis and extended in a curvilinear fashion distally along the medial edge of the patella.

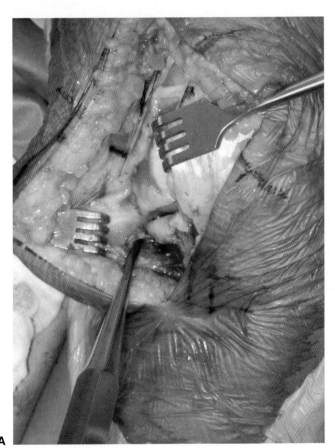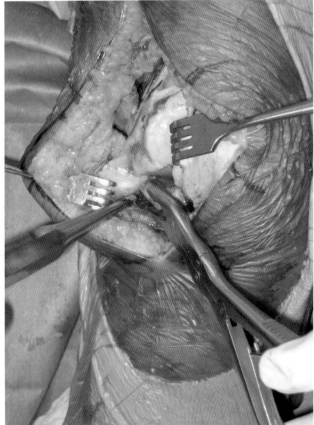

A   B

FIGURE 1-6

(A) A sharp rake is placed on the cut edge of the medial segment of the meniscus and gently retracted. **(B)** With the foot externally rotated, a small Cobb elevator or an osteotome is placed under the medial tibial osteophyte, allowing safe and rapid removal of the osteophytes on the medial tibial plateau and medial femoral condyle with a rongeur.

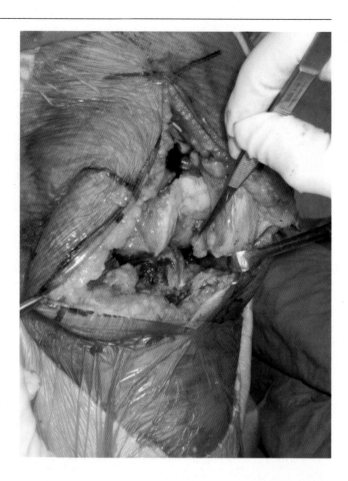

FIGURE 1-7

A right-angle retractor is placed into the bursa posterior to the patellar fat pad, and dissection is carried across the anterior aspect of the lateral tibial plateau exposing the entire anterior lateral aspect of the knee.

implant and to avoid notching the anterior cortex. We then tension the extensor mechanism with a laterally placed right-angle knee retractor, release the lateral patellofemoral ligaments, and clear the lateral gutter with the knee in extension. Any osteophytes on the lateral femur are also removed at this juncture. Dissection is then carried across the anterior aspect of the lateral tibial plateau (Fig. 1-7). A right-angle retractor is placed into the bursa posterior to the patellar fat pad, exposing the entire anterior lateral aspect of the knee. The fat pad is detached from the lateral meniscus, and the anterior horn of the lateral meniscus is incised vertically. In some knees, the lateral mensicus can be detached at this stage along the lateral margin of the tibial plateau into the meniscal popliteal hiatus. These maneuvers allow the patella to be readily mobilized for eversion. The ligamentum mucosa, if present, should also be sectioned. Although we personally prefer patellar eversion, others have had a great deal of success with patellar subluxation, without everting it.

The patella is everted with the knee in extension, and the knee is slowly flexed. We carefully observe the insertion of the patellar tendon to avoid avulsion. The medial flap of the quadriceps must slide medially off the face of the femur. If the patella will not evert, we revisit the dissection in a systematic fashion, particularly the dissection across the lateral tibial plateau. If we believe the patellar tendon is at risk, a smooth pin can be driven through the insertion on the tibial tubercle to secure it until further bone cuts and soft tissue releases are performed. If the knee will not flex with safe patellar eversion, the patella can also be allowed to sublux laterally without eversion until further bone cuts and soft tissue releases are performed, or for the duration of the case. We rarely consider a more extensile approach, such as the quadriceps snip or tibial tubercle osteotomy discussed later. These options are usually only considered in revision or complex primary surgery.

With the knee flexed and the patella safely everted, we address the fat pad. We prefer to leave the fat pad or resect only as much as is needed to allow for proper visualization medially and laterally. We then excise the anterior cruciate ligament. Complete anterior subluxation of the tibia from beneath the femur can be accomplished at this stage with gentle flexion and external rotation of the knee. Depending on surgeon preference, the menisci and posterior cruciate ligament can also be removed at this stage. It is our preference to perform the distal and posterior femoral bone cuts at this stage to facilitate tibial exposure (Fig. 1-8A–C). Other surgeons, as reflected in other chapters in this text, prefer to resect the proximal tibia before preparing the distal femur. We take

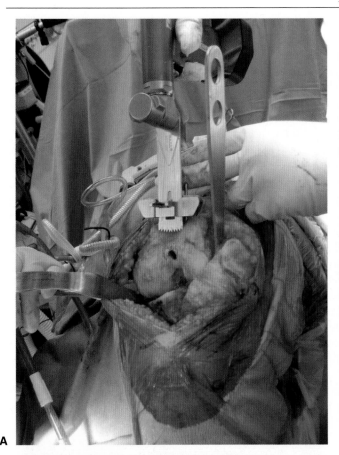

A

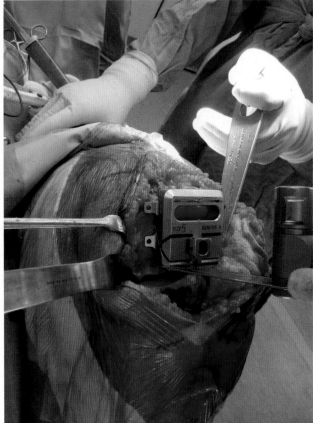

B

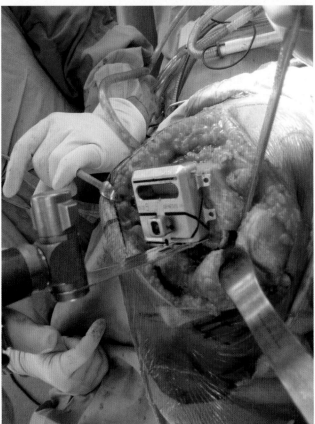

C

FIGURE 1-8

(A) A lateral retractor is placed along the lateral tibial plateau peripheral to the lateral meniscus at the junction between its anterior and middle thirds, and the distal femoral bone cut is made. **(B)** A medial blunt Homan retractor is placed around the medial femoral condyle during posterior medial femoral condylar resection to protect the medial collateral ligament. **(C)** The same retractor is then transferred around the lateral femoral condyle during posterior lateral femoral condylar resection to protect the popliteus and lateral collateral ligament complex.

advantage of minimally invasive cutting blocks available to minimize the length of initial skin incisions and extent of our soft tissue exposure.

A lateral retractor is placed along the lateral tibial plateau peripheral to the lateral meniscus at the junction between its anterior and middle thirds. If the lateral meniscus has not been dissected off to this level, a 1- to 2-cm slit needs to be made with electrocautery or a scalpel. This retractor is used through the entire operation for lateral exposure when the knee is flexed. A blunt Homan retractor is placed medially then laterally to safely expose the medial and lateral femoral condyles during posterior femoral condylar resection (Fig. 1-8B,C).

We have found a series of four retractors extremely valuable for the remainder of the exposure (Fig. 1-9). An intramedullary Mikhail retractor can be placed into the femoral canal while an assistant pulls up on the prepared distal femur to assist in exposure of the posterior aspect of the knee. Alternatively, a laminar spreader can be used to elevate the femur with the knee flexed 90 degrees (see Fig. 5-21A). We routinely excise the posterior cruciate ligament at this stage (Fig. 1-10A), given our standard practice of using a posterior stabilized knee. A single or double prong posterior cruciate ligament retractor can be placed behind the tibia to assist in anterior subluxation of the tibia beneath the femur and during removal of the medial and lateral menisci with electrocautery (Fig. 1-10B). The inferior lateral geniculate artery is often encountered laterally and should be identified and cauterized. A thin medial meniscal rim should be retained to ensure there has been no violation of the medial collateral ligament, to which it is attached (Fig. 1-10C). Excellent exposure of the tibia can be achieved using a lateral Mikhail retractor and a single-prong posterior cruciate ligament retractor for tibial bone preparation (Fig. 1-11). After tibial preparation, we routinely remove all posterior femoral osteophytes from the back of the knee prior to flexion-extension gap assessment (Fig. 1-12).

The remainder of the total knee arthoplasty is then performed. After alignment, stability, range of motion, kinematics, and patellar tracking have been thoroughly checked, definitive implants are inserted with cement.

PEARLS

We have found that a systematic approach to exposure has allowed us to rapidly and safely expose even the most complex patients and deformities. In obese patients, we have found it extremely helpful to create a subcutaneous pocket on the dorsal surface of the patella to allow a place for the patella to sit during knee flexion (Fig. 1-4A,B). If this is not done, the large envelope of subcutaneous fat tends to prevent the patella from everting or pushes it into the wound, compromising visibility. We sometimes also allow the patella to slide without eversion.

We have also found that proper retractor placement can greatly facilitate the performance of safe and expeditious bone cuts. Specifically, we have found that placement of a blunt Homan retractor along the medial femoral condyle during bone preparation with a saw can prevent inadvert damage or transection of the medial collateral ligament (Fig. 1-8B). Similarly, a blunt Homan retractor placed along the lateral femoral condyle anterior to the popliteus during posterior lateral femoral condylar resection can prevent damage or inadvertent transection of the popliteus or lateral collateral

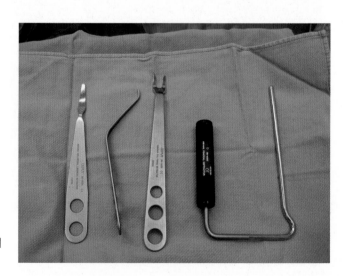

FIGURE 1-9

From left to right, we routinely use a "lateral" Mikhail retractor, a single-prong PCL retractor, a double-prong PCL retractor (for PCL-retaining knees), and an "intramedullary" Mikhail retractor to assist with our total knee arthroplasty exposure.

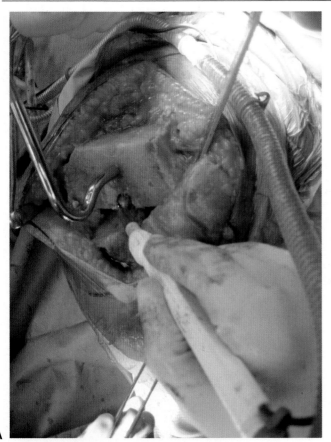

A

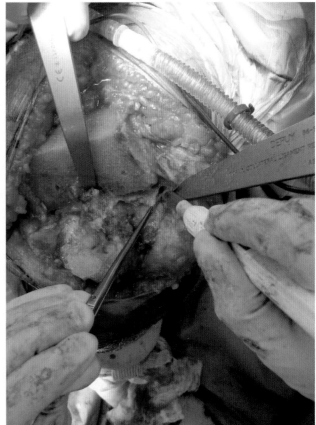

B

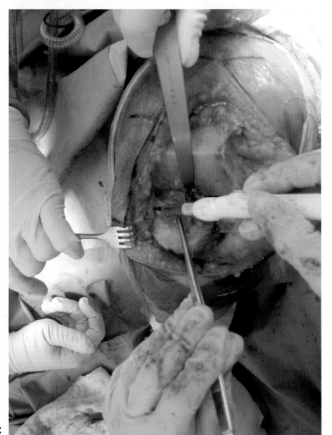

C

FIGURE 1-10

(A) An intramedullary Mikhail retractor can be placed
into the femoral canal while an assistant pulls up on
the prepared distal femur to facilitate excision of the
posterior cruciate ligament. **(B)** A single-prong
posterior cruciate ligament retractor can be placed
behind the tibia to assist in anterior subluxation of the
tibia beneath the femur. Removal of the lateral
meniscus is performed with electrocautery, and the
inferior lateral geniculate artery should be identified
and cauterized. **(C)** A thin medial meniscal rim should
be retained during removal of the medial meniscus to
ensure there is no violation of the medial collateral
ligament.

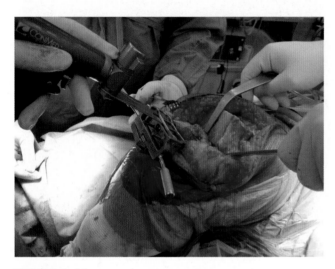

FIGURE 1-11

Excellent exposure of the tibia can be achieved using a lateral Mikhail retractor and a single-prong posterior cruciate ligament retractor during tibial bone preparation.

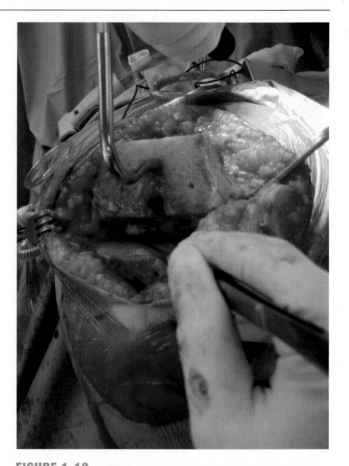

FIGURE 1-12

A large posterior femoral osteophyte is removed from the back of the femur with the assistance of an intramedullary Mikhail retractor.

ligament complex (Fig. 1-8C). Finally, a well-placed posterior and lateral retractor can greatly assist in proper visualization of the tibial plateau for tibial resection (Fig. 1-11).

Limited Exposures

A short medial arthrotomy incision is appropriate for medial unicompartmental arthroplasty, allografts to articular defects, and treatment of osteochondritis dissecans. This method uses the distal segment of the approach to the knee described previously (Fig. 1-13A). The incision is made from the superomedial pole of the patella to the top of the tibial tubercle. It is taken through the skin and subcutaneous tissue and down through the deep fascia. The skin can be undermined with Metzenbaum scissors. The arthrotomy is taken through the medial capsule and synovium approximately 5 mm from the medial border of the patella. The quadriceps can be spared, or for wider exposure, the quadriceps incision can be extended above the superior pole of the patella, or a "mini" midvastus incision can be performed (Fig. 1-13B). This mini-midvastus incision gives excellent visualization of the medial condyle and medial proximal tibia without patellar eversion, and it can be used effectively for exposure for performing TKA (see Chapter 4).

Extensile Exposures

In complex primary and revision TKA, adequate exposure can be challenging. Fortunately, with a systematic approach, even the most complex revisions can be exposed without the need for any extensile exposure (see Chapter 4) (Fig. 1-14A,B). In such cases, we spend considerable time clearing the medial, suprapatellar, and lateral gutters, allowing good mobilization of the extensor mechanism. A generous subperiosteal medial soft tissue release from the proximal tibia will allow

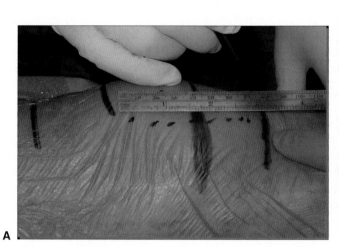

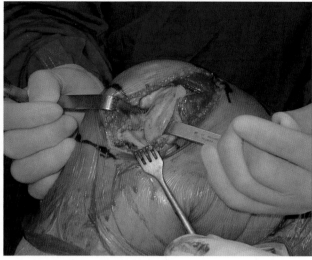

A

B

FIGURE 1-13

(A) A short medial arthrotomy incision drawn from the superomedial pole of the patella to the top of the tibial tubercle can be employed for medial unicompartmental arthroplasty. **(B)** A "mini" midvastus incision into the quadriceps can be performed and gives excellent visualization of the medial condyle and medial proximal tibia without patellar eversion.

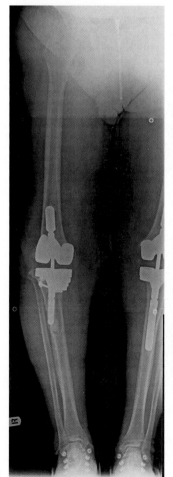

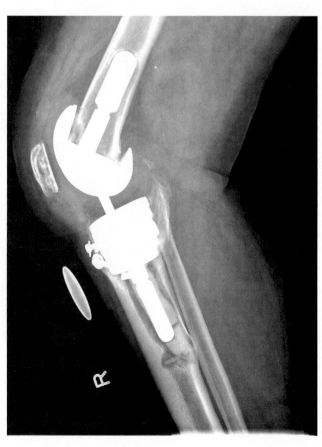

A,B

FIGURE 1-14

(A,B) Anteroposterior and lateral radiographs of a failed revision right total knee arthroplasty (performed at another institution) prior to re-revision. A tibial tubercle osteotomy would be relatively contraindicated in this circumstance given the amount of proximal tibial bone loss.

external rotation and anterior translation of the tibia. This maneuver relaxes tension on the patellar tendon attachment at the tibial tubercle and decreases the risk of patellar tendon avulsion. We also try to remove the polyethylene in modular tibial trays before attempting patella eversion and knee flexion. In most revision cases, we place a prophylactic pin in the patellar tendon to avoid peel-off. If unsatisfactory or undue tension is on the patellar tendon, then an extensile approach (such as a quadriceps snip or tibial tubercle osteotomy) is indicated and should be performed. This decision must be made before avulsion of the tibial tubercle or patellar tendon rupture occurs.

Quadriceps Snip

The quadriceps snip has evolved from traditional descriptions of the V-Y quadriceps turndown (9). The quadriceps snip is easily incorporated into the medial parapatellar arthrotomy (Fig. 1-15A). To allow the patella and extensor mechanism to be mobilized laterally, the quadriceps is incised in a lateral oblique fashion from distal to proximal at a 45-degree angle into the vastus lateralis. This allows the patella to be mobilized distally and laterally on the lateralis muscle and gives excellent visualization (Fig. 1-15B). The oblique incision has an advantage in that it is directed in line with the vastus lateralis muscle and remains within the substance of the quadriceps tendon. This avoids coming out into the medialis muscle and leaves good tissue to reapproximate during closure. After completion of the quadriceps snip, the vertical and oblique portions of the quadriceps tendon are repaired in a side-to-side fashion with interrupted sutures. Postoperative physical therapy can begin without delay and is not altered because of the surgical exposure.

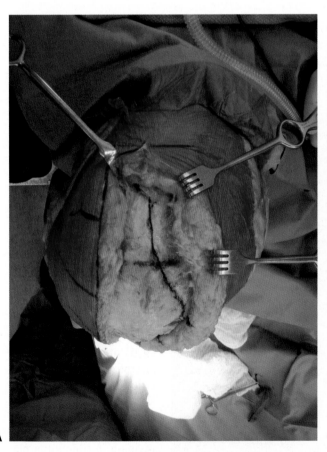
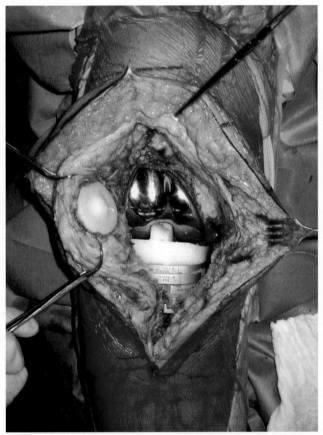

A   B

FIGURE 1-15

(A) A standard medial parapatellar arthrotomy with a proximal quadriceps snip marked with a sterile marking pen in the event that it would be required for exposure.
(B) Successful exposure and patellar eversion of this complex revision case with a limited proximal quadriceps snip.

Tibial Tubercle Osteotomy

The tibial tubercle osteotomy was first described by Dolin in 1983 and has been subsequently popularized by Whiteside (10–12). In addition to allowing adequate exposure to be obtained, use of this technique can also be helpful in providing access to the tibial canal. This may be required in cases in which previous components with well-fixed long tibial stems need to be extracted. A tibial tubercle osteotomy is contraindicated in cases with severe anterior tibial bone loss or osteolysis because of concerns of compromised healing (Fig. 1-14B). The skin is incised an additional 5 cm distally. Just proximal to the tibial tubercle, a transverse osteotomy is made perpendicular to the long axis of the tibia using an osteotome. This will serve as a buttress against proximal displacement of the tibial tubercle after closure. The osteotomy is carried distally for 5 to 7 cm using an oscillating saw. Proximally, the osteotomized segment should measure approximately 1 cm deep. Distally, the depth of the fragment is tapered to 1 to 2 mm to minimize a stress riser. The thickness of the osteotomy should be strong enough to hold the wires (or screws) used in closing the osteotomy, without risking fracturing the tubercle when tensioning the wires (Fig. 1-16A–E). The osteotomy typically is performed from medial to lateral. The oscillating saw is taken up to, but not through the lateral cortex. Several straight osteotomes are inserted across the osteotomy, and the lateral cortex is scored. The osteotomes are then rotated anterolaterally to complete the osteotomy of the lateral cortex, without disrupting the soft tissue attachments of the anterior compartment muscles. The lateral soft tissues are kept intact to serve as a soft tissue hinge and vascular pedicle as the extensor mechanism is folded laterally. The use of stemmed tibial component is recommended to bypass the distal stress riser. If rigid fixation is obtained, the patient is allowed full weight bearing and unrestriced range of motion with the use of a hinged knee brace. In selected cases, postoperative immobilization may be required until radiographic evidence of union is noted.

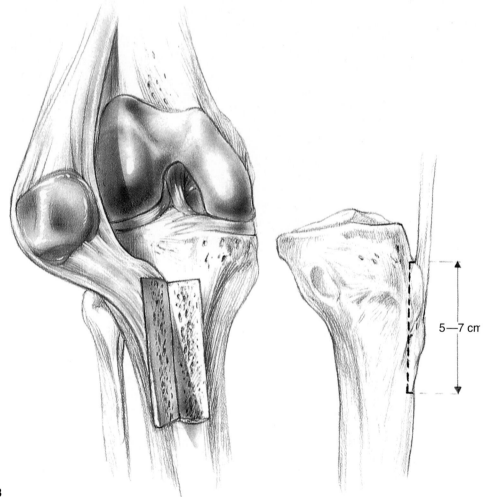

5—7 cm

FIGURE 1-16

(A,B) A 5- to −7-cm tibial tubercle osteotomy is made. At the proximal extent of the osteotomy, the bone depth is approximately 1 cm deep; at its distal edge, it tapers to 1 to 2 mm, to avoid a stress riser. *(continued)*

A,B

FIGURE 1-16 *(Continued)*

(C) A distally tapered tibial tubercle osteotomy performed from medial to lateral, keeping the soft tissues attached laterally as a vascular pedicle. **(D,E)** Repair of the osteotomy can be performed with cerclage wires passed through drill holes. The wires are tensioned, twisted, and cut for stable closure.

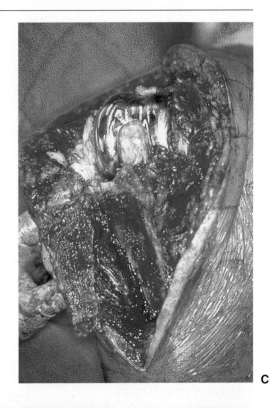

C

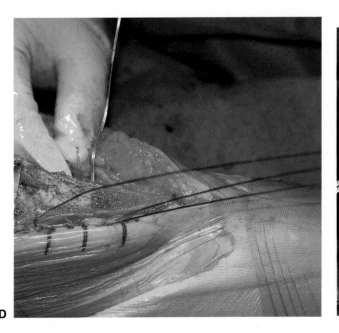

D

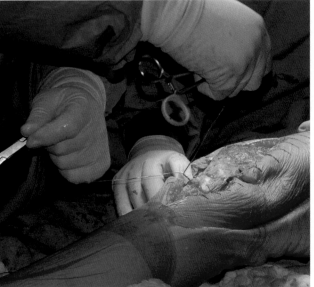

E

POSTOPERATIVE MANAGEMENT

The postoperative management of the medial arthrotomy depends on the underlying procedure for which the arthrotomy was completed. With a short anterior medial incision, such as for unicompartmental arthroplasty, the recovery time is very brief. With long arthrotomies and extensile exposures, the course can be more prolonged. In general, patients are allowed to fully bear weight immediately with unrestricted motion. Patients can expect to return to usual activities within 6 weeks. Postoperative rehabilitation protocols are unchanged when a quadriceps snip is performed. In patients treated with a tibial tubercle osteotomy, weight bearing may be protected for 6 weeks, and range of motion may be restricted for several weeks, depending on the stability of the fixation while it heals.

COMPLICATIONS

The most common complications of medial parapatellar arthrotomies are associated with wound healing. Unless adequate soft tissue closure is achieved, areas of wound separation or drainage can occur. The combination of swelling, a long incision, and early mobilization can contribute to delayed healing. Therefore, careful management of the closure is important. There is no substitution for good surgical technique during deep and superficial wound closure.

Lesser complications include the sacrifice of the infrapatellar branch of the saphenous nerve. Depending on the size of this nerve, there will be an area of numbness or dysesthesia on the skin antero-lateral in the proximal tibia. This gradually becomes less noticeable but can be permanent. It is noteworthy because some patients confuse the associated dysesthesia and numbness with a problem resulting from the intra-articular procedure.

An uncommon but potentially devastating complication results from overzealous eversion of the patella during flexion of the knee, which can avulse the patellar tendon from the tibial tubercle. This can be an extremely disabling problem, and every effort should be made to avoid it. Techniques to avoid this complication are alluded to earlier in this chapter and are described later in the text. It is important to realize that the more difficult the exposure is, the greater the risk of avulsion of the patellar tendon from the tibial tubercle will be.

Tibial tubercle osteotomies can fracture during exposure or closure. When rotating the intact lateral hinge anterolaterally with osteotomes, the bone can fracture. It can also fracture when securing it at the end of the procedure during tensioning of the cerclage wires or compressive screws. Nonunion or proximal migration of the tubercle can also occur. This risk is reduced with the proximal transverse "shelf." Finally, tibia fracture at the distal edge of the tibial tubercle can occur, particularly if the osteotomy is not tapered distally and if a stemmed tibial component is not used.

RESULTS

The medial parapatellar approach and its modifications remain the most commonly employed approaches to TKA. While having the advantages of being simple to perform, utilitarian, and extensile, these methods also have the potential disadvantages of disrupting muscle fibers, destabilizing the extensor mechanism, and interrupting the blood and nerve supply. Lateral and minimally invasive approaches have been developed and will be the topic of subsequent chapters.

Several studies have compared the minor variations on the traditional medial parapatellar approaches. Engh and associates were the first group to compare groups of patients who underwent knee arthroplasty using a standard medial parapatellar and a midvastus surgical arthrotomy (13). They found that there was a reduction in the percentage of lateral retinacular releases performed in the midvastus group. Kelly and associates also found a significantly higher rate of lateral release and greater blood loss with the median parapatellar approaches compared to the midvastus approach (14). These investigators, however, also identified electromyographic abnormalities in the quadriceps muscle in the midvastus group. Other groups have also compared these approaches and supported evidence that the midvastus approach may offer advantages over the standard parapatellar arthrotomy in the early rehabilitation period (15).

Some studies have compared the subvastus approach for total knee replacement with the standard medial parapatellar approach and concluded that although the subvastus approach may have early advantages over the standard parapatellar arthrotomy, such as more limited compromise of early quadriceps strength, this limited benefit comes at the expense of a longer operation and a higher risk of complications (16–18).

One study has gone so far as to compare the midvastus with the subvastus approaches to determine their influence on quadriceps femoris muscle function in TKA (19). This study concluded that the subvastus approach does not provide any advantages compared with the midvastus approach with respect to the quadriceps femoris muscle strength in the early postoperative period, and actually caused significantly more pain postoperatively.

REFERENCES

1. Langenbeck B von. Uber die Schussverietzungen des Huftgelenks. *Arch Klin Chir* 1874;16:263.
2. Insall JN. A midline approach to the knee. *J Bone Joint Surg* 1971;53:1584.
3. Hofmann AA, Plaster RL, Murdock LE. Subvastus (Southern) approach for primary total knee arthroplasty. *Clin Orthop* 1991;269:70–77.

4. Engh GA, Holt BT, Parks NL. A midvastus muscle-splitting approach for total knee arthroplasty. *J Arthroplasty* 1997;12:322–331.
5. Haertsch PA. The blood supply of the skin of the leg: a postmortem investigation. *Br J Plast Surg* 1981;34:470.
6. Hempfing A, Schoeniger R, Koch PP, et al. Patellar blood flow during knee arthroplasty surgical exposure: intraoperative monitoring by laser Doppler flowmetry. *J Orthop Res* 2007;25:1389–1394.
7. Jojima H, Whiteside LA, Ogata K. Anatomic consideration of nerve supply to the vastus medialis in knee surgery. *Clin Orthop Relat Res* 2004;423:157–160.
8. Dalury DF, Snow RG, Adams MJ. Electromyographic evaluation of the midvastus approach. *J Arthroplasty* 2008;23:136–140.
9. Coonse K, Adams JD. A new operative approach to the knee joint. *Surg Gynecol Obstet* 1943;77:344–347.
10. Dolin MG. Osteotomy of the tibial tubercle during total knee replacement. A report of twenty-six cases. *J Bone Joint Surg* 1983;72:706.
11. Dolin MG. Osteotomy of the tibial tubercle in total knee replacement. A technical note. *J Bone Joint Surg* 1983;65:704–706.
12. Whiteside LA, Ohl MD. Tibial tubercle osteotomy for exposure of the difficult total knee arthroplasty. *Clin Orthop Relat Res* 1990;260:6–9.
13. Engh GA, Parks NL, Ammeen DJ. Influence of surgical approach on lateral retinacular releases in total knee arthroplasty. *Clin Orthop Relat Res* 1996;331:56–63.
14. Kelly MJ, Rumi MN, Kothari M, et al. Comparison of the vastus-splitting and median parapatellar approaches for primary total knee arthroplasty: a prospective, randomized study. *J Bone Joint Surg Am* 2006; 88:715–720.
15. Bäthis H, Perlick L, Blum C, et al. Midvastus approach in total knee arthroplasty: a randomized, double-blinded study on early rehabilitation. *Knee Surg Sports Traumatol Arthrosc* 2005;13:545–550.
16. Cila E, Güzel V, Ozalay M, et al. Subvastus versus medial parapatellar approach in total knee arthroplasty. *Arch Orthop Trauma Surg* 2002;122:65–68.
17. Roysam GS, Oakley MJ. Subvastus approach for total knee arthroplasty: a prospective, randomized, and observer-blinded trial. *J Arthroplasty* 2001;16:454–457.
18. Jung YB, Lee YS, Lee EY, et al. Comparison of the modified subvastus and medial parapatellar approaches in total knee arthroplasty. *Int Orthop* 2008 Jan 15 [epub ahead of print].
19. Berth A, Urbach D, Neumann W, Awiszus F. Strength and voluntary activation of quadriceps femoris muscle in total knee arthroplasty with midvastus and subvastus approaches. *J Arthroplasty* 2007;22:83–88.

2 Lateral Approach to the Valgus Total Knee

James B. Stiehl

HISTORICAL PERSPECTIVE

Surgical techniques evolve to create easy, reproducible methods that simplify a procedure and reduce complications. These objectives were the guidelines of Dr. Peter A. Keblish, the originator of the lateral retinacular or valgus approach to the knee in total knee arthroplasty (TKA). The surgical problem in this case was how to do an adequate and complete release of contacted lateral ligaments often combined with articular deformity and lateral femoral condyle hypoplasia in valgus-deformed knees (Figs. 2-1 and 2-2). This approach was further necessitated by the fact that early extension ligament balancing was needed for the "tibia cut first method" adopted around the world for mobile-bearing TKA. Following the principles of Insall, the ligaments had to be completely balanced before the femoral bone cuts could be initiated; otherwise, potential flexion space instability could arise if balancing was altered after trials had been implanted. The most efficient method of balancing the lateral ligaments was to go directly at them through a lateral skin and fascial incision. This approach is desirable for any valgus-deformed knee but is optimal in cases of severe valgus deformity and patellar dislocation when extensile lateral releases are mandated. The experienced surgeon should use the approach on simpler cases such that the difficult case is not magnified by unfamiliarity with the approach.

ANATOMICAL CONSIDERATIONS

The direct lateral approach (1–3) is a technique that offers many advantages in correction of fixed valgus deformity, as well as other challenges that confront the knee surgeon, primarily, patella alignment and soft tissue considerations. It is less commonly used (and understood) than the standard medial approaches but has been shown to improve stability and patella results in fixed valgus TKA (4–7). Fixed contractures in valgus TKA require sequential releases that include the lateral capsule, iliotibial band (I-TB), vastus lateralis tendon, and very occasionally, the lateral collateral ligament (LCL), the popliteus, lateral gastrocnemius, and inner aspect of the fibular head (preserving and lengthening the LCL). These releases are best addressed by the direct access using the lateral approach.

Fixed valgus deformity is usually associated with lateral femoral condyle hypoplasia, femoral-tibial malrotation, resorption of the lateral femoral condyle and tibial plateau, and a relatively large medial condyle. Lateral structures are tight, and the patella is frequently deformed and subluxed over the deformed lateral condyle. The valgus knee deformity is most prevalent in females (9:1), and rheumatoid arthritis is more common. Prosthetic cover and joint seal can be a problem because the skin and soft tissue are often deficient. Excessive undermining, increased tension, or lack of a soft tissue layer between the skin and the prosthesis can lead to skin necrosis, a potentially devastating complication of TKA.

The fascia lata extension envelops the quadriceps with attachment to the posterior aspect of the femur. The distal lateral confluence becomes the iliotibial band with distinct insertion into Gerdy's

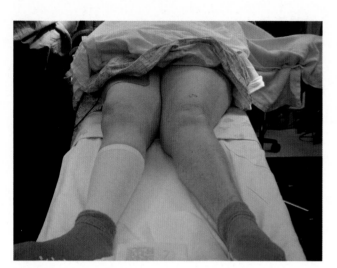

FIGURE 2-1

Severe valgus deformity in a 74-year-old female.

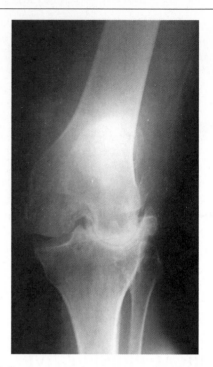

FIGURE 2-2

Valgus deformity noted with lateral femoral hypoplasia and severe erosion of the lateral tibial plateau with a mechanical axis alignment of 23 degrees valgus.

tubercle and the lateral tibial plateau. Transverse and oblique fibers extend to the patellar mechanism (lateral retinaculum), and longitudinal fibers attach to bone via Sharpey's fibers and extend to the myofascia of the anterior compartment. The I-TB and the lateral retinaculum are deforming factors in the fixed valgus knee. The I-TB attachment to the upper tibia produces a valgus moment with external rotation, and the oblique and transverse extensions produce a lateral (subluxing) moment to the patella. The extra-articular (superficial) layer also includes the lateral hamstring, the fabellofibular ligament, the lateral head of the gastrocnemius, and the popliteus. These structures may be contracted secondary to long-standing valgus. Bony deformity may further increase concave side contractures.

The lateral superficial layer differs from the (compliant) medial oblique retinaculum of the vastus medialis in that the lateral retinaculum is relatively noncompliant. This noncompliant lateral fascial extension to the patellar mechanism, coupled with contractures of the deeper layer, becomes a major determinant of the soft tissue deformity in the valgus knee.

The popliteus tendon, LCL, fabellofibular ligament, arcuate ligament, and capsule form the posterolateral complex. Anteriorly, the vastus lateralis inserts at the proximal patellar facet. The tendon of the vastus lateralis is usually of substantial thickness and joins the lateral aspect of the central quadriceps (rectus tendon). This structure is covered by a capsular and/or synovial layer in the joint. The muscles, by definition, have an extra-articular origin. The LCL differs from the medial collateral ligament in that its distal insertion is at the fibular head. The deep anterior and posterior lateral soft tissue layers are usually contracted to different degrees, depending on factors such as the underlying pathology, longevity of the deformity, and bony pathology. Management of superficial and deep layer contractures in valgus TKA must be understood and represents a key to correction of tibial rotation, centralization of the patella, and achieving proper flexion/extension gap balancing. In either case, the direct lateral approach enhances exposure and provides other advantages that will be discussed in the Technique section.

INDICATIONS

The standard medial parapatellar and subvastus/midvastus variations are the most commonly used approaches in TKA (8). There is a general consensus that sequential releases should be performed from the medial side prior to or after prosthetic insertion in fixed valgus (5–10). However, the medial approach in valgus TKA fails to address the pathologic anatomy directly, and releases may be overdone because exposure is limited after patella relocation and trial testing. Patella maltracking is more common (10), and there is increased potential for inaccurate flexion-extension gap balancing and less than optimum femoral-tibial stability. Other technical disadvantages include (a) increased external rotation of the tibia, (b) access to the posterolateral corner is more difficult, (c) an extensive lateral release is still required, (d) joint seal and prosthetic soft tissue coverage is difficult, (e) vascularity to the quadriceps patella tendon mechanism and lateral skin (beneath the extensive lateral release) is decreased (12), (f) it does not allow for optimal correction of the external rotation contracture of the tibia, and (g) it may encourage over-release of deep soft tissues.

The lateral approach in valgus deformity, by contrast, addresses the pathologic anatomy in a rational and sequential manner (17,18). The approach (a) is direct, (b) accomplishes the extensive "lateral release" with the exposure, (c) decreases skin undermining, (d) internally rotates the tibia with improved access to the pathologic posterolateral corner, (e) allows for better titration of sequential releases based on flexion-extension gap balance requirements, (f) preserves vascularity because the medial side is untouched, (g) allows for planned soft tissue gap and prosthetic coverage, (h) centralizes the quadriceps patella tendon mechanism, which optimizes patella tracking, (i) improves femoral-tibial alignment stability, and (j) rehabilitation is unimpeded because the medial quadriceps remains intact.

CONTRAINDICATIONS

There are few contraindications to this approach, although it may not be advisable in the presence of a nearby scar if the distance between the incision and prior scar is less than 6 to 8 mm, because the viability of the intervening skin bridge could be compromised. Additionally, given the more limited access and exposure of the medial side of the knee compared to medial approaches, this surgical approach is relatively contraindicated in the presence of a fixed varus deformity, because it is difficult to release medial side contractures through the lateral approach.

TECHNIQUE

The surgical technique of the direct lateral approach differs substantially from the standard medial parapatellar approach (14,17,18). The surgeon is less familiar with the lateral side of the knee; orientation is reversed, and more careful handling of the soft tissues is required. The recommended skin incision in the virgin knee follows the Q-angle and is slightly lateral to the patella, lateral border of the patellar tendon, and the tibial tubercle. Long incisions are preferred, especially in short, large legs (Fig. 2-3). It is important to avoid unnecessary undermining. In previously operated knees, the existing incision should be incorporated and extended proximally and distally. If multiple incisions are present, select the most direct or latest.

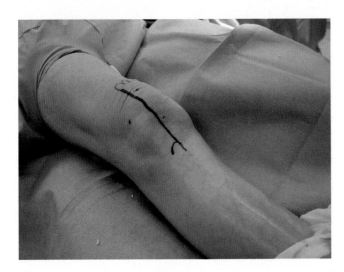

FIGURE 2-3

Skin incision follows the Q-angle and is slightly lateral to the midline.

Six major steps of the direct lateral approach are as follows:

- Step 1: I-TB release/lengthening
- Step 2: Lateral arthrotomy, coronal plane Z-plasty
- Step 3: Patella dislocation, joint exposure
- Step 4: Deep concave side releases (options)
      Tibial sleeve release, osteoperiosteal
      Distal LCL lengthening
      Proximal LCL lengthening
      Sleeve or osteoperiosteal
      Sliding lateral condyle osteotomy
- Step 5: Instrumentation/prosthetic insertion
- Step 6: Soft tissue closure deep to superficial layer

I-TB Release/Lengthening

Classically, the I-TB is exposed proximally by separating the inner fascial sleeve from the vastus lateralis muscle. The band is released from the posterior femur and "finger stripped" to the postero-lateral corner. A varus stress at the knee joint will "bowstring" the tight fascial bands, allowing for a multiple puncture "pie-crusting" lengthening under visual and digital control. The release is performed approximately 10 cm proximal to the joint line. The peroneal nerve can be palpated or explored, but this is seldom required and not recommended except in very severe cases. A simpler method preferred by the author is to expose the distal insertion of the I-TB into Gerdy's tubercle and either sharply incise or use a periosteal elevator to elevate the distal fascial insertion (Fig. 2-4). The simple I-TB release with subsequent lateral capsular release will allow the anatomical correction of all but the most severe deformities (>90%).

Lateral Retinacular Incision (Superficial Layer)

The lateral parapatellar incision begins proximally in the central quadriceps patella tendon along the vastus lateralis insertion to the lateral retinaculum where a coronal Z-plasty is performed (Fig. 2-5). The course of the lateral parapatellar incision extends 2 to 3 cm lateral to the patella and extends distally into the fat pad adjacent to the patellar tendon. The lateral incision penetrates only the dense superficial layer, leaving the underlying synovial later intact; therefore, proceed cautiously through the outer layers.

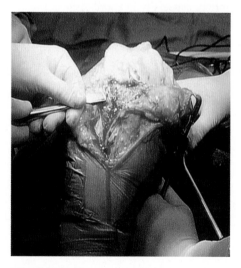

FIGURE 2-4
The ITB is elevated from Gerdy's tubercle in the frontal plane.

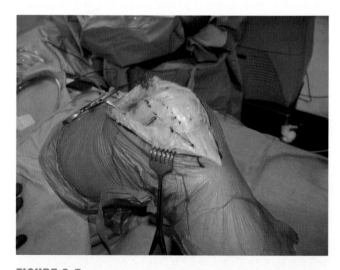

FIGURE 2-5
Incision of the lateral retinaculum is the more lateral straight line, followed by the incision of the deeper capsular synovial layer (*dotted line*) for the coronal Z-plasty.

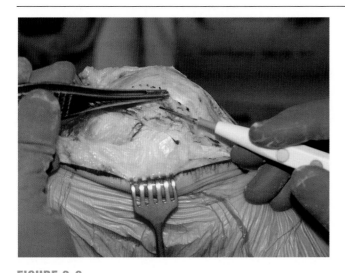

FIGURE 2-6

Note dissection of the lateral retinaculum to the rim of the patella exposing the underlying capsular synovial layer.

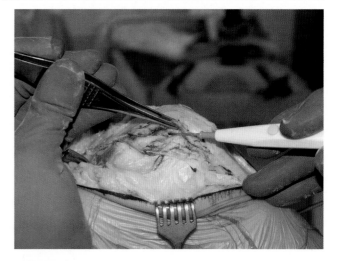

FIGURE 2-7

Incision of the deeper capsular synovial layer from the rim of the lateral patella.

Lateral Arthrotomy (Deep Layer)

The superficial dense lateral retinaculum layer adjacent to the patella is separated from the deep capsular synovial layer (Fig. 2-6). The deep synovial layer is incised from the patellar rim, performing the so-called coronal plane Z-plasty. This allows a lateral layer of synovial tissue that may be reattached to the medial portion of the lateral retinaculum, thus lengthening the lateral closure (Fig. 2-7). The fat pad incision distally continues obliquely to the intermeniscal ligament, retaining about 50% of the fat pad with the patella tendon and 50% with the lateral sleeve, which includes the lateral meniscus rim for increased soft tissue stability (Figs. 2-8 and 2-9).

Distal Tubercle Elevation or Osteotomy

The distal extension of the retinacular incision ends at Gerdy's tubercle and continues distally into the anterior compartment fascia. The osteoperiosteal sleeve release (utilizing a sharp osteotome) begins medial to Gerdy's tubercle and extends to, but stops at the tibial tubercle (Fig. 2-10). As the osteoperiosteal sleeve is elevated, the elevation stops at the lateral border of the patella tendon, protecting the tendon insertion and dissipating stresses to the anterior compartment sleeve (Fig. 2-11). A formal

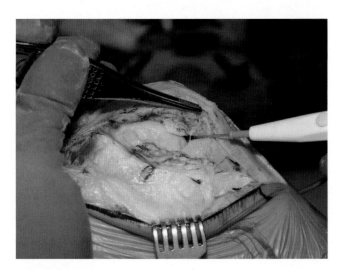

FIGURE 2-8

Incision of the fat pad creates a lateral flap for later closure.

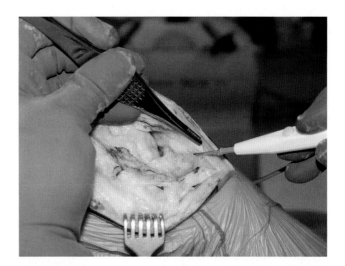

FIGURE 2-9

The incision extends into the lateral meniscal tibial ligament.

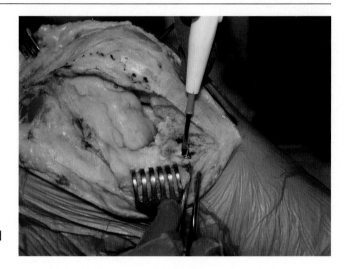

FIGURE 2-10

Incision of anterior Gerdy's tubercle iliotibial band insertion.

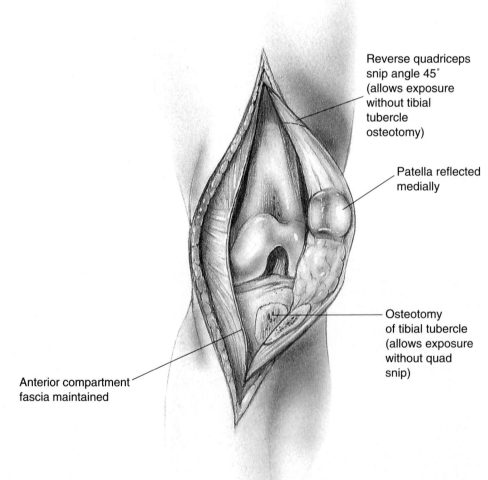

Reverse quadriceps snip angle 45° (allows exposure without tibial tubercle osteotomy)

Patella reflected medially

Osteotomy of tibial tubercle (allows exposure without quad snip)

Anterior compartment fascia maintained

FIGURE 2-11

Elevation of the tibial tubercle and medial displacement of the patella.

lateral-to-medial tibial tubercle osteotomy can be performed to enhance exposure in most difficult cases or as the surgeon's choice (13,15).

Patella Dislocation/Joint Exposure

Classically, the patella is dislocated/everted medially as the knee is flexed with a varus stress (Fig. 2-12) (11). Grasping the patella with a towel clip can be helpful. In recent years, an equally effective method is to simply translate the patella medially without eversion. Often, patellar and femoral condyle osteophytes must be removed to enhance the translation. Extending the proximal quadriceps incision may enhance this exposure further. Rarely, a lateral-to-medial rectus snip may be needed. Following patella displacement, a 90-degree Homan retractor is placed medially through the periphery of the medial meniscus and over the medial cortical rim.

Tibial Sleeve Release

Osteoperiosteal release from Gerdy's tubercle to the posterolateral tibia begins in extension (before joint exposure) and is completed in flexion (Fig. 2-13, see also Fig. 2-4). The combined release of the I-TB and the lateral capsule back to the posterolateral corner is extensile and will usually correct most deformities (Figs. 2-14 and 2-15). Osteophytes and the posterior capsule are released, and flexion/extension correction is checked with lamina spreaders or computer navigation. The posterior cruciate ligament (PCL) can be released at this time (if required because of non-correctable

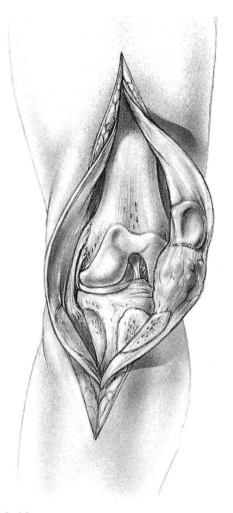

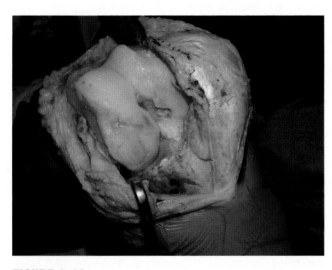

FIGURE 2-12

The patella is dislocated over the medial condyle to complete the initial exposure.

FIGURE 2-13

The anterior compartment muscle and the iliotibial tract from the Gerdy tubercle are elevated. (See also Fig. 2-4.)

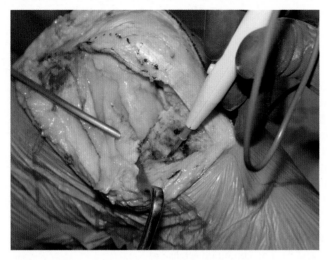

FIGURE 2-14

Incision of the lateral capsular insertion extends along the lateral tibial plateau.

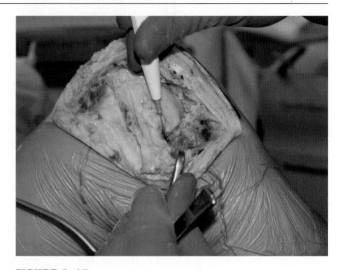

FIGURE 2-15

Important release of the lateral capsule from the "posterolateral" corner. Note that the Blount retractor protects the popliteus and lateral collateral ligaments.

contractures or if the surgeon chooses PCL-substituting prostheses) and will provide a modest amount of correction. Most importantly, these releases allow for anterior translation of the lateral tibial plateau, which dramatically increases exposure of the joint.

Distal LCL Release

When required, direct exposure and removal of the inner proximal fibula (with retention of the outer periosteum and ligament attachments) allows for medial translation and a relative lengthening of the LCL, without the need for fixation. Using this maneuver may provide enough length, avoiding the need for femoral side releases.

Femoral Sleeve Release

If required, two options are possible: osteoperiosteal release of the popliteus and LCL (limited osteotomy) or soft tissue sleeve release, beginning under the popliteus insertion and extending proximally (Fig. 2-16A,B). This is a classically recommended method, but it can lead to compromised ligament attachment with resultant instability and should probably be avoided in most cases.

COMPUTER NAVIGATION WITH VALGUS RELEASE

The author has been a strong advocate of computer navigation, particularly in cases of severe preoperative deformity. For the valgus approach, the author recommends placing the distal femoral array with two pins lateral to medial through the transepicondylar axis and posterior femoral shaft (19). This method allows placement of intramedullary femoral instrumentation, avoids soft tissue entrapment, and places the optical trackers out of the way in the sagittal plane. The valgus release should allow extension correction of the mechanical axis to 0 degrees. This is best done with computer monitoring. One consideration is that if there is significant medial joint laxity, correct balancing should allow even a bit more release beyond 0 degrees.

PERFORMANCE OF BONE CUTS AND TRIAL COMPONENT INSERTION

Lateral soft tissue release, tibial plateau translation, and patellar dislocation allows for excellent exposure of the anterior joint compartment for arthroplasty performed in the usual fashion. The initial bone resections are most difficult and are done with "mirror reverse" of the medial approach (Figs. 2-17 to 2-23). As the operation proceeds, the exposure becomes easier and final component insertion is straightforward. The goal of implant insertion should be to create anatomical mechanical axis alignment of

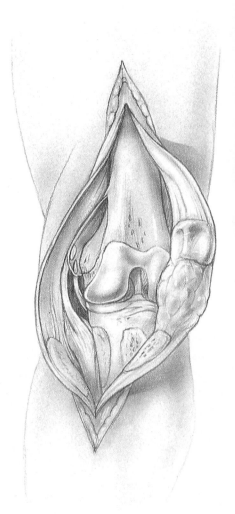

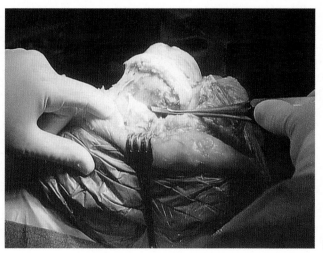

A

FIGURE 2-16

(A) The lateral collateral ligament (LCL) and popliteus tendon (PT) are elevated. **(B)** The LCL, PT, and periosteum are elevated from the lateral femoral condyle.

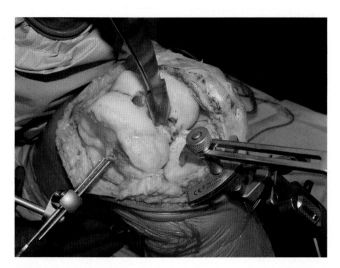

FIGURE 2-17

The tibial extramedullary cut guide is applied referencing the lateral tibial plateau. Note the placement of the distal femoral computer navigation array, with a transepicondylar double pin placement.

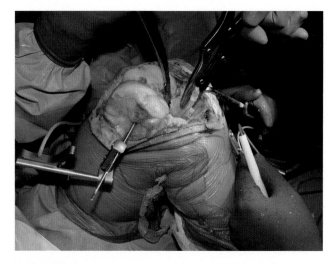

FIGURE 2-18

The tibial plateau remnant is removed. Note that the anterior translation of the lateral tibial plateau enhances medial exposure.

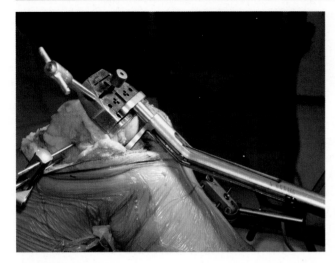

FIGURE 2-19

Anterior/posterior cut guide is applied with a tensor spacer instrument.

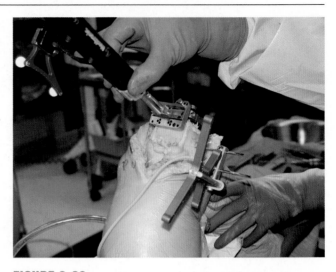

FIGURE 2-20

Computer navigation of the distal femoral cut guide.

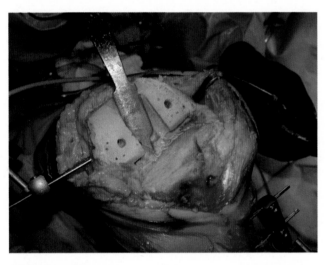

FIGURE 2-21

Excellent exposure of the femur and tibia for final prosthetic insertion. Note that the patella has not been everted but only dislocated medially.

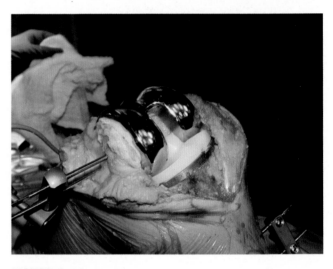

FIGURE 2-22

The final implantation demonstrates placement of a 10-mm polyethylene spacer with excellent flexion stability.

FIGURE 2-23

Note the position of the prosthesis in full extension.

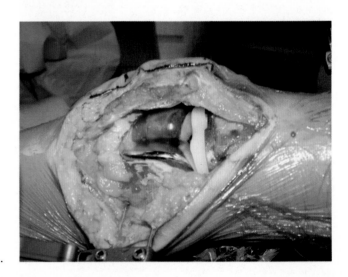

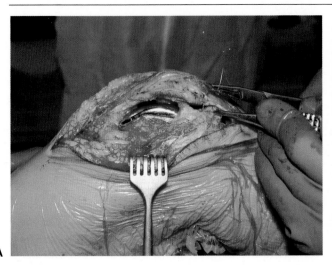
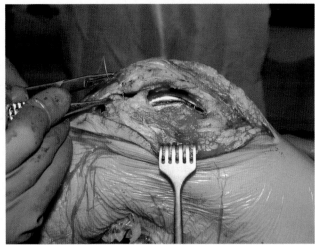

A   B

FIGURE 2-24

(A,B) Closure is done in flexion starting distally with the fat pad and lateral meniscal remnant.

0 degrees, perfect extension/flexion gap balancing under 3 degrees, correct femoral rotation for physiological patellar tracking, and limited bone resection and release to allow use of a 10-mm tibial polyethylene insert. Tibial component rotational alignment can be determined so that its center is aligned with the medial third of the tibial tubercle or mated to the femoral component in extension.

SOFT TISSUE SLEEVE CLOSURE

Closure is accomplished in flexion (Fig. 2-24). Depending on the amount of medial patellar translation with joint reconstruction, lateral wound closure begins proximally repairing the vastus lateralis split and then closing the coronal Z-plasty over the lateral joint, adjusting tension as needed (Fig. 2-25A,B). Distally, the lateral fat pad and lateral ligament sleeve is sewn to the lateral patellar tendon. A watertight closure of the lateral approach is possible in most cases (Fig. 2-26A,B).

TIPS AND PEARLS

The lateral tibial release from Gerdy's tubercle to the posterolateral corner can be performed before or after joint exposure. An osteoperiosteal technique with a sharp osteotome and/or electrocautery

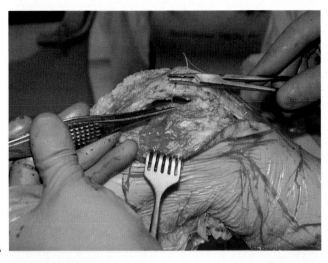
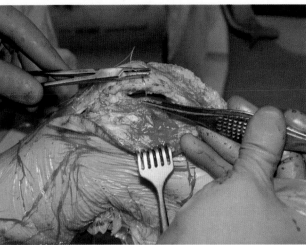

A   B

FIGURE 2-25

(A,B) Note that the closure of the lateral retinacular superficial layer to the deeper capsular synovial layer allows 2- to 3-cm advancement with the coronal Z-plasty.

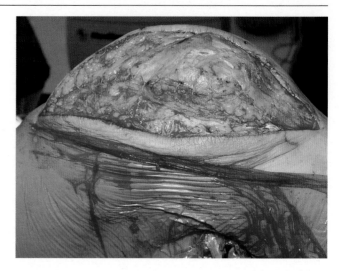

FIGURE 2-26
Final closure allows a "watertight" seal of the lateral compartment.

allows for exposure/release of the posterolateral corner and the posterior capsule (Fig. 2-27). If satisfactory correction is accomplished following the tibial sleeve and PCL releases, proceed with bony resections and fine-tune the ligament releases at the time of trial reduction. If the lateral structures remain tight and do not allow for satisfactory varus/valgus balance, proceed with distal LCL lengthening (fibula or proximal lengthening femoral side). Keep in mind that the LCL affects both the flexion and extension gap stability, whereas the popliteus tendon affects only flexion and rotation stability. Therefore, avoid cutting the popliteus, as increased flexion laxity is a potential liability. The sliding lateral condyle osteotomy with a more extensive bone segment is a newer concept that has the advantage of maintaining a strong proximal soft tissue ligament attachment.

When correcting a valgus deformity, distal femoral resection of 6 to 7 degrees is recommended because it allows for improvement of extension gap balancing and tensioning of "intact" medial structures. Slight residual valgus (mechanical axis 1 to 2 degrees) is cosmetically acceptable in the patient with long-standing valgus deformity.

Type II valgus with stretch-out of the medial structures can create instability in the M-L and rotational planes. Most preexisting instabilities represent pseudolaxity and are corrected with the direct lateral approach (when the medial side is left untouched) and a minimal medial tibial resection. True medial instabilities caused by incompetent soft tissue structures can be treated with a combination of prosthetic implants such as the posterior stabilized, constrained condylar, and/or proximal medial collateral ligament advancement.

Long-standing posterolateral contractures with severe rotation deformities require more prospective releases and concern for peroneal nerve stretch and/or compression injury. The peroneal nerve

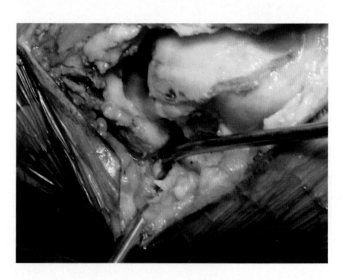

FIGURE 2-27
The sucker tip is directed to the "posterolateral" corner that has been released by the periosteal elevator.

can be exposed and decompressed proximally, and/or a partial proximal fibulectomy can be performed. When performing extensive soft tissue dissection in a high-risk rheumatoid type (thin-skinned) patient, splinting in extension for 2 to 3 days should be considered. In general, the rehabilitation is less intensive in this high-risk group.

Patella technique is a significant problem for most surgeons and continues to be a point of controversy (16). The author's experience has been that patella tracking is a rare problem of the lateral approach, as the entire lateral side has been released, and the patella easily floats to the midline if the medial ligamentous structures remain untouched. However, the surgeon must account for a correct femoral component rotation and implant positioning in the coronal and sagittal planes, as these may all affect patellar stability. With current implant designs, the author routinely leaves the patella unresurfaced, especially if the native patella is small or has fairly normal cartilage surface.

RESULTS

The author has studied a group of valgus deformed knees in patients who had undergone TKA with computer navigation from September 2003 until November 2004. Of this group of 85 patients, the lateral surgical approach was used in 15 (17%). The preoperative long-standing radiographs revealed a mean of 6.7 degrees of valgus to the mechanical axis with a range of 1 to 14 degrees valgus. The postoperative radiographic review showed a mean of 0.1 degrees valgus (95% confidence interval, 0.72 degrees) with a range of 2 degrees valgus to 2 degrees varus (Fig. 2-28). Finally, the thickness of polyethylene inserts was assessed and was 10 mm in nine cases, 12 mm in four cases, and 14 mm in one case. None of these cases required release of the LCL, and all alignment corrections were possible with the IT-B resection from Gerdy's tubercle, the lateral capsular release to the posterior/lateral corner of the knee, and PCL resection. Finally, the transepicondylar axis in relation to the tibial shaft axis usually mirrored the preoperative mechanical axis deformity with a comparable valgus position.

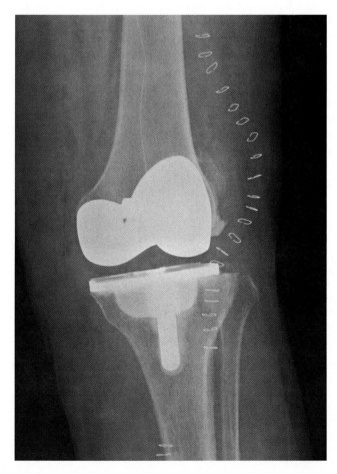

FIGURE 2-28

Final alignment of 2 degrees valgus to the mechanical axis was accomplished using a 12-mm polyethylene tibial insert and a standard lateral tibial sleeve release.

COMPLICATIONS

Performed well, the risk of complications related to this exposure should be limited. Component alignment has proven accurate in numerous published reports (1–3). Patella tracking is optimized through this approach; therefore, patella instability is uncommon. Peroneal palsy is a risk in the setting of severe fixed valgus knees, regardless of the surgical approach. The risk to the peroneal nerve may be increased with inadvertent surgical dissection or overzealous retraction but should not be significantly increased when sound surgical technique and principles are followed. Hematoma can be a potential source of compressive neuropathy and can be minimized with hemostasis. Patients who develop postoperative peroneal nerve palsy should be evaluated for the possible presence of an expanding hematoma, and evacuation of the hematoma should be performed if necessary. Most peroneal palsies after correction of a severe fixed valgus deformity, however, are transient traction phenomena or are related to external compression. When observed in the immediate postoperative period, the circumferential cotton and wrapping should be loosened and the knee flexed slightly for 24 hours to relieve pressure or tension on the peroneal nerve. If a foot drop is present, an ankle-foot orthosis should be applied to reduce the risk of development of an equinus contracture. Although most peroneal palsies improve over a 6- to 12-month period, an electromyelogram and neurological consultation may be prudent if there is limited improvement at 6 weeks.

CONCLUSIONS AND FUTURE PERSPECTIVES

Fixed valgus deformity presents a major challenge in TKA. The literature suggests that correction of fixed valgus deformities via the standard medial parapatellar approach leads to higher failure rates, primarily at the patellofemoral joint. Another important concern for the patella is the avascularity caused by the combination of the medial parapatellar approach when combined with the typical lateral release that is required in most severe lateral valgus deformities (12). The literature supporting the lateral approach for valgus deformity demonstrates outcomes similar to medial approaches for varus preoperative deformities. The surgeon should be familiar with and should consider the direct lateral approach in challenging total knee replacements, including (a) fixed valgus deformity with patella subluxation, (b) partially correctable valgus deformity with lateral orientation and/or patella subluxation, (c) previous lateral incisions in multiply operated knees—when skin is at risk (with undermining), (d) lateral unicompartmental replacement, and (e) high tibial osteotomy conversion to TKA, especially if lateral incision and/or retained metal is present (14,17,18).

Those who have gained experience with this method feel strongly about its validity and necessity in certain unusual cases such as the severe valgus knee and the chronic dislocated patella. One surgeon has suggested that "the driver can enter his car from either door, but it is easiest to enter on the side where the steering wheel is located." This comparison can be made regarding the lateral approach in the valgus deformed knee. The author suggests that to be ready for that once-in-a-while disaster deformity, any knee with a valgus angulation over 8 degrees should be approached laterally. If you follow this method, the lateral approach is as easy and routine as the medial approach requiring a mirror image of techniques.

REFERENCES

1. Buechel FF. A sequential three-step lateral release for correcting fixed valgus knee deformities during total knee arthroplasty. *Clin Orthop* 1990;260:170–175.
2. Keblish PA. The lateral approach to the valgus knee: surgical technique and analysis of 53 cases with over two-year follow-up evaluation. *Clin Orthop* 1991;271:52–62.
3. Keblish PA. Valgus deformity in TKR: the lateral retinacular approach. *Orthop Trans* 1985;9:28.
4. Lootvoet L, Blouard E, Himmer O, Ghosez JP. Complete knee prosthesis in severe genu valgum. Retrospective review of 90 knees surgically treated through the anterio-external approach. *Acta Orthopaedica Belgica* 1997;63:278–286.
5. Fiddian NJ, Blakeway C, Kumar A. Replacement arthroplasty of the valgus knee. A modified lateral capsular approach with repositioning of vastus lateralis. *J Bone Joint Surg [Br]* 1998;80:859–861.
6. Tsai CL, Chen CH, Liu TK. Lateral approach without ligament release in total knee arthroplasty: new concepts in the surgical technique. *Artificial Organs* 2001;25:638–643.
7. Whiteside LA. Correction of ligament and bone defects in total arthroplasty of the severely valgus knee. *Clin Orthop* 1993;288:234–245.
8. Insall JN, Scott WN, Keblish PA, et al. Total knee arthroplasty exposures and soft tissue balancing. In Insall JN, Scott WN, eds. *VideoBook of Knee Surgery*. Philadelphia: JB Lippincott; 1994.

9. Krackow KA, Jones MM, Teeny SM, et al. Primary total knee arthroplasty in patients with fixed valgus deformity. *Clin Orthop* 1991;273:9–18.
10. Ranawat CS. Total-condylar knee arthroplasty for valgus and combined valgus-flexion deformity of the knee. *Tech Orthopaedics* 1988;3:67–76.
11. Merkow TL, Soudry M, Insall JN. Patellar dislocation following total knee replacement. *J Bone Joint Surg* 1985;67A:1321.
12. Scapinelli R. Blood supply of the human patella. *J Bone Joint Surg* 1967;49B:563.
13. Wolff AM, Hungerford DS, Krackow KA, et al. Osteotomy of the tibial tubercle during total knee replacement. *J Bone Joint Surg [Am]* 1989;71:848–852.
14. Keblish PA, Boldt J, Varma C, Briard JL. Soft-tissue balancing in fixed valgus TKA: methods of achieving concave side releases. Presented at AAOS 2002 Scientific Exhibit, Dallas, Texas.
15. Burki H, von Knoch M, Heiss C, et al. Lateral approach with osteotomy of the tibial tubercle in primary total knee arthroplasty. *Clin Orthop* 1999;362:156–161.
16. Arnold MP, Friederich NF, Widmer H, et al. Patellar substitution in total knee prosthesis—is it important? *Orthopade* 1998;27:637–641.
17. Keblish PA, Stiehl JB, Boldt JA. The direct lateral approach. *Techniques in Knee Surgery* 2003;2:250–266.
18. Keblish PA, Briard JL. Surgical Approaches: Lateral Approach or Approaching the Valgus Knee. In Hamelynck KJ, Stiehl JB, eds. *LCS Mobile Bearing Knee Arthroplasty: 25 Years of Worldwide Experience.* Heidelberg: Springer Verlag; 2002:150–160.
19. Stiehl JB. Transepicondylar distal femoral pin placement in computer assisted surgical navigation. Journal of Computer Assisted Surgery. In press.

3 Minimally Invasive Total Knee Arthroplasty

David Watson and Steven Haas

INDICATIONS

Innovative techniques and alteration in instrument design have facilitated the safe and accurate place-ment of a total knee arthroplasty (TKA) while utilizing smaller incisions and less dissection/disruption of the extensor mechanism and joint capsule. Several techniques have been popularized, including the mini-medial parapatellar, mini-subvastus, quadriceps-sparing, and mini-midvastus approaches with a unifying theme of minimal disruption of the extensor mechanism. These techniques were developed to minimize the surgical insult and allow for an earlier return to function and in no way alter the indica-tions for TKA. Regardless of which particular minimally invasive surgical approach is used, the general philosophy and approaches to the knee are similar, and outcomes similar, despite only subtle variations in the arthrotomies and capsular incisions (Fig. 3-1).

The advantages of minimally invasive knee arthroplasty are as follows:

- Earlier return of quadriceps function
- Earlier return of motion
- Improved flexion
- Decreased postoperative narcotic usage
- Improved cosmesis
- Equal complication rate to standard techniques

TKA is a highly successful operation, rewarding for both the surgeon and patient when performed well, in well-selected individuals. It is indicated in the situation of significant disability arising from an underlying arthritic condition of the knee that has been refractory to nonoperative measures. Before surgical consideration, a patient should have an appropriate diagnosis and participated in a trial of conservative measures including activity modification, nonnarcotic analgesics/anti-inflammatory medication, physical therapy, and weight reduction when appropriate.

The decision to proceed with a minimally invasive technique depends on the surgeon, instrumen-tation, and patient factors.

Surgeon

Although the underlying principles of appropriate bony cuts and soft tissue balancing are un-changed, the techniques used in minimally invasive (MIS) TKA are different, and the execution of a well-placed and balanced knee is more technically demanding than the more traditional extensile arthrotomy. Specialized training sessions, in addition to a thorough understanding and technical mastery of standard knee arthroplasty techniques are recommended before attempting these techniques.

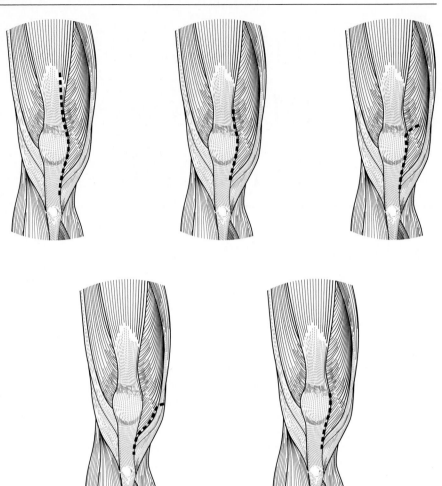

FIGURE 3-1

Standard arthrotomy, mini-parapatellar, mini-midvastus, mini-subvastus, and quadriceps-sparing incisions.

Instrumentation

In the development of minimally invasive techniques, instrumentation was adapted to facilitate use through smaller operative windows. A minimally invasive set with significantly smaller, side-specific guides, and cutting blocks is very advantageous and certainly recommended if MIS TKA is to be undertaken. Specialized saw blades are also recommended (Fig. 3-2).

Patient

In the day of direct-to-consumer advertising and Internet access, patients often request MIS techniques. If the surgical expertise and appropriate instrumentation are available, I believe it is reasonable to proceed if the patient is an appropriate candidate. Although there are no absolute contraindications to MIS TKA, the relative contraindications are patient related. Patients, particularly those requesting the techniques, are advised that incisions are increased in size, and dissections are made more extensile at any time during the reconstruction should safety, visualization, or quality be felt to be compromised. Early in a surgeon's experience, MIS approaches to the knee are typically reserved for the simplest of cases; as the surgeon's experience and comfort level improve, the indications for MIS approaches expand.

Relative contraindications to MIS TKA are as follows:

- Men with substantial quadriceps muscle mass
- Men with very large bone dimensions
- Significant obesity (body mass index [BMI] >40)
- Severe coronal plane deformity
- Flexion contracture >25 degrees

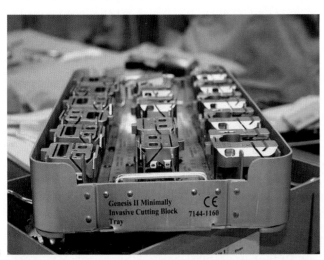

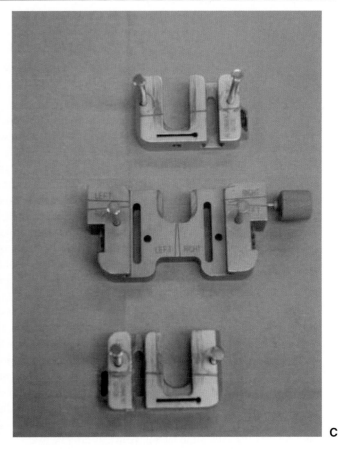

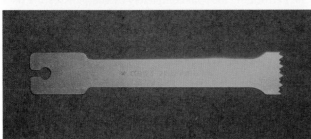

FIGURE 3-2

(A) A dedicated minimally invasive set is necessary for successful MIS technique.
(B) Appropriate saw blades facilitate resection through the mini-jigs and allow bony
resection in a safe manner with less side-to-side saw excursion. **(C)** A comparison of
older guides (middle) with new "sided" mini-guides—the significantly reduced bulk
enables smaller operative windows.

- Passive flexion <80 degrees
- Severe patella baja
- Significant scarring of the quadriceps mechanism

Thin female patients tend to be the easiest candidates for MIS TKA, particularly those with a
"loose knee" and an underdeveloped vastus medialis obliquus (VMO) inserting high on the patella.
Patients with a well-developed VMO (muscular men) and those in whom the VMO inserts lower on
the patella at a more oblique angle are more challenging and may warrant standard technique until
considerable experience is gained.

Preoperative Planning

Planning proceeds as per standard knee arthroplasty. The author obtains standing anteroposterior
(AP), lateral, flexed PA, and merchant views. Full-length views are not obtained unless otherwise
indicated by history or physical examination. In cases of deformity, anticipating an appropriate
valgus cut angle and height of tibial resection can be helpful.

TECHNIQUE

Positioning

Appropriate leg positioning is crucial when performing minimally invasive TKA. I prefer to use a
tourniquet if there is no contraindication, although it may be done without one. A sandbag is placed

under the drapes at the level of the opposite ankle so that the knee can sit flexed at approximately 70 to 90 degrees. The majority of the procedure is done in this position. Hyperflexion is sometimes required to prepare the proximal tibia and insert the definitive tibial tray. A lateral support is used so that the leg sits without being held by an assistant (Fig. 3-3).

Exposure

Landmarks for the skin incision are the borders of the patella and the tibial tubercle. These are marked, and a longitudinal incision line is drawn at the junction of the middle and medial thirds of the patella. The incision extends from 1 cm above the superior pole of the patella to the proximal half of the tibial tubercle on its medial side. A typical skin incision length is between 8.5 and 12 cm; however, the technique is not defined by incision length, and there should be no hesitation to extend this at any stage if there appears to be undue tension, especially at the distal apex of the incision (Fig. 3-4).

A medial arthrotomy is performed. This extends from the superior pole of the patella to the level of the tibial tubercle. We leave a 5-mm cuff of tissue adjacent to the tubercle to aid in closure later on. The VMO is identified, and an oblique split is made in the muscle in the line of its fibers at the level of the superior pole of the patella (Fig. 3-5).

The first centimeter of the muscle split is started sharply, but the remainder is performed bluntly with a finger, gently separating the muscle fibers. Performing the split completely by sharp dissection risks damaging the distal innervation of the vastus musculature. The muscle split is generally between 2 and 4 cm in length. We have found from experience that this usually does not propagate any further with this technique. The suprapatellar pouch is preserved except in cases of severe inflammatory disease.

With the knee extended, a subperiosteal dissection is carried around the medial pretibial border, releasing the meniscotibial attachments. The patella is then retracted laterally, and a partial excision of the infrapatellar fat pad is performed. We also excise the medial fat pad at this stage. Excision of the fat pad is a crucial maneuver at this point, as it releases a distal tether of the patella allowing for lateral subluxation. The tibial attachments of the anterior cruciate ligament and the anterior horn of the lateral meniscus are released. This allows placement of a thin bent Homan retractor laterally to sublux the patella. A small synovial window is made over the antero-lateral femoral cortex to aid in our initial anterior femoral resection.

In patients with tight extensor mechanisms, large patellae, or an abundance of patellar osteophytes, the patella can be cut first. Initial patellar resection is usually not required, however.

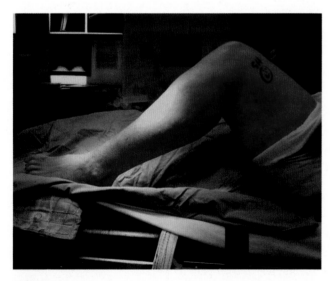

FIGURE 3-3

Appropriate setup is critical. Notice the bump is placed across from the contralateral ankle allowing for a resting position of the operative extremity at less than 90 degrees of flexion. A padded tourniquet is placed high on the operative thigh.

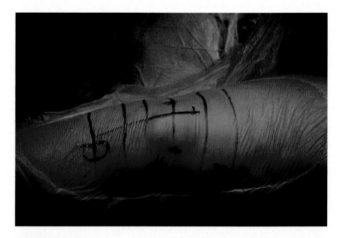

FIGURE 3-4

The tibial tubercle is represented by the circle, and the borders of the patella have been marked. The skin incision is then drawn at the junction of the medial third and lateral two thirds of the patella extending from just above the superior pole to the medial aspect of the tibial tubercle.

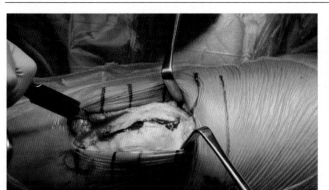

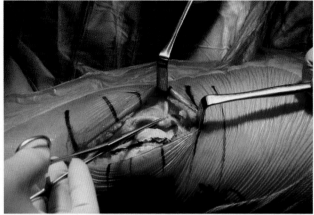

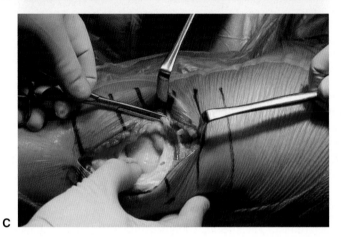

FIGURE 3-5

(A) The intended arthrotomy is depicted. A 5-mm cuff of tissue is left along the medial border of the patella for ease of repair. At the superior pole of the patella, the dissection turns medial and enters the VMO at a 45-degree angle. **(B)** The initial 1-cm split of the VMO is performed sharply. **(C)** After the initial split, the rest of the vastus dissection is performed bluntly to minimize the risk of distal denervation.

Femoral Preparation

Femoral preparation is performed first to relax the extension space. This is done with the knee in 70 degrees of flexion. Limiting knee flexion places the soft tissue window over the distal and anterior femur. Hyperflexion must be avoided, as it not only tightens the extensor mechanism but also limits exposure. A thin, bent Homan retractor is placed laterally around the margin of the femoral condyle without excessive lateral traction to hold the patella subluxed.

The AP axis (Whiteside's line) is marked on the distal femur and is used as our major landmark for establishing component rotation. The posterior condylar axis is used as a secondary reference in varus knees where it is most reproducible. The transepicondylar axis is more difficult to assess, as it requires excessive retraction of the patella laterally.

A 9.5-mm drill is used to enter the femoral canal at a starting point in the notch just anterior to the posterior cruciate ligament insertion on the femur. The canal is then suctioned of its marrow contents to reduce fat embolization risk. An intramedullary alignment guide set at 5 degrees of valgus relative to the anatomic axis is inserted. We only use posterior paddles for additional referencing when there is concern about rotational alignment. An AP axis guide inserted over the rod is placed in line with the marking of the AP axis, and the block is pinned in place. An anterior referencing guide is then slid under the quadriceps mechanism touching the antero-lateral femoral cortex, which usually represents the highest point. Maintaining the knee in approximately 70 to 90 degrees of flexion with minimal use of retractors is important to keep the extensor mechanism relaxed enough to allow for accurate anterior referencing without struggling (Fig. 3-6).

The preliminary anterior resection guide is then pinned in place, and the preliminary cut is performed. We prefer to use an anterior resection first technique so that later corrections in rotational or sagittal placement can be made if we are not satisfied with our initial position. This cut also relaxes the extensor mechanism before placing the distal cutting guide and allows the guide to sit more evenly on a flat surface.

We then perform our distal femoral resection. Additional retraction is not required at this point, as the guide's wedge shape usually retracts the proximal tissues adequately. The block is secured with two headed pins, the intramedullary rod is removed, and the distal resection is performed.

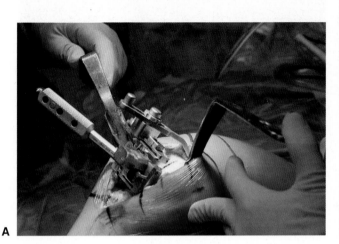

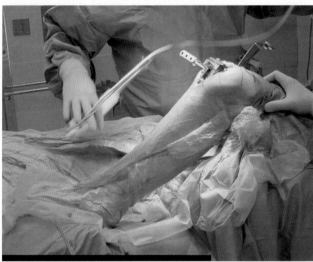

A   B

FIGURE 3-6

Femoral preparation. **(A)** The left 5 degrees valgus guide is in place, and the initial anterior resection is being planned. Note that the retractors are being maintained in a neutral position to minimize tension on the soft tissues and that no proximal retractors are needed after the stylus has been slid under the soft tissues. **(B)** The position of the limb for femoral preparation is critical. Maintaining the knee at 70 to 90 degrees of flexion relaxes the soft tissues sufficiently to allow safe and accurate placement of guides under the extensor mechanism proximally.

The femoral component size is then determined. The knee may require further flexion so that the posterior paddles can be passed behind the posterior condyles. In tight knees, an initial pass with the saw to remove the tibial eminences will often facilitate sizer placement without the need for hyperflexion. If we are between sizes, we prefer to choose the smaller component size so as not to overtighten the flexion space. We then pin the appropriate four-in-one cutting guide in place and once again assess our rotation. It is critical at this stage that a thin bent Homan retractor is placed deep to the medial collateral ligament for protection. The femoral resection is performed in the following order: posterior condyles, posterior chamfer, anterior resection, and anterior chamfer.

Tibial Preparation

The proximal tibial resection is then performed. We prefer extramedullary referencing, but both techniques are capable of being used with this technique. The knee is flexed to approximately 90 degrees. Excessive external rotation, which is often used in the standard approach, must be avoided, as this decreases visualization of the lateral compartment by rotating the lateral tibial plateau under the femur. A thin bent Homan retractor is then placed medially and laterally, to once again protect the medial collateral ligament and the extensor mechanism. Any overhanging anteromedial osteophytes are removed at this stage with a rongeur so that the tibial resection guide can sit in direct contact with the margin of the tibia. The tibial guide is placed parallel to the tibial crest proximally. We also use the tibialis anterior tendon over the ankle and the second metatarsal as reference points distally. Posterior slope is then adjusted so that the alignment guide is parallel to the fibular shaft. We aim for an 11-mm resection off the intact side. The guide is then pinned in place. An Aufranc retractor is placed posteriorly to protect the posterior neurovascular structures without changing the position of the knee (Fig. 3-7).

We then perform the proximal tibial resection. In order for the blade to be captured by the cutting guide, the saw must initially be angled at 45 degrees aiming posterolaterally. Once within the bone, the medial resection can be safely completed directing the blade in an anterior-to-posterior direction. We then direct the blade laterally to complete the resection. If we are in any doubt of the depth of the resection, we prefer to leave a small rim of bone. It is much safer to remove this later during the procedure as exposure increases, than aiming to remove the bone in one piece and causing an iatrogenic injury to the ligaments or potentially, the neurovascular bundle. The alignment of our tibial cut is then rechecked using an alignment rod connected to a spacer block.

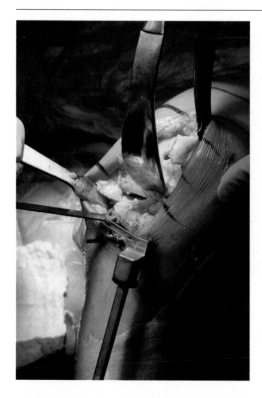

FIGURE 3-7

Tibial preparation. Retractors are placed to protect the soft tissues. The tibia is subluxed (minimally) anterior without any external rotation. In this case, a left extramedullary tibial cutting guide has been applied. Again, retractors are maintained in a neutral position to minimize soft tissue tension. Note the initial pass with the saw starts from an anteromedial angling posterolateral. Once captured within bone resection, it may be turned medially.

The knee is then placed in 90 degrees of flexion. Using laminar spreaders, we assess the posterior condyles for any retained osteophytes. These are removed with a curved osteotome and aid in re-establishing flexion capability. The meniscal remnants are excised at this stage along with the posterior cruciate ligament (if a posterior stabilized system is being used). We then place spacer blocks into both the flexion and extension spaces to ensure we have obtained symmetrical spaces with adequate resection levels. Additionally, it is a useful tool to predict later soft tissue releases.

The knee is then flexed to 120 degrees and an Aufranc retractor is once again placed posteriorly. This is the only time before component insertion that hyperflexion is used. An appropriately sized tibial component is pinned in place with one pin. Using an asymmetric tibial tray facilitates appropriate placement. The proximal tibia is then prepared to accept the definitive prosthesis, taking care to remove posteromedial osteophytes if needed (Fig. 3-8).

Final Preparation

Once we have confirmed that no further bone resection is required, we complete our femoral preparation. A trial femoral component designed to allow femoral box preparation is positioned. Using this technique rather than a standard box cutting guide saves a step and allows more accurate mediolateral placement of the component. Over all, we aim for slight lateral position to optimize

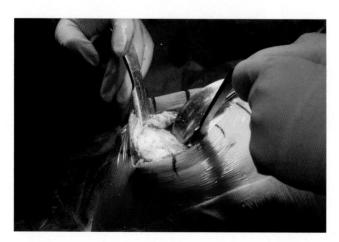

FIGURE 3-8

Final tibial preparation requires anterior subluxation. This is achieved by hyperflexion and is the only time this maneuver is necessary prior to cementing the real tibial tray. The bent Homan retractor laterally has been placed on the anterior third of the tibia to prevent soft tissue from draping on the plateau.

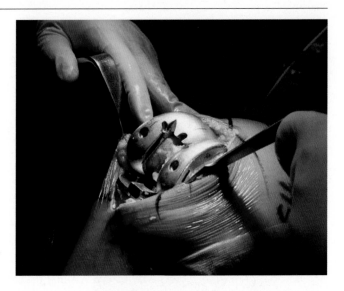

FIGURE 3-9

The proximal tibia has been prepared, and the ream through the trial femoral component is in place. After preparation of the box, the knee can be trialed.

patellar tracking. Medial overhang should be avoided, as this is a cause of capsular pain (Fig. 3-9). A cam is then placed in the box of the femoral component and trialing can proceed.

If the patella is being resurfaced, it is usually done at this stage. It is easier to wait until both femoral and tibial cuts have been performed, as the extensor mechanism is at its most relaxed and allows it to be turned 90 degrees. The patella is then prepared for a trial component. Once the trial is in place, we chamfer the lateral margin with a saw to minimize lateral retinacular impingement (Fig. 3-10).

We then perform a trial reduction with a variety of inserts and assess for coronal plane stability with the knee in both extension and at 90 degrees of flexion. Soft tissue releases are then performed until satisfactory balance is achieved. Patellofemoral tracking is then observed. If this is found to be suboptimal, it is rechecked with the tourniquet deflated to ensure that a lateral retinacular release is not required.

Component Insertion

We prefer to use cemented implants, however, noncemented devices may be used. Before cementing, the bone surfaces are lavaged under pulsatile pressure to achieve a bloodless and dry bone bed. A bone plug is fashioned and impacted into the femoral hole of the intercondylar notch. Occasionally, sclerotic bone requires drilling with a 2.5-mm drill to enhance cement interdigitation.

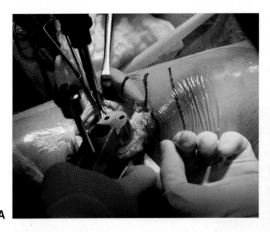
A

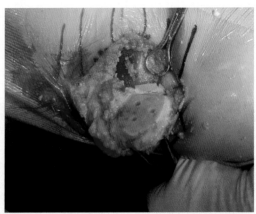
B

FIGURE 3-10

(A) After appropriate bony cuts the extension space is relaxed, and the patella can be everted for preparation. Patellar eversion with a fully tensed extension space should be avoided as it risks unnecessary propagation of the vastus split. **(B)** The lateral margin of the patellar button has been noted, and lateral bony overhang is beveled to minimize the risk of lateral patellar impingement.

The tibial component is inserted first. Exposure is obtained using an identical technique to that employed when inserting the trial component. The posterolateral overhang, which frequently occurs with symmetric tibial implants, can lead to difficulty with implant insertion and cement removal. For this reason, we prefer to use an asymmetric tibial base plate to facilitate clearance of the femoral condyle during implantation and subsequent cement removal. Once the tibial component has been implanted, the femoral and patellar components are inserted along with a trial polyethylene insert.

Cement removal from the posterior margins of the tibia can be aided by placing the knee in extension and applying traction prior to the femoral component implantation. A small curved curette can then be swept posteriorly along the margin of the tibial component to help remove any additional cement. On the femoral side, initial excessive proximal retraction should be avoided to remove cement when the component is being implanted at 90 degrees of flexion. It is best to only remove the cement extruded into the intercondylar notch and the condylar margins at this stage. A trial liner is then inserted, and the knee is taken in to extension. The mobile window will then easily deliver the anterior femoral cortex in view to remove the remaining extruded cement without the need for retraction.

The patellar component is then placed and clamped, and the cement is allowed to harden. Any additional cement is removed at this stage. The definitive polyethylene insert is next inserted. If using a posterior stabilized insert, the surgeon should begin inserting the polyethylene in 90 degrees of flexion. The knee should then be brought into full extension to engage the locking mechanism.

Closure

The tourniquet is deflated at this stage, and bleeding is controlled. The knee is copiously lavaged with normal saline solution, and two drains are inserted. The capsular layer is closed by placing three to five 0–0 Vicryl sutures into the VMO tendon and perimuscular fascia. The remainder of the arthrotomy and the subcutaneous tissues are closed with interrupted sutures as well. The authors prefer to use 0–0 Vicryl sutures for the capsular layer and deep fat and 3–0 Vicryl for the subcutaneous layers. Clips are used to oppose the skin edges (Fig. 3-11).

PEARLS AND PITFALLS

- Pearl: During setup, ensure the foot-positioning device allows a resting position of 70 to 90 degrees of knee flexion, as hyperflexion effectively contracts the mobile window by tightening the extensor mechanism.
- Pearl: The need for proximal retraction is minimal. Generally, proximal access when the knee is in flexion can be gained by mild anterior retraction of the soft tissues with a right angle retractor allowing the instruments to be slid under the extensor after which further retraction is unnecessary.
- Pearl: In muscular patients, a 60 degrees split of the vastus from the superior pole of the patella rather than the standard 45 degrees minimizes the muscle bulk draping over the distal femur thereby improving exposure while still maintaining the integrity of the quadriceps tendon.
- Pearl: Appropriate lateral Homan retractor placement improves visualization. For femoral preparation, it should be placed on the posterior third of the tibia where it can maintain the patella out of the way while resting on the lateral femoral condyle. Moving this more anterior for tibial preparation protects the tendon and retracts the soft tissues from falling onto the plateau.
- Pitfall: Simultaneous retraction in both the medial and lateral direction counter-intuitively decreases working space by tightening the operative window. Retractors should be maintained in a neutral position with maximal retraction only on the side where the surgeon is currently working.
- Pitfall: Patellar eversion places too much tension on the extensor mechanism as it necessitates greater excursion to achieve the same exposure. This effectively tightens the working space in flexion and risks unnecessary propagation of the vastus split. Work with the patella subluxed.

REHABILITATION

All patients are started on a continuous passive motion machine in the recovery room, and flexion is increased as pain allows. Weight bearing is started on the first postoperative day. All patients receive thromboembolic prophylaxis, and foot- compressive devices are used until the patient is ambulating unassisted. A patient- controlled epidural is continued until the second postoperative day, when it is removed and the patient is placed on oral analgesics.

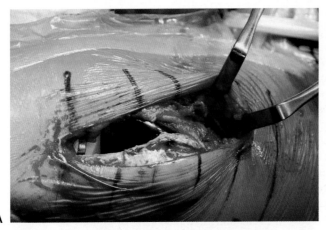

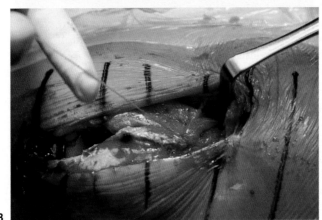

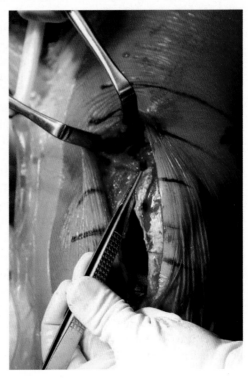

FIGURE 3-11

(A) The final split in the vastus is visualized extending approximately 2.5 cm proximally. **(B)** The apex of the split is identified and replaced anatomically. **(C)** With the apical stitch in place, the vastus split is visualized and will require two or three more sutures for it to close proximally.

COMPLICATIONS

The typical risks of TKA exist with minimally invasive approaches. However, given the smaller incisions and more limited exposure, some of these can occur with increased frequency. For instance, some investigators have reported a tendency for increased component malalignment, particularly with instrumentation that is not necessarily modified and miniaturized for a minimally invasive approach (8). Fractures, soft tissue imbalance, iatrogenic ligament, tendon, or bone injury, neurovascular injury, and improper cementing technique can be minimized with adequate exposure, attention to details, patience, and use of sound surgical technique and instrumentation.

RESULTS

Currently, no studies have the statistical power to provide a strong rationale for favoring any specific minimally invasive approach to TKA over another. Studies show that when performed well, however, in appropriate patients, early functional recovery is improved after TKA performed with minimally invasive techniques compared to those performed with a more traditional approach.

In one study, the results of 40 consecutive minimally invasive TKAs performed with a modified midvastus approach in which the patella was subluxed, but not everted, were compared to the results of 40 standard TKAs. Patients in both groups were matched for age, gender, preoperative range of motion, weight, Knee Society scores, implant, and anesthesia. There were no significant overall differences in alignment of either the tibial or femoral components, although there were several outliers in terms of femoral alignment in the MIS patient group. The range of knee flexion at 6 weeks,

12 weeks, and 1 year was all significantly greater in the MIS TKA patient group than in the standard TKA patient group. At 1 year after surgery, the mean Knee Society knee and function scores were significantly greater in the MIS group compared to the standard group ($p < 01$ for both parameters), despite comparable preoperative scores (2).

The short-term clinical results were reported in a prospective, observer-blinded study comparing TKAs performed using either the mini-subvastus approach without patella eversion (60 patients) or the standard medial parapatellar approach with patellar eversion (60 patients). Patients were matched according to age, gender, preoperative knee flexion, alignment, and BMI. There was significantly less blood loss, less postoperative pain, and shorter time to achieving straight leg raise and 90 degrees of flexion in patients treated with the mini-subvastus approach compared to the standard approach. The range of motion at all intervals measured, including 1 month and 3 months, was also significantly greater in the mini-subvastus patient group. Of concern, there was one case of tibial malalignment (3 degrees) as well as one patellar tendon rupture and one fracture of the lateral femoral condyle, leading the authors to express some caution regarding the minimally invasive technique (7).

The results of a prospective multicenter study comparing 27 matched groups of TKAs performed with either a standard medial parapatellar approach or the various minimally invasive approaches— the mini-medial parapatellar, mini-midvastus, quadriceps-sparing, and mini-subvastus. Patients were all matched by height, weight, BMI, and preoperative range of motion, alignment, pain, and function. The average age was 68 years for each group, and the BMI was 31 for each group. Outcomes were assessed weekly for 6 weeks and then at 3 months, 6 months, and 12 months postoperatively. There were no identifiable significant differences in any of the outcome measures or complications occurring up to 1 year postoperatively between any of the MIS approaches. At 6 weeks, the range of motion in the MIS cohort was greater than in the standard arthroplasty cohort (116 vs. 109 degrees); and at 6 months, it was 123 degrees versus 116 degrees in the MIS group and standard group, respectively. Within the first 4 to 6 weeks after arthroplasty, there was significantly less pain among those who underwent a minimally invasive approach compared to those who had a standard approach (6).

REFERENCES

1. Engh GA, Parks NL. Surgical technique of the midvastus arthrotomy. *Clin Orthop Relat Res* 1998;351: 270–274.
2. Haas SB, Cook S, Beksac B. Minimally invasive total knee replacement through a mini midvastus approach: a comparative study. *Clin Orthop Relat Res* 2004;428:68–73.
3. Laskin RS. Minimally invasive total knee arthroplasty: the results justify its use. *Clin Ortho Relat Res* 2005;440:54–59.
4. Trousdale R, McGrory B, Berry D, Becky M, Harmsen W. Patients concerns prior to undergoing total hip and total knee arthroplasty. *Mayo Clinic Proceedings* October 1999;74:978–982.
5. Bonutti PM, Mont MA, McMahon M, et al. Minimally invasive total knee arthroplasty. *J Bone Joint Surg* 2004;2:(86A suppl):26–32.
6. Lonner JH. Minimally invasive approaches to total knee arthroplasty: results. *Am J Orthop* 2006;7S:27–29.
7. Boerger TO, Aglietti P, Mondanelli N, Sensi L. Mini-subvastus versus medial parapatellar approach in total knee arthroplasty. *Clin Orthop* 2005;440:82–87.
8. Dalury DF, Dennis DA. Mini-incision total knee arthroplasty can increase risk of component malalignment. *Clin Orthop* 2005;440:77–81.
9. Tenholder M, Clarke HD, Scuderi GR. Minimal incision total knee arthroplasty. The early clinical experience. *Clin Orthop* 2005;440:67–76.

4 Exposing the Revision Total Knee Arthroplasty: Patellar Inversion Method

Thomas K. Fehring

INDICATIONS/CONTRAINDICATIONS

Adequate exposure is an essential part of revision total knee surgery. However, adequate exposure is frequently difficult to obtain because of scarring and lowered tissue resiliency in these cases. Quadriceps tendon thickening and contraction of the patella tendon compound exposure problems. Preserving patella tendon integrity is of paramount importance and must be prioritized, as results following avulsion are dismal. Various strategies to safely expose a revision total knee have been described including tibial tubercle osteotomy, quadriceps snip, and V-Y quadricepsplasty (1–9). Each of these methods compromises the extensor mechanism to some degree and should be used only if necessary.

This chapter describes a stepwise approach to exposing the revision total knee without using the traditional extensile measures involving the extensor mechanism (see Chapter 1). Our preferred method of exposure—the so-called patella inversion method—does not violate the extensor mechanism (10). In our experience, this method of exposure is applicable in 95% of revision cases and reduces the risk of patellar tendon avulsion. It may be difficult to apply this technique alone in cases of extreme patella baja or ankylosed knees, in which cases more extensile exposure options, such as a quadriceps snip, modified V-Y plasty, or tibial tubercle osteotomy may be necessary to gain adequate exposure, while protecting the attachment of the patellar tendon.

PREOPERATIVE PLANNING

Preoperative planning for a revision total knee involves a careful evaluation of the following issues:

● Previous skin incisions
● Current degree of range of motion
● Previous surgical complications
● Presence of osteolysis

Previous Skin Incisions

It is not unusual to be confronted by multiple incisions in performing revision total knee surgery. Therefore, it is important for the surgeon to understand the vascular anatomy of the anterior aspect of the knee before making an incision. The blood supply to the skin on the anterior aspect of the knee comes in from medial to lateral. If there are pre-existing medial and lateral incisions, the lateral incision must be used to avoid skin complications. Very large flaps can be raised safely without risk

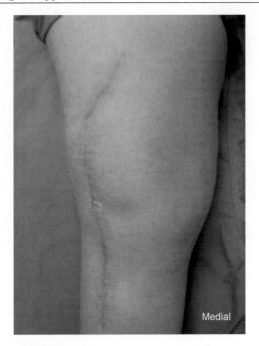

FIGURE 4-1

Large lateral flap used to safely expose the revision knee.

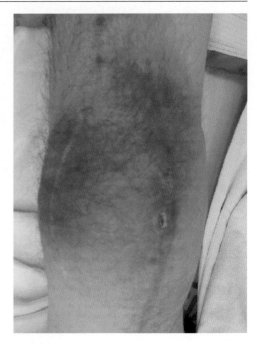

FIGURE 4-2

Medial wound breakdown following use of medial rather than lateral incision.

of skin necrosis, provided the dissection occurs in the subfascial plane (Fig. 4-1). Taking the fascia up with the subcutaneous tissue preserves the vasculature of the flap that runs between the fascia and the subcutaneous tissue.

Failure to adhere to the rule of using the most lateral incision risks skin necrosis in the bridge of tissue between the two previous incisions. Little comfort should be taken by the operating surgeon by measuring 6 to 8 cm between incisions and then using the most medial incision. This measurement technique may occasionally jeopardize the whole reconstruction if the medial incision is chosen (Fig. 4-2).

Current Range of Motion

The pre-revision range of motion is an important determinant of exposure selection. If the patient has greater than 70 to 80 degrees of range of motion, extensile exposure methods are usually unnecessary. The patellar inversion technique described here can be routinely used. However, if the patient has less than 70 degrees of motion, an "early" quadriceps snip is usually used to safely expose the knee. The quadriceps snip is usually performed approximately 6 cm above the top of the patella. An incision is made from distal medial to proximal lateral at a 45-degree angle within the quadriceps tendon (Fig. 4-3). In extremely tight knees, this incision is carried into the vastus lateralis to facilitate safe exposure.

Previous Surgical Complications

A careful history must be taken to determine if there were any complications related to the extensor mechanism during the primary arthroplasty. Radiographs are helpful in this regard. The presence of suture anchors or staples in the tibial tubercle area should alert the surgeon to be extremely careful in exposing this joint, as the attachment of the previously repaired tendon may be tenuous. In this situation, an "early" quadriceps snip should be done if the surgeon notes that the tissue in the tubercle area tends to peel during routine exposure.

Osteolysis

When revising any knee, a careful inspection of the pre-revision radiographs is essential to search for areas of lysis that may weaken structurally important bone. In no area is this more important than the

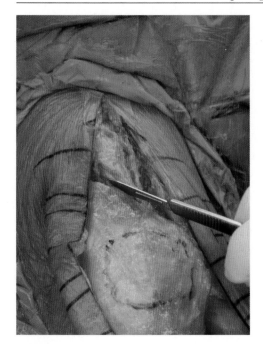

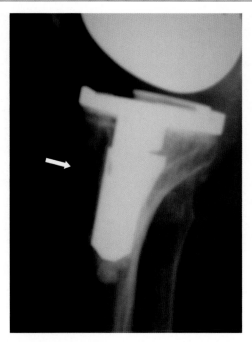

FIGURE 4-3

Snip quadricepsplasty used for extensile exposure.

FIGURE 4-4

Retrotubercle osteolysis.

area of the tibial tubercle (Fig. 4-4). If lysis has undermined the tibial tubercle, then an "early" quadriceps snip is mandatory to avoid a fracture in this area. Additionally, for surgeons inclined to perform a tibial tubercle osteotomy, osteolysis in the region of the tibial tubercle limits its applicability.

PATELLA INVERSION SURGICAL TECHNIQUE

The patient is placed supine on the operating table. A knee positioner with a lateral support is placed at the level of the tourniquet with the knee flexed 90 degrees. A transverse foot piece that holds the leg at 90 degrees without any support is used at the lower aspect of the table. The knee is then prepped and draped in the standard orthopedic fashion, and the surgeon takes care to keep the tourniquet well above the previous incision. As discussed, if there are multiple incisions, the lateral incision is chosen, and a subfascial flap is raised. If a midline incision was used initially, this incision is utilized. The incision is usually extended an inch or two proximally so that no scar tissue will be encountered, and the level of the quadriceps tendon can be easily identified. The surgeon raises the medial and lateral skin flaps by hand using gentle retraction rather than with sharp instruments to minimize skin trauma. While the initial skin incision is made with the knee at 90 degrees of flexion, after the skin incision has been made, the flap dissection is performed in extension. Every attempt is made to make these flaps full thickness, which is facilitated by the proximal extension of the incision into virginal territory so that the depth of the quadriceps tendon can be easily identified. The dissection proceeds distally keeping tension on the skin flap exposing Sharpey's fibers and scar tissue, which are identified and cut from the dorsal aspect of the extensor mechanism (Fig. 4-5). Laterally, the flap is raised to the lateral edge of the patella. Medially, the flap is raised until the vastus medialis musculature has been exposed.

Once the flaps have been developed adequately from the tibial tubercle up into the quadriceps, the knee is then flexed, and an arthrotomy is made. With the knee at 90 degrees of flexion, the surgeon makes an incision from the midportion of the patella proximally into the quadriceps expansion being careful to stay within the medial aspect of the tendon. The knee is then placed in extension, and an incision is made from just medial to the tibial tubercle to the midportion of the patella where the previous arthrotomy has ended. It is important to leave a cuff of tissue about 5 mm in width medial to the tibial tubercle for later repair and to strengthen the attachment of the tibial tubercle.

Once the arthrotomy has been made, fluid cultures, tissue cultures, and frozen sections are sent to the laboratory before continuing the procedure. A knife is then used to expose the antero-lateral aspect of the tibia by sliding the knife into the bursa proximal to the tubercle and cutting in a

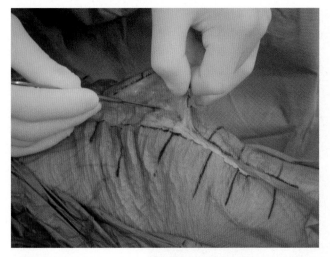

FIGURE 4-5

Gentle handling of tissue to expose Sharpey's fibers and scar tissue.

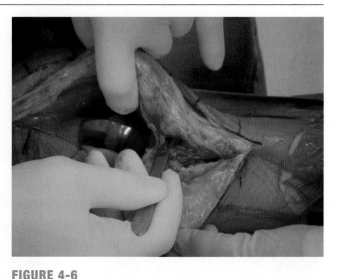

FIGURE 4-6

Bursa released between the proximal tibia and patella ligament.

cephalad direction (Fig. 4-6). The knee is then flexed up to 90 degrees merely subluxing the patella and laterally exposing the suprapatellar pouch and the medial gutter. A complete synovectomy is then performed in the medial gutter and in the anteromedial and antero-lateral suprapatellar pouch (Fig. 4-7). The surgeon then walks around to the other side of the table where he performs a peripatellar dissection and takes down some of the scarred tissue in the area of the fat pad. The lateral gutter is then debrided, as an assistant pulls up on the extensor mechanism and subluxed patella. After this complete synovectomy has been done, a lateral retinacular release is performed. The surgeon attempts to find the lateral superior genicular artery in the lateral gutter usually at a level 1 to 2 cm distal to the top of the femoral implant. This structure is frequently encased in scar and difficult to identify. The surgeon performs an inside out lateral retinacular release from the joint line proximally (Fig. 4-8). Proximally, the muscle is stripped off the inside surface of the iliotibial band and raised up with a Homan retractor allowing the lateral retinacular release to be extended far superiorly.

Once this has been accomplished, the next step is to deliver the tibia out from under the femur. A posteromedial dissection is carried out similar to the way in which the surgeon would perform an extensive medial release for a varus knee in a primary situation. Initially, a rake is used on the

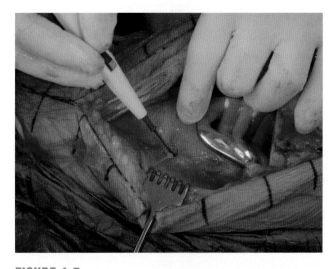

FIGURE 4-7

Debridement of the medial gutter.

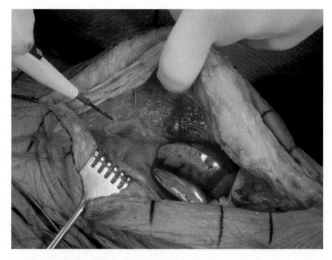

FIGURE 4-8

Inside out lateral retinacular release.

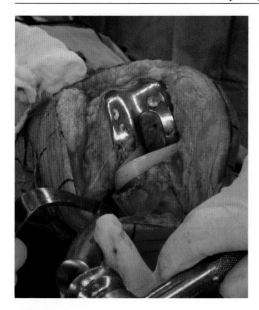

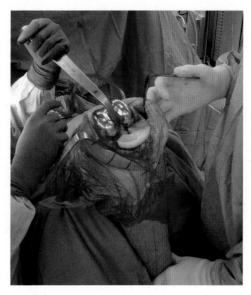

FIGURE 4-9
Posteromedial corner release

FIGURE 4-10
Expose without patellar eversion.

capsular tissues. Once the surgeon reaches the midcoronal plane, a bent Homan retractor is placed around the posteromedial aspect of the tibia, and a 1/2-inch osteotome is taken around the proximal medial tibia exposing the posteromedial aspect of the tibia (Fig. 4-9). At this point, the knee is hyperflexed, and the foot is externally rotated while a two-pronged Homan retractor is placed in the intercondylar area. While the assistant levers on the femur, the surgeon delivers the tibia out from under the medial femoral condyle. As tension is placed on the two-prong retractor, dissection is carried around the proximal medial tibia to the area of the posterior cruciate ligament's insertion. Gradual external rotation of the tibia in a slow, patient fashion with anterior pressure on the posterior tibia usually facilitates this exposure (Fig. 4-10). The previously performed lateral retinacular release diminishes the tension on the extensor mechanism and facilitates exposure without jeopardizing the patellar tendon insertion on the tibial tubercle. Throughout this maneuver, the surgeon should keep an eye on the tibial tubercle area to make sure that no peeling of this area is occurring. If he notices that there is too much tension on the area or if it begins to peel, a snip should be performed. However, if a complete lateral retinacular release and the external rotation maneuver of the tibia are performed slowly and cautiously, this step is rarely necessary.

Once the tibia has been exposed, the modular polyethylene insert is removed, and the surgeon removes the existing implants in the following order:

- Femoral component
- Patellar component
- Tibial component

Once the implants have been removed, the tibia is cut first, building the reconstruction on a stable tibial base. Conventional external alignment guides are placed on top of the soft tissue anteriorly and pinned to the bone (Fig. 4-11). No attempt is made to slide a tibial cutting jig onto the anterolateral bony tibia under the patellar tendon. The guide is placed merely over the tibial tubercle and tendon with the patella not everted. The tibia is then cut only on the exposed medial tibial plateau from front to back (Fig. 4-12). The saw blade is then angled from anteromedial to posterolateral to cut the posterolateral aspect of the tibia. Finally, the surgeon walks to the other side of the table, directing the saw in a medial-to-lateral direction using the medial tibial plateau as a cutting block to cut the anterolateral aspect of the proximal tibia (Fig. 4-13). This three-step tibial cutting technique is accurate, safe, and does not jeopardize the extensor mechanism.

The three-step tibial cutting technique is as follows:

- The tibial cutting jig is placed directly on the soft tissues laterally.
- The medial tibial plateau is cut perpendicular to the mechanical axis.
- The medial tibial plateau is then used as the cutting guide for the lateral tibial plateau.

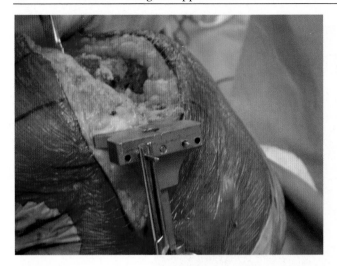

FIGURE 4-11

Tibial guide placed on top of lateral soft tissue.

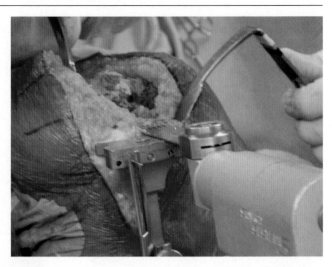

FIGURE 4-12

Medial tibial plateau cut.

POSTOPERATIVE MANAGEMENT

Postoperative management is routine when using the patella inversion technique. The extensor mechanism does not need to be protected in any way. Range of motion and isometric quadriceps exercises begin immediately.

RESULTS

In one published series, the patella inversion method provided adequate exposure in 397 of 420 revision total knee arthroplasties (95%). In the remaining 5% of cases, alternative exposures were necessary to protect the patellar tendon insertion or medial collateral ligament (MCL). In that consecutive series, there were no cases of patellar tendon avulsions (10).

COMPLICATIONS

Provided adequate exposure is achieved, with appropriate soft tissue releases and attention to the tension on the patellar tendon attachment or the MCL, damage to these structures should be avoidable. The exposure may be particularly difficult in the presence of patella baja. In circumstances when the patellar tendon or MCL appear at risk, ancillary exposure options should be used, such as proximal releases (quadriceps snip or a modified V-Y quadricepsplasty) or a tibial tubercle osteotomy, all of which can be easily combined with the patella inversion technique.

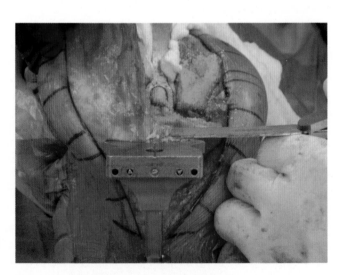

FIGURE 4-13

Using the medial plateau as a cutting block, the lateral tibia is cut from medial to lateral.

CONCLUSION

Exposing a revision total knee arthroplasty should proceed in a logical stepwise fashion:

- Use the most lateral incision.
- Raise the subfascial skin flaps gently.
- Debride the entire suprapatellar pouch and the medial and lateral gutters.
- Perform an early lateral retinacular release.
- Gradually externally rotate the tibia by dissecting the posteromedial corner of the tibia.
- Slowly deliver the tibia from under the femur by externally rotating the tibia continuing the posterior medial dissection to the midline.
- Make no attempt to evert the patella!
- If the patella tendon insertion or MCL insertion appear to be in jeopardy, perform a quadriceps snip.
- Remove the tibial polyethylene, followed by the femoral component, the patellar component once the joint has been decompressed, and finally, the tibial component.

Although multiple exposure options are available to the revision knee surgeon, the vast majority of cases can be managed without violating the extensor mechanism using the patellar inversion technique. In revision cases in which full function is inherently difficult to obtain, extensile exposures may slow the rehabilitative process unnecessarily and add to the morbidity of the procedure. Although more extensile exposures need to be used on occasion, they are the exception rather than the rule in revision total knee arthroplasty.

REFERENCES

1. Coonse K, Adams JD. A new operative approach to the knee joint. *Surg Gynecol Obstet* 1943;77:344.
2. Scott RD, Sikiski JM. The use of a modified V-Y quadricepsplasty during total knee replacement to gain exposure and improve flexion in the ankylosed knee. *Orthopedics* 1985;8:45.
3. Trousdale RT, Hanssen AD, Rand JA, Cahalan TD. V-Y quadricepsplasty in total knee arthroplasty. *Clin Orthop* 1993;286:48.
4. Garvin KL, Scuderi G, Insall JN. Evolution of the quadriceps snip. *Clin Orthop* 1995;321:131.
5. Dolin MG. Osteotomy of the tibial tubercle in total knee replacement. *J Bone Joint Surg Am* 1983;65:704.
6. Whiteside LA, Ohl MD. Tibial tubercle osteotomy for exposure of the difficult total knee arthroplasty. *Clin Orthop* 1990;26:6.
7. Ries MD, Richman JA. Extended tibial tubercle osteotomy in total knee arthroplasty. *J Arthroplasty* 1996;11:964.
8. Ritter MA, Carr KE, Keating M, et al. Tibial shaft fracture following tibial tubercle osteotomy. *J Arthroplasty* 1996;111:117.
9. Wolf AM, Hungerford DS, Krackow KA, Jacobs MA. Osteotomy of the tibial tubercle during total knee replacement. *J Bone Joint Surg Am* 1989;71:848.
10. Fehring TK, Odum S, Griffin WL, Mason JB. Patella inversion method for exposure in revision total knee arthroplasty. *J Arthroplasty* 2002;17:101.

PART TWO

PRINCIPLES IN PRIMARY TOTAL KNEE ARTHROPLASTY

5 Primary Total Knee: Standard Principles and Technique

Paul A. Lotke

INDICATIONS AND CONTRAINDICATIONS

A total knee arthroplasty (TKA) is indicated for severe disability resulting from pain, deformity or limited function as a result of osteoarthritis, rheumatoid arthritis, or any other type of arthritic deformity around the joint. Surgery should be considered only after adequate trials of conservative therapy, including anti-inflammatory medications and modifications in daily activities. In addition, both pain and deformity should be present. Pain alone should make the physician look for other diagnoses and treatment alternatives. Structural deformities without significant pain or disability may be well tolerated, especially in the elderly, and should not alone be an indication for surgery. The patient should also have realistic goals. A well-placed total knee will neither feel nor function like a normal knee. Younger patients should be advised about overuse and activity leading to failure or pain. Older patients should realize that reconstructing the joint alone will not alter their overall functional abilities. When the disease involves a single compartment, other surgical alternatives should be considered. A unicompartmental arthroplasty can offer excellent results, less bone loss, and lower morbidity then a TKA. This procedure is especially useful for younger patients with unicompartmental disease who engage in high-level activities.

When there is deformity in both knees, arthroplasty may be performed in either one or two stages. If both knees are operated on at the same stage, we must compensate for the blood loss. The amount of blood loss is frequently unrecognized and underestimated. In the elderly, acute lowering of the red cell mass is not well tolerated and can lead to medical problems.

There are relatively few contraindications of TKA and include inactive or latent infection. The relative contraindications include Charcot joint, poor skin coverage, and ankylosis. Although it sounds simplistic, a good history and examination are the most effective ways to ensure that the patient meets the criteria and recommendations for a TKA. Once it is established that the patient is a satisfactory candidate for a TKA, the specific details of the procedure can be addressed.

PREOPERATIVE EVALUATION

The standing anterior posterior (AP) radiograph is usually the most important study for evaluating the preoperative status of the knee. However, lateral and patella views are also relevant in assessing the preoperative knee. Some surgeons consider having a full-length radiograph taken from hip to ankle. However, without a history of prior trauma, I do not routinely obtain a full-length film and feel that most of the necessary information can be obtained on a 17-inch cassette. If the patient has a history of surgical procedures or trauma to the hip or lower leg, he or she should have a radiograph taken of that site to rule out unrecognized bone pathology. The standing AP radiograph will allow us to determine joint space, bone loss requiring augmentation, ligamentous laxity, and alignment. In addition, observations are made as to the size and position of the osteophytes that should be removed to reconstruct the anatomical contours of the knee and avoid impingement.

The lateral and patella views are also important for preoperative planning. The patella view will show if there are erosive changes, thinning, or subluxation of the patella. The lateral radiographs are important assessments for patella baja, which may occur from previous surgery, osteotomy, or arthroscopic procedures. In addition, we can assess if the posterior compartment of the knee contains large osteophytes that require removal during the surgical procedure.

The preoperative examination should document the condition of the skin and the location of previous scars. Any prior incision or scar is important, especially if parallel to your planned arthrotomy. Every effort should be made to incorporate the old scar into the new incision. In general, if two scars are present, I choose the longer of two scars and extend it as necessary. Parallel incisions should be assiduously avoided. The presence of psoriasis should be noted. This is not a contraindication for surgery, but the skin condition should be optimized before surgery.

SURGERY

Arthrotomy

The patient is placed in the supine position and carefully prepped and draped. I fold a cuff into the sterile drape, under the thigh, so that the drapes will not be disturbed or restrictive when I move or flex the knee (Fig. 5-1A,B). I use an anterior medial incision of approximately 12 to 15 cm. It may begin 3 cm above the patella and end 1 cm below the top of the tibial tubercle (Fig. 5-2). The length of the incision is not important as long as it allows adequate exposure to perform the procedure efficiently and safely. Proximally, the margins of the quadriceps tendon are identified with a right angle retractor slid on the quadriceps tendon and beneath Scarpa's fascia. I make a median parapatellar incision, which is extensile and can be extended, if necessary, in obese, muscular, or stiff joints. (Fig. 5-3). The knee joint is entered and briefly inspected. Some of the fat pad is removed (Fig. 5-4). The surgeon enters the bursa below the retroperitoneal fat pad and incises the anterior lateral capsule (Fig. 5-5). Medially, the soft tissue sleeve is dissected from the proximal medial tibial metaphysic, on top of the periosteum, and follows within the natural plane of the pes anserinus bursa (Fig. 5-6). This dissection is extended back to the posterior corner of the knee. The only structure that requires sharp dissection in this plane is the meniscal tibial ligament. The edge of the medial soft tissue sleeve is kept intact so that a watertight closure can be obtained at the end of surgery. With this approach into the knee, the blood supply in the periosteum on the anterior and medial side of the tibia is essentially left undisturbed.

The knee is extended, and the patella is everted in extension. With a Lahey clamp holding the eversion, and a Homan retractor stabilizing the patella, the retropatellar osteotomy is carried out (Figs. 5-7A,B, 5-8, and 5-9).

The knee is then flexed, and the surgeon excises the anterior cruciate ligament. If the surgeon is preserving the posterior cruciate ligament (PCL), it should be left undisturbed. I release the lateral meniscus and place a Homan retractor under the meniscus retracting the meniscus and extensor

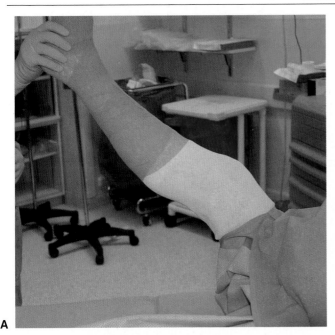

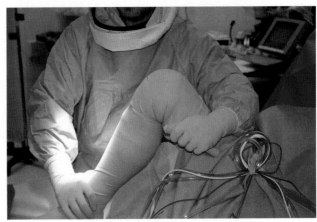

A

B

FIGURE 5-1

(A) Prepping and draping the leg with a large cuff under the thigh to prevent migration of the drapes and restriction of motion. **(B)** The leg is flexed prior to inflating the tourniquet to relax the quadriceps muscles.

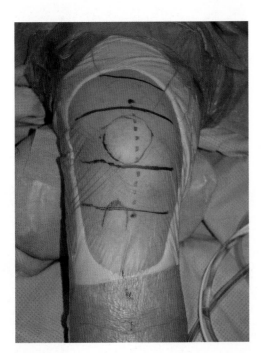

FIGURE 5-2

The incision starts just proximal to the patella and extends 1 cm below the medial side of the tibial tubercle. It may measure 12 to 15 cm but can be extended if needed.

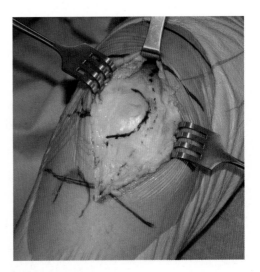

FIGURE 5-3

The incision into the deep fascia is as straight as possible and runs alongside the patella with enough of a cuff to suture. A right angle retractor slides proximal on the quadriceps tendon and exposes as much of the tendon as needed.

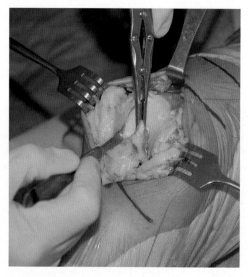

FIGURE 5-4

The posterior half of the patella fat pad may be excised for exposure.

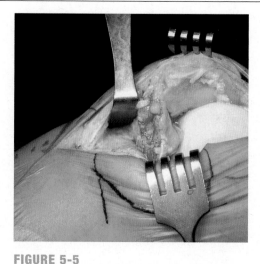

FIGURE 5-5

A right angle retractor slides within the bursa, under the remaining fat pad, and exposes the anterior and lateral aspects of the tibia without cutting a vessel.

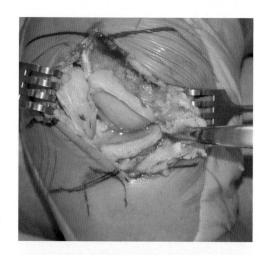

FIGURE 5-6

The medial sleeve is developed on the periosteum and within the pes anserinus bursa. Again, no vessel needs to be cut in this plane, and the bursa is preserved.

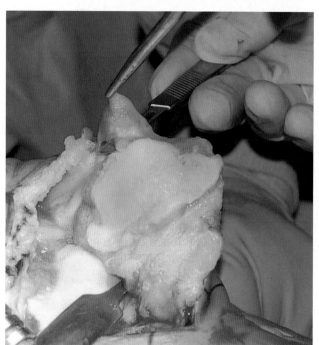

A

B

FIGURE 5-7

(A) The leg is extended, and the patella is everted in preparation for the retropatellar osteotomy. **(B)** The fat/synovium on the proximal pole of the patella is excised to reduce the risk of clunk syndrome.

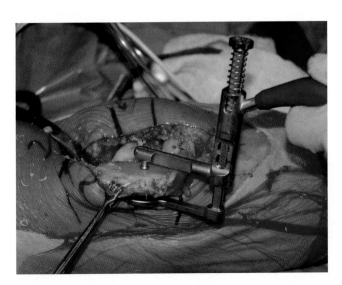

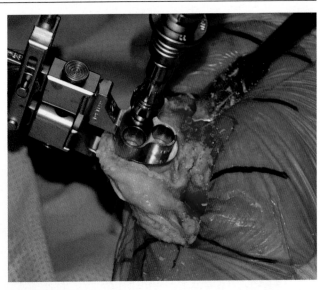

FIGURE 5-8

The thickness of the patella can be measured before and after the osteotomy. As the surgeon gains experience, this step becomes less essential.

FIGURE 5-9

Drill holes are placed in the retropatellar surface.

mechanism laterally. The patella is not everted, as it is not necessary for good exposure of the knee. With flexion, external rotation, and anterior displacement, the tibia can be subluxed forward, and excellent exposure of the tibial plateau and femoral condyles can be obtained (Fig. 5-10). If there is too much tension on the skin, I lengthen the incision as needed.

Bone Cuts

In the total knee procedure, the surgeon uses the same five bone cuts whether the prosthesis is cemented in place, fixed with porous ingrowth, and/or if the PCL is saved or preserved (Fig. 10B). The only difference is the sixth step for removing the intercondylar notch for posterior cruciate-substituting prosthesis. These essential bone cuts are made regardless of the amount of bone loss, ligament imbalance, or osteophytes present around the joint. For a routine TKA, I perform a measured resection technique in which the osteotomies are calculated to reproduce the joint lines with the thickness of the metal prosthesis. I will make the bone cuts, remove all osteophytes, and then evaluate and compensate for any soft tissue imbalance. In general, after the osteophytes are removed and normal anatomic boundaries have been re-established, no specific releases or additional balancing is necessary. For knees with severe deformities, or when soft tissue imbalances are a major problem, however, only then soft tissue releases are considered (see Chapter 7).

The five essential cuts for any TKA are as follows (Fig. 5-10B):

1. Retropatellar osteotomy
2. Transverse osteotomy of the proximal tibia
3. Resection of distal femoral condyles angulated 4 to 6 degrees of valgus alignment
4. Anterior and posterior condylar resections to accept prostheses of the appropriate size and rotated to make equal flexion gaps medially and laterally
5. Chamfers from the distal femur anteriorly and posteriorly to conform to the internal prosthetic configuration
6. (This cut is optional.) Resection of the intracondylar notch for a posterior cruciate-substituting prosthesis

Patellar Osteotomy

The retroperitoneal osteotomy is completed early in the case with the knee in extension (Fig. 5-7). This debulks the patella and allows it to be subluxed without eversion and reduces the tension on the tibial tubercle. It almost eliminates the risk of patellar tendon peel from the tubercle. I try to reproduce the native thickness of the patella with 10 to 15 mm of patella remaining. A caliper can be used

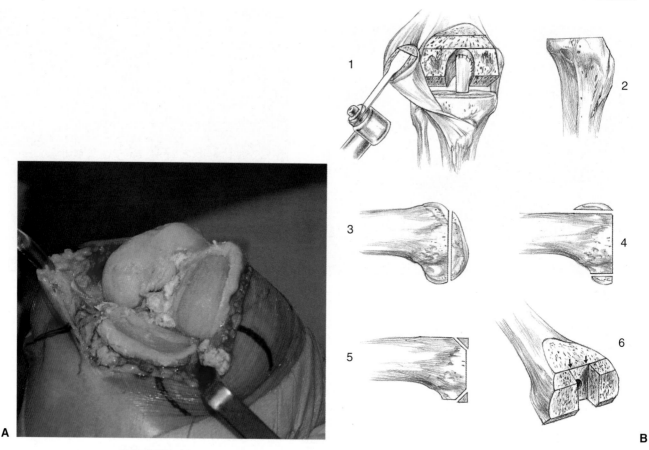

A   B

FIGURE 5-10

(A) The knee is flexed, externally rotated, and subluxed forward. This step should allow the necessary exposure. **(B)** A total knee procedure comprises the same five cuts whether the prosthesis is fixed by methylmethacrylate, porous ingrowth, or press fit technique. A sixth step is added if the PCL is to be substituted. The six steps are as follows: *(1)* retropatellar osteotomy; *(2)* transverse osteotomy in the proximal tibia, titled 5 degrees posteriorly; *(3)* resection of the distal femoral condyles in 4 to 6 degrees of valgus; *(4)* anterior and posterior condylar resections; *(5)* chamfers of the anterior and posterior condyles; and *(6)* (optional) resection of the intercondylar notch and the PCL for posterior cruciate-sacrificing prostheses.

to determine the thickness of the patella before and after the osteotomy (Fig. 5-8), however, with experience, this becomes less necessary. There are clamps that can be used to guide in this retroperitoneal osteotomy. Again, with experience, the guides become less necessary. The synovial/fat soft tissue mass at the superior pole of the patella should be excised to avoid a postoperative "clunk syndrome" (Fig. 5-7A). After the osteotomy has been completed, drill holes can be placed into the retroperitoneal surface to accept the patellar button (Fig. 5-9). I generally use a patellar button in my total knee replacements.

Osteotomy of the Proximal Tibia

The femoral and tibial osteotomies are independent of each other, so either may be performed first. I recommend that the tibia be osteotomized first, however, to accurately determine the femoral rotation and establish equal medial and lateral gaps in flexion by tension. Rarely, if the knee is tight or if good exposure is difficult to obtain, will I osteotomize the femoral condyles first.

I osteotomize the tibia with an extramedullary guide (Fig. 5-11). Before the surgery, I will make ink lines on the tibial spline. If the lower leg is very obese and bony landmarks cannot be readily appreciated, I will use an intramedullary guide to ensure a transverse osteotomy on the proximal tibia. The depth of the tibial cut should correspond to the thickness of the tibial insert. In general, I prefer about a 10-mm combined thickness of the tray and polyethylene insert. To achieve this, I

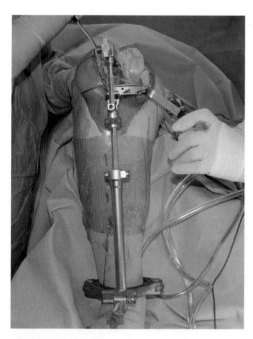

FIGURE 5-11

The external tibial alignment guide is placed on the tibia. I try to make this guide parallel to the tibial spline.

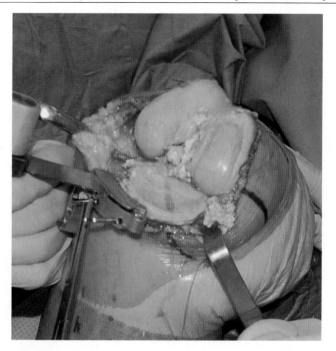

FIGURE 5-12

The osteotomy is taken within or on the guide. A retractor should be placed to protect the MCL.

look at the more normal side, and I will target for a 10-mm osteotomy below what I perceive to be the normal lateral tibial plateau or a 7-mm osteotomy below what I perceive to be the normal medial tibial plateau (Figs. 5-12 and 5-13). This accounts for a 3-degree varus of many tibias. Because of the arthritic deformities in the native contours, the precise distance for making this osteotomy cannot be determined. Some surgeons prefer a marking stylus to assist in this "guesstimate."

I do not try to remove all bone defects with one cut. If a bone defect is very shallow, an additional 1- to 2-mm resection is easy and can completely eliminate the defect. On the other hand, if it is very deep and steep, some augmentation may be required and can be better visualized after the first pass. This decision is made at the time of surgery.

It is very important that a retractor be placed beneath the MCL to prevent damage to the ligament with a power saw (Fig. 5-12). I generally place a bent Homan retractor laterally to displace the extensor mechanism. With the tibia subluxed, an additional Homan retractor can be placed posteriorly to protect the vessels. I do not attempt to advance the saw blade entirely across the tibial plateau but stop a few millimeters short of the posterior margin, then raise the blade and crack the last bit of the tibial plateau (Fig. 5-13). In this manner, I again protect the saw from going too posteriorly and damaging the neurovascular structures. A Bovie is used to release the posterior horns of the lateral and medial meniscus and the anterior fibers of the PCL. This allows the proximal tibial osteotomy to be brought forward readily and removed from the knee (see Fig. 1-3). After the osteotomy segment has been removed, osteophytes on the medial and/or lateral margins of the knee can be removed to anatomic contours. The tibia is then placed posteriorly under the femoral condyle, and the surgeon directs his attention to the next series of cuts on the femur.

Osteotomy of the Distal Femur

An intramedullary guide is used for the femur. A large drill hole is placed in the mid-portion of the medial condylar notch just anterior and medial to the PCL attachment (Fig. 5-14). After the drill is placed through the cortex, the canal is irrigated with antibiotic solution (Fig. 5-15). This step is very important, as it reduces the risk of fat emboli after the tourniquet is removed.

A preliminary estimate of rotation is determined at this time with one or more of the techniques noted (information to follow). This allows us to make the anterior cut on the femur in proper rotation (Figs. 5-16 and 5-17A,B). The intramedullary guide, adjustable to 4 to 6 degrees of valgus,

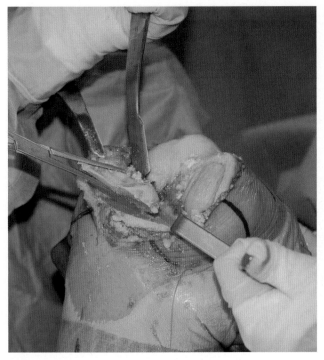

FIGURE 5-13

The proximal tibial segment can be lifted off the tibia. It is made easier if the insertion of the PCL and posterior meniscal horn attachments have been precut.

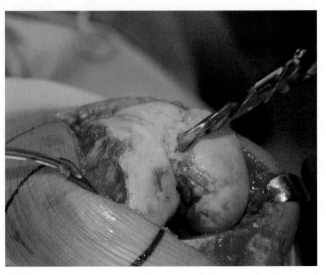

FIGURE 5-14

A pilot hole is drilled into the distal femur.

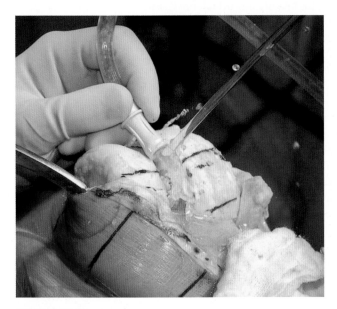

FIGURE 5-15

The femoral canal is irrigated with a long tip irrigator. This reduces the risk of marrow emboli and the fat embolus syndrome.

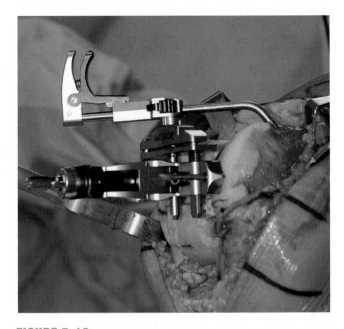

FIGURE 5-16

A stylus locates the anterior cortex for an anterior referencing guide.

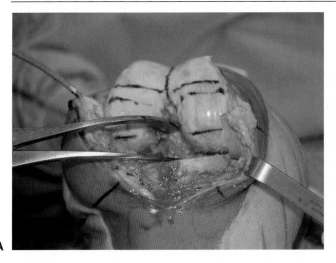

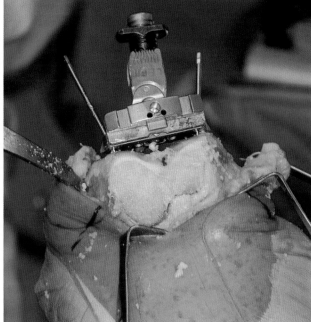

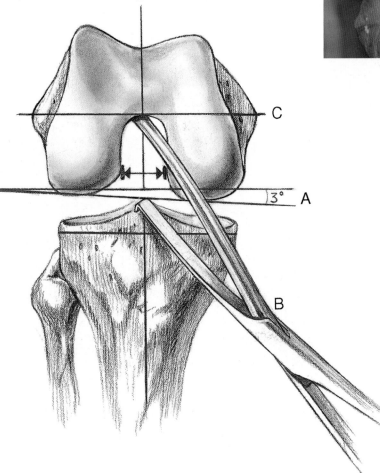

FIGURE 5-17

(A) Correct rotation of the femur is determined at this time. A laminar spreader is used in the center of the knee to look for an equal gap medially and laterally. If rotation is correct, the lines should be parallel to the tibial osteotomy. **(B)** There are four methods to estimate correct femoral rotation. (*A*) Measured 3 degrees of external rotation by removing 2 to 3 mm more bone from the medial posterior condyle. (*B*) Putting tension in the flexion space and resecting parallel to the transverse tibial osteotomy. (*C*) Resecting the posterior condyles parallel to the transepicondylar axis. (*D*) Resecting the condyles transverse to the trochlear Whiteside's line (from the center of the condyles to the center of the patellar groove). **(C)** If the anterior osteotomy has a "grand piano" shape, the rotation is correct.

is placed in the shaft of the femur. In general, I choose 5 degrees of valgus alignment for most knees. The anterior cortical cut is completed and checked for appropriate rotation with the "grand piano sign" (Fig. 5-17C).

A distal femur-cutting guide is fixed to the anterior osteotomy, and the distal femur is resected (Fig. 5-18A). The amount of bone resected should be that which is going to be replaced by the thickness of the prosthesis measured from the lateral condyle (generally between 8 to 12 mm). I find that the appropriate resection depth corresponds to the lowest portion of the trochlear groove. I like to

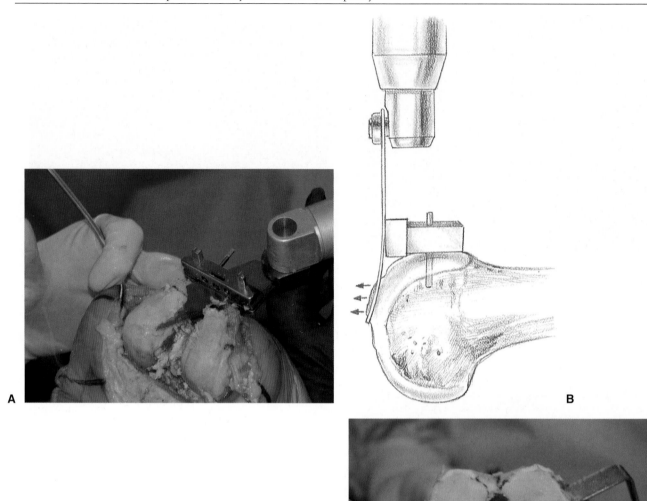

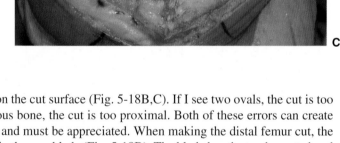

FIGURE 5-18

(A) The osteotomy of the distal femur. **(B)** Care should be taken to avoid distortions that sclerotic bone will cause in a flexible saw blade. **(C)** If the distal femoral osteotomy has a figure eight shape, the distal location of the osteotomy is correct.

see a "figure eight" configuration on the cut surface (Fig. 5-18B,C). If I see two ovals, the cut is too far distal. If the surface is continuous bone, the cut is too proximal. Both of these errors can create flexion/extension space imbalance and must be appreciated. When making the distal femur cut, the sclerotic bone can cause distortion in the saw blade (Fig. 5-18B). The blade has the tendency to bend away from the sclerotic bone and therefore alter the alignment.

Anterior and Posterior Femoral Condylar Osteotomies

These cuts are very important because they determine size and rotation. The anterior osteotomy continues along the line of the anterior femoral cortex. It should not be too high, which tightens the retinaculum, and it should not be too low, notching the femur and creating a potential stress riser for fracture. The posterior femoral condyle cuts set the rotation of the prosthesis. It is important to avoid internal rotation of the prosthesis, as this can lead to a lateral position of the patella and potential for dislocation.

Appreciating the importance of femoral rotation and the effects it has on patellar tracking has significantly improved the results of TKA and has reduced patellar complications. In general, there are now four techniques to judge rotation, none of which is perfect, so familiarity with all of them is important (Fig. 5-17B). The techniques are (a) measured degrees of external rotation, (b) tension technique to obtain a rectangular flexion space, (c) transepicondylar axis, and (d) the anteriaposterior line of Whitesides.

We now appreciate that the posterior medial femoral condyle of a normal knee generally extends below the anatomic transepicondylar axis further than the lateral condyle. This means that more of the posterior femoral condyle should be removed than the lateral condyle. There is a large variation in the size differences in these two condyles; consequently, no precise measures can prescribe the amount of bone to be removed from each side. In general, one can estimate that 2 to 3 mm more should be removed from the posterior femoral condyle on the medial side than the lateral side. Therefore, when the AP cutting guide is placed on the distal femur, it should be rotated 2 to 3 degrees so that additional bone is taken from the medial side of the knee. We must compensate for erosive change, especially in the lateral femoral condyle. After setting the distal femoral cutting block in an "estimated" rotational position, I will check the medial and lateral flexion gaps with tension. By separating the femur and the tibia with tension at 90 degrees of flexion, the gap should be rectangular (Fig. 5-17B). If so, I proceed with the osteotomy. If not, I will check the epicondylar axes by palpating the medial and lateral epicondyles. If the knee is deformed or if there has been considerable soft tissue stretching or dissection, none of these lines are in perfect conformity; therefore, the surgeon must then choose which would seem to be the best axis. Fortunately, this situation does not arise too often, and most of the time, the 3 degrees rotation and tension technique conform to each other.

The size of the prosthesis must then be determined. The situation is best when the size corresponds exactly to available stock; however, this is rarely the case. In general, I choose the smaller size. If the surgeon saves the PCL, resecting more bone from the posterior femoral condyles will loosen this ligament. Conversely, by removing too little condylar bone, the PCL may be made too tight and must be reassessed or balanced. By substituting for the ligament, the surgeon avoids the PCL balancing problem.

After the femoral size and rotation are determined, I use the appropriate size distal femoral cutting block. The ideal position and rotation are those in which the cutting block will align directly with the anterior surface of the femur, and the posterior condylar resections will produce a rectangular flexion gap after approximately 8 mm of bone has been resected from the posterior lateral condyle.

Anterior and Posterior Chamfers

These osteotomies are made with the distal cutting block (Fig. 5-19).

Intercondylar Notch Cut

The PCL can be saved, resected, or substituted. Up until this point, the PCL could have been saved. The surgeons who prefer to save the PCL can proceed with debriding the posterior femoral condyles and fitting the prosthesis. They should then balance the PCL.

I generally substitute for the PCL; therefore, I use the intercondylar cutting guide and resect the bone from the intercondylar notch (Fig. 5-20).

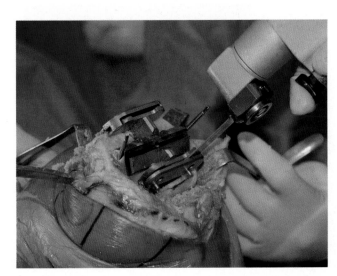

FIGURE 5-19

A distal cutting block allows the anterior/posterior osteotomies to be completed and integrated with their chamfer cuts.

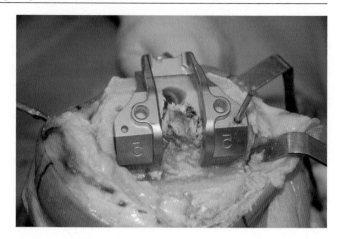

FIGURE 5-20
The central box can be removed for posterior cruciate-substituting designs.

Soft Tissue Debridement and Balancing

The most difficult part of a TKA is achieving appropriate soft tissue balance. I do this after the osteotomies have been completed. The first step in achieving such balance is to remove all the osteophytes to an anatomic border. Exposure to the back of the joint can be achieved with a laminar spreader (Fig. 5-21A). With the spreader in place, I can remove the osteophytes and also the

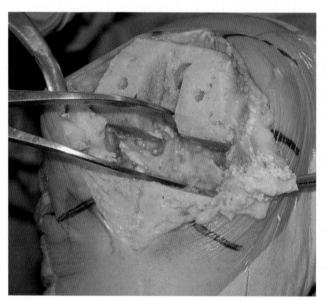

A

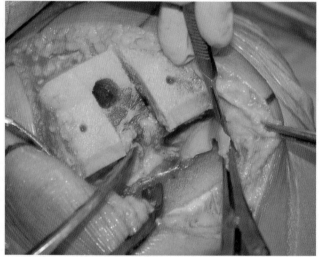

B

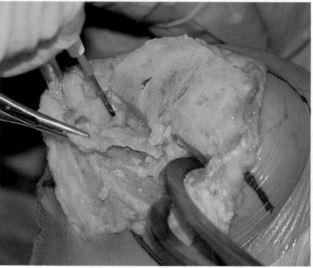

C

FIGURE 5-21

(A) The laminar spreader can give exposure to aid in removing the meniscal remnants and the osteophytes in the back of the knee. **(B)** The medial meniscus is removed within its substance. **(C)** The lateral meniscus is removed at the junction with the popliteal hiatus.

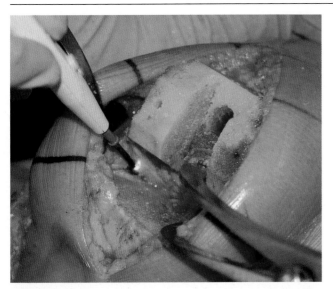

FIGURE 5-22

The lateral geniculate artery can be cauterized at this time.

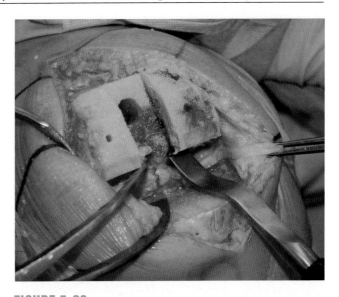

FIGURE 5-23

Osteophytes can be removed from the back of the knee with a reverse-angle osteotome.

remnants of the menisci (Fig. 5-21B,C). When I remove the lateral meniscus, I also Bovie the lateral geniculate artery (Fig. 5-22). The posterior femoral condylar osteophytes can be removed with a reverse curved osteotome (Fig. 5-23).

Trial Reduction

After the osteotomies have been completed and the osteophytes have been debrided, the knee is now ready for a trial reduction. In theory, the amount of bone removed is equivalent to the thickness of the components. Theoretically, additional balancing should not be required. If the flexion gap is equal medially and laterally, the tibial plateau component should go in with equal tension on both sides of the knee.

With flexion and extension, the tibial plateau should remain stable and not lift off from the anterior tibial surface in flexion. By applying a varus and valgus stress in extension, the surgeon can determine the stability of the knee and the appropriate thickness of the tibial insert (Fig. 5-24). With the knee in full extension, it should be very secure. With a few degrees of flexion, which relaxes the posterior capsule, the knee should open 1 to 2 mm on the medial side. There may be some natural lateral laxity, which is acceptable.

If there is preoperative valgus deformity, which is associated with stretching of the MCL, I will release the tight structures along the lateral capsule to achieve tension, which is equal to the MCL. The management of excessive varus/valgus deformity and ligament balance is described in Chapter 7.

The tibial component must be placed on the tibial plateau in the correct rotation. There are very few scientifically established guidelines for positioning this tibial component. By experience, we generally place the center of the tibial plate on the medial one third of the tibial tubercle. It is important to avoid internally rotating the tibial component (Fig. 5-25). Good exposure in the posterior lateral corner of the knee is important so that the femur does not push the tibial plate into internal rotation.

The knee is taken through a range of motion (ROM) to be sure the patella tracks centrally. If the rotation of the femoral component is appropriate, the patella remains seated squarely in the trochlea. If there is any tilting of the patella, I release the patella femoral ligament in the retinaculum. I do this in extension, by pulling anteriorly on the patella, feel the tight band, and release the ligament.

COMPONENT FIXATION

The components of the prosthesis can either be press fit with ingrown surfaces or cemented in place with methylmethacrylate. To cement the components, I irrigate the bone completely. I insert the tibia tray first, trimming excess cement. I frequently use a vacuum suction through one of the pin holes to pull the cement down into the tibial metaphyseal bone (Figs. 5-26 and 5-27A,B). I place the

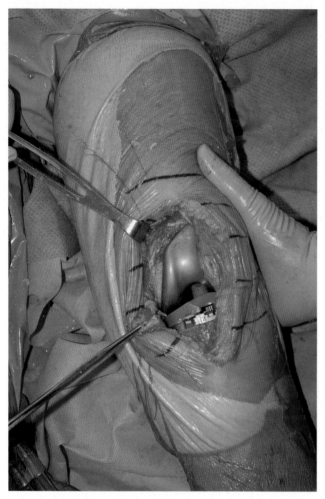

FIGURE 5-24

A trial prosthesis is inserted, and ligament tension is tested. In full extension, the knee should be very stable. With a few degrees of flexion, the knee should have a degree of medial laxity.

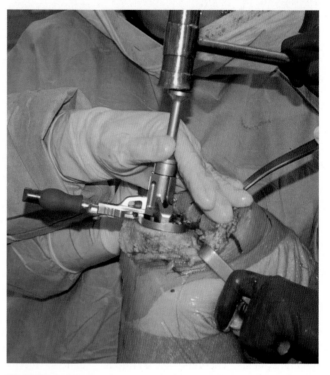

FIGURE 5-25

A central box or hole is made for the tibial component. Care should be taken to avoid internal rotation of the tibial component.

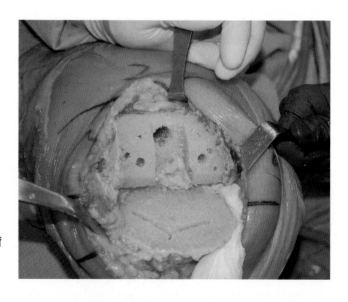

FIGURE 5-26

The bone has been irrigated, and a sponge has been placed medially to assist in retraction and removal of cement. The knee is now ready for placement and/or cementation.

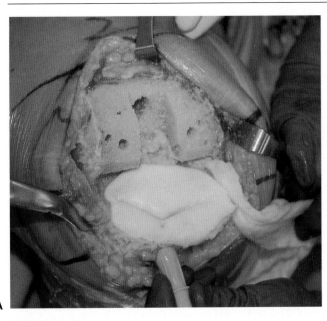
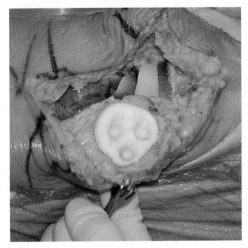

A

B

FIGURE 5-27

(A) Suction can be applied to a tibial pinhole to assist in drawing the cement into the tibia. **(B)** Patellar peg holes can be identified with pressure or a rim of blue marker in the hole.

femoral component and remove the excess cement exuding from the prosthesis. Then, I place the tibial polyethylene onto the tibia and extend the knee. Any excess cement will extrude from beneath the prosthesis and can be removed (Fig. 5-28). With the knee in full extension, the pressurization of the cement into the femur is quite dramatic. After it is assembled, the knee is taken through ROM, carefully assessing stability and patellar tracking (Fig. 5-29). Necessary changes can be made at this time, and extension must also be achieved (Fig. 5-30).

Closure

The knee is irrigated, and the wound is closed. I use two running sutures (Fig. 5-31). I place two figure eight sutures at the top corner of the patella and then run distally and proximally. I perform a

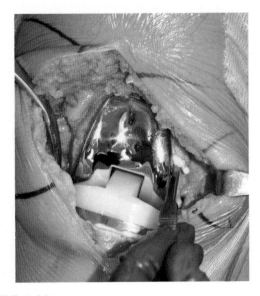

FIGURE 5-28

The knee is extended, and the excess cement can be removed as it is expressed.

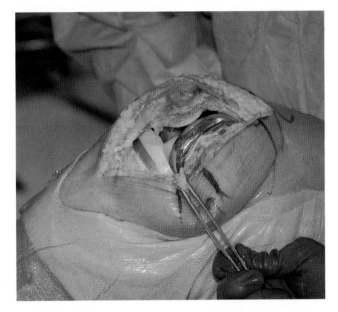

FIGURE 5-29

The patella must track without subluxation or tilting. If not perfect, a short lateral release can be done.

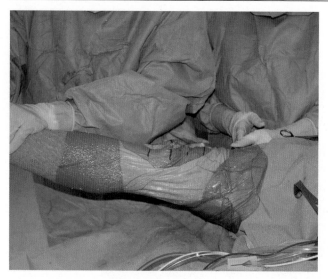

FIGURE 5-30

The knee should reach full extension at this time.

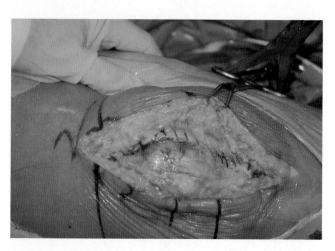

FIGURE 5-31

A careful deep fascia closure is necessary.

very careful subcutaneous closure, attempting to approximate the subcutaneous tissues without undue tension (Fig. 5-32). If the closure is watertight, we can use an analgesia cocktail injected into the knee. I generally use Marcaine with epinephrin, and long-acting morphine (Fig. 5-32). One of the most common problems after total knee replacements is wound healing, and extra care must be taken with the subcutaneous closure, especially in obese patients (Fig. 5-33). For the skin closure, I use staples (Fig. 5-34).

POSTOPERATIVE MANAGEMENT

I routinely place the patient on continuous passive motion (CPM) with a CPM machine set in flexion running slowly from 70 to 100 degrees in the recovery room. I have found that this is a particularly effective method to obtain good motion before discharge. It does not benefit the final result of flexion. If no CPM machines are available, then I start the patient with a "drop and

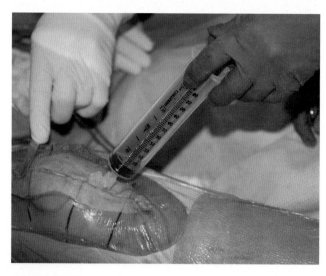

FIGURE 5-32

If the closure is watertight, a local anesthetic cocktail can be injected.

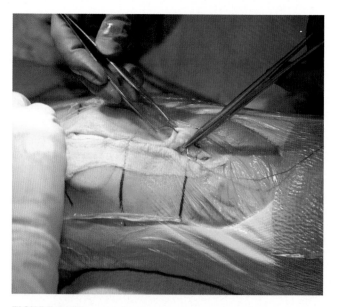

FIGURE 5-33

A careful subcutaneous closure is important to prevent delayed wound healing.

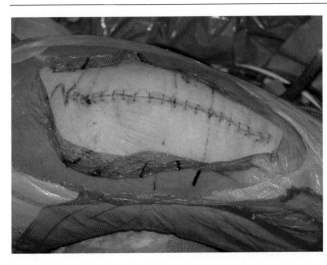

FIGURE 5-34

The patients appreciate a careful skin closure.

dangle" at 90 degrees the next day. Either way, I change the blood-stiffened dressing the morning after surgery and mobilize the patient with physical therapy on the first postoperative day. The patients do not do much on this day, but on the second day, they are walking reasonably comfortably, and on the third day, they are discharged. I generally remove the staples before discharge and replace them with Steri-Strips with benzoin. These strips will remain in place for the next 7 to 10 days. Patients can avoid a separate visit for staple removal, and they are less likely to develop cross marks.

I carefully monitor hemoglobin levels after surgery. Elderly patients do not tolerate acute blood loss very well and can develop arrhythmias. This is particularly important in patients receiving bilateral implants. We should appreciate that the unrecognized blood loss is between 1200 to 1400 mL per knee.

I do not recommend using suction drainage after a TKA. There does not appear to be any scientific basis for the use of drains, and most of the literature suggests that there is no benefit and some disadvantages in using drains in total knee replacements. They have been shown to increase blood loss, to occasionally be sewn into place, and do not seem to be associated with risk of infection.

I advise patients to gradually increase activities on crutches or a walker during the first 3 weeks, which allows the bone around the prosthesis to adapt to the new stresses being applied and/or allow in-growth to occur. After 3 weeks, patients can progressively increase activities as tolerated. I generally advise a slow course after surgery and tell my patients to try to avoid aggressive physical therapy or activity. I caution them that the new knee will not reach its full healing and rehabilitation plateau for many months.

The functional results of the TKA do not replicate the function of a normal knee. The average ROM will be 125 degrees, which is less than normal flexion. Patients will notice a sense of tightness or achiness with prolonged activity, and there are some restrictions with vigorous activity. The chief benefit of a total knee replacement, however, is pain relief, and most patients will experience this goal. I tell my patients that they will be able to perform all normal activities compatible with their age. These activities include dancing, swimming, golfing, walking unlimited distances, and light tennis. I suggest that patients avoid any impact sports or activities that require squatting or kneeling. With these guidelines, I hope to obtain survival of 20 years or longer in more than 90% of my patients.

REHABILITATION

Specific rehabilitation after TKAs is somewhat controversial. In general, I take a laissez-faire approach, encouraging patients to work on ROM and gradually increase their activities as tolerated. I tend to avoid overzealous physical therapy or vigorous attempts to build muscles in the immediate postoperative period. I have found more problems from a swollen stiff knee after overexertion than from a lack of immediate muscle strength.

Physical therapists play an important role in supervising the postoperative course of patients who have undergone total knee replacements. They can supervise and encourage gentle ROM exercises and extend our ability to observe progress. Excessive activity and stress should be avoided, however.

COMPLICATIONS

TKA is a complex operation with several potential complications. The following is a discussion of the five most common problems directly related to surgical technique:

Wound Healing

Problems with wound healing may be a direct result of surgical technique. Many patients are obese, elderly, poorly nourished, or immunosuppressed. Therefore, attention to details and special closure techniques are especially necessary. In general, I advise residents and fellows to avoid sutures that are too tight and to use suture materials of the appropriate size for the tissue to be repaired, to make sharp open incisions with edges that lend themselves for easy repair and to approximate tissues into their anatomic planes to avoid shear across the incision surfaces. It appears that attention to surgical technique and detail reduces problems with wound healing in the postoperative period.

Malrotation and Patellar Subluxation

At one time, the patella was associated with more than 50% of the problems requiring additional surgery after a TKA. In the past decade, appreciating the problems in the femoral rotation has reduced patella complications to less than 1%. One of the most important aspects in achieving consistent patella tracking has been the appreciation of correct external rotation of the osteotomy of the posterior distal condyles. The medial posterior femoral condyle usually extends further below the transepicondylar axis than the lateral condyle, and therefore, more of the medial femoral condyle needs to be resected in order to achieve appropriate rotation. In addition, keeping the anterior patella flange at the level of the anterior femoral cortex avoids excessive tension on the patellar retinaculum and reduces the tendency to dislocate the patella.

Flexion Extension Imbalance

One of the more common causes of failure of a TKA is the instability in the flexion space as related to the extension space (flexion laxity). In full extension, the knee feels secure because of the tightness of the posterior capsule. When the knee is flexed a few degrees, however, the capsule is relaxed, and the instabilities can be appreciated. If this occurs, a larger-sized femoral component could be considered, or replacing the distal femur more proximally and at the same time increasing the thickness of the tibial insert may help. Understanding the mechanics of achieving equal flexion and extension balance is important for preventing this common complication.

Patella Tendon Avulsion

Avulsion of the patella tendon is potentially a disaster after TKA. Therefore, attention to protect the attachment to the patella tendon is essential throughout the entire treatment and rehabilitation program. There is a tendency to hyperflex the knee and laterally sublux an everted patella. This can peel the patella tendon from its insertion. This can be protected by not everting the patella and subluxing it while the knee is in flexion.

Stiffness

One of the most perplexing problems after total knee surgery is the tendency to develop limited motion in 1.3% of the patients. In some of these patients, the stiffness may result from technical problems such as overthick polyethylene, oversized prosthesis, the femoral component set too far anteriorly, an excessively thick patella, or careless surgical technique. More often than not, the exact cause of the loss of motion cannot be identified, and some patients have a biologic response to increased scar formation and inflammation. The best way to prevent this complication is to avoid these errors, mobilize the patient rapidly after surgery, and avoid excessive painful physical therapy.

6 Cruciate-Retaining Total Knee Arthroplasty

Michael E. Berend and Trevor R. Pickering

The decision to retain and balance the posterior cruciate ligament (PCL) or remove it and substitute it with a prosthetic interface is an important and somewhat controversial choice in total knee arthroplasty (TKA). PCL substitution in general has been associated with increased articular constraint in TKA. Kinematics in a cruciate-retaining (CR)-TKA are not directed by the prosthesis but rather by the ligaments and dynamic forces about the knee and have been shown to facilitate long-term survivorship of knee replacements with a very low incidence of aseptic loosening (1–4). We believe that retaining the PCL is possible in almost all TKAs and highly depends on surgical technique to sufficiently "balance" the kinematics of the knee. This chapter describes the principles behind a CR-TKA.

INDICATIONS AND CONTRAINDICATIONS

CR-TKA can be considered for virtually all primary TKAs. Although a knee that has sustained a "dashboard"-type injury in a motor vehicle accident and has an incompetent PCL may require a posterior-stabilized implant to achieve stability in the anterior/posterior (AP) plane, we have found this scenario to be quite rare. We have no firm contraindications for using a CR implant in a primary TKA. It was once thought that patients with inflammatory arthropathies should be excluded from consideration for a CR implant. Our vast experience with this population, however, has shown CR-TKA to have an excellent long-term outcome (see Results section below). Even knees with a lax PCL to start with can be balanced with a CR-TKA. Surgeons can use a CR implant for revision TKA as long as soft tissue balancing is meticulous and stability is rigorously evaluated during trialing. Many revisions require a greater degree of constraint secondary to ligamentous laxity or bony deficiency on the tibia and femur. Obviously, CR-TKA is not an option in these patients.

PREOPERATIVE PREPARATION

Preoperative planning includes determining coronal deformity on standing radiographs. Further, a detailed assessment of range of motion, flexion contracture, and ligament balance should be undertaken. Our surgical plan begins with marking a tibial cut that is perpendicular to the anatomic axis on the AP radiograph of the knee (Fig. 6-1). The location of the anatomic axis relative to the tibial spines becomes a proximal landmark for the extramedullary tibial cutting jig (Fig. 6-2). This helps prevent a varus tibial cut. Preoperative radiographs can also help the surgeon assess the need for augments, screws, or bone graft in cases with significant tibial defects. Sizing of the components with templates can also be done preoperatively on radiographs, although we have not found this to be as accurate as intraoperative assessment using osseous landmarks.

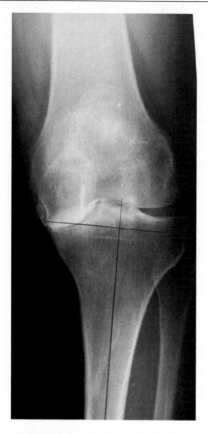

FIGURE 6-1

Preoperative AP radiograph demonstrating a planned tibial cut that is perpendicular to the anatomic axis. The cut piece of proximal tibia can be compared to the template to check that the cut is not in varus.

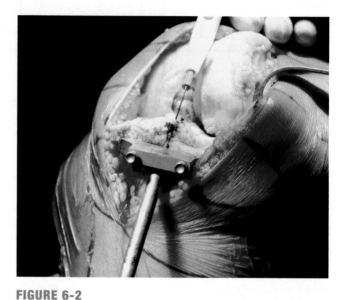

FIGURE 6-2

Intraoperative view of the frontal plane of the tibia. The mark on the proximal tibia corresponds to the vertical line on the preoperative radiograph and serves as a reference point intraoperatively for proper rotational placement of the tibial cutting jig and rotation of the final component.

Knees with significant coronal and sagittal deformity often necessitate ligament releases of the concave side of the deformity. This may include combined releases of the medial or lateral and posterior structures, including the PCL. Preoperative planning for these deformities may better prepare the surgeon for the intraoperative findings.

Surgical technique is critical for the short- and long-term performance of a TKA, regardless of design (5). The principles of exposure, deformity correction, bone preparation, collateral ligament balancing, implant positioning, PCL balancing emphasizing flexion kinematics, and implantation are discussed in this chapter.

SURGICAL TECHNIQUE

Exposing the knee is the first step to effective deformity correction and appropriate implant position. A CR-TKA can be implanted with traditional and proven approaches such as a medial parapatellar arthrotomy of various lengths of quadriceps tendon split or with so-called, less invasive, techniques such as midvastus and sub-vastus exposures (6). We believe visualization can be adequately achieved with retention of the PCL in all knees.

We reflect the medial sleeve of the knee including the deep medial collateral ligament (MCL) in the vast majority of knees with a periosteal elevator. This is done with care to protect the superficial MCL and the pes anserine insertion. The surgeon excises the fat pad, which facilitates exposure. Fat pad removal has little effect on long-term outcome of TKA (7). Knee flexion follows with division of the anterior cruciate ligament (ACL) and the anterior horn of the lateral meniscus to facilitate patellar subluxation. We have made smaller incisions over the past few years, as instruments have been refined for smaller exposures, and we now utilize patellar subluxation rather than patellar eversion.

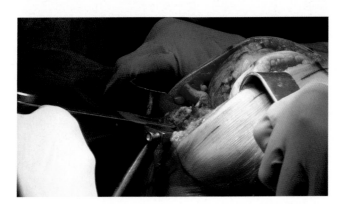

FIGURE 6-3

Extramedullary tibial cutting guide. The external rod should overlie the center of the ankle distally.

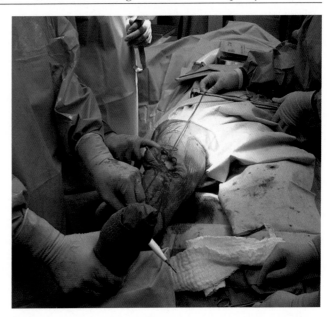

FIGURE 6-4

This system uses the ASIS bilaterally to locate the center of the hip on the operative side, which is then used to establish the mechanical axis of the knee.

We cut the tibia first in most primary PCL-retaining TKAs. The surgeon uses an extramedullary guide to check the tibial cut with reference to the center of the ankle (Fig. 6-3). Tibial alignment has been shown to be an important factor in the long-term survivorship of TKA tibial components (5,8,9). Preoperative planning may help aid in determining the relative resection level of the medial and lateral tibial plateaus based on preoperative deformity. This may vary for varus and valgus patterns of arthrosis. A 90-degree templated resection level may help not only with positioning of the central portion of the cutting jig but also with determining tibial component rotation (Fig. 6-2). A pelvic-based reference system may also aid in external alignment of the center of the hip (Fig. 6-4) (10). Most CR-TKA implant systems have a greater amount of tibial slope built in relative to PCL-sacrificing systems. If not, we recommend increasing the slope of the tibial cut by 2 to 3 degrees in order to ensure that the flexion gap will not be too tight. Once the tibial cut is completed, we have found that a confirmatory check of alignment with a flat tibial plate and an extramedullary rod helps identify and prevent a varus tibial cut (see Fig. 6-6).

We use intramedullary femoral cutting jigs when possible. With retained hardware or significant distal femoral deformity, we use extramedullary jigs and a soft tissue tensioning device. Smaller distal cutting jigs are available, which facilitate less invasive surgical approaches. We cut the distal femoral valgus angle between 4 to 6 degrees in most knees with a measured resection technique, which correlates with the distal thickness of the implant (Fig. 6-5). In the presence of significant flexion contracture, an additional 2 mm of bone is removed for each 9 degrees of flexion contrac-

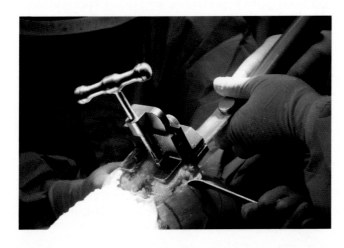

FIGURE 6-5

Measured resection of the distal femur correlates with the distal thickness of the implant.

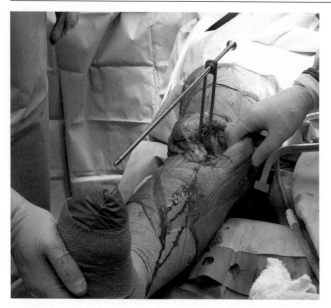

FIGURE 6-6

The mechanical alignment of the leg is checked after the tibial and distal femoral cuts are made by using an external alignment rod. If the tibia is cut in varus, the distal end of the rod will be lateral to the center of the ankle.

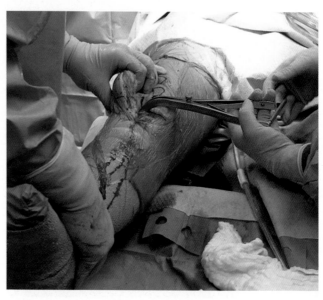

FIGURE 6-7

Lamina spreaders can help assess the extension gaps after the tibia and distal femur are cut.

ture, as described by Bengs and Scott (11). With the tibial and distal femoral cuts completed, the knee can be extended, and a spacer block or flat tibial plate with an extramedullary rod is used to check the mechanical alignment of the leg (Fig. 6-6). Medial and lateral osteophytes on the femur and tibia should be removed with an osteotome or a rongeur before evaluating the extension gaps, as large osteophytes can cause collateral ligaments to appear tightened. Lamina spreaders placed with the knee in extension are used to evaluate extension gap balance (Fig. 6-7). Gap balancing with soft tissue release is undertaken as needed to achieve equal medial and lateral gaps.

The rotational axis of the femoral component may be based on a number of landmarks including (a) the flexion gap referencing from the resected tibial surface, (b) the posterior condyles, (c) the epicondylar axis, or (d) the AP axis (also known as Whiteside's line). We mark the epicondylar and the AP axes with methylene blue in each case (Fig. 6-8A–C). The goal of all femoral component rotational references should be to establish a symmetric flexion gap in the medial and lateral compartments and equal to that seen in extension. Accurate rotational alignment of the femoral component ensures proper patellofemoral joint kinematics and avoids subluxation, as well as corrects any deformity of the flexion axis that is commonly seen in valgus deformity of the knee (12). In valgus deformity, erosion of the posterior lateral condyle is important to consider, as there is often rather severe deficiency of the posterior lateral femoral condyle. If the posterior condylar reference is used for rotating the femoral component in a valgus knee, a relative internally rotated position of the femoral component will result. A good way to check the flexion axis in any primary knee is to place the patella relocated in the trochlea with the knee flexed 90 degrees and assess the flexion gap before final posterior condylar femoral resection. In the same position and with distraction on the tibia to tighten the soft tissues, the cut tibial plane should be parallel to the epicondylar axis or perpendicular to Whiteside's line. The remaining cuts on the femur are then made, orienting the jig according to the previously mentioned references, thus ensuring proper rotation of the femoral component. In PCL-retaining knee arthroplasty, it is important to avoid raising the joint line, as this can severely alter the kinematics of the PCL during flexion extension of the knee. With CR implants, the posterior resection off the medial femoral condyle should equal the medial distal resection, which restores the joint line to the proper location. The rotational position of the femoral component is important at this point to recreate the normal flexion and extension axis of the knee.

The rotational position of the tibial component is equally important for the same reason. Final tibial component rotation may be based on this landmark as well. The rotational position of the flexion axis of the knee should coincide with the rotational position of the tibial cutting jig as

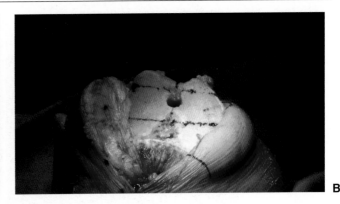

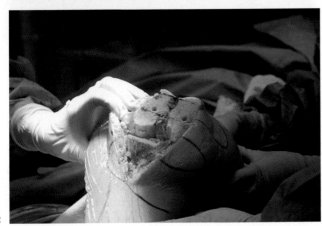

FIGURE 6-8

(A) Methylene blue and a protractor are used to mark the epicondylar axis and the AP axis (the line drawn from the low point on the trochlear to the high point of the intercondylar notch). **(B)** The lines are normally perpendicular to each other. **(C)** The femoral rotation (indicated by the lug holes) is typically established perpendicular to the AP axis or parallel to the epicondylar axis.

previously marked (Fig. 6-9). The prearthroplasty wear pattern on the tibial surface helps indicate the proper rotational jig position so that the slope of the newly cut surface matches the native slope in the AP dimension. During tibial resection, the tibial insertion of the PCL can be protected using a one-quarter or one-half-inch osteotome between the PCL and the posterior tibia. Furthermore, when the tibial resection is completed, the removed surface fragment can be compared to the preoperative plan to ensure that the appropriate amount of medial and lateral bone (which varies greatly in the varus and valgus deformities) is removed. This step helps to ensure that the cut is not placed in varus.

Balancing the PCL

Assessing flexion kinematics is the most crucial portion of PCL-retaining knee arthroplasty. This step can greatly enhance postoperative function and long-term performance of the knee and can decrease polyethylene wear and failure (13). Proper balancing of the PCL remains the hallmark of long-term success of PCL-retaining TKA. The POLO (pull-out, lift-off) test popularized by Richard

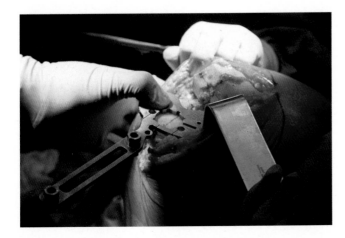

FIGURE 6-9

The jig for the tibial punch is rotationally aligned in the frontal plane according to the preoperative template (see also Figs. 6-2 and 6-3).

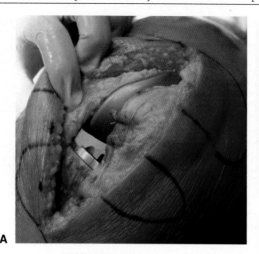
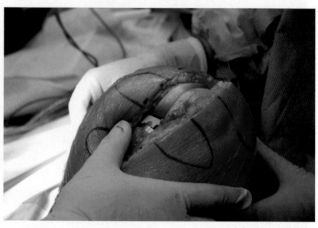

A **B**

FIGURE 6-10

(A) A PCL that is too tight in flexion will cause the femur to rest posterior to the anterior lip of the polyethylene trial and "lift off" the tibia. **(B)** A balanced PCL will sit in the middle of the polyethylene and will closely approximate the curve of the anterior lip.

Scott, MD, describes either laxity or tightness of the PCL in flexion, respectively. We traditionally examine the position of the trial tibial component beneath the posterior condyles of the trial femur in flexion and desire to have the posterior condyles in the central portion of the tibial plateau in this position (80 to 100 degrees of flexion). If during a posterior drawer test the tibia tends to sag or displace posteriorly relative to the femur in flexion, the PCL is lax. This displacement is corrected by increasing the thickness of the polyethylene to achieve a neutral and stable anterior and posterior drawer test with the knee in flexion. More often, the PCL will be too tight, particularly in knees that had no anterior cruciate ligament and in those with more severe deformity, and will require recession. A tight PCL will cause the femur to roll back onto the posterior lip of the polyethylene which will "lift off" the tibia. A well-balanced PCL will slide as well as roll when the knee is flexed, remaining centered in the polyethylene, with no significant anterior tray exposed (Fig. 6-10A,B).

Several techniques can be used during trialing of the components in order to balance a tight PCL:

1. Posterior drawer or "dashboard" technique: The surgeon applies a posteriorly directed force to the proximal tibia while the knee is flexed 90 degrees to stretch the PCL (Fig. 6-11).
2. Tibial insertional recession: With the knee flexed and the tibia pulled anteriorly, electrocautery is used to release anterior fibers of the PCL from the posterior tibia (Fig. 6-12).
3. Femoral insertional recession: With the knee flexed, the anterior fibers of the PCL are released from the distal femur with electrocautery (Fig. 6-13).
4. V-wedge tibial osteotomy: With the knee flexed and the tibia pulled anteriorly, a one-half-inch osteotome is used to osteotomize a V-shaped wedge of bone to which the PCL attaches at the proximal posterior tibial plateau.

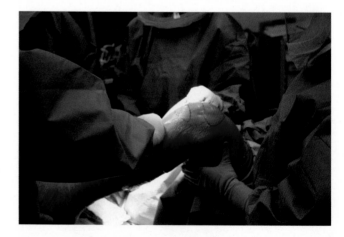

FIGURE 6-11

The "dashboard" technique is used to balance a tight PCL. With the knee flexed 90 degrees, a posterior force is applied to the proximal tibia.

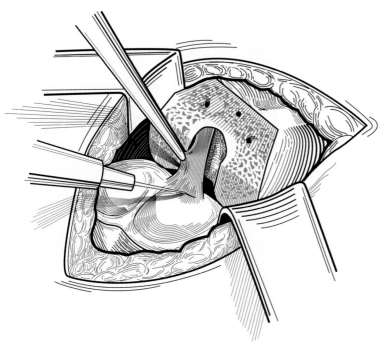

FIGURE 6-12

A tight PCL can be recessed by carefully transecting anterior fibers from the posterior of a subluxated tibia.

When the knee is flexed, if the PCL is too tight, any of these techniques can be used and must be followed by visualization of the flexion kinematics with the trial components in place. We generally use a "dashboard" technique and proceed to tibial or femoral insertion recession if necessary. Even with full PCL release off of the tibia, excellent flexion balance can be achieved uniformly in primary knee arthroplasty utilizing CR-TKA implants.

MODULARITY AND CR KNEE ARTHROPLASTY

We have found that exposure and insertion of a nonmodular (monoblock polyethylene/metal back) tibial component is achievable uniformly during primary knee arthroplasty. The advantages of non-modular components include proven wear reduction through compression molding techniques and elimination of locking mechanism problems associated with wear and lysis in modular knee arthroplasties (14,15). This type of implant should not be confused with an all-polyethylene tibial

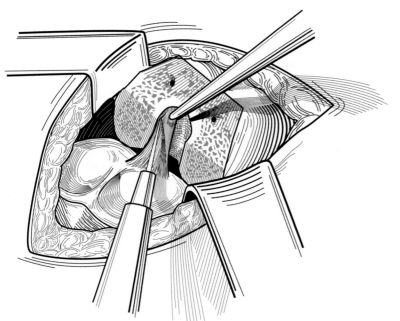

FIGURE 6-13

The PCL can be recessed from the medial side of the femoral notch with the knee in flexion.

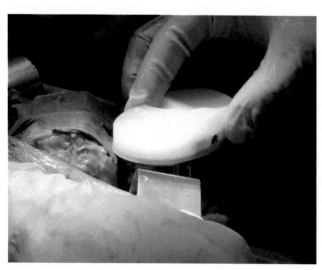

FIGURE 6-14

A monoblock tibial component can be easily used in CR-TKA (Vanguard, Biomet, Inc., Warsaw, IN)

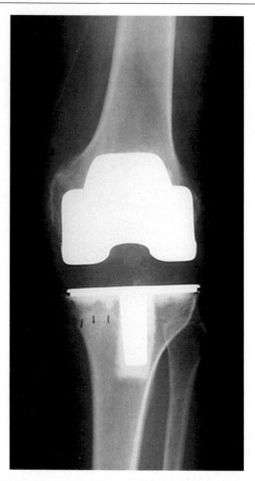

FIGURE 6-15

Radiograph of a tibial component placed in varus. Varus positioning is associated with early failure in CR-TKA.

component, which is associated with early failure in some CR-TKA designs, as discussed later. Non-modular implants can be inserted through some less invasive techniques, provided the tibia can be subluxed adequately to clear the posterior lateral femoral condyle (Fig. 6-14). Insertion of the components follows standard cementation principles including bony preparation with pulsatile lavage and drying, cement pressurization, and appropriate cement removal to prevent third-body wear.

PEARLS AND PITFALLS

- In CR knee arthroplasty, avoiding a varus aligned tibial component is critical (Fig. 6-15). Furthermore, if there is isolated tibial component loosening, revision with a well-fixed revision to a second CR implant with retention of the femoral component has proven durable in a series from our institution (16).
- Planovalgus deformity of the foot, which is often associated with preoperative and postoperative valgus alignment of the knee has been a harbinger of failure (17). In cases with severe planovalgus deformity, a more conforming articulation may be indicated to eliminate late posterior lateral rotational instability that has been observed with the flat on flat CR articulation (AGC, Biomet, Warsaw, IN).
- Surgeons should avoid inserting a CR implant when ligament balance and symmetric flexion/extension gaps have not been achieved or with a PCL that remains too tight at the conclusion of the arthroplasty.

POSTOPERATIVE MANAGEMENT

Standard rehabilitation techniques with early mobilization, pain control, deep vein thrombosis prophylaxis, and antibiotic regimens are used with all forms of knee arthroplasty. Weight bearing as tolerated is the standard at our institution with progressive weight bearing and weaning off of any assist device during the ensuing 4 to 6 weeks after discharge. The average length of stay has been dramatically reduced with perioperative pain protocols and now is less than 3 days at our institution.

COMPLICATIONS

We have seen early loosening of CR-TKA components in knees that employ an all-polyethylene tibial design and with the use of metal-backed patellar components (17,18). A lateral retinacular release can be best avoided through proper femoral and tibial component rotation as described previously and soft tissue balancing of the tibiofemoral articulation, as well as medialization of the patellar component. Rupture of the PCL following CR-TKA is rare and is usually the result of a dashboard-type injury in a motor vehicle accident or fall. There is often injury to collateral ligaments as well, and the result is a knee with multiplanar instability. In these cases, a revision using implants with a significantly greater degree of constraint is usually necessary.

RESULTS

The long-term survivorship of CR knees has been excellent and durable out to 15- to 20-year follow-up (3,4). Modes of failure have been well established, and further refinement of surgical technique, implant design, polyethylene manufacturing, and patient selection will further enhance this survivorship. In patients with osteoarthritis and rheumatoid arthritis, 10- to 15-year implant survivorship remains greater than 98% (3,4,20). Some investigators have suggested that in patients with severe deformity or inflammatory arthropathies, an implant, which substitutes for the PCL, a posterior stabilized design, should be used (21). Survivorship data from our institution suggests that a CR implant is excellent even in the presence of severe deformity and regardless of diagnosis (22,23).

REFERENCES

1. Rand JA, Trousdale RT, Ilstrup DM, et al. Factors affecting the durability of primary total knee prostheses. *J Bone Joint Surg Am* 2003;85-A(2):259–265.
2. Ritter MA, Herbst SA, Keating EM, et al. Long-term survival analysis of a posterior cruciate-retaining total condylar total knee arthroplasty. *Clin Orthop* 1994;309:136–145.
3. Ritter MA, Berend ME, Meding JB, et al. Long-term follow-up of anatomic graduated components posterior cruciate-retaining total knee replacement. *Clin Orthop* 2001;388:51–57.
4. Ritter MA, et al. Proceedings of the International Symposium on Current Topics in Knee Arthroplasty, June 13–15, 2007, Marbella, Spain. *J Bone Joint Surg Br* 2008;90:1–44.
5. Berend ME, Ritter MA, Meding JB, et al. Tibial component failure mechanisms in total knee arthroplasty. *Clin Orthop* 2004;428:26–34.
6. Schroer WC, Diesfeld PJ, LeMarr A, et al. Applicability of the mini-subvastus total knee arthroplasty technique: an analysis of 725 cases with mean 2-year follow-up. *J Surg Orthop Adv* 2007;16(3):131–137.
7. Meneghini RM, Pierson JL, Bagsby D, et al. The effect of retropatellar fat pad excision on patellar tendon contracture and functional outcomes after total knee arthroplasty. *J Arthroplasty* 2007;22(6 suppl 2):47–50.
8. Lotke PA, Ecker ML. Influence of positioning of prosthesis in total knee replacement. *J Bone Joint Surg Am* 1977;59A:77–79.
9. Ritter MA, Fans PM, Keating EM. Postoperative alignment of total knee replacements. Its effect on survival. *Clin Orthop* 1994;299:153–156.
10. Ritter MA, Campbell ED. A model for easy location of the center of the femoral head during total knee arthroplasty. *J Arthroplasty* 1988;3 Suppl:59–61.
11. Bengs BC, Scott RD. The effect of distal femoral resection on passive knee extension in posterior cruciate ligament-retaining total knee arthroplasty. *J Arthroplasty* 2006;21(2):161–166.
12. Newbern DG, Faris PM, Ritter MA, et al. A clinical comparison of patellar tracking using the transepicondylar axis and the posterior condylar axis. *J Arthroplasty* 2006;21(8):1141–1146.
13. Yamakado K, Worland RL, Jessup DE, et al. Tight posterior cruciate ligament in posterior cruciate-retaining total knee arthroplasty: a cause of posteromedial subluxation of the femur. *J Arthroplasty* 2003;18(5):570–574.
14. Berend ME, Ritter MA. The pros and cons of modularity in total knee replacements. *J Bone Joint Surg Am* 2002;84-A(8):1480–1481.
15. Weber AB, Worland RL, Keenan J, et al. A study of polyethylene and modularity issues in >1000 posterior cruciate-retaining knees at 5 to 11 years. *J Arthroplasty* 2002;17(8):987–991.

16. Berend ME, Ritter MA, Meding JB, et al. Clinical results of isolated tibial component revisions with femoral component retention. *J Arthroplasty* 2008;23(1):61–64.
17. Meding JB, Keating EM, Ritter MA, et al. The planovalgus foot: a harbinger of failure of posterior cruciate-retaining total knee replacement. *J Bone Joint Surg Am* 2005;87 Suppl 2:59–62.
18. Faris PM, Ritter MA, Keating EM, et al. The AGC all-polyethylene tibial component: a ten-year clinical evaluation. *J Bone Joint Surg Am* 2003;85-A(3):489–493.
19. Crites BM, Berend ME. Metal-backed patellar components: a brief report on 10-year survival. *Clin Orthop* 2001;388:103–104.
20. Berend ME, Ritter MA, Keating EM, et al. The failure of all-polyethylene patellar components in total knee arthroplasty. *Clin Orthop* 2001;388:105–111.
21. Ritter MA, Lutgring JD, Davis KE, et al. Total knee arthroplasty effectiveness in patients 55 years old and younger: osteoarthritis vs. rheumatoid arthritis. *Knee* 2007;14(1):9–11.
22. Laskin RS, O'Flynn HM. The Insall Award. Total knee replacement with posterior cruciate ligament retention in rheumatoid arthritis. Problems and complications. *Clin Orthop* 1997;345:24–28.
23. Meding JB, Keating EM, Ritter MA, et al. Long-term follow-up of posterior cruciate-retaining TKR in patients with rheumatoid arthritis. *Clin Orthop* 2004;428:146–152.
24. Ritter MA, Faris GW, Faris PM, et al. Total knee arthroplasty in patients with angular varus or valgus deformities of > or = 20 degrees. *J Arthroplasty* 2004;19(7):862–866.

7 Soft Tissue Balancing Technique for Posterior Stabilized Total Knee Arthroplasty

Hari P. Bezwada and Robert E. Booth Jr.

INDICATIONS

Total knee arthroplasty (TKA) is indicated for end-stage arthritis involving the knee. It is often tricompartmental in nature and may be the result of a variety of arthritides. The majority of knee arthroplasties are performed for "garden-variety" osteoarthritis; however, inflammatory arthritis, avascular necrosis, and posttraumatic arthritis are other conditions that can be treated with TKA. Knee arthroplasty is currently being performed in younger and higher-demand patients than in previous decades, with a decline in the average patient age. Obesity is commonplace. The majority of patients in our practice have a body mass index ≥30, with an evolving group of patients with a body mass index ≥50. Advanced tricompartmental arthritis is often associated with substantial deformity and reduced range of motion, both of which need to be addressed at the time of surgery. Many of these patients have also typically failed an attempt at nonoperative treatment, such as viscosupplementation, physical therapy, nonsteroidal anti-inflammatory medications, weight loss, and steroid injections.

CONTRAINDICATIONS

Medically infirm patients with severe comorbidities may not be candidates for TKA because of a substantial risk of medical complications. Active knee sepsis, osteomyelitis, severe peripheral vascular disease, severe and profound neuropathy or neurologic disease (Parkinson's disease, cerebrovascular accident), deficient extensor mechanism, and severely traumatized soft tissues may be contraindications to knee arthroplasty.

PREOPERATIVE PREPARATION

With this technique of knee replacement surgery, the soft tissue balancing is done early and progressively because bone preparation based on poorly balanced and improperly tensioned soft tissues can be flawed. This is different than the measured resection technique, in which the bone cuts are made independent of the soft tissues. After the trial components are inserted, the tissues are then balanced.

Evaluation

If the coronal alignment of the knee is "passively correctable" to neutral in 5 degrees of flexion, a smaller incision and no initial soft tissue release other than osteophyte removal should be necessary to balance the knee. If it is not, the surgeon should anticipate a longer incision and more extensive soft tissue balancing.

X-ray assessment may or may not show osteophyte formation. If there are substantial osteophytes on the concavity of the deformity, minimal dissection other than the osteophyte excision is necessary. If there is minimal correction passively and little arthrosis (such as in the mesomorphic middle-aged male), a soft tissue release is probably necessary (Figs. 7-1 and 7-2). Assess limb alignment and pattern of arthritis on preoperative x-rays to help determine roughly what may be needed in terms of osteophyte removal and ligament balancing. Regarding special situations, mild valgus knees may be passively correctable and need no early soft tissue release, whereas those with a developmental valgus and a hypoplastic lateral femoral condyle need soft tissue releases early to facilitate alignment. Laterally subluxated patellae in valgus knees—and even in some varus knees—require preoperative awareness such that femoral and tibial components can be lateralized or rotated to their maximal safe limit during the procedure and thus avoid patellar problems at the end of the case. Pure patellofemoral arthritis, without maltracking, often requires little soft tissue correction but may require strategies to avoid overstuffing the patellofemoral compartment, such as slight posterior displacement of the femoral component (which would cause a small notch in the anterior cortex) and overresecting the patella (which could result in fracture or avascular necrosis).

TECHNIQUE

Skin Incision

The surgical steps are as follows (Figs. 7-3 and 7-4).

The patient is placed in the supine position, and a bump is placed to hold the knee at 90 degrees. The leg is marked, prepped, and draped. Typically, a midline incision is used. The length of the skin incision should be proportional to the difficulty of the case. A well-padded pneumatic tourniquet is applied and insufflated to 350 mm Hg following Esmarch exsanguination. The midline skin incision should be proportionate to the body habitus, with knee in flexion for obese patients. Create minimal skin flaps, yet enough to fully identify the quadriceps mechanism.

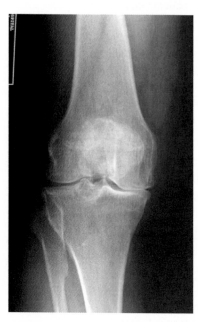

FIGURE 7-1

Anteroposterior radiograph of the right knee in a 63-year-old man with severe osteoarthritis.

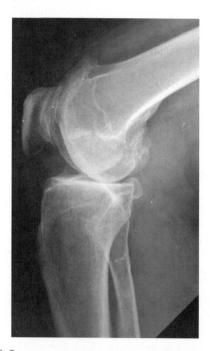

FIGURE 7-2

Lateral radiograph of the right knee in a 63-year-old man with severe osteoarthritis.

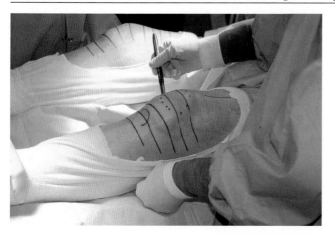

FIGURE 7-3

Bilateral knees are marked for skin incisions with crosshatches. The tibial tubercle, patella, and quadriceps tendon are outlined.

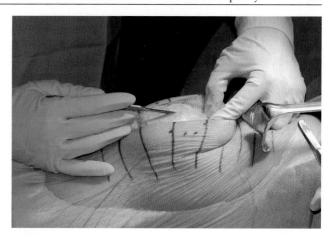

FIGURE 7-4

Skin incision with dissection to the level of the quadriceps tendon and medial retinaculum, with minimal skin flaps.

Surgical Approach

The initial arthrotomy should include the medial patellar capsule distally, extending subperiosteally down to the pes anserinus tendons. After osteophyte removal, subperiosteal dissection should extend posteriorly to but not through the semimembranosus tendons. Proximal to the patella, multiple arthrotomy options can be used, including a traditional quadriceps tendon incision (medial parapatellar), subvastus, midvastus (see Chapter 1). All osteophytes that are accessible (excluding those in the posterior part of the femur and tibia) should be excised early on to avoid oversizing the prosthetic components and to facilitate earlier soft tissue balancing.

An initial evaluation, perhaps with a central lamina spreader in extension, will help determine whether the soft tissue balance is approximately correct at this point, although it need not be precise. When releases are necessary, the surgeon needs to determine whether the tightness is in flexion or extension, or both. Static stabilizers such as ligaments may require release, whereas dynamic stabilizers such as tendons should generally be left to stretch after the arthroplasty. The primary issue is to avoid overreleasing in an attempt to gain full correction at this time, although approximate correction allows the soft tissues to contribute to the alignment of the parts. At this point, moving the knee between flexion and extension creates an opportunity for assessment regarding the need for future soft tissue releases.

The surgical steps are as follows (Figs. 7-5 to 7-15).

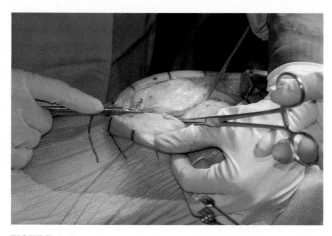

FIGURE 7-5

Medial parapatellar arthrotomy.

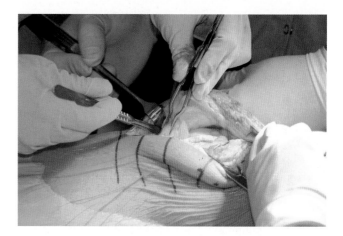

FIGURE 7-6

An infrapatellar fat pad excision is made with care to protect the patellar tendon.

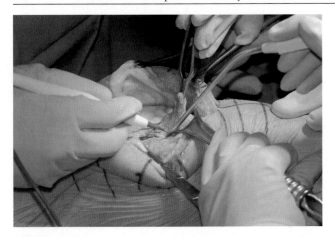

FIGURE 7-7

Minimal anterior femoral synovectomy defines the anterior femur, which is important in an anterior referencing system.

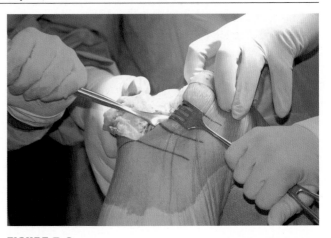

FIGURE 7-8

The medial release is performed with a sharp Cobb elevator.

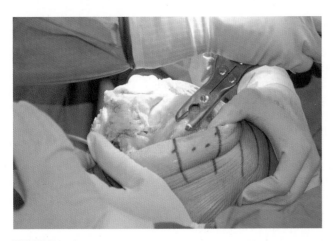

FIGURE 7-9

Overhanging osteophytes are excised with a rongeur.

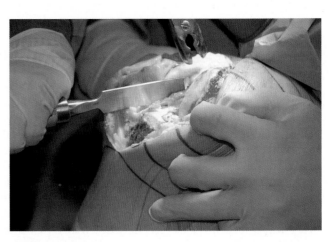

FIGURE 7-10

Notch osteophytes are excised with a curved osteotome.

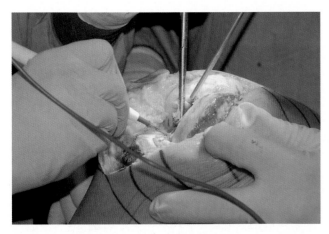

FIGURE 7-11

The cruciate ligaments are excised with electrocautery.

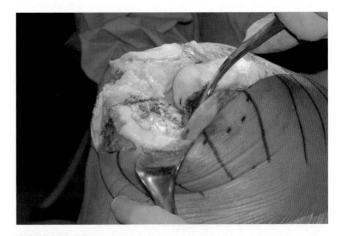

FIGURE 7-12

A Homan retractor is placed along the posterior border of the tibia forcing the tibia to sublux anteriorly.

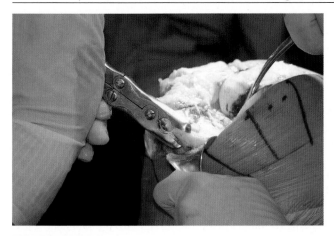

FIGURE 7-13

Medial osteophytes from the tibia are removed.

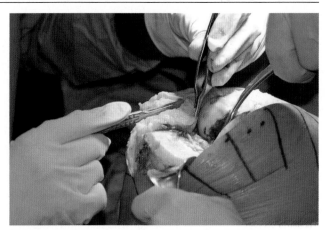

FIGURE 7-14

The remaining fat pad is excised and a lateral Homan retractor is placed.

We prefer to perform a medial parapatellar arthrotomy, leaving a 2-mm tendon cuff to repair on the medial border of the patella. The surgeon must take care with fat pad excision to protect the patellar tendon.

An anterior femoral synovectomy is performed to identify the anterior margin of the femur. Medial soft tissue release is initiated with electrocautery or a scalpel and then continued with a Cobb elevator with the knee in a figure-four position.

The patient's knee is flexed, the patella is everted, and the foot is placed on the bump.

Osteophytes from the anteromedial tibia and femur are excised, and overhanging femoral notch osteophytes are removed with a curved osteotome. Next, the anterior and posterior cruciate ligaments are removed with a Kocher and electrocautery.

The surgeon places a Homan retractor along the midline posterior border of the tibia, and the tibia is externally rotated and subluxed anteriorly. A Richardson retractor is placed along the medial soft tissue sleeve, and the medial meniscus is removed. Additional medial releases may be performed in a tight varus knee after the remaining medial tibial osteophytes are removed. Sequential release of the semimembranosus is typically all that is necessary, followed by subperiosteal slide of the superficial medial collateral ligament. Release of the pes anserinus tendons is almost never necessary. An additional fat pad may be removed to visualize lateral tibia, and a lateral Homan retractor is placed. The lateral meniscus excised, and the lateral inferior geniculate vessels are identified and cauterized.

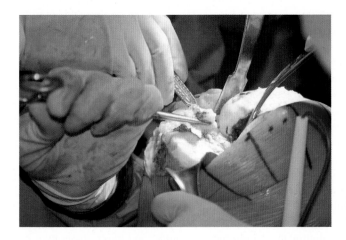

FIGURE 7-15

The lateral meniscus is removed.

BONE CUTS

The tibial cut is performed first. The resection is made such that the coronal alignment is oriented 90 degrees relative to the long axis of the tibia; the sagittal cut should be between 3 and 7 degrees as dictated by the intrinsic posterior slope of the prosthetic tibial components. We prefer to resect the tibia first because it is a single cut, which is easiest to make and easiest to correct. If the resection is performed correctly, it is the base and the reference point for all future femoral cuts. It creates space, it partially determines the thickness of the subsequent components, it facilitates estimation of future soft tissue releases, and most importantly, it determines femoral rotational alignment once the soft tissues are balanced. After balancing the tissues in flexion, a rectangular flexion gap is the goal. A varus tibial cut will cause internal rotation of the femur when a tensioned rectangular flexion gap is made; a valgus tibial cut will cause the femoral component to be excessively externally rotated based on a tensioned and balanced flexion gap. This highlights the importance of a perfect tibial cut when using the soft tissue balancing technique in a posterior-stabilized total knee. "Flexion first": Once the tibial base has been established, the surgeon should next balance the knee in flexion. The transepicondylar axis and/or Whiteside's line can be inscribed on the femur, the knee can be "tensed" at 90 degrees of flexion, and the anterior and posterior femoral resections can be made after appropriate sizing of the femoral component. Precise flexion balance is critical to empower the cam mechanism, optimize patella tracking, and ensure appropriate flexion kinematics. Therefore, a tensed joint in flexion should show the transepicondylar axis to be parallel (and Whiteside's line to be perpendicular) to the tibial cut. If this occurs, no further releases or balancing should be necessary. If there is disagreement between the soft tissue and the bony arbiters of alignment, selective releases should be performed, or the reason for this disagreement should be determined. Again, this approach is only accurate if the tibial resection is accurate; therefore, it must be scrupulously confirmed.

Therefore, tightness on the medial side suggests the need for more release of the semimembranosus or subperiosteal slide of the medial collateral ligament. The surgeon can address lateral tightness by releasing the iliotibial band and the posterolateral capsule, typically in a pie crust fashion, with the limb distracted in flexion. More severe cases of valgus may require release of the popliteus tendon and lateral collateral ligament. In femoral anteroposterior (AP) measuring, the patient is often in between sizes, and the surgeon should choose the larger size femoral component in a posterior stabilized knee, unless using the larger size causes medial-lateral overhang or excessive flexion tightness. Downsizing may require a requisite increase in distal femoral resection to balance flexion extension gaps.

After AP femoral bone cuts have been made, four parallel lines should be observed when the knee is tensioned in flexion: the cut surface of the tibia; the resected posterior femoral condylar surface; the transepicondylar axis; and the anterior cut surface of the femur. Spacer blocks or other confirmatory devices may be used to ensure this orientation and balance.

In the distal femoral cut, once flexion has been established, the limb should be put in extension, and distal femoral bone should be resected. Posterior femoral (and occasionally tibial) osteophyte removal should precede this step, to eliminate a source of persistent flexion contracture or impingement. With the limb in full extension and the soft tissues tensed with tensors, both the bony anatomy and soft tissues again have a voice in the final alignment. An extramedullary alignment rod is attached to the anterior aspect of the tensor (see Fig. 7-27). It should be directed roughly two finger breadths medial to the anterior superior iliac spine, which represents the center of the femoral head. If, at this juncture, the bony landmarks and the soft tissue tensions suggest the identical distal femoral cut, then it is undoubtedly correct. If there is disagreement between the determination of the cut based on soft tissue tension and bony alignment, the surgeon must either perform further soft tissue releases to modulate tension in the soft tissues and in effect change the direction of the distal femoral cut, or make bone cuts based on the extramedullary or intramedullary bony cues and further balance the soft tissues later in the case after the trial components have been implanted. Although the former path is preferable, the latter is acceptable and occasionally necessary.

The surgical steps are as follows (Figs. 7-16 to 7-33). Retractors are placed around the proximal tibia, and it is osteotomized perpendicular to the long axis using an oscillating saw and a 3-degree posterior sloped cutting guide. The tibial cut is checked with an alignment rod and provisionally sized. A laminar spreader is placed in extension to ensure that adequate releases have been performed and the knee is in appropriate alignment. Additionally, a valgus and varus stress may be

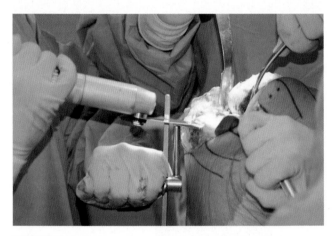

FIGURE 7-16

The proximal tibia is osteotomized perpendicular to the long axis using an oscillating saw and a cutting guide with a 3-degree posterior slope.

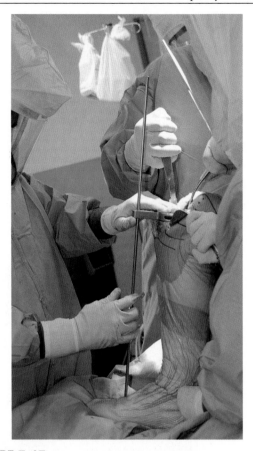

FIGURE 7-17

The tibial cut is checked to be perpendicular to the long axis.

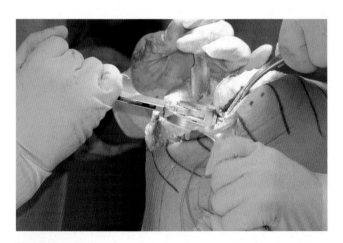

FIGURE 7-18

The tibia is provisionally sized.

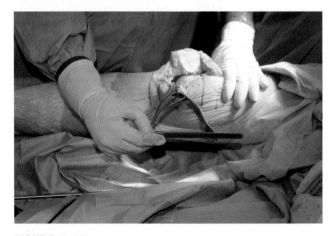

FIGURE 7-19

A laminar spreader is placed in extension to ensure that adequate releases have been performed and the knee is in appropriate alignment.

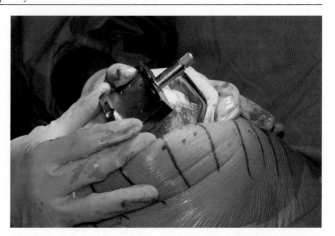

FIGURE 7-20

An anterior referencing AP cutting block is placed to establish the flexion gap.

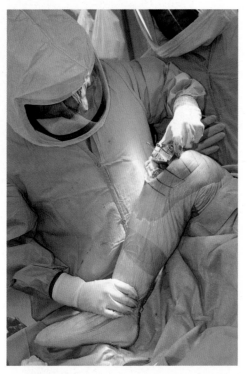

A

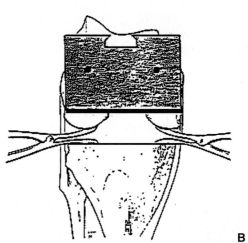

B

FIGURE 7-21

(A,B) Femoral rotation may be based on the AP axis and the epicondylar axis. The flexion space is rectangular when distracted in 90 degrees of flexion.

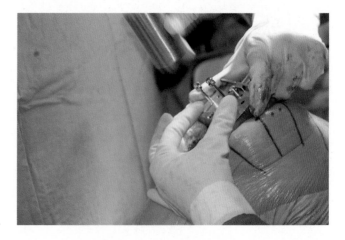

FIGURE 7-22

The AP cutting block is then pinned into place.

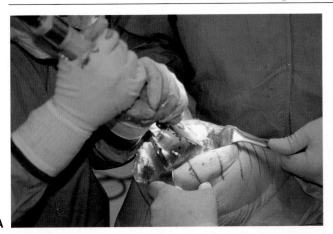
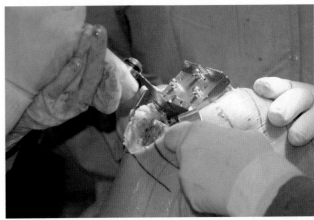

A   B

FIGURE 7-23

(A,B) The anterior and posterior femoral cuts are made with special care to protect the collateral ligaments.

placed on the knee to doubly check, and the gapping should be similar. The surgeon selects an AP anterior referencing cutting block based on the medial-lateral dimensions. It is then applied to the distal femur to establish the flexion gap. Femoral rotation may be roughly determined, applied perpendicular to the AP axis and parallel to the epicondylar axis. The flexion gap is manually tensioned in 90 degrees of flexion. The AP cutting block is then pinned into place when confirmed to have a rectangular gap. The surgeon makes the anterior and posterior femoral cuts with special care to protect the collateral ligaments and soft tissues with retractors. The posterior compartment is decompressed, removing osteophytes, loose bodies, and any remaining menisci. A Cobb elevator is used to perform an adequate posterior capsular release, and a spacer block is placed in flexion to assess the flexion gap.

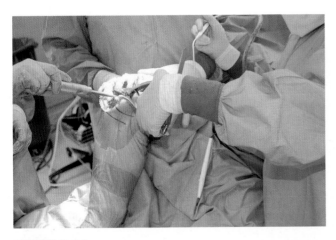

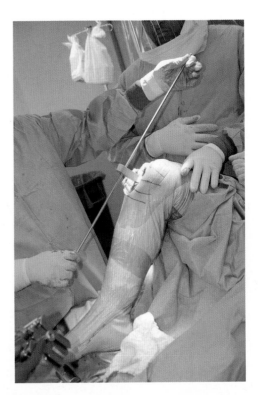

FIGURE 7-24

An osteotome is needed to remove posterior osteophytes, and a Cobb elevator is used to perform an adequate posterior capsular release.

FIGURE 7-25

A spacer block is placed in flexion to assess the flexion gap.

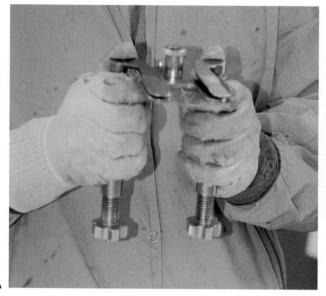
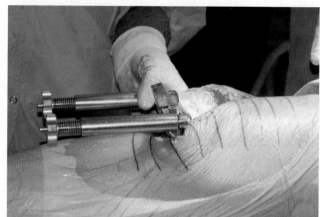

A

B

FIGURE 7-26

(A,B) A soft tissue tensor is used to create an equivalent extension gap.

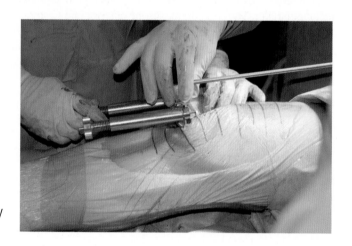

FIGURE 7-27

Limb alignment is assessed with a long extramedullary guide rod.

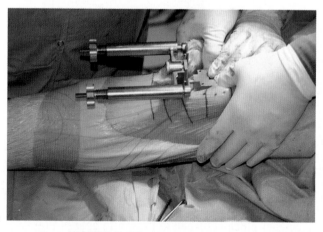
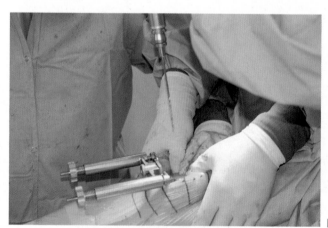

A

B

FIGURE 7-28

(A,B) Distal femoral cutting guide is drilled in place.

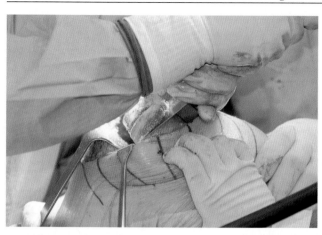

FIGURE 7-29

Distal femoral cut is made in flexion.

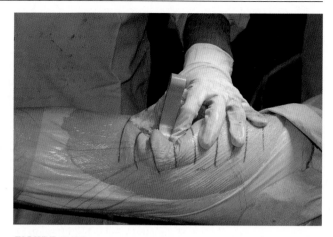

FIGURE 7-30

The same flexion block is placed in extension to ensure equal flexion and extension gaps.

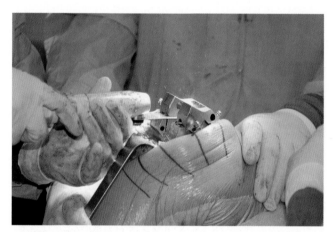

FIGURE 7-31

A femoral finishing block is placed for lug holes, chamfer cuts, and notch cut.

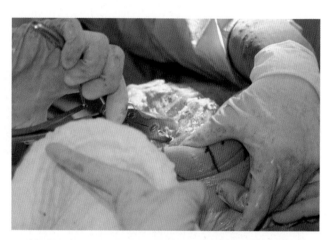

FIGURE 7-32

A rongeur is used to finish femoral preparation.

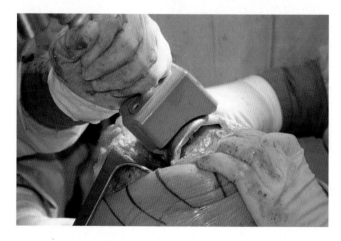

FIGURE 7-33

A provisional femoral trial is placed.

A soft tissue tensor is used to create an equivalent extension gap and tensed to 30 lbs of pressure. The overall limb alignment is assessed with a long extramedullary guide rod. The rod should point two finger breadths medial to the anterior superior iliac spine, which corresponds to the center of the femoral head. Once the orientation of the block is established, the distal femoral cutting guide is pinned in place to resect an amount of bone that will equalize the extension and flexion gaps. The distal femoral cut is made in flexion with a retractor to elevate the distal femur and protect the tibia. It is also important to protect the medial collateral ligament. The same flexion block is placed in extension to ensure equal gaps.

A femoral finishing block is pinned into place for lug holes, chamfer cuts, and notch cut. Finally, a provisional femoral trial is placed and checked for fit and position.

Tibial Placement

Once the femoral provisional component has been applied, a "floating tibial tray" can be inserted, testing the knee in both flexion and extension to determine the preferential rotation of the tibial component as driven by the soft tissue balance and the surface geometry of the prostheses. A mark can be placed on the anterior tibial surface to show the desired rotation.

With the floating trial removed and the tibial surface fully exposed, the tibial tray can be aligned using bony guide marks: the medial third of the tibial tuberosity; occasionally, the second metatarsal; and the exposed posteromedial tibial bone. If this position matches the mark dictated by the soft tissues, then tibial rotation is correct. If these two marks do not match, the reason should be ascertained. If that is not forthcoming, the general preference is to honor the bony landmarks in varus knees and the soft tissue landmarks in valgus knees. Persistent patellar subluxation suggests the need to further lateralize or externally rotate the tibial component.

The surgical steps are as follows (Figs. 7-34 to 7-37).

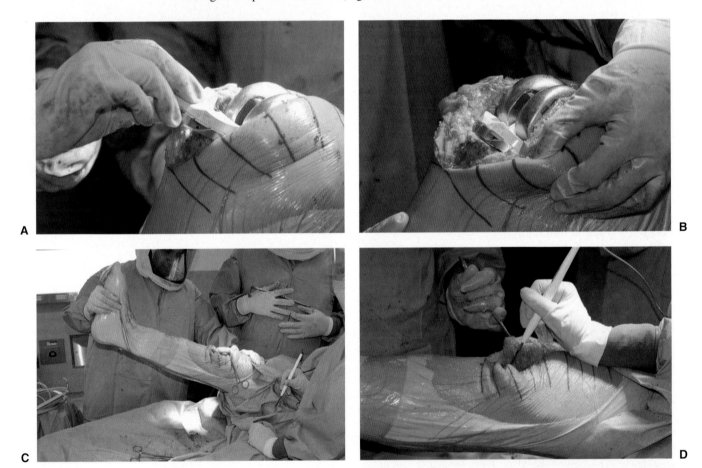

FIGURE 7-34

(A–D) A floating tibial tray is placed, and the knee is taken through a range of motion. The center of rotation is marked with electrocautery matching rotation with the femur after self-centering.

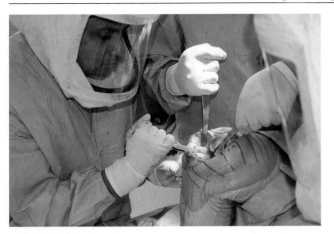

FIGURE 7-35
The tibia is prepared for a stemmed trial using the mark and tibial tubercle for tibial rotation.

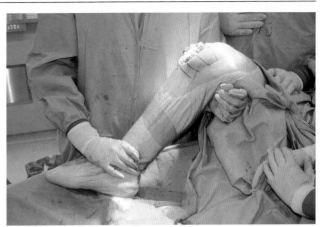

FIGURE 7-36
Flexion stability is assessed with a lift-off test or distraction.

With the trials in place, flexion and extension stability are also assessed. The knee should reduce snugly in flexion. The tibia is then reamed and broached in the proper rotation for a stemmed trial ensuring that it externally rotates to mate with the femoral component in extension and the medial one third of tibial tubercle. The surgeon assesses flexion stability for either lift-off of the tibial component in flexion (i.e., the flexion gap is too tight) or distraction (i.e., the flexion gap is too loose). Full extension should be obtained. If it is too tight in extension, release the posterior capsule or resect more distal femur, depending on its severity.

Patellar Resurfacing

Our preferred technique for the patellar cut is to evert the patella and to identify the patellar nose within the substance of the patellar tendon. A saw blade placed on this inferior surface of the patella will determine the appropriate thickness of resection, such that a cut from the posterior edge of the patellar tendon to the posterior edge of the quadriceps tendon is made from medial to lateral chondral facets, leaving a symmetrical patella surface. A patellar button is placed on the medial edge of the prepared surface, leaving some exposed lateral bone on the "odd" facet, and making sure that it is sized so that it does not overhang beyond the edges of the bone. Typically the composite patellar thickness should be the same size as or 1 mm thinner than the original patella.

The surgical steps are as follows (Figs. 7-38 to 7-41). The surgeon uses the patellar nose as a guide for patellar resection. It is the intratendinous portion of the patella in the patellar tendon. A portion

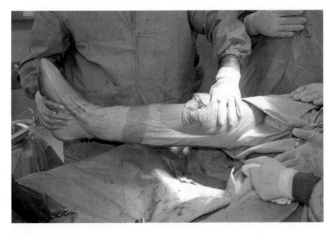

FIGURE 7-37
Full extension should be obtained.

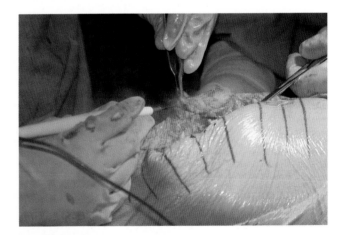

FIGURE 7-38
The patellar nose is used as a guide for patellar resection.

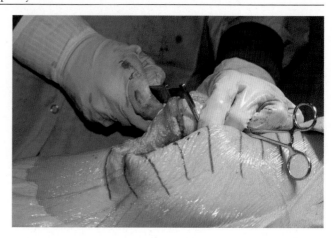

FIGURE 7-39

The patellar thickness is assessed with calipers.

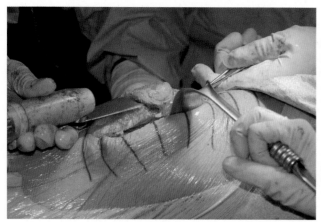

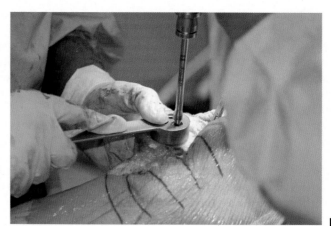

A   B

FIGURE 7-40

(A,B) The patella is prepared.

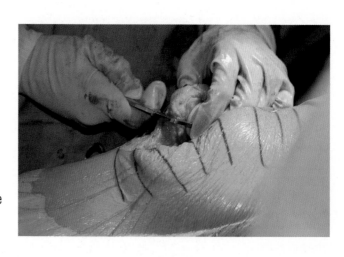

FIGURE 7-41

The composite thickness is assessed and should be approximately 1 to 2 mm less than the original thickness.

of the fat pad may need to be released to identify it. The surgeon assesses the patellar thickness with calipers, and the patella is then prepared. The composite thickness is assessed and should be approximately 1 to 2 mm less than the original thickness. Synovium from the undersurface of the quadriceps is routinely removed.

FINAL ASSESSMENT

Tracking of the patella by the "no-thumbs" technique is optimal, and lateral subluxation of the patella prompts a re-examination of the prosthetic alignment before routinely performing a lateral retinacular release (Fig. 7-42).

The final evaluation should show central tracking of the patella. In full extension, the limb should have approximately 2 mm of medial-lateral play; in 90 degrees of flexion, the knee should be slightly tighter (but not too tight that it causes lift-off of the tibial tray in flexion). The cut bony surfaces are prepared for cementation with copious irrigation and thorough drying. The cement is applied in a doughy state, first on the patella. The femoral component is cemented, and the excess cement is trimmed away. Bone cement is then finger pressed into the tibia. The tibial tray and modular polyethylene insert are assembled at the back table and implanted as a monoblock (Fig. 7-43). The tibial assembly is carefully inserted and pressurized. Excess cement is removed posteriorly first and swept out with bayonet forceps. The knee is reduced and placed in full extension, which forces cement out anteriorly. The patellar component is cemented and pressurized with a clamp. The knee is again copiously irrigated to remove any debris.

Wound closure is performed in layers with absorbable no. 1 sutures to repair the arthrotomy and absorbable 2–0 sutures for the subcutaneous tissues. Skin staples are used on the skin followed by compressive sterile dressings and tourniquet deflation (Figs. 7-44 and 7-45).

PEARLS AND PITFALLS

Soft tissue balancing is critical to this technique. Imbalance may lead to prosthetic component overload and premature failure. Also when using this technique, a varus tibial cut will lead to internal rotation of the femoral component. The tibial cut must be checked with an alignment guide, and secondary

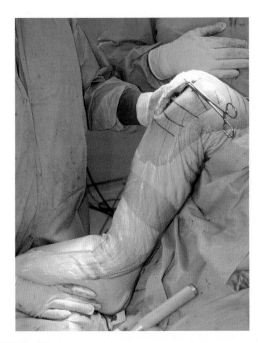

FIGURE 7-42

Patellar tracking is assessed with a no-thumbs technique.

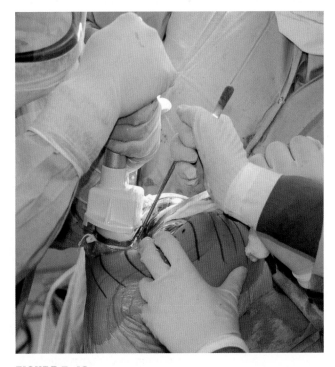

FIGURE 7-43

The tibial component is inserted as a monoblock after being assembled at the back table.

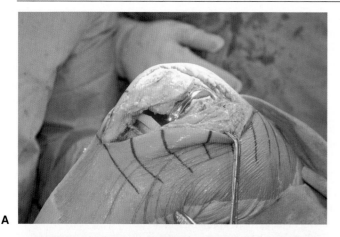

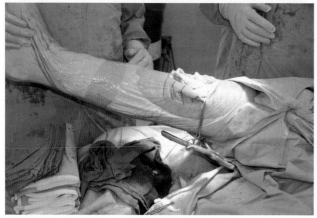

FIGURE 7-44

(A,B) Once the cement hardens, a final check of patellar tracking is performed, and flexion and extension are checked as well. Any remaining excess cement is removed.

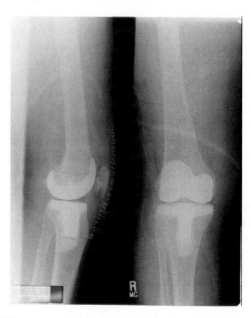

FIGURE 7-45

Postoperative anteroposterior and lateral radiographs of the right knee.

checks of femoral rotation including the AP axis and epicondylar axis should be used. The surgeon must also pay careful attention to patellar tracking. When patellar subluxation is occurring, the surgeon must recheck femoral rotation, appropriate femoral lateralization, tibial rotation and lateralization, and patellar thickness and patellar medialiation. The rate of lateral release is low when component position is precise.

POSTOPERATIVE MANAGEMENT

Postoperative management is routine including 24 hours of parenteral antibiotics. Deep venous thrombosis prophylaxis is used with an adjusted dose of warfarin with a goal international normalized ratio of ~2 or enteric coated aspirin and pneumatic compression pumps. Continuous passive motion machines are routinely used except in morbidly obese patients, because of concerns regarding skin breakdown. Patients receive twice-daily physiotherapy.

COMPLICATIONS

Rotational malalignment of the femur can occur with the balanced tissue technique if the tibial cut is in varus or valgus alignment. This risk is minimized by carefully ensuring that the tibial cut is accurate and using secondary rotational landmarks before resecting the distal femur, such as the epicondylar axis or the AP axis of the femur. Additionally, the resection of the distal femur can be inaccurate if the tibial cut is inaccurate if the soft tissue tension is strictly relied on without using secondary alignment cues, such as an intramedullary rod or extramedullary alignment check (the latter is our preference).

General complications may be divided into systemic and local complications. Systemic complications include thromboembolism, bleeding, and anesthetic complications. Local complications include hematoma, wound problems, skin necrosis, vascular complications, nerve palsy, fracture, contractures (stiffness), extensor mechanism failure, and infection. Prosthesis-related complications include instability, osteolysis, loosening (septic and aseptic), and patellar clunk.

REFERENCES

1. Insall J, Scott WN, Ranawat CS. The total condylar knee prosthesis. A report of two hundred and twenty cases. *J Bone Joint Surg Am* 1979;61:173–180.
2. Insall JN, Lachiewicz PF, Burstein AH. The posterior stabilized condylar prosthesis: a modification of the total condylar design. Two to four-year clinical experience. *J Bone Joint Surg Am* 1982;64:1317–1323.
3. Scuderi GS, Insall JN. The posterior stabilized knee prosthesis. *Orthop Clin North Am* 1989;20:71–78.
4. Stern SH, Insall JN. Posterior stabilized prosthesis. Results after follow-up of nine to twelve years. *J Bone Joint Surg Am* 1992;74:980–986.
5. Font-Rodriguez, Scuderi GR, Insall JN. Survivorship of cemented total knee arthroplasty. *Clin Orthop Rel Res* 1997;345:79–86.

8 Navigation in Total Knee Arthroplasty

Alfred J. Tria Jr.

INDICATIONS

Navigation is a technology that assists the surgeon in checking the position and alignment of the total knee arthroplasty (TKA) to help decrease the number of outliers and, hopefully, extend the longevity of the implant. There is good scientific support for the use of the technology; however, there are reports in the literature that refute its efficacy and indicate that it increases the operative time for the procedure without additional accuracy for the experienced surgeon. Line-of-sight navigation remains the gold standard for the technology. Electromagnetic navigation has been introduced, and it does eliminate the problems of the line of site in the operating room; however, iron-containing instruments tend to interfere with the generated magnetic field and lead to associated inaccuracies.

CONTRAINDICATIONS

Most navigation techniques use percutaneous pins that are placed away from the operative site (Fig. 8-1). The pins can lead to fractures and can introduce infection into the area (Fig. 8-2). If the bone is particularly osteoporotic, such as in a severe rheumatoid patient, it may be difficult to stabilize the array with the pins. As the technology has improved, the pin diameter has been decreased, and most of the frames use two pins for greater stability. In an attempt to address the pin sites, some of the arrays are set within the operative incision, and there are now plates that can be attached to the metaphysis of the medial femur and tibia with small- diameter screws (Fig. 8-3). The plates form a base for the attachment of the arrays, and the arrays can be removed from the operative site when the navigation is not being used (Fig. 8-4). Navigation adds time to the operative procedure; and, if the anesthetic time is critical for a given patient, it may not be advisable to include it in the operative procedure.

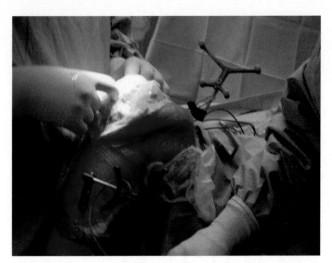

FIGURE 8-1

The percutaneous pins are placed outside the incision, and the arrays are attached to them.

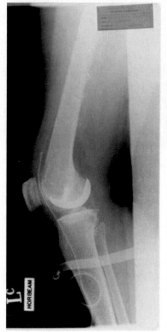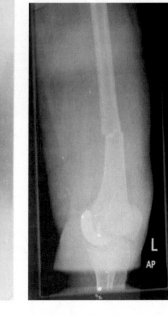

A   B

FIGURE 8-2

(A) Lateral x-ray of a knee after a unicondylar arthroplasty performed with percutaneous pins for navigation with a pin tract in the diaphyseal area of the femur. **(B)** Fracture through the pin site 10 days after the surgical procedure.

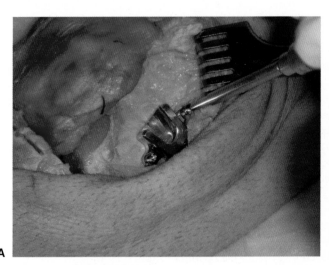

A   B

FIGURE 8-3

(A) Navigation plate attached to the medial side of the femoral metaphysis in a cadaver dissection. **(B)** The navigation plate is attached to the medial side of the femur in a right varus knee with the completed tibial array fully attached.

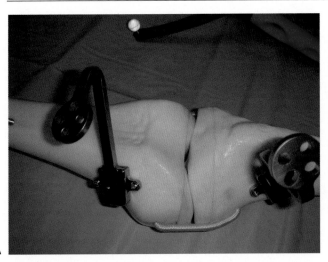

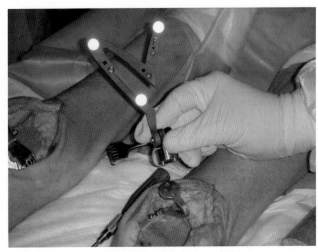

A

B

FIGURE 8-4

(A) The base is attached to the plate. **(B)** The array is then attached to the base.

PREOPERATIVE PREPARATION

The preparation for the navigated knee arthroplasty should include the setup of the computer in the operating room so that this does not interfere with the usual procedure (Fig. 8-5). One or more of the instruments for landmarking will need to be calibrated with the computer and this step should also be completed before starting (Fig. 8-6). If percutaneous pins are going to be used, the area of preparation and draping should be extended both superiorly and inferiorly to include these areas in the sterile field. It saves time and effort if all of the instruments are prepared for the insertion of the pins or plates before beginning (Fig. 8-7).

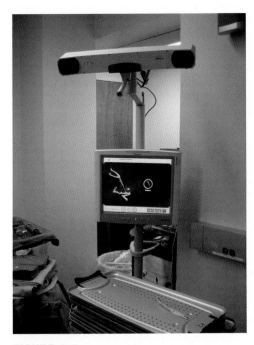

FIGURE 8-5

The navigation screen is positioned at the foot of the table with the camera aimed at the operative arrays.

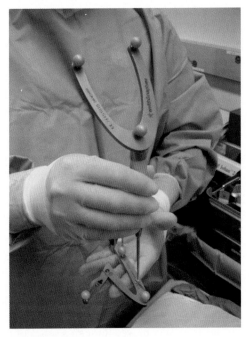

FIGURE 8-6

The calibration of the pointer for landmarking is completed before the start of the operation. In this case, there is a site on the array for the pointer for the calibration.

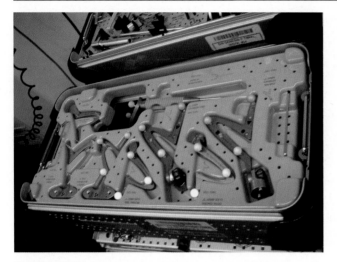

FIGURE 8-7

The navigation instruments are set up completely before the operation begins to decrease the time needed for the procedure.

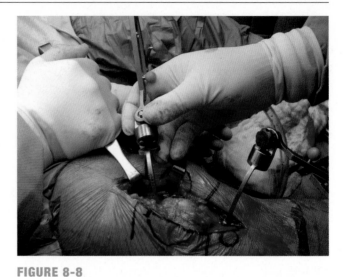

FIGURE 8-8

It is best to set up the entire array and estimate the position for the plate on the medial aspect of the femur before pinning the plate in position. This allows for the array-camera relationship and for the relationship of the array arm to the surrounding soft tissues.

TECHNIQUE

Before the patient is brought into the operating room, it is best to have the computer screen and associated camera set at a convenient location in the room that will allow good access to the camera with as little repositioning as possible. The best location is typically at the foot of the operating room table or opposite the side of the table where the surgeon stands.

After the anesthetic has been stabilized, the lower leg will require preparation for proper sterility of the field, which must include the area for placement of the pins for the arrays. Dual-pin configurations are best applied outside the operative incision but not too far beyond the metaphyseal area to avoid pin-site fractures. Single-pin arrays usually require larger-diameter pins to ensure stability. This type of configuration can be placed more readily into the operative field but can interfere with the standard instruments used for the surgical procedure. The author favors using base plates for the arrays. These devices are placed within the operative incision, and the standard incision can be used for all cases (Fig. 8-3).

After the arthrotomy is completed, the medial femoral and tibial metaphyses are cleared as part of the standard approach. The femoral array is completely constructed including the base plate, the curved arm, and the array itself (Fig. 8-8). The plate is placed along the medial femoral metaphysis as a trial to see if it will lie in an area that will not interfere with the knee's capsule and the standard instrumentation. After confirming the freedom of the surrounding soft tissues, the plate is fixed to the cortical bone surface with two locking screws. The tibial plate is attached next in a similar fashion. After both plates are in place, the full array is attached to both of the plates with the knee in full extension (Fig. 8-9). The arrays can still be rotated on the magnetic base and can also be moved from flexion to extension. Once the position is set in full extension, the knee should be taken through the full range of motion to check line of sight with the camera through the entire range of motion of the knee. It is much easier to check the visibility at this time before proceeding with the landmarking.

After the array positions are confirmed, the anatomic landmarks of the knee must be identified. The leg is usually moved through a series of positions with the hip and knee slightly flexed to identify the center of the femoral head in the hip joint (Fig. 8-10). Each system has a routine number of points that must be identified on the femur and the tibia. It is critical to identify these points as accurately as possible. This step requires time and patience; however, if the points are well identified, the navigation will be much more accurate and reliable.

Before proceeding with the surgery, the alignment of the knee should be established with reference to the mechanical axis. A routine mechanical axis x-ray is performed on each patient before the

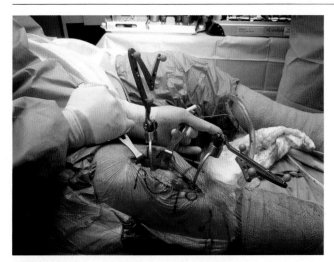

FIGURE 8-9

Once both arrays are set in position, it is important to place the knee in full extension and document that the camera can see the arrays. Then, the knee should be flexed to 120 degrees while checking that the camera sees the arrays throughout the entire range of motion.

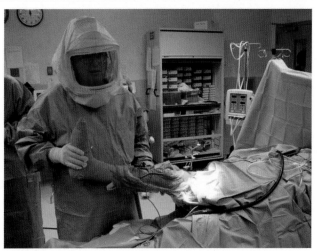

FIGURE 8-10

The center of the hip is established first by holding the limb with the hip and knee slightly flexed and changing the position by a few degrees at a time while the camera records the data.

surgery, which is used to confirm the accuracy of the intraoperative navigation. In most cases, the two numbers for the mechanical axis should be within 1 to 2 degrees of each other. If there is a great discrepancy, the land-marking is fully repeated, and the x-ray is measured again and checked for abnormal rotation. Once these parameters have been fully confirmed, the surgery can commence.

At the present time, the author combines the navigation with traditional instrumentation, including intramedullary referencing on the femoral side (Fig. 8-11). One of the benefits of the navigation is that there is no need to instrument the femoral canal. This step presumes, however, that the navigation is completely accurate. If bicortical percutaneous pins are used for the arrays, it is not possible to use intramedullary instrumentation on either side of the knee. The plates allow this type of referencing because the screws do not penetrate the canal enough to obstruct intramedullary rod positioning. Thus, the surgeon can use instruments and navigation throughout the operation.

After the mechanical axis is confirmed, the surgery proceeds with the femoral cuts first. The anterior and distal cuts are navigated and confirmed with the navigation and the standard instruments. If there is a discrepancy of greater than 3 degrees between the two references, the surgeon must recheck both references before proceeding. The navigation can be checked by going back to the reference points that were marked on the femoral and tibial sides in case the arrays loosened. The instruments are replaced back on the bone, and the landmarks for their positioning are rechecked.

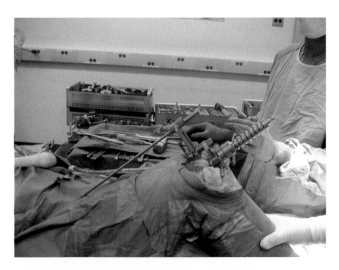

FIGURE 8-11

The navigation plates do not violate the intramedullary canal, and the cuts can be confirmed with both intramedullary and extramedullary instrumentation.

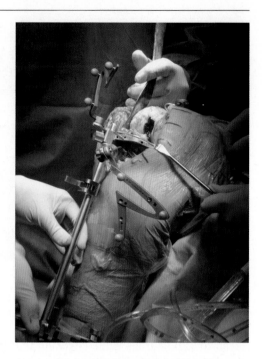

FIGURE 8-12

The extramedullary tibial cutting guide can be set with navigation and also can be checked clinically.

Usually, this step will identify which reference is inaccurate, and the surgeon can correct the problem before proceeding.

The proximal tibial cut is made using an extramedullary guide that can be navigated and also positioned clinically (Fig. 8-12). This cut is a critical one because many TKA failures are a result of malaligned tibial resections. The cut must be set in all three planes respecting the depth, the anteroposterior slope, and the coronal plane varus and valgus. After the cut is completed, it is checked with the navigation and also with a standard spacer block with an extramedullary rod. The flexion and extension gaps are then compared to confirm that the two gaps are symmetric and equal. With the spacer block in the extension gap, the overall alignment of the knee can be checked to be sure that the mechanical axis is zero. If this is not the case, the femoral and tibial cuts should be checked individually, and the gaps are reconfirmed for symmetry and balance.

After confirming the overall alignment, the femur and tibia can be finished to accept the specific design of femoral component and tibial tray. The overall alignment is checked one last time after the final components are cemented in place. This alignment should be the same as the alignment of the trial components.

The arrays are removed at this point. If the holes are in the operative field, they can be examined to be sure there are no associated fracture lines that can propagate after the surgery. The plates use small fragment screws and do not tend to encourage stress risers. If the arrays have been placed percutaneously, it is not possible to check the holes, and this step will not be possible.

PEARLS AND PITFALLS

Percutaneous pins perform best if they penetrate both cortices but care must be taken not to insert the pin a significant distance beyond the distal cortex with possible injury to the surrounding soft tissues and neurovascular structures. It is best to perform a trial positioning of the complete array before drilling the cortices to be sure that the chosen position does not interfere with the operative field and that the array is visible throughout the range of motion of the knee.

The plates must be at least 15 mm proximal to the femoral joint line and distal to the tibial joint line to avoid interference with the instruments and the surface resections. On the femoral side, it is important to place the plate on the medial aspect of the metaphysis below the level of the anterior resection in the coronal plane. On the tibial side, the plate usually extends a few millimeters underneath the proximal margin of the pes tendon insertion. In a small knee, the tibial plate should be placed between the joint line and the superior margin of the pes and not more distal, or the stem of the tibial component may strike one of the attaching screws with subsequent motion of the array and loss of navigational accuracy.

COMPLICATIONS

There are very few complications from the use of navigation, and most are related to the percutaneous pins. The possibility of fracture can be decreased by avoiding insertion too far from the joint lines with less invasion of the diaphysis of the bone. The pin diameters should be less than 4 mm, and the most stable configuration uses two pins that are locked together with a frame. Infection is not very common, and proper preparation of the insertion sites with inclusion in the sterile operative field gives the greatest protection.

RESULTS

The author moved from a line-of-sight navigation system to an electromagnetic (EM) system to try to avoid the difficulties of the percutaneous pins and the line of sight in the operating room. The EM system uses an emitter (Fig. 8-13) as a substitute for the camera, and there are sensors (dynamic reference frames) attached to the medial femoral and tibial metaphyses, similar to the navigation plates used for line-of-sight navigation (Fig. 8-14). The instruments are guided with a paddle that can be inserted into the cutting slots of the instruments (Fig. 8-15). EM navigation was used in 60 consecutive patients, and data were available for analysis in 57 patients. EM surveillance was abandoned in three operative procedures because the data from the navigation was grossly incorrect when compared to the clinical presentation in the operating room. In one case, the initial EM mechanical axis alignment was 37 degrees of varus when the knee clinically measured only 5 degrees. In the second case, the rotation of the anterior femoral cut was 20 degrees internally rotated by the EM, and it was 5 degrees externally rotated with clinical reference to the epicondylar femoral axis. In the third case, the EM indicated 8 degrees of varus in the tibial cut when the clinical measurement was neutral. In all three cases, the landmarking was repeated, and the results were exactly the same. In one of the operations, a reference plate was noted to be loose. Data from five preoperative x-rays were not used for analysis because of rotation. Therefore, 52 knees were available for preoperative comparisons. All of the knees had acceptable post-operative radiographs, thus leaving 57 knees for the postoperative measurements. Two knees did not have archived data for the tibial component alignment; therefore, only 55 knees were available for the postoperative measurement of the tibial component. Table 8-1 summarizes the patient data.

The distribution of paired differences for preoperative alignment and postoperative tibial alignment was not Gaussian (Shapiro-Wilk test <0.05); therefore, the p value for the non-parametric (Wilcoxon log-rank) test was used to determine significance. Criteria were met for the paired t-test

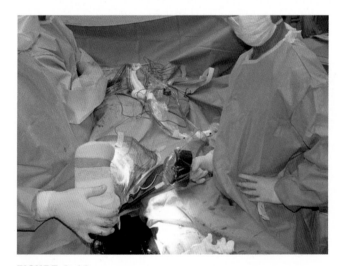

FIGURE 8-13

The emitter for the EM must be covered for proper sterility and can be left in the operating field.

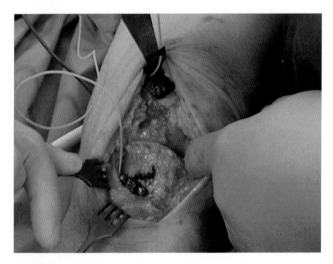

FIGURE 8-14

The EM dynamic reference frames can be screwed into position on the medial aspect of the femur and the tibia similar to the position for the plates for the line-of-sight navigation. The sterile wires connect to USB ports on the computer.

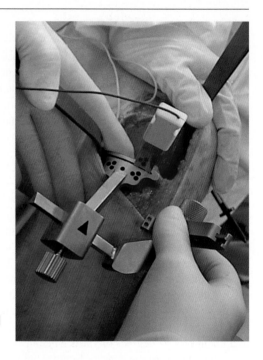

FIGURE 8-15

The sterile paddle can be set into the cutting slots of the standard instruments to check the clinical position with navigation.

for postoperative limb alignment; therefore, the *p* value for the paired t-test was used to determine significance. Table 8-2 summarizes the statistical analysis.

There were no significant differences in preoperative alignment when measured radiographically and by EM navigation. There was a significant difference of 1.8 degrees in postoperative limb alignment and a significant difference of 0.7 degrees in postoperative tibial component alignment when measured by the two techniques.

The alignment measured by EM was within 3 degrees of the predicted preoperative alignment in 63% (33/52) of cases. The alignment measured by EM was within 3 degrees of the predicted postoperative alignment in 67% (38/57) of cases. The alignment of the tibial component measured by EM was within 3 degrees of the predicted postoperative x-ray alignment in 87% (48/55) of cases.

Although there is some inherent variability in x-ray measurement, it is currently the standard for evaluating limb alignment after TKA. In this experience with EM navigation, there were no complications secondary to the navigation. It was not difficult to adapt to the system, and the average tourniquet time was 69 minutes for the entire operative procedure. There were no surgical delays caused by interruption in camera line of site and no difficulties with debris interfering with arrays. The reference plates are small enough to be attached to the bone within the operative field.

TABLE 8-1. Patient Data	
Mean Age	70 (range, 43–86)
Mean BMI	30.6 (range, 21.2–52.5)
Gender	38 female
	22 male
Approach	22 QS
	38 mini
Side	28 right
	32 left
Deformity	59 varus
	1 valgus
Mean blood loss	247
Mean tourniquet time	69 (range, 47–108)
Mean Preop TFA	182.9 degrees
Mean Preop EM Alignment	7.4 degrees mechanical varus
Mean Postop TFA	174.9 degrees
Mean Postop EM Alignment	2.2 degrees mechanical varus

BMI, body mass index; EM, electromagnetic; QS, quadriceps sparing; TFA, tibiofemoral angle.

TABLE 8-2. Statistical Analysis		
Measurement		**Difference**
Preoperative Alignment	N	52
	Mean	−1.5
	Median	−1.0
	Standard deviation	3.20
	Min	−6.5
	Max	5.0
	Paired t-test p value	.0015
	Shapiro-Wilk p value	.0002
	Nonparametric p value	.0563
Postoperative Alignment	N	57
	Mean	1.8
	Median	2.0
	Std dev	2.95
	Min	−4.0
	Max	9.0
	Paired t-test p value	<.0001
	Shapiro-Wilk p value	.1998
	Nonparametric p value	<.0001
Postoperative Tibial Alignment	N	55
	Mean	−0.7
	Median	2.07
	Std dev	−1.0
	Min	−6.0
	Max	4.0
	Paired t-test p value	.0117
	Shapiro-Wilk p value	.0231
	Nonparametric p value	.0142

The preoperative measurements for alignment showed no significant difference between the radiographic examination and the EM navigation data. Despite the fact that the postoperative knee alignment and tibial component alignment measurements showed significant differences, the differences of 1.8 and 0.7 degrees, respectively, are within the examiner's ability to measure the x-rays. The three outliers from the EM navigation are of some concern. This represents a 3% incidence, and the author was unable to correct the discrepancies despite attempts to repeat the landmarking and the measurements. The only explanation available is the presence of extraneous metal in the operative field that leads to incorrect readings.

Because of the outliers in the EM technology, the author returned to a line-of-sight technique using the base plates. Forty consecutive cases have been studied with mechanical axis films for comparison. The maximum difference was never more than 1.5 degrees between the x-ray studies and the navigation results. Although these are early data, there have been no outliers and no plate loosenings.

The assumption of most articles about navigation is that the alignment determined by the computer is absolutely accurate. This assumption is not entirely correct, and the operating surgeon must be aware of the limitations of any system that is used for operative support. All systems that rely on kinematic hip center determination may have some error in assessing alignment. Victor and Hoste reported a mean deviation between the kinematic and radiographic hip center of 1.6 mm with a range of 0 to 5 mm. They also suggested that other systems may have even more variability. It is sometimes difficult to accurately identify all of the anatomic landmarks that are necessary for navigation. Variability in landmarking will affect the accuracy of navigation. Motion in the referencing frames adversely effects computer measurement of alignment, and anatomic variation makes it difficult for any one software program to calculate the alignment correctly on every occasion. Navigational alignment is determined with the knee joint in the non–weight-bearing position on the operating room table with the patella subluxed laterally and with a portion of the deep medial collateral ligament released. The radiographs are taken with the knee in the weight-bearing position and without any opening or laxity of the capsule of the knee. These factors can contribute to differences in alignment when measured by navigation and x-rays.

Navigation is still in an early phase of development. It is not actively embraced by most clinical surgeons in the United States because of the associated financial costs and loss of time in the operating rooms. Although there are articles both in favor and against the technology, navigation does force the surgeon to think more about the procedure, which should result in greater accuracy. It will take time to perfect navigation, but it should lead to improved results and greater longevity for TKAs.

RECOMMENDED READING

Bargren JH, Blaha JD, Freeman MA. Alignment in total knee arthroplasty. Correlated biomechanical and clinical observations. *Clin Orthop Relat Res* 1983;(173):178–183.

Bathis H, Perlick L, Tingart M, et al. Radiological results of image-based and non-image-based computer-assisted total knee arthroplasty. *Int Orthop* 2004;28:87–90.

Bathis H, Perlick L, Tingart M, et al. Alignment in total knee arthroplasty. A comparison of computer-assisted surgery with the conventional technique. *J Bone Joint Surg Br* 2004;86:682–687.

Cates HE, Ritter MA, Keating EM, Faris PM. Intramedullary versus extramedullary femoral alignment systems in total knee replacement. *Clin Orthop Relat Res* 1993;(286):32–39.

Chauhan SK, Scott RG, Breidahl W, Beaver RJ. Computer-assisted knee arthroplasty versus a conventional jig-based technique. A randomized, prospective trial. *J Bone Joint Surg Br* 2004;86:372–377.

Decking R, Markmann Y, Fuchs J, et al. Leg axis after computer-navigated total knee arthroplasty: a prospective randomized trial comparing computer-navigated and manual implantation. *J Arthroplasty* 2005;20:282–288.

Dennis DA, Channer M, Susman MH, Stringer EA. Intramedullary versus extramedullary tibial alignment systems in total knee arthroplasty. *J Arthroplasty* 1993;8:43–47.

Evans PD, Marshall PD, McDonnell B, et al. Radiologic study of the accuracy of a tibial intramedullary cutting guide for knee arthroplasty. *J Arthroplasty* 1995;10:43–46.

Hankemeier S, Hufner T, Wang G, et al. Navigated intraoperative analysis of lower limb alignment. *Arch Orthop Trauma Surg* 2005;125:531–535.

Hsu RW, Himeno S, Coventry MB, Chao EY. Normal axial alignment of the lower extremity and load-bearing distribution at the knee. *Clin Orthop Relat Res* 1990;(255):215–227.

Hvid I, Nielsen S. Total condylar knee arthroplasty. Prosthetic component positioning and radiolucent lines. *Acta Orthop Scand* 1984;55:160–165.

Ishii Y, Ohmori G, Bechtold JE, Gustilo RB. Extramedullary versus intramedullary alignment guides in total knee arthroplasty. *Clin Orthop Relat Res* 1995;(318):167–175.

Jeffery RS, Morris RW, Denham RA. Coronal alignment after total knee replacement. *J Bone Joint Surg Br* 1991;73:709–714.

Laskin R. Alignment of total knee components. *Orthopedics* 1984;7:62–72.

Laskin RS. Instrumentation pitfalls: you just can't go on autopilot! *J Arthroplasty* 2003;18(3 suppl 1):18–22.

Lotke PA, Ecker ML. Influence of positioning of prosthesis in total knee replacement. *J Bone Joint Surg Am* 1977;59:77–79.

Perlick L, Bathis H, Tingart M, et al. Navigation in total-knee arthroplasty: CT-based implantation compared with the conventional technique. *Acta Orthop Scand* 2004;75:464–470.

Petersen TL, Engh GA. Radiographic assessment of knee alignment after total knee arthroplasty. *J Arthroplasty* 1988;3:67–72.

Plaskos C, Hodgson AJ, Inkpen K, McGraw RW. Bone cutting errors in total knee arthroplasty. *J Arthroplasty* 2002;17:698–705.

Ritter MA, Faris PM, Keating EM, Meding JB. Postoperative alignment of total knee replacement. Its effect on survival. *Clin Orthop Relat Res* 1994;(299):153–156.

Robinson M, Eckhoff DG, Reinig KD, et al. Variability of landmark identification in total knee arthroplasty. *Clin Orthop Relat Res* 2006;442:57–62.

Sparmann M, Wolke B, Czupalla H, et al. Positioning of total knee arthroplasty with and without navigation support. A prospective, randomized study. *J Bone Joint Surg Br* 2003;85:830–835.

Stockl B, Nogler M, Rosiek R, et al. Navigation improves accuracy of rotational alignment in total knee arthroplasty. *Clin Orthop Relat Res* 2004;(426):180–186.

Stulberg DS. How accurate is current TKR instrumentation? *Clin Orthop Relat Res* 2003;(416):177–184.

Teter KE, Bregman D, Colwell CW Jr. The efficacy of intramedullary femoral alignment in total knee replacement. *Clin Orthop Relat Res* 1995;(321):117–121.

Victor J, Hoste D. Image-based computer-assisted total knee arthroplasty leads to lower variability in coronal alignment. *Clin Orthop Relat Res* 2004;(428):131–139.

PART FOUR

COMPLEX ISSUES IN PRIMARY TOTAL KNEE ARTHROPLASTY

9 Varus and Valgus Deformities

William J. Long and Giles R. Scuderi

INDICATIONS/CONTRAINDICATIONS

Fixed angular deformity about the knee necessitates special consideration to restore normal alignment during a total knee arthroplasty (TKA). With fixed angular deformity, one ligament is shortened or contracted while the opposite ligament is usually elongated. Particularly with varus deformity, there is often an associated flexion contracture with involvement of the posterior capsule. The cruciate ligaments, being in the center of the knee, usually retain their normal length; however, it may be difficult to elongate the contracted side without releasing the cruciate ligaments. The ideal postoperative alignment is independent of the original anatomy and should not be compared to that of the opposite, "normal knee," because it most likely has a similar angular deformity. This ideal alignment, which is achieved by balancing the soft tissues and placing the prosthetic components in proper position, is 5 to 9 degrees of anatomic valgus. The tibial component should be placed at 90 degrees (perpendicular) to the mechanical axis of the tibia in the coronal plane, while the posterior slope in the sagittal plane is dictated by the implant design. The ideal placement of the femoral component is 5 to 7 degrees of valgus angulation in the coronal plane and 0 to 5 degrees of flexion in the sagittal plane (1). When the alignment is not sufficiently corrected, the components will be unequally loaded and subjected to excessive stress, resulting in eventual loosening of the prosthesis (2). Intraoperatively, it is imperative to reassess each step of the soft tissue release as it is performed so as not to overcorrect the deformity and create an unwanted instability. When using cruciate-retaining or posterior stabilized knee prostheses, the intact collateral ligaments and not the prosthesis alone give stability to the knee (3).

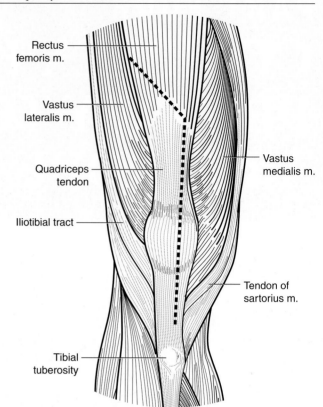

Rectus femoris m.

Vastus lateralis m.

Quadriceps tendon

Iliotibial tract

Vastus medialis m.

Tendon of sartorius m.

Tibial tuberosity

FIGURE 9-1

Varus deformity is usually caused by medial tibial bone loss and contracture of the medial supporting structures. (Redrawn and reprinted with permission from Collizza W, Insall JN, Scuderi GR. The posterior stabilized total knee prosthesis: assessment of polyethylene damage and osteolysis. Ten-year minimum follow-up. *J Bone Joint Surg* 1995;77A:1713–1720.)

Varus deformity is usually caused by medial tibial bone loss with contracture of the medial collateral ligament, posterior medial capsule, pes anserinus, and semimembranosus muscle (Fig. 9-1). Medial femoral bone loss, which may be present, is usually minimal. Elongation of the lateral collateral ligament is a late event, and rupture of the ligament is rare.

A fixed valgus deformity is caused by contracture of the iliotibial band and biceps femoris, lateral collateral ligament (LCL), popliteus, and posterolateral capsule (Fig. 9-2A,B). Elongation of the medial collateral ligament (MCL) is a late secondary event. Knees with rheumatoid arthritis and valgus deformity usually have an external rotation deformity of the tibia caused by contracture of the iliotibial band. Because of the articulation of the lateral femoral condyle with the posterior aspect of the tibia, valgus deformity usually includes a posterior lateral tibial defect with sparing of the anterior tibial margin. The lateral femoral condyle, which is often hypoplastic, is eroded in a valgus deformity because of its articulation with the tibia and wear from a laterally tracking patella.

PREOPERATIVE PLANNING

A careful physical examination should determine the degree of deformity, whether or not it is correctable, range of motion, muscle strength, and condition of the soft tissue envelope surrounding the knee. Ligamentous instability is rarely a problem in the degenerative knee with a fixed angular deformity. The anterior cruciate ligament is usually deficient or degenerative, particularly in younger patients with osteoarthritis, but this is not a problem in TKA (4). The integrity of the posterior cruciate ligament (PCL), however, will determine the choice of prosthesis. If the PCL is deficient or needs to be released or resected to correct the fixed deformity, then a PCL-substituting prosthesis should be implanted. For cases with severe contracture requiring extensive ligamentous release and difficulty in balancing the soft tissues, a constrained condylar prosthesis should be available.

Although limited weight-bearing knee views may provide sufficient templating ability for mild deformities (<15 degrees) (5), we continue to use a full-length standing anteroposterior radiograph, including the hip, knee, and ankle for more severe or complex deformities. The objective in correcting fixed angular deformities is to restore the mechanical axis of the leg to 0 degrees. This mechanical axis consists of a straight line from the center of the femoral head through the center of the knee and to the center of the ankle. Preoperative radiographs should also demonstrate any bony defects that may need augmentation, while the tangential (merchant) view allows for an assessment of patellar alignment and wear.

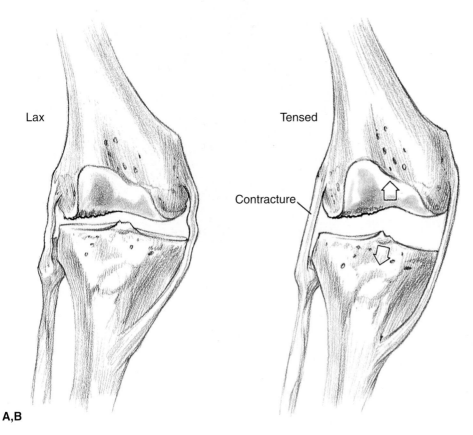

Lax

Tensed

Contracture

FIGURE 9-2

(A,B) Valgus deformity is usually caused by lateral femoral bone loss and contracture of the lateral supporting structures. (Reprinted with permission from Collizza W, Insall JN, Scuderi GR. The posterior stabilized total knee prosthesis: assessment of polyethylene damage and osteolysis. Ten-year minimum follow-up. *J Bone Joint Surg* 1995;77A:1713–1720.)

A,B

TECHNIQUE

Surgical Exposure

The anterior midline approach allows full exposure of the distal femur and proximal tibia (6). It is an extensile approach and can be extended proximally or distally as needed. This anterior incision also allows exposure of the medial and lateral supporting structures.

Following the skin incision, a limited medial parapatellar arthrotomy is performed through a straight incision extending over the medial one third of the patella and continuing along the medial border of the tibial tubercle (Fig. 9-3). The quadriceps expansion is peeled from the anterior surface of the patella by sharp dissection until the medial border of the patella is exposed (Fig. 9-4). The synovium is divided, and the fat pad is split in line with the capsular incision. The patella is then subluxed

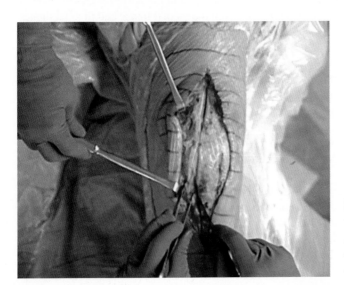

FIGURE 9-3

The medial parapatellar arthrotomy extends from the quadriceps tendon over the medial one third of the patella and continues along the medial border of the tibial tubercle.

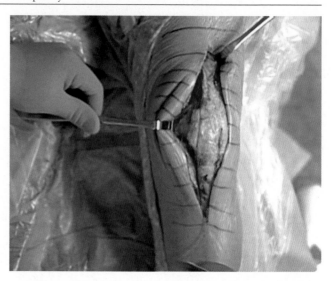

FIGURE 9-4

The quadriceps expansion is sharply dissected from the medial border of the patella.

laterally. To avoid avulsion of the patellar tendon, it can be subperiosteally dissected to the crest of the tibial tubercle, releasing tension while the knee is flexed (6). This approach is the most versatile, allows the broadest exposure to the knee joint, and can be extended proximally into a quadriceps snip, or distally with a tibial tubercle osteotomy.

Varus Deformity

To correct a fixed varus deformity, progressive release of the tight medial structures is performed until they reach the length of the lateral supporting structures (7). With the knee in extension, soft tissues are dissected from the anteromedial tibia, as a continuous subperiosteal sleeve progressing medially (Fig. 9-5A,B). A periosteal elevator can be used to develop this plane approximately 3 to 4 cm distal to the medial joint line (Fig. 9-6). Retraction for better exposure during the release is performed with a sharp bent Homan retractor (Fig. 9-7). Placement of this retractor also allows traction on the medial soft tissues, facilitating the subperiosteal release around to the posteromedial corner distal to the joint line.

The cruciate ligaments may inhibit the correction and should be resected if they do (8). Attempts to retain the PCL in cases of severe varus deformity usually result in an inability to correct the deformity. Although conceptually it would be appealing to progressively release the PCL or perform a recession from the tibial spine, we prefer to resect it and insert a PCL-substituting prosthesis. In addition to preventing the correction of a fixed varus deformity, a tight PCL will limit motion and cause the knee to open like a book, preventing the more normal gliding and rolling motion that occurs with knee flexion (8).

The knee can now be flexed and the tibia externally rotated. The insertion of the semimembranosus muscle is released from the posterior medial corner (Fig. 9-8A,B), and the posterior and medial osteophytes are removed at this time. Excising osteophytes from the medial femur and tibia facilitates the release as they tent the medial capsule and ligamentous structures, and their removal can produce a minimal amount of correction by relaxing tension on the superficial MCL, before the soft tissue release is begun. Further trimming of posteromedial osteophytes may need to be performed after the proximal tibia is resected and the trial tibia is applied.

At this point, and following each further step in the release, gap and alignment balance can be assessed by removing retractors and applying a valgus movement across the knee in extension or inserting lamina spreaders within the medial and lateral joint space and judging alignment with respect to the mechanical axis.

A medial release is performed with the knee in extension and a Homan retractor in place. A ¾-inch osteotome is used to progressively release medial soft tissues including the superficial MCL and pes insertion from proximal to distal along the tibia. Palpation of tight structures facilitates a focused release. Complete release extends up to 15 cm distal to the medial joint line.

In marked fixed varus deformities, the medial subperiosteal dissection is continued posteriorly and distally, including the deep fascia of the soleus, while maintaining continuity of the medial soft tissue sleeve (Fig. 9-9A,B). When a flexion contracture is present, it may be necessary to resect

(text continues on p. 117)

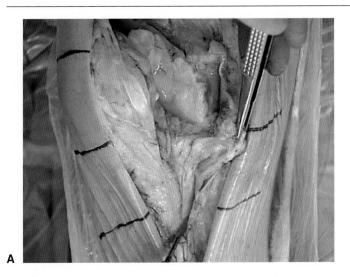

A

Patella displaced laterally

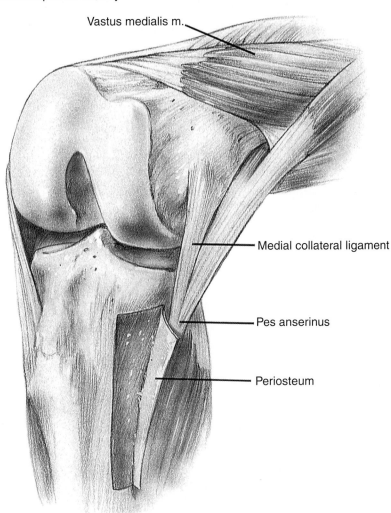

Vastus medialis m.

Medial collateral ligament

Pes anserinus

Periosteum

B

FIGURE 9-5

(A) Initially, the varus release is begun with sharp subperiosteal dissection of the deep and superficial medial collateral ligament, along with the insertion of the pes anserinus tendons. **(B)** Representation of the initial varus release. (Reprinted with permission from Collizza W, Insall JN, Scuderi GR. The posterior stabilized total knee prosthesis: assessment of polyethylene damage and osteolysis. Ten-year minimum follow-up. *J Bone Joint Surg* 1995;77A:1713–1720.)

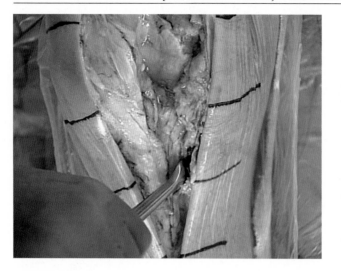

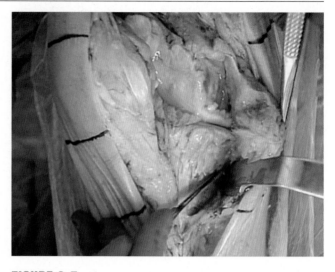

FIGURE 9-6

The subperiosteal sleeve is continued posteriorly, using a periosteal elevator for further release.

FIGURE 9-7

A Homan retractor is placed beneath the subperiosteal sleeve for better exposure.

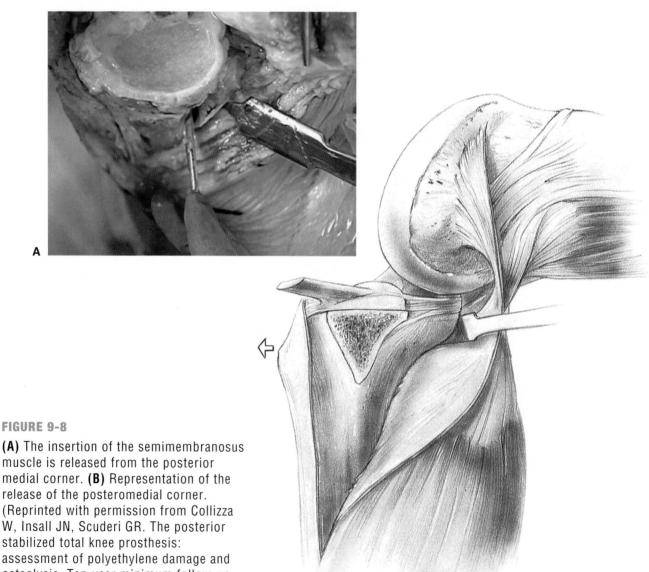

FIGURE 9-8

(A) The insertion of the semimembranosus muscle is released from the posterior medial corner. **(B)** Representation of the release of the posteromedial corner. (Reprinted with permission from Collizza W, Insall JN, Scuderi GR. The posterior stabilized total knee prosthesis: assessment of polyethylene damage and osteolysis. Ten-year minimum follow-up. *J Bone Joint Surg* 1995;77A:1713–1720.)

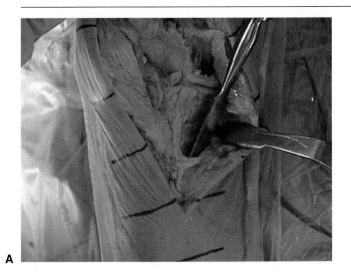

A

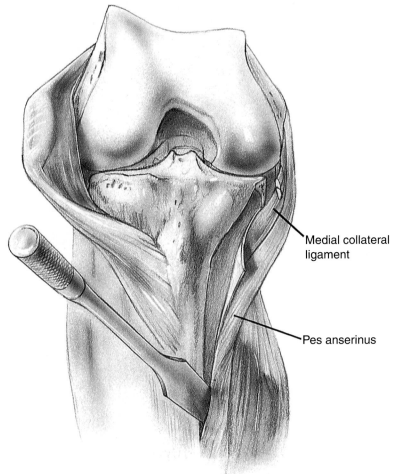

Medial collateral ligament

Pes anserinus

B

FIGURE 9-9

(A) In severe varus deformity, the medial subperiosteal dissection is continued posteriorly and distally, maintaining continuity of the medial structures.
(B) Representation of more distal medial release. (Reprinted with permisison from Collizza W, Insall JN, Scuderi GR. The posterior stabilized total knee prosthesis: assessment of polyethylene damage and osteolysis. Ten-year minimum follow-up. *J Bone Joint Surg* 1995;77A:1713–1720.

posterior tibial osteophytes and further release the posterior capsule, which can be stripped subperiosteally from the femur and/or the tibia, after the bone cuts are made. In severe cases with extensive subperiosteal dissection, the proximal medial tibia appears skeletonized (Fig. 9-10).

When the medial release is complete and normal alignment has been achieved, the standard bone cuts are made (9). The level of the tibial cut is constant, conservative, and perpendicular to the long axis of the tibia. In a knee with a varus deformity, more bone is resected from the lateral than from the medial tibial plateau. Once the tibia is cut, resection of the femur is undertaken. The flexion gap produced should be rectangular rather than trapezoidal in shape (Fig. 9-11A,B), and to achieve this, the femoral component is rotationally set along the epicondylar axis. This results

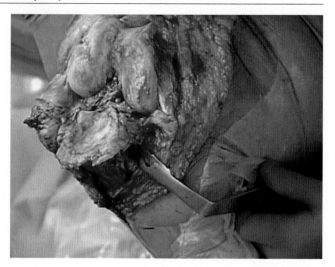

FIGURE 9-10

In severe cases of varus deformity, with extensive subperiosteal dissection, the proximal medial tibia appears skeletonized.

in more bone resection from the posterior medial femoral condyle than from the posterolateral femoral condyle.

When a large tibial bone defect is present after the bone cut, several options are available and are reviewed in Chapters 19, 20, and 21 of this text.

Valgus Deformity

The surgeon approaches the knee in a fashion similar to that described for the varus knee; however, for the valgus knee, the bone cuts are usually made before the ligament release to facilitate exposure. By comparison with that of a varus release, the principle of a valgus release is to stretch the contracted lateral structures to the length of the medial structures. Although lateral osteophytes may be present and should be removed, they do not bowstring the lateral collateral ligament in the same manner as osteophytes on the medial side, as the distal insertion of the lateral collateral ligament into the fibular head carries the ligament away from the tibial rim.

With the knee in extension and distracted with a laminar spreader (Figs. 9-12 and 9-13), the arcuate ligament and posterolateral capsule are transversely cut at the joint line with a no. 15 blade.

FIGURE 9-11

(A,B) The flexion and extension gaps should be equal and rectangular in shape. (Reprinted with permission from Collizza W, Insall JN, Scuderi GR. The posterior stabilized total knee prosthesis: assessment of polyethylene damage and osteolysis. Ten-year minimum follow-up. *J Bone Joint Surg* 1995;77A:1713–1720.)

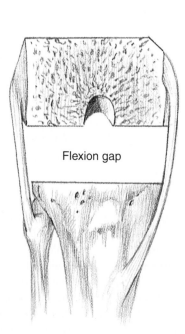

Flexion gap

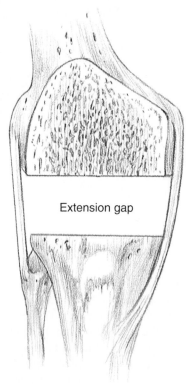

Extension gap

A,B

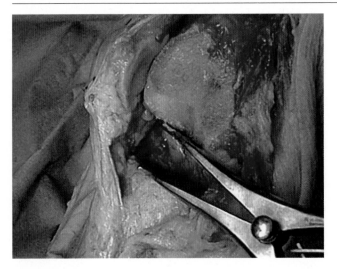

FIGURE 9-12

With the knee in extension, the joint is distracted with laminar spreaders.

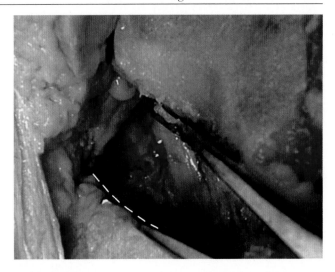

FIGURE 9-13

With the knee in extension, the posterolateral capsule and arcuate ligament are cut transversely at the joint line (*dashed line*). The popliteus tendon is preserved.

Take care not to cut or detach the popliteus tendon, as it is important in maintaining stability in flexion. Then the iliotibial band, lateral retinaculum, and LCL are pierced with the no. 15 blade in a "pie crust" fashion, both proximal to the joint and distally within the joint (Fig. 9-14) (10,11). Care must be taken not to penetrate the soft tissues beyond 1 cm in depth particularly in the posterolateral corner where the peroneal nerve lies at an average 1.49 cm from the bone edge (12). The lateral side is then progressively stretched using a second laminar spreader, and further "pie crusting" is performed until the gaps are balanced. This technique allows lengthening of the lateral side while preserving a continuous soft tissue sleeve and creating a rectangular extension space. Ligament balance in flexion and extension is confirmed with spacer blocks.

For a severe fixed valgus deformity, it may be necessary to perform a complete release of the lateral supporting structures including the LCL, lateral capsule, arcuate complex, and popliteus tendon. This step can be performed by sharp dissection of the popliteus tendon, LCL, and posterolateral capsule from the lateral femoral epicondyle (Fig. 9-15), although our current preferred method in these cases is to perform an osteotomy of the lateral femoral epicondyle (Fig. 9-16).

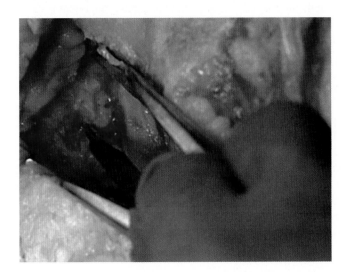

FIGURE 9-14

The iliotibial band and the lateral retinaculum are pierced with a no. 15 blade in a "pie crust" fashion.

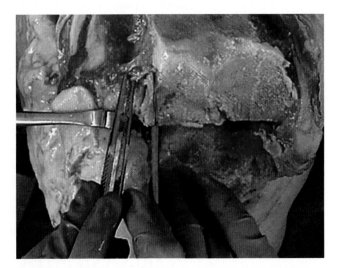

FIGURE 9-15

For severe deformities, the lateral collateral ligament, popliteus tendon, and posterolateral capsule are sharply detached from the lateral femoral condyle.

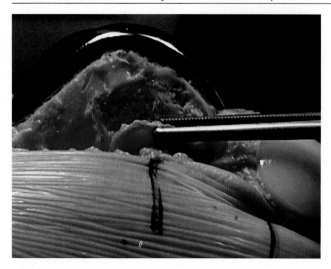

FIGURE 9-16

The lateral collateral ligament and popliteus tendon can be osteotomized from the lateral epicondyle.

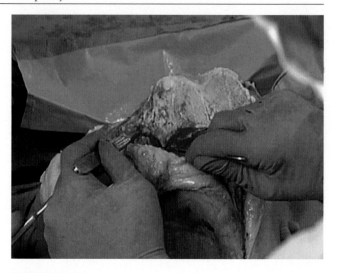

FIGURE 9-17

Occasionally, the lateral head of the gastrocnemius requires release.

The bone shingle created has the aforementioned soft tissue structures attached and affords the appropriate release. This detached fragment is not fixed down but is allowed to float freely on the remaining soft tissue attachments. The release can be extended around the posterolateral aspect of the femur, and occasionally, the lateral head of the gastrocnemius requires division (Fig. 9-17). Division of the biceps femoris is rarely required. We do not routinely recommend MCL advancement, but there may be some specific cases in which it can be applied when refractory medial laxity exists, despite appropriate releases (13).

When more marked valgus deformities are encountered, a decision must be made as to whether pie crusting will provide sufficient release, or if a lateral epicondylar osteotomy is required. We prefer to make this decision before beginning the release, as we prefer not to perform both procedures in combination. In most cases, a noncorrectible deformity greater than 20 degrees requires an osteotomy. Stiff knees with a flexion contracture may require an osteotomy with a lesser deformity. Knees with hyperextension and a full range of motion are often fully corrected with pie crusting despite a significant valgus deformity.

Following a valgus release, the resultant space between the femur and tibia is usually larger than it normally is when the MCL is tensed, and for this reason, a thicker tibial component is usually needed. Occasionally, overrelease of the lateral side may cause flexion instability, particularly when the popliteus is released. If this occurs, a constrained implant should be used (14). A hypoplastic or deficient lateral femoral condyle may require modular augmentation of the femoral component. In these cases, we use the epicondylar axis to assess appropriate femoral component rotation, as a standard posterior condylar referencing system can result in internal rotation of the femoral component (15).

Special consideration should also be given to the alignment of the patella, because subluxation usually exists preoperatively in cases of valgus deformity. A lateral retinacular release may be necessary to restore normal patellar alignment and tracking. This is accomplished by incising the lateral retinaculum in line with its fibers, at 1 cm from the patella and should be done in stages, extending the incision as necessary. If possible, the lateral superior geniculate vessels should be preserved to avoid avascular necrosis of the patella. If the patella still appears to be tracking laterally after lateral release, a proximal patellar realignment may be performed during closure of the arthrotomy. Recurrent patellar subluxation or dislocation following TKA is generally caused by errors in surgical technique (16).

PEARLS AND PITFALLS

General

- Maintain a low threshold for extending incisions and using a quadriceps snip, as exposure and visualization are paramount in accurately achieving a balanced knee.

- Avoid overresecting bone before achieving appropriate balancing of soft tissues. Conservative bone resections, particularly on the tibial side, are often sufficient following soft tissue release.
- Do not complete the case with unconstrained components and an unbalanced knee. Incomplete correction leads to increased focal stresses and early failure.

Varus

- Carefully titrate the medial release. At each stage, palpate the remaining medial soft tissue envelope and assess particular areas of tightness. Interval reassessment of gaps is important to avoid overrelease.
- Preoperative lateral translation of the tibia may indicate significant lateral laxity. A conservative bone resection in this case will prevent the creation of an excessive flexion/extension gap.

Valgus

- Removing a portion of the retropatellar fat pad and release of the lateral patellofemoral ligaments facilitates exposure to lateral structures.
- Carefully protect the MCL and popliteus during bone resection.
- Particular attention to component rotation and bony cuts must be made in cases with hypoplasia of the lateral femoral condyle.
- A distal femoral cut at 4 to 5 degrees of valgus is used to decrease strain on the attenuated MCL.
- Excessive medial soft tissue stripping can damage already-attenuated medial structures.
- Excessive lateral soft tissue releases that involve the iliotibial band, lateral collateral ligament, popliteus tendon, and posterolateral capsule can result in rotatory instability, which can predispose to knee dislocations in deep flexion. In these rare circumstances, use of an implant that provides varus-valgus constraint, such as an LCCK-type implant may be necessary to stabilize the joint.

POSTOPERATIVE MANAGEMENT

After appropriate ligament balancing is achieved and the flexion and extension gaps are equal, the components of the prosthesis are fixed into place. The tourniquet is released, and major vascular sources of bleeding are cauterized. The tourniquet is then reinflated and the wound is copiously irrigated and closed in a routine manner.

Postoperatively, patients who have undergone ligament releases for fixed deformities of the knee are managed in a manner similar to those who have had routine TKAs. A light pressure dressing is applied, and the patient is immediately placed in a continuous passive motion (CPM) machine in the recovery room. We have found CPM to be a useful adjunct to rehabilitation, which has reduced the time required to achieve 90 degrees of flexion. Some patients are unwilling to participate aggressively in their postoperative therapy and have difficulty obtaining 90 degrees of flexion by the second to third week postoperatively. These patients are seen in the clinic and are evaluated regarding motion and pain levels, and in some cases, ongoing therapy is insufficient, and early manipulation under general or epidural anesthesia is required (17).

A complex multimodal pain protocol is followed beginning preoperatively and continued with pain team management throughout the hospitalization. Patients are instructed to stand and begin walking full weight bearing with the assistance of the physical therapist on the evening of surgery or on the first postoperative day. Care is taken with early mobilization, as quadriceps weakness can occur secondary to the femoral block, and thus an assistant (and crutches or a walker) is used during this period. Patients usually remain in the hospital until they walk independently with crutches or a cane, can climb stairs, and have achieved 90 degrees of flexion. These tasks are generally accomplished by the third postoperative day.

CLINICAL RESULTS

Our surgical technique for releasing the medial structures of the knee, balancing the collateral ligaments, and restoring normal alignment has been successful since we began performing TKAs. The results of our survivorship analysis (18) and clinical studies (7,19–24) have supported our technique for correcting fixed varus deformities and have proven enduring and predictable. In our series of total condylar replacements, 63 knees had a varus deformity, including 23 with more than 10 degrees of fixed deformity (24). Stability was maintained at 10 to 12 years of follow-up, with 88% of the knees continuing to have good or excellent results. In one case, proper balancing of the soft tissues was not achieved, and varus instability recurred. Although initially rated as showing a good result, this knee deteriorated to yield a poor result because of progressive instability and required revision at 8.5 years after the original TKA.

Although we believe that complete excision of the cruciate ligaments and use of a PCL-substituting prosthesis is helpful in correcting a fixed varus deformity (8), Tenney et al have found that routine excision of the PCL is unnecessary (25). Instead, they advocate using a PCL-retaining prosthesis, which has been shown to be stable even when a PCL recession is performed.

An earlier report of the results of TKA in valgus knees with lateral ligamentous release from the femur showed that they are comparable to the results of arthroplasty in knees with lesser deformity (26). A review of 168 arthroplasties for valgus deformity demonstrated 91% good and excellent results, 6% fair results, and 3% poor results, with an average follow-up of 4.5 years. There were no revisions for recurrent instability, and the postoperative tibial femoral alignment was maintained at an overall average of 7 degrees of valgus. Although valgus deformities represented a greater challenge in terms of intraoperative balancing, the results showed TKA to be a reliable and durable procedure.

A more recent review of our results using the lateral "pie crust" technique for valgus knees showed excellent results (10). Twenty-four consecutive patients with valgus knees treated with the described protocol combined with a cemented posterior stabilized prosthesis were examined at a mean 54 months and had an average Knee Society score of 97 and range of motion of 121 degrees. There were no known complications or revisions.

In selected cases of elderly, low-demand patients with a significant valgus (average, 17.6 degrees) deformity, a primary constrained implant has been used without performing lateral releases. Thirty-seven patients underwent 44 primary TKAs using this protocol. Results at a mean 7.8-year follow-up showed an average 5.3 degrees weight-bearing anatomic alignment, with no radiographic loosening, prosthetic failures, peroneal nerve palsies, or flexion instabilities (14).

COMPLICATIONS

Several complications may arise from the correction of fixed angular deformities. These are discussed in the following sections.

Instability

Instability in extension can be either symmetric or asymmetric. Symmetric extension instability occurs when the extension gap is incompletely filled by the components of the prosthesis and there is residual laxity of the collateral ligaments in extension. This problem can result from the resection of too much bone from the distal femur because of miscalculation or from improper soft tissue balancing. Inserting a thicker tibial component can sometimes solve the problem, but when the flexion gap is too tight to accommodate such a thicker component, it may be necessary to augment the distal femur. This can be achieved with distal femoral modular augments. Another option may be to downsize the femoral component and use the thicker tibial component.

Symmetric flexion instability is encountered when the flexion space is greater than the extension space. This condition may result from undersizing of the femoral component with over-resection of the posterior condyles in which case upsizing of the femoral component with possible posterior modular augmentation is required. Alternatively, underresection of the distal femur may be responsible for the mismatch, in which case further distal resection and a thicker tibial insert will achieve appropriate balancing.

Asymmetric instability can occur when the contracted ligament is not completely released. In extension, the underreleased contracted ligaments act as a tether and lead to recurrence of the preoperative deformity. Performing the appropriate ligamentous release and equalizing the collateral ligaments corrects this imbalance.

While the knee may be balanced in extension, asymmetric instability may occur in flexion if the femoral component rotational position is not appropriate. The preferred method for determining femoral component rotation is the epicondylar axis, but secondary references include the anteroposterior axis, the tibial shaft, and balanced soft tissues (27). Overrelease to correct a fixed axial deformity, especially a valgus knee, may cause the knee to spring open asymmetrically on the released lateral side. This can lead to flexion instability. If significant, a constrained implant may be necessary.

Rotatory instability can occur because of instability in flexion or more commonly from malposition of the tibial component causing a mismatch at the femoral-tibial articulation. Apparent malrotation of the tibial component is seen when the popliteus is too tight and flexing of the knee causes internal rotation of the tibia. The simple solution to this problem is to divide the popliteus tendon, allowing the lateral tibial plateau to drop back in flexion and restoring congruent tracking.

Apart from the special case of inadvertent division of the medial collateral ligament, the absence of collateral ligaments is unusual, even in rheumatoid arthritis or following trauma. Although the collateral ligaments may appear incompetent prior to arthroplasty, they tend to be present and elongated. Sometimes, stretching of the collateral ligaments to obtain a tight fit is impractical because of the degree of leg lengthening needed to equalize the ligaments. In such cases, it is more practical to use a constrained condylar prosthesis (14).

Patellar Instability

Recurrent subluxation or dislocation of the patella following ligamentous release to correct a fixed deformity, especially with a fixed valgus deformity, is caused by errors in surgical technique. Internal rotation of the tibial component with respect to the tibia leads to external rotation of the tibia when the knee is reduced, resulting in lateral displacement of the tibial tubercle. This displacement increases the valgus vector and the tendency of the patella to sublux laterally. Correct rotational positioning of the tibial component is best achieved by aligning the intercondylar eminence of the tibial component with the tibial crest. External rotation of the femoral component will also improve patellar tracking. Other sources of patellar instability are a tight lateral retinaculum or malalignment of the extensor mechanism. In these cases, a lateral retinacular release is necessary to restore normal patellar tracking. If possible, preservation of the lateral superior geniculate vessels should be attempted in an effort to maintain the patellar and lateral skin circulation. This may sometimes be impossible because the vessels and soft tissue bridge may continue to tether the patella and keep it tracking laterally, and in these extreme cases, the vessels should be sacrificed. If the patella still appears to be tracking laterally after a lateral retinacular release, the surgeon should perform proximal patellar realignment during closure.

Avulsion of the Patellar Tendon

Avulsion of the patellar tendon can easily occur during exposure of the stiff knee with a fixed angular deformity. When the patella is subluxed laterally, considerable traction is exerted on the patellar tendon at the tibial tubercle. Repairing a transverse tear of the patellar tendon and periosteum is a difficult process, and the best way to avoid this intraoperative complication is with meticulous technique during knee exposure. The joint is exposed through a medial parapatellar arthrotomy that is continued onto the tibia to a point within 1 cm of the medial border of the tibial tubercle. This allows a cuff of periosteum to be dissected subperiosteally to the crest of the tibial tubercle, along with the insertion of the patellar tendon. As the knee is flexed and the patella is subluxed laterally, this periosteal sleeve may pull further away from the tibial tubercle, along with the patellar tendon similar to a banana peel. This technique permits distal continuity of the soft tissue and prevents a horizontal tear. If there is a chance of patellar tendon avulsion, a quadriceps snip should be performed. This technique provides excellent exposure and allows eversion of the patella (Fig. 9-18).

Peroneal Nerve Injury

The risk of inadvertent and unavoidable stretching of the peroneal nerve as it courses around the fibular neck is an issue of concern in valgus release and lengthening of the lateral side of the knee, because the leg is being lengthened. Peroneal nerve palsy remains a significant worry with a valgus knee and has been seen postoperatively in 3% of patients (26). The peroneal nerve can be injured with either undercorrection or overcorrection of the valgus deformity. Inadequate soft tissue release necessitates forceful manual correction, which will stretch the nerve, while overcorrection creates a "bowstring" effect with possible nerve injury. Direct injury to the nerve is a concern, although with careful use of the "pie crust" technique, the nerve is safely protected (10,12). Ischemic injury to the peroneal nerve can also occur and may be the source of injury in patients with arteriosclerotic disease. To avoid the deleterious affects of peroneal nerve injury, it had been previously suggested that the nerve be exposed, freeing it from the fascial sheath behind the head of the fibula. However, we do not advocate routine exploration of the peroneal nerve.

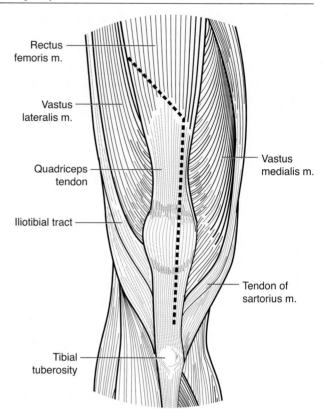

FIGURE 9-18
The quadriceps snip.

The use of CPM machines in the recovery room, which tends to keep the knee in a flexed position, avoids stretching of the peroneal nerve and reduces the incidence of this complication. To avoid excessive stretching of the lateral side in severe deformities, we also suggest consideration of a constrained prosthesis with a tibial polyethylene thickness slightly smaller than the one that will fully elongate the medial structures. The constrained prosthesis provides inherent stability and can be used for primary implantation (14).

Bleeding

Because of the increased amount of soft tissue dissection required to balance these knees, there is a higher risk of postoperative bleeding both intra-articularly and into the calf. We have adopted a technique of injection prior to arthrotomy. Following subcutaneous dissection, 20 mL of lidocaine 1% with epinephrine is injected along the planned arthrotomy line. Before closure, a single reinfusion drain is inserted in most cases, although a second drain may be added if necessary. The tourniquet is released, and bleeders are addressed prior to closure. Postoperatively, thromboprophylaxis includes foot pumps, TED stockings, early mobilization, and Acetylsalicylic acid (ASA) or coumadin.

In cases of significant bleeding, CPM and mobilization are held. A pressure dressing, ice, and elevation are used, and the knee is allowed to rest. Only in very rare cases is a return to surgery required for hematoma evacuation and repeat closure.

REFERENCES

1. Scuderi GR, Insall JN. The posterior stabilized knee prosthesis. *Orthop Clin North Am* 1989;20:71–78.
2. Windsor RE, Scuderi GR, Insall JN, et al. Mechanism of failure of the femoral and tibial components in total knee arthroplasty. *Clin Orthop* 1989;248:15–20.
3. Insall JN. Total knee replacement. In: Insall JN, ed. *Surgery of the Knee.* New York: Churchill Livingstone; 1984:587–696.
4. Cushner FD, La Rosa DF, Vigorita VJ, et al. A quantitative histologic comparison: ACL degeneration in the osteoarthritic knee. *J Arthroplasty* 2003;18:687–692.
5. McGrory JE, Trousdale RT, Pagnano MW, et al. Preoperative hip to ankle radiographs in total knee arthroplasty. *Clin Orthop Relat Res* 2002;(404):196–202.
6. Tenholder M, Clarke HD, Scuderi GR. Minimal-incision total knee arthroplasty: the early clinical experience. *Clin Orthop Relat Res* 2005;440:67–76.

7. Collizza W, Insall JN, Scuderi GR. The posterior stabilized total knee prosthesis: assessment of polyethylene damage and osteolysis. Ten year minimum follow-up. *J Bone Joint Surg* 1995;77A:1713–1720.

8. Baldini A, Scuderi GR, Aglietti P, et al. Flexion-extension gap changes during total knee arthroplasty: effect of posterior cruciate ligament and posterior osteophytes removal. *J Knee Surg* 2004;17:69–72.

9. Scuderi GR, Insall JN. Cement technique in primary total knee arthroplasty. *Techniques Orthop* 1991;6:39–43.

10. Clarke HD, Fuchs R, Scuderi GR, et al. Clinical results in valgus total knee arthroplasty with the "pie crust" technique of lateral soft tissue releases. *J Arthroplasty* 2005;20:1010–1014.

11. Clarke HD, Scuderi GR. Correction of valgus deformity in total knee arthroplasty with the pie-crust technique of lateral soft-tissue releases. *J Knee Surg* 2004;17:157–161.

12. Clarke HD, Schwartz JB, Math KR, et al. Anatomic risk of peroneal nerve injury with the "pie crust" technique for valgus release in total knee arthroplasty. *J Arthroplasty* 2004;19:40–44.

13. Krackow K. Medial and lateral ligament advancement. In: Scuderi GR, Tria AJ Jr, eds. *Surgical Techniques in Total Knee Arthroplasty*. New York: Springer-Verlag; 2002:205–209.

14. Easley ME, Insall JN, Scuderi GR, et al. Primary constrained condylar knee arthroplasty for the arthritic valgus knee. *Clin Orthop* 2000;380:58–64.

15. Griffin FM, Insall JN, Scuderi GR. The posterior condylar angle in osteoarthritic knees. *J Arthroplasty* 1998;13:812–815.

16. Merkow RL, Soudry M, Insall JN. Patella dislocation following total knee replacement. *J Bone Joint Surg* 1985;67A:1321–1327.

17. Keating EM, Ritter MA, Harty LD, et al. Manipulation after total knee arthroplasty. *J Bone Joint Surg Am* 2007;89:282–286.

18. Scuderi GR, Insall JN, Windsor RE, et al. Survivorship of cemented knee replacements. *J Bone Joint Surg* 1989;71B:798–803.

19. Fuchs R, Mills EL, Clarke HD, et al. A third-generation, posterior-stabilized knee prosthesis: early results after follow-up of 2 to 6 years. *J Arthroplasty* 2006;21:821–825.

20. Insall JN, Hood RW, Flawn LB, et al. The total condylar knee prosthesis in gonarthrosis. *J Bone Joint Surg* 1983;65A:619–628.

21. Laskin RS. Soft tissue techniques in total knee replacement. In: Laskin RS, ed. *Total Knee Replacement*. New York: Springer-Verlag, New York; 1991:41–54.

22. Scuderi GR, Insall JN. Total knee arthroplasty. Current clinical perspectives. *Clin Orthop* 1992;276:26–32.

23. Stern SH, Insall JN. Posterior stabilized prosthesis. Results after follow-up of nine to twelve years. *J Bone Joint Surg* 1992;74A:980–986.

24. Vince KG, Insall JN, Kelly MA. The total condylar prosthesis 10 to 12 year results of a cemented knee replacement. *J Bone Joint Surg* 1989;71B:793–797.

25. Tenney SM, Krackow KA, Hungerford DS, et al. Primary total knee arthroplasty in patients with severe varus deformity. *Clin Orthop* 1991;273:19–31.

26. Stern SH, Moeckel BH, Insall JN. Total knee arthroplasty in valgus knees. *Clin Orthop* 1991;273:5–8.

27. Griffin FM, Insall JN, Scuderi GR. Accuracy of soft tissue balancing in total knee arthroplasty. *J Arthroplasty* 2000;15:970–973.

10 Correction of Flexion Contractures in Total Knee Arthroplasty

Adolph V. Lombardi, Keith R. Berend, and Bradley S. Ellison

INDICATIONS

The success of total knee arthroplasty (TKA) has been well established. The clinical success, however, depends on the surgical correction of the deformity, attainment of optimal mechanical alignment, and meticulous soft tissue balancing. Flexion contractures are inherent in the pathophysiology of severe articular degeneration of the knee, either as a consequence of previous traumatic injury, advanced osteoarthritis, or inflammatory arthritis. Commonly, flexion contractures are related to an inability to maintain full knee extension secondary to the presence of painful synovitis, large joint effusion, prominent osteophytes at the posterior aspect of the femoral condyles, posterior adhesive capsulitis, as well as contractures of the posterior capsule, cruciate ligaments, and hamstrings (1). Fixed flexion contractures affect the gait cycle at initial contact, midstance, and the terminal stance phases. To compensate for the flexed posture of the knee during gait, this disorder necessitates recruitment of the quadriceps, leading to additional energy expenditure (2,3). The pathologic gait pattern associated with a knee flexion contracture results in inefficient locomotion, accelerated fatigue, and compromises the clinical outcome of TKA.

To ensure optimal postoperative range of motion (ROM) and functional outcome, we believe that full correction of any flexion contracture should be performed at the time of surgical intervention. The specific approach depends on the degree of flexion contracture present, which is classified according to severity. A mild contracture is considered to be 15 degrees or less and is classified as grade I (Fig. 10-1). A moderate contracture is considered to be between 15 and 30 degrees and is classified as grade II. A severe contracture is considered to be greater than 30 degrees and is classified as grade III. Each grade requires a slightly different surgical approach, and accurately assessing the degree of flexion contracture will guide the surgeon as the contracture is addressed with a combination of soft tissue releases and bony resection.

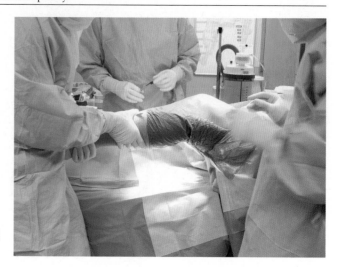

FIGURE 10-1

Grade I flexion deformity represents mild flexion contracture of 15 degrees or less and is the most commonly encountered type in primary total knee arthroplasty. Note the posterior adhesive capsulitis and posterior osteophytes.

CONTRAINDICATIONS

Although the surgical management of fixed flexion contracture in TKA is technically challenging and associated with a higher rate of complications, the technique can be performed reliably and is successful in providing improved postoperative function, ROM, and pain relief. One of the potential complications in correcting severe flexion contractures, especially in the setting of an associated valgus deformity, is peroneal nerve palsy. Fixed flexion contracture, however, regardless of severity, is not a contraindication to TKA, insofar as the patient meets all other criteria for surgery and does not have another identifiable contraindication for the operation.

PREOPERATIVE PREPARATION

Once the patient is determined to be a suitable candidate for TKA, a detailed assessment of coronal and sagittal deformity, flexion contracture, extensor lag, and preoperative ROM should be obtained. Accurate measurement of these patient-specific variables allows the surgeon to enter into an individualized discussion with each patient regarding surgical technique, clinical expectations, and associated risks and complications. When present, a flexion contracture can be classified according to severity as measured during clinical examination using a goniometer. A grade I contracture is considered mild and 15 degrees or less. A grade II contracture is considered moderate and between 15 and 30 degrees. A grade III contracture is considered severe and is greater than 30 degrees. With each increasing grade, there is a concomitant increase in the complexity of deformity.

Once the flexion contracture has been appropriately classified, the next step is to identify the structures contributing to the deformity, as determined by clinical examination and standard preoperative radiographic studies. Typically, standard radiographic views will reveal abnormalities in the bony anatomy, including prominent posterior osteophytes, condylar deficiency, and significant coronal or sagittal malalignment. Attention should be directed toward the bony deficiency of the posterior condyles that may affect rotation of the femoral component when using a measured resection technique or posterior referencing system. Occasionally, large bone deficits may require the use of augmentation with allograft or modular inserts. Additionally, various soft tissue structures commonly contribute to a flexion contracture, including an adherent or taut posterior capsule, as well as a contracted posterior cruciate ligament (PCL), collateral ligaments, and/or hamstrings. The authors believe that full correction of flexion contractures should be attempted at the time of surgical intervention and further suggest that the best chance of correction may only be obtained at the time of surgery. All components of the deformity must be addressed intraoperatively, and each grade of flexion contracture requires a slightly different surgical approach to soft tissue release, bony resection, and degree of prosthetic constraint.

As the severity of the flexion contracture increases, a corresponding amount of bony resection and soft tissue releases will be needed. To compensate for bone deficits and attenuated soft tissue structures, the surgeon may employ various options in prosthetic constraint for the chosen implant design. Thus, it is expected that with increased severity of flexion contracture, an increased level of constraint in prosthetic design will be needed. Depending on the grade of flexion contracture, the authors have developed an algorithm based on pathologic criteria to assist in the decision to implant a posterior cruciate-retaining (PCR), posterior stabilized (PS), posterior stabilized constrained (PSC), or linked hinge component. Based on the preoperative evaluation, measures should be taken to ensure the necessary implants and accessories are available at the time of surgery.

TECHNIQUE

Management of Flexion Contractures—An Algorithmic Approach

Once the decision to move forward with surgery has been made, and all the necessary preoperative plans have been developed and surgical implants and materials assembled, the patient will be escorted to the operative suite. A pneumatic tourniquet is applied to the proximal thigh and will be activated prior to incision. Following the use of regional anesthesia supplemented with mild sedation, the operative leg is prepared and draped in standard fashion. An anterior longitudinal midline skin incision is used beginning 4 to 6 cm proximal to the suprapatellar pole and extended distally to the medial border of the tibial tubercle. A medial parapatellar arthrotomy is performed allowing sufficient exposure of the medial and lateral condyles while everting the patella. Once adequate visualization is obtained, elementary correction of the coronal deformity with appropriate osteophyte removal and soft tissue release is performed.

The key to successful management of flexion contracture is addressing the contracture by a combination of soft tissue releases and bony resection to restore coronal and sagittal stability. Every effort should be undertaken to completely correct the flexion deformity during the operation while maintaining adequate stability and motion through meticulous soft tissue balancing. There are several different approaches to soft tissue balancing in TKA. The first approach is referred to as the classic Insall technique (1,4–6) and involves creating a balanced flexion gap by resecting the posterior condyles about a rotational axis that changes based on soft tissue balance. The corresponding extension gap is matched to the flexion gap via tensioning devices or spacer blocks. The second approach to soft tissue balancing is referred to as the measured resection technique (7,8) and involves replacing the exact thickness of resected bone from the distal femur and proximal tibia with a prosthetic implant of matched thickness. Assuming correct alignment of the resections, the knee is then balanced by ligamentous release. A third approach is a hybrid technique, which balances the knee with ligamentous releases first, and then the surgeon performs measured resections of the distal femur and proximal tibia. The flexion gap is then balanced with a tensioner device to establish femoral rotation (1).

Regardless which technique is used as the method of soft tissue balancing, the posterior recess of the knee should be the focus of attention. The posterior capsule should be released in all cases of flexion contracture and possibly in all primary TKAs, as this maneuver positively enhances final postoperative ROM (9). If the tightened capsule is not released and posterior osteophytes are not removed, then an erroneous distal femoral resection will be performed in an effort to obtain full extension and balanced flexion/extension gaps. An error of this kind can result in elevation of the joint line and midflexion instability, negatively affecting the function of an intact PCL and further altering patellofemoral kinematics.

Newer prosthetic designs allow for increased flexion, which is obtained by increasing the distance that the tibial insert travels behind the femur before impinging on the posterior femur. These designs often require an increased posterior condyle resection, which should facilitate debridement of the posterior aspect of the knee, indirectly increasing correction of the fixed flexion deformity. Additionally, the posterior condyles of the femoral prosthesis do not edge load at higher angles. The propensity for a PS design to dislocate at higher flexion angles is reduced by these prosthetic design modifications. It may be possible to conceive that "high-flexion" prosthetic designs may allow for improved motion and facilitate the correction of fixed flexion contractures. Even when using a "high-flexion" prosthesis, meticulous soft tissue balancing and bony resection must still be performed (10). More importantly, if these designs are to be successful in allowing increased ROM, the posterior recess must be devoid of osteophytes, and the posterior capsule should be subperiosteally released from the femur.

Grade I Flexion Contracture

For contractures of 15 degrees or less, the decision between the implantation of either a PCR or PS device depends on the correctability of the deformity, surgeon preference, and competency of the PCL. Using the principles of measured resection, the distal femur and proximal tibia are cut with the

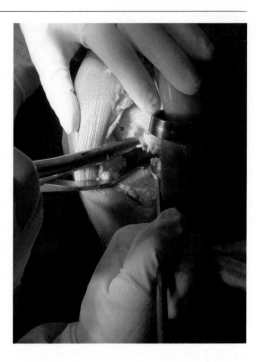

FIGURE 10-2

Appropriate bony resections, meticulous removal of osteophytes, and re-establishment of the posterior recess will correct the majority of grade I flexion contractures. With the knee in flexion, a rongeur and curette are used to remove posterior osteophytes.

goal of obtaining appropriate alignment in the coronal and sagittal planes. The rotational alignment for the femur and tibia is determined by using the appropriate landmarks. For femoral landmarks, the anteroposterior axis, epicondylar axis, and posterior condylar axis are used. For tibial landmarks, the insertions of the PCL and patella tendon are used, along with a trial ROM.

Removal of overhanging bone at the posterior femoral condyle and osteophytes at the posterior femoral condyle is mandatory to obtain full correction of flexion contracture (Fig. 10-2). An intramedullary rod may be used to elevate the femur and tense the posterior capsule while a Cobb elevator or dull curved 0.5-inch osteotome is used to establish a posterior recess. Alternatively, a specialized laminar spreader may be utilized to separate the condyles from the tibia and tense the posterior capsule, thereby facilitating a thorough debridement of the posterior capsule (Fig. 10-3). A trial reduction with PCR implants is performed to identify perceivable tension imbalances in the medial collateral ligament, lateral collateral ligament, and PCL, as well as symmetry of the flexion and extension gaps. If the extension gap is less than the flexion gap, further release of the

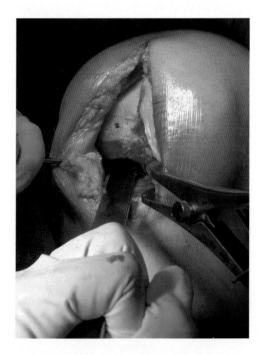

FIGURE 10-3

A specialized laminar spreader may be used to separate the condyles from the tibia and tense the posterior capsule, thereby facilitating a thorough debridement of the posterior capsule. The spreader is placed on the medial side to facilitate debridement of the lateral side, and it is then switched to the lateral side to facilitate debridement of the medial side. The posterior adhesive capsulitis is addressed by subperiosteal stripping of the posterior capsule with a curved osteotome, thereby re-establishing the posterior recess of the knee.

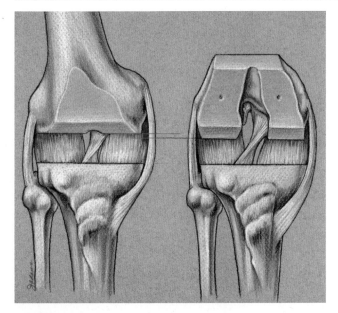

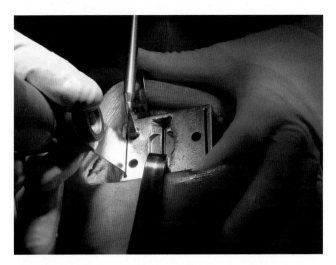

FIGURE 10-4

On occasion, despite meticulous attention to the removal of posterior osteophytes and release of the posterior capsule, the extension gap will remain smaller than the flexion gap. (Reprinted with permission from Joint Implant Surgeons, Inc.)

FIGURE 10-5

An additional 2 mm of bone can be removed from the distal femur without alteration of the kinematic function of the posterior cruciate ligament.

posterior capsule must be performed. This step can be combined with resection of an additional 2 mm of the distal femoral condyles, which represents the maximum amount of joint elevation tolerated by the PCL (Figs. 10-4 and 10-5). Trial reduction with PCR implants is performed again. If the extension gap exceeds the flexion gap secondary to a tight PCL, the tibial trial may lift off anteriorly, the femoral component may not roll back appropriately, or the femur may be forced forward on the tibial trial. If this situation exists, the posterior slope of the tibia should be evaluated to ensure it is approximately 5 to 8 degrees. A slight increase in the posterior slope can balance flexion-extension gaps with equal tension in the PCL and collateral ligaments (Fig. 10-6).

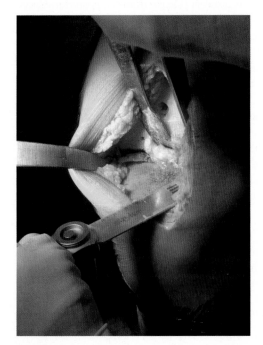

FIGURE 10-6

With preservation of the posterior cruciate ligament, the tibia should be sloped posteriorly 5 to 8 degrees. If tibial resection has not been carried out with a posterior slope of 5 to 8 degrees, adjustment of the slope may assist in balancing the flexion/extension gap.

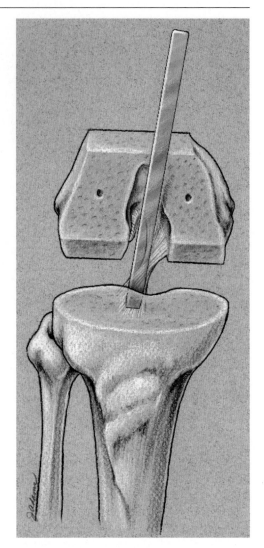

FIGURE 10-7

The posterior cruciate ligament (PCL) attaches to an area 2 cm in length, distal to the tibial articular surface. Approximately 8 to 10 mm of tibial bone have been removed, leaving approximately 1 cm of PCL insertion. In the presence of a tight PCL, an osteotome can be used to perform a partial release of the PCL from the posterior aspect of the tibia. (Reprinted with permission from Joint Implant Surgeons, Inc.)

If tension in the PCL seems excessive, a partial recession of the ligament can be performed. Three methods of PCL release have been described. The first is a direct release from the posterior aspect of the proximal tibia (Fig. 10-7). The PCL insertion spans 2 cm distal to the joint line. Because 1 cm of proximal tibia has been resected, approximately 1 cm of attachment remains, which can be carefully recessed. A second method of PCL release is a "V"-shaped osteotomy of the posterior tibia at the PCL insertion, which leaves an intact periosteal sleeve that slides and establishes an appropriate balance (Fig. 10-8). A third release is a partial release of the posterior fibers at the origin off the medial femoral condyle (Fig. 10-9).

After completion of a PCL release, the PCR implants should be trialed again. If there is balance between the flexion-extension gaps, the prosthesis is ready for implantation. If the PCL is excessively taut or has been rendered incompetent, the authors recommend resection of the PCL and conversion to a PS device. If full extension is not possible and the extension gap is less than the flexion gap, then 2 mm of additional femur should be resected to equalize the flexion-extension gaps. At this point, a PS prosthesis would be appropriate for implantation.

Grade II Flexion Contracture

In most cases, the key distinction between treating grade I and grade II flexion contractures commonly involves leaving or removing the PCL, respectively. The decision to implant a CR or PS design when addressing grade II flexion contractures may be a function of surgeon preference, however, as recent studies have suggested that satisfactory results can be reliably achieved with CR designs when correcting flexion contractures greater than 20 degrees (11,12). In these reports, the flexion contracture was corrected by addressing associated varus or valgus contractures with soft tissue releases from the

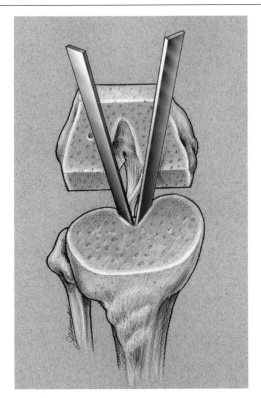

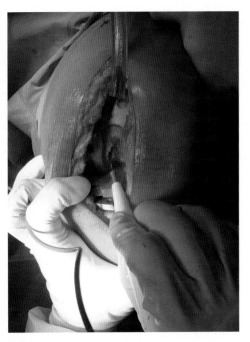

FIGURE 10-8

Release of the posterior cruciate ligament can be accomplished by performing a "V"-shaped osteotomy of the posterior tibia and allowing the posterior cruciate ligament to slide on a periosteal sleeve. (Reprinted with permission from Joint Implant Surgeons, Inc.)

FIGURE 10-9

Tension in the posterior cruciate ligament results in excessive rollback of the femur with respect to the tibia. Partial release of the insertional fibers of the posterior cruciate ligament on the medial femoral condyle is performed with electrocautery.

contracted side of the deformity. Arguably, the decision to implant a CR or PS design will need to be weighed on a patient-dependent basis, as correction of a grade II flexion contracture may result in compromise of the PCL or collateral soft tissue structures, therein requiring a PS design.

The proximal tibia is resected perpendicular to the long axis and removes 8 to 10 mm of bone, as referenced off the more intact tibial plateau to restore the joint line. The distal femoral resection is performed, removing 2 mm thicker than the design to be implanted. Next, the anterior, posterior, chamfer, and intercondylar resections are performed. Overhanging posterior femoral condyle osteophytes and the remaining portion of the PCL are debrided from the posterior recesses of the knee. A curved osteotome is used to establish the posterior recess by releasing the posterior capsule off the posterior aspect of the distal femur. A trial reduction is performed, and the flexion-extension gaps are evaluated. If any residual flexion contracture persists, the authors recommend further release of the posterior capsule, followed by trial reduction. In some cases, 2 mm of additional distal femur may need to be resected to obtain full extension. Once balance in the flexion-extension gaps has been achieved, a PS prosthesis is prepared for implantation.

Grade III Flexion Contracture

Grade III flexion contractures are 30 degrees or more and are typically observed in patients with severe inflammatory arthritis or chronic neuromuscular disorders. In general, such patients are non-ambulatory with advanced arthrosis and substantial contractures of the surrounding soft tissues, making the task of balancing the flexion-extension gaps extremely difficult, if not impossible. Therefore, a varus/valgus constrained or rotating hinge prosthesis should be considered if instability results from correcting the flexion contracture.

The key to obtaining full extension is generous release of the posterior capsule combined with aggressive resection of the distal femur. With severe flexion contractures, the medial and lateral soft

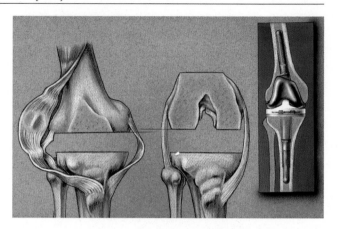

FIGURE 10-10

Grade III contractures are treated with extensive, meticulous removal of posterior osteophytes and release of the posterior capsule. Additionally, a generous amount of distal femoral resection is required, resulting in a relative laxity of all structures anterior to the midcoronal plane. This is best treated with utilization of a varus/valgus constrained implant. (Reprinted with permission from Joint Implant Surgeons, Inc.)

tissue structures will also be substantially contracted, as often a significant varus or valgus contracture will also be present. Thus, the appropriate soft tissue release from the contracted side of the coronal deformity should be performed initially. Next, the tibial resection is performed with the authors recommending a proximal tibial resection 2 mm from the more deficient tibial plateau, unless the bony deficiency is exorbitant. If the deficiency is excessive, the resection should be minimized to approximately 10 mm from the more intact tibial plateau. A preliminary resection of the distal femur is 2 mm greater than the thickness of the femoral component. Anterior, posterior, chamfer, and intercondylar resections are made based on appropriate femoral sizing and rotation. Generous reestablishment of the posterior recess of the knee is performed by elevating the posterior capsule. If necessary, a release of the gastrocnemius can be performed with a recession extending 5 to 6 cm proximal to the joint line at the posterior aspect of the femur. The flexion gap is then measured. Next, the extension gap is equalized to the flexion gap by resecting the distal femur. Trial reduction with a PS design and implantation of the prosthesis is performed.

The degree of ligamentous instability and inequality of the flexion-extension gaps dictate the level of constraint required. A posterior-stabilized varus/valgus constrained condylar design (PSC) should be used if instability persists with a PS design or if midflexion instability results in dysfunction dislocation of the extensor mechanism (Fig. 10-10). If there is a gross disparity between flexion-extension gaps or if substantial ligamentous instability persists, a rotating hinge design should be considered. In these severe cases, a redundancy of the extensor mechanism may be present and is best treated by distal and lateral advancement of the vastus medialis obliquus (Fig. 10-11).

Operative Algorithm for Correction of Grade I, II, and III Flexion Contractures

Step 1: Medial exposure, osteophyte removal, and posterior capsule release (Fig. 10-12).

Step 2: Distal femoral resection using the measured resection technique and additional distal femoral resection of 2 mm. CR trial with complete ligament balancing.

Step 3: If full correction of flexion contracture is not accomplished, the PCL is released, and a PS is trialed.

Step 4: If contracture persists, additional distal femoral resection of 2 mm is performed, and a PS is trialed.

Step 5: If contracture persists, additional soft tissue releases from the contracted side of the coronal deformity are performed until full extension is achieved. If this step results in ligamentous instability, a PSC device is used.

Step 6: If instability persists after achieving full extension, the surgeon uses a rotating hinge design.

PEARLS AND PITFALLS

- Preoperative evaluation should include careful measurement and classification of the flexion contracture as either grade I, II, or III.
- The grade of flexion contracture has a direct impact on the level of constraint necessary for the prosthesis to maintain optimal ROM and stability.
- Removal of the overhanging posterior femoral condyle and posterior femoral osteophytes is critical.

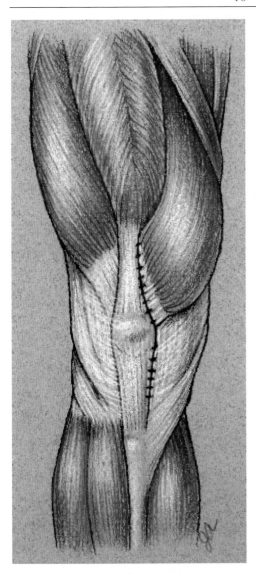

FIGURE 10-11

In combination with the use of a constrained device to treat ligamentous laxity, distal and lateral advancement of the extensor mechanism may enhance stability. (Reprinted with permission from Joint Implant Surgeons, Inc.)

- Careful establishment of the posterior recess should be performed before the distal femur is resected.
- If a PCR design is selected, no more than 2 mm should be resected from the distal femur to avoid compromise of PCL function. If more than 2 mm of distal femur is resected, a PS design should be considered.
- Grade II flexion contractures should be treated with a PS prosthesis design.
- Grade III flexion contractures warrant consideration of a constrained or rotating hinge prosthesis.
- Postoperative rehabilitation programs should emphasize extension exercises with consideration of extension night splinting for 6 weeks.

Postoperative Management

Routine postoperative rehabilitation may be used for patients with grade I flexion contractures. A splint or knee immobilizer may be worn at night in patients who lack extension at the time of discharge. Additionally, in obese patients, a night splint should be considered, as these patients tend to lie with the limb externally rotated at the hip and flexed at the knee. The authors do not routinely use continuous passive motion machines, as these devices give a false impression of full extension. Instead, early active quadriceps strengthening is encouraged with isotonic contraction exercises.

For patients with more severe preoperative flexion deformities (grade I and II), various modifications to the routine postoperative rehabilitation program are advised. Typically, these patients have a problem in obtaining and maintaining full extension, despite achieving this during surgery. The postoperative rehabilitation program must aggressively encourage full extension of the knee. Participation

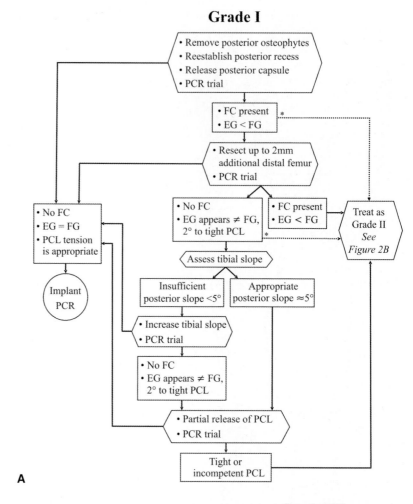

Grade I

- Remove posterior osteophytes
- Reestablish posterior recess
- Release posterior capsule
- PCR trial

- FC present
- EG < FG

- Resect up to 2mm additional distal femur
- PCR trial

- No FC
- EG = FG
- PCL tension is appropriate

Implant PCR

- No FC
- EG appears ≠ FG, 2° to tight PCL

- FC present
- EG < FG

Treat as Grade II *See Figure 2B*

Assess tibial slope

Insufficient posterior slope <5°

Appropriate posterior slope ≈5°

- Increase tibial slope
- PCR trial

- No FC
- EG appears ≠ FG, 2° to tight PCL

- Partial release of PCL
- PCR trial

Tight or incompetent PCL

A

FIGURE 10-12

Algorithms for treating **(A)** grade I, **(B)** grade II, and **(C)** grade III flexion contractures. EG, extension gap; FC, flexion contracture; FG, flexion gap; PCL, posterior cruciate ligament; PCR, posterior cruciate retaining.
(**A** reprinted with permission from Lombard AV Jr, Berend KR. Soft tissue balancing of the knee—Flexion contractures. *Techniques in Knee Surgery* 2005;4:193–206; **B,C** reprinted with permission from Lombardi AV Jr. Soft tissue balancing of the knee—Flexion. In: Callaghan JJ, Rosenberg AG, Rubash HE, et al, eds. *The Adult Knee*. Philadelphia: Lippincott Williams & Wilkins; 2003:1223–1232.)

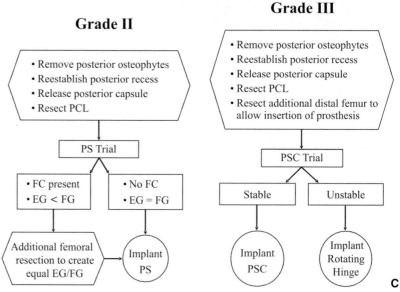

Grade II

- Remove posterior osteophytes
- Reestablish posterior recess
- Release posterior capsule
- Resect PCL

PS Trial

- FC present
- EG < FG

- No FC
- EG = FG

Additional femoral resection to create equal EG/FG

Implant PS

B

Grade III

- Remove posterior osteophytes
- Reestablish posterior recess
- Release posterior capsule
- Resect PCL
- Resect additional distal femur to allow insertion of prosthesis

PSC Trial

Stable

Unstable

Implant PSC

Implant Rotating Hinge

C

in three to four sessions of stretching is recommended on a daily basis. This is important to emphasize with the patient and family, as many of these patients were accustomed to maintaining the knee in a flexed position. Additionally, these patients should be discouraged from placing pillows behind the knee or sitting in recliner-type chairs that maintain the knee in a flexed posture. Frequently, these patients sleep in a fetal position with their knees flexed, thus night splints may be used for at least the first 6 weeks postoperatively.

During the postoperative period, the flexion deformity should be followed closely so that a plateau in motion or a recurrence in deformity can be recognized early. Patients should be examined at 6 weeks, 3 months, and 1 year if progression is acceptable. More frequent postoperative evaluation may be needed if the patient is slow to progress or experiences a restriction in ROM. In these cases, manipulation under anesthesia may be necessary. During manipulation, flexion is more easily gained than extension, and caution is needed, as fracture of the distal femur may occur if excessive force is applied.

COMPLICATIONS

Recurrent Flexion Contracture

In the majority of cases, if the flexion contracture is corrected completely intraoperatively, there will be no recurrence for up to 1 year after surgery. However, 15% of grade I and II flexion contractures may recur by 1 year (12). For grade III contractures, 25% to 30% of patients may develop residual grade I flexion contractures despite complete correction at the time of surgery.

Loss of ROM

The authors advocate complete correction of flexion deformity at the time of surgery. However, the main determinant of postoperative ROM is preoperative ROM (9,13–15). Additionally, patients with grade II/III flexion contractures have adapted to these deformities, and although complete correction is obtained intraoperatively, results may deteriorate in the postoperative period. Bad habits including placing pillows behind the knee, and recliner chairs should be avoided. Aggressive physical therapy aimed at obtaining and maintaining full extension with supplementation of extension splinting at night should be instituted as standard postoperative protocol.

Flexion-Extension Imbalance

Persistent inequality may exist in the flexion-extension gap despite performing the steps outlined in this chapter. This scenario demands increased prosthetic constraint, and a varus-valgus–constrained or rotating-hinge prosthesis should be considered.

Peroneal Nerve Injury

Commonly, flexion contractures are observed in combination with a concomitant valgus deformity. The peroneal nerve is at increased risk when the valgus-flexion deformity is corrected with an effective relative lengthening of the lower extremity. Additionally, the medial collateral ligament may be attenuated and necessitate the use of a constrained prosthetic design to compensate for coronal instability. In the acute postoperative setting, a continuous passive motion device may be used to keep the knee in a flexed posture to avoid stretching of the peroneal nerve and minimize the incidence of nerve injury.

RESULTS

In this chapter, we have outlined an algorithm that allows full intraoperative correction of flexion contractures during TKA. The key to successful management of flexion contracture is first characterizing the severity of the deformity, which subsequently directs the specific approach necessary for correction and combining the use of soft tissue releases, bony resection, and prosthetic constraint. In our practice, we observed 732 TKAs over a 3-year period with patients stratified according to the severity of flexion contracture (16). For 627 knees with grade I flexion contracture, 539 knees (86%) maintained full extension, and 88 knees (14%) had a residual flexion contracture of less than 15 degrees. None of the grade I flexion contractures worsened. For 52 knees with grade II flexion contractures, full extension was maintained in 42 knees (81%). The remaining 10 knees (19%)

maintained significant improvement but still had residual contractures of less than 10 degrees. In a recent report, we applied our stepwise algorithm to 52 knees with severe preoperative flexion contractures greater than 20 degrees (grade II and III). At final examination, 33 knees (67%) maintained full extension, and 13 knees (27%) had a residual contracture less than 10 degrees. A CR device was used in 31 knees (60%), and a PS device was used in 14 knees (27%). A PSC device was used in five knees (10%), but only two knees (4%) required implantation of a rotating hinge.

As the technique of TKA has continued to evolve, the understanding of the pathology responsible for flexion contracture has also improved. In an early study, Laskin et al observed overall less favorable results in treating flexion contractures with CR designs with an average residual flexion contracture of 11 degrees for PCR designs in knees with severe flexion contractures (17). From these early results, many experts concluded the PCL needed to be resected to successfully treat flexion contractures. We have recently shown, however, that a clinically successful result can be obtained in 97% of knees treated with a CR design when the deformity is corrected intraoperatively without creating sagittal or coronal instability (16). Posterior-stabilized designs were warranted if the deformity was not eliminated after the initial steps of correction with successful results obtained in 93% of PS TKA.

Other investigators advocate similar steps in addressing flexion contractures during TKA. Bellemans et al reviewed 924 knees with flexion mild to severe contractures (11). These authors concluded that 98.6% of cases could be satisfactorily corrected with resection of all osteophytes, overresection of the distal femur by 2 mm, adequate medial-lateral soft tissue balancing, and establishing the posterior capsular recess. Clearly, flexion contractures often coexist with concomitant contractures of the medial or lateral structures. Definitive correlations exist between the severity of flexion contracture and the degree of coexistent varus or valgus deformity. In reviewing, 552 knees with flexion contractures that underwent TKA, Whiteside and Mihalko were able to obtain complete correction through adequate bony resection and medial-lateral soft tissue balancing (18). In 98% of their cases, correction of the coronal deformity was associated with correction of the flexion contracture, therein averting the need for resection of the PCL and additional resection of the distal femur (18,19).

REFERENCES

1. Freeman MAR. *Arthritis of the Knee: Clinical Features and Surgical Management.* Berlin: Springer-Verlag; 1980:31–56.
2. Perry J. Pathologic Gait. *Instr Course Lect* 1990;39:325–331.
3. Tew M, Forster IW. Effect of knee replacement on flexion deformity. *J Bone Joint Surg Br* 1987; 69-B:395–399.
4. Insall JN. Technique of total knee replacement. *Instr Course Lect* 1981;30:324–341.
5. Insall JN. Choices and compromises in total knee arthroplasty. *Clin Orthop Relat Res* 1988;226:43–48.
6. Insall JN, Easley ME. Surgical techniques and instrumentation in total knee arthroplasty. In: Insall JN, Scott WN, eds. *Surgery of the Knee*, 3rd ed. Philadelphia: Churchill Livingstone; 2001:1553–1620.
7. Hungerford DS, Krackow KA. Total joint arthroplasty of the knee. *Clin Orthop Relat Res* 1985;192: 23–33.
8. Martin JW, Whiteside LA. The influence of joint line position on knee stability after condylar knee arthroplasty. *Clin Orthop Relat Res* 1990;259:146–156.
9. Ritter MA, Harty LD, Davis KE, et al. Predicting range of motion after total knee arthroplasty. *J Bone Joint Surg Am* 2003;85-A:1278–1285.
10. Li G, Most E, Sultan PG, et al. Knee kinematics with a high-flexion posterior stabilized total knee prosthesis: an in vitro robotic experimental investigation. *J Bone Joint Surg Am* 2004;86-A:1721–1729.
11. Bellemans J, Vandenneuker H, Victor J, et al. Flexion contracture in total knee arthroplasty. *Clin Orthop Relat Res* 2006;452:78–82.
12. Berend KR, Lombardi AV, Adams JB. Total knee arthroplasty in patients with greater than 20 degree flexion contracture. *Clin Orthop Relat Res* 2006;452:83–87.
13. Harvey IA, Barry K, Kirby SPJ, et al. Factors affecting range of movement of total knee arthroplasty. *J Bone Joint Surg Br* 1993;75-B:950–955.
14. Lizaur A, Marco L, Cebrian R. Preoperative factors influencing the range of movement after total knee arthroplasty for severe osteoarthritis. *J Bone Joint Surg Br* 1997;79-B:626–629.
15. Ritter MA, Stringer EA. Predictive range of motion after total knee replacement. *Clin Orthop Relat Res* 1979;143:115–119.
16. Lombardi AV, Berend KR. Soft tissue balancing of the knee—flexion contractures. *Tech Knee Surg* 2005; 4:193–206.
17. Laskin RS, Rieger M, Schob C, et al. The posterior-stabilized total knee prosthesis in the knee with severe fixed deformity. *Am J Knee Surg* 1988;1:199–203.
18. Whiteside LA, Mihalko WM. Surgical procedure for flexion contracture and recurvatum in total knee arthroplasty. *Clin Orthop Relat Res* 2002;404:189–195.
19. Mihalko WM, Whiteside LA. Bone resection and ligament treatment for flexion contracture in knee arthroplasty. *Clin Orthop Relat Res* 2003;406:141–147.

11 Genu Recurvatum in Total Knee Arthroplasty

Trevor R. Pickering, John B. Meding, and E. Michael Keating

INDICATIONS

A recurvatum deformity in patients prior to total knee arthroplasty (TKA) is relatively rare and has received little attention in the literature (1–6). Hyperextension deformities greater than 5 degrees occur in only 0.5% to 1% of TKA candidates (2,5). Because satisfactory postoperative function may be difficult in patients with neuromuscular disorders, the primary goal when determining the appropriateness of TKA in a patient with genu recurvatum is to identify the etiology of the patient's deformity. If the etiology does not affect the patient's quadriceps function, the surgeon can proceed with performing TKA. A contracture of the iliotibial (IT) band can result in recurvatum in knees with a fixed valgus deformity (Fig. 11-1) (6). The IT band is anterior to the axis of rotation of the knee when the knee is in extension. In the absence of a knee flexion contracture, an IT band contracture can cause hyperextension. At the time of surgery, erosions will be found on the antero-lateral aspect of the tibial plateau (Fig. 11-2). Patients with rheumatoid arthritis can present with significant ligamentous laxity about the knee, which, in turn, can lead to a hyperextension deformity as well (7). Finally, anterior sloping of the tibial plateau, which may be found secondary to trauma or in patients who have undergone a high tibial osteotomy, can predispose to genu recurvatum. In such cases, there is no neuromuscular compromise, and TKA is indicated in the setting of degenerative disease of the knee.

CONTRAINDICATIONS

Recurvatum in individuals with a neuromuscular disorder, as may be seen with poliomyelitis, for example, is common. The outcome of TKA in these patients is generally poor secondary to bone deformity and quadriceps degeneration or paralysis (4,8). In these patients, TKA is generally contraindicated because of the high rate of recurring hyperextension and knee instability after surgery (8).

PREOPERATIVE PREPARATION

Preoperative full-length standing anteroposterior and lateral non–weight-bearing radiographs should be obtained. This provides a preliminary evaluation of coronal and sagittal plane deformities as well as evaluation of the knee's joint space. A measurement of the recurvatum deformity in the clinic using a goniometer with the patient in a supine position will further characterize its severity. Most importantly, any patient with genu recurvatum who presents for TKA evaluation must undergo a complete assessment of quadriceps, hamstring, and gastrocnemius complex strength and function. Paralysis or significant weakness of the quadriceps may lead a patient to lock the knee in

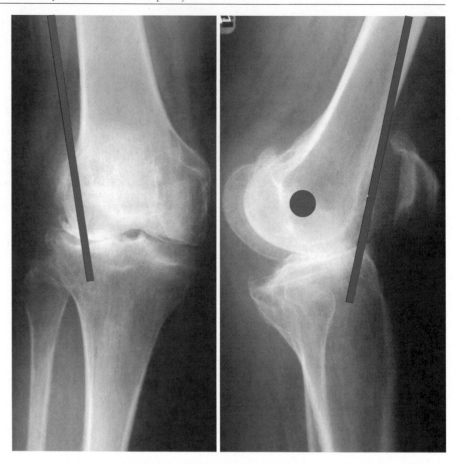

FIGURE 11-1

Anteroposterior and lateral radiographs of a knee with valgus deformity. Note that the iliotibial band (*solid line*) lies anterior to the center of rotation (*solid circle*) in the hyperextended knee.

hyperextension to ambulate. If such locking is inhibited with a knee replacement, these individuals can lose the ability to ambulate completely. Also important is the functional position of the foot and ankle. A plantar flexion contracture of the ankle and weak dorsiflexors will predispose the knee to hyperextension, especially at heel strike and should be corrected before surgery (Fig. 11-3).

The degree of constraint must be carefully considered when selecting an implant to use in patients with a neuromuscular disorder undergoing a TKA. Varying degrees of constraint have been suggested to prevent the high rate of recurrent paralytic recurvatum observed in this population (3,7). Even arthrodesis has been advocated in the most severe cases. However, in any patient who needs to hyperextend the knee to ambulate, all constrained prostheses will undergo significant stresses, which can lead to pain, loosening, and wear. If conservative treatment is unsuccessful, and if the high risk of failure is unacceptable to the patient or surgeon, a knee fusion must be considered.

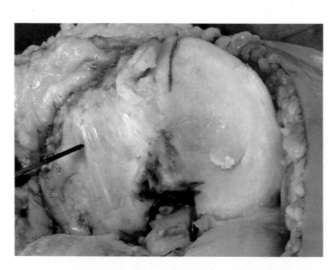

FIGURE 11-2

Erosion of the antero-lateral aspect of the tibial plateau is common in the knee with recurvatum (electrocautery tip).

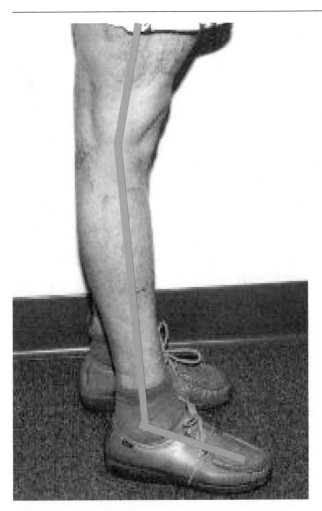

FIGURE 11-3

Plantar flexion deformity in a patient with genu recurvatum is associated with recurrence of hyperextension postoperatively and is a contraindication to TKA.

In patients without a neuromuscular etiology for their recurvatum, constrained implants are not indicated unless significant ligamentous laxity would otherwise dictate the use of such implants. Prostheses should be chosen as they normally would, based on any residual knee instability that is not corrected with ligament balancing at the time of surgery.

TECHNIQUE

Numerous techniques have been proposed to correct recurvatum during TKA. Cutting less distal femur and proximal tibia can tighten the extension gap, as can using thicker components (2,3). Other methods include plication of the posterior capsule (1), using thicker femoral and tibial components (3), and transferring the collateral ligaments proximally and posteriorly (2), which tightens the collateral ligament as the knee goes into extension. These techniques depend on intact collateral ligaments to achieve stability and prevent recurrence of knee hyperextension. In the absence of a satisfactory soft tissue envelope, constrained implants have been suggested. In patients with nonneuromuscular etiologies for their recurvatum, however, such measures are typically not needed (5).

A standard medial parapatellar incision can be used to approach the knee. We prefer to use a posterior cruciate ligament-retaining prosthesis if the ligament is intact and competent. Standard bone cuts are made on the femur, and tibia and ligament balancing and posterior cruciate ligament recession are undertaken as needed. The surgeon takes care to avoid instability in the coronal plane after the prosthesis is implanted. In addition, it is important to select a femoral component that has a progressively increasing radius of curvature from posterior to anterior to limit the ability to hyperextend a well-balanced knee without hindering flexion (Fig. 11-4A–G). If such a component is not available, less distal femur can be cut to achieve similar results. Thus, the surgeon must know what components will be available before surgery so that appropriate planning of bone cuts can be undertaken.

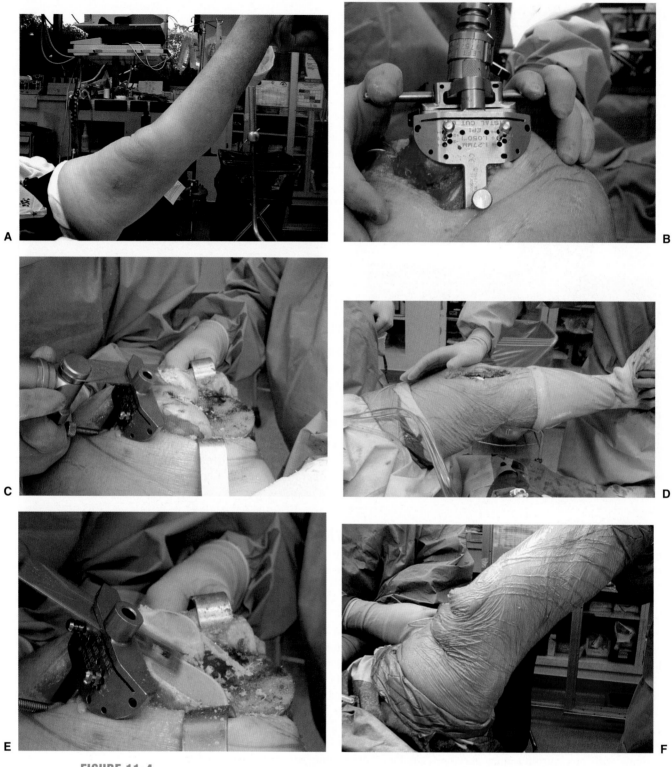

FIGURE 11-4

(A) Preoperative knee with a 10-degree hyperextension deformity. **(B)** A distal femoral resection jig that allows multiple-depth cuts is useful. **(C)** A minimal distal femoral resection was tried initially. **(D)** The minimal distal femoral cut did not allow full extension, which is unsatisfactory in patients with a nonneuromuscular etiology for their recurvatum. **(E)** The distal femur was re-cut using the standard cutting depth. **(F)** Postoperatively, the extension was normal. Standard prostheses and bone cuts are used without the need to plicate the posterior capsule or increase the size of the polyethylene. Ligament balancing must be meticulous. *(continued)*

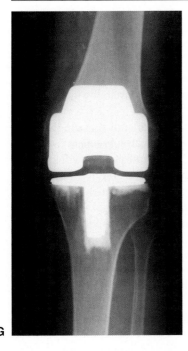

G

FIGURE 11-4 *(Continued)*

(G) Postoperative radiograph at 5 years shows good position of the nonconstrained, cruciate-retaining prosthesis. Standard bone cuts were used in conjunction with meticulous soft tissue balancing. The patient has had no recurrence of recurvatum.

Recurvatum deformity is commonly associated with a fixed valgus deformity, which necessitates a sequential release of the lateral capsular complex to straighten and balance the knee. This treatment includes the progressive release of the IT band, the lateral capsule, and the arcuate complex, with or without the popliteal tendon, as needed to achieve balance. Release should be performed in a controlled, stepwise manner, beginning with "pie crusting" or a controlled shallow incision through the meniscal remnant and progressing to additional lateral structures at the level of the joint line as needed. Extension and flexion gaps should be checked frequently after each step of release to assess the knee's balance and overall integrity of the soft tissue envelope. If necessary, the lateral collateral ligament can be released subperiosteally from its epicondylar attachment (beginning at the distal femur and elevating tissue proximally along the lateral femur) if the knee is still tight laterally. Additional details of release of the lateral soft tissue structures are provided in Chapter 9.

PEARLS AND PITFALLS

- Genu recurvatum found in association with neuromuscular disorders is a relative contraindication to TKA.
- Patients require the ability to dorsiflex the foot at least to neutral.
- Nonneuromuscular recurvatum should be approached similarly to other TKAs, making sure to balance the flexion and extension spaces.
- Constrained prostheses are generally not needed to correct nonneuromuscular recurvatum.
- Avoid any residual collateral ligament instability.
- Underresection of bone and thicker components are generally not needed.

POSTOPERATIVE MANAGEMENT

Postoperative rehabilitation and follow-up are the same as those used for TKA patients without recurvatum. Ambulation with full weight bearing is undertaken on postoperative day one and range of motion is begun the following day. Postoperative thickening of the joint capsule restricts radical changes in knee flexion, allowing progressive range of motion and strengthening (9). Knee extension remains stable, and recurrent recurvatum is unlikely as long as preoperative evaluation adequately screened for neuromuscular etiologies and muscular weakness (5). Follow-up is the same as for standard TKA postoperative follow-up.

COMPLICATIONS

Recurring recurvatum is the risk specific to patients who present with hyperextension prior to surgery, in addition to the complications typically associated with any TKA. As stated previously, however, patients with nonneuromuscular etiologies for their recurvatum have excellent results from TKA and do not hyperextend postoperatively as long as there is no residual instability in the knee at the time of surgery.

Postoperative complications are far more common when neuromuscular etiologies are involved. Patients in this group are more likely to experience recurring instability with subsequent functional deterioration and less pain relief. If hyperextension is corrected by TKA, these patients will lose their ability to ambulate if their quadriceps strength will not support their weight. A Mayo Clinic study showed this in four of 16 TKAs performed in patients with poliomyelitis. These patients experienced recurring instability, and their pain relief was directly related to quadriceps strength. The investigators concluded that progressive functional loss is possible in all knees affected by poliomyelitis (8).

RESULTS

Patients with nonneuromuscular etiologies for their recurvatum have excellent results after TKA. Our institution retrospectively examined 57 TKAs performed in patients with nonneuromuscular recurvatum using standard techniques and not tightening the extension gap (5). Only two (3.5%) knees had a hyperextension deformity after surgery (10 degrees each). Notably, these knees had residual medial instability at the time of surgery, thereby underscoring the importance of avoiding any instability in the coronal plane in these patients. Overall, Knee Society knee, function, and pain scores improved by 40, 37, and 30 points, respectively, at 4.5 years. No knee replacement has been revised for any reason. In patients with a nonneuromuscular etiology, therefore, a recurvatum deformity does not preclude a successful total knee replacement.

REFERENCES

1. Krackow KA. *The Technique of Total Knee Arthroplasty*. St. Louis: CV Mosby; 1990.
2. Krackow KA, Weiss A. Recurvatum deformity complicating performance of total knee arthroplasty: a brief note. *J Bone Joint Surg* 1990;72-A:268–271.
3. Insall JN. Surgical techniques and instrumentation in total knee arthroplasty. In: Insall JN, Windsor RE, Scott WN, et al, eds. *Surgery of the Knee*. New York: Churchill Livingstone; 1993:739–804.
4. Insall JN, Haas SB. Complications of total knee arthroplasty. In: Insall JN, Windsor RE, Scott WN, et al, eds. *Surgery of the Knee*. New York: Churchill Livingstone; 1993:891–934.
5. Meding JB, Keating EM, Ritter MA, et al. Total knee replacement in patients with genu recurvatum. *Clin Orthop* 2001;393:244–249.
6. Tew M, Forster IW. Effect of knee replacement on flexion deformity. *J Bone Joint Surg* 1987; 69-B:395–399.
7. Laskin RS, O'Flynn HM. The Insall award. Total knee replacement with posterior cruciate ligament retention in rheumatoid arthritis. Problems and complications. *Clin Orthop* 1997;345:24–28.
8. Giori NJ, Lewallen DG. Total knee arthroplasty in limbs affected by poliomyelitis. *J Bone Joint Surg* 2002;84-A:1157–1161.
9. Schurman DJ, Parker JN, Ornstein D. Total condylar knee replacement: a study of factors influencing range of motion as late as two years after arthroplasty. *J Bone Joint Surg* 1985;67-A:1006–1014.

12 The Stiff Knee: Ankylosis and Flexion

Chitranjan S. Ranawat and William F. Flynn Jr.

INDICATIONS/CONTRAINDICATIONS

Knees with less than a 50° arc of motion are considered "stiff," but there is a wide variation in presentation. One may be faced with a knee ankylosed in extension or one with flexion of 0° to 50°. The surgeon who is to successfully correct such problems with an arthroplasty must have a clear plan in mind.

The approach to total knee arthroplasty (TKA) in the patient with a stiff knee is similar to planning the revision of a TKA. One must first identify the reason for the lack of motion. Some of the most common causes are previous surgery on the knee; previous injury to the knee; ankylosis, particularly in rheumatoid or psoriatic arthritis; reflex sympathetic dystrophy; severe pain; neuromuscular disorder; and previous infection.

The underlying cause of stiffness of the knee can have a profound effect on the success of the proposed surgery. Mechanical problems (bony deformity and ligamentous and capsular contracture) can usually be addressed successfully. Severe pain may limit motion with an alert patient; the same patient anesthetized may have a much better range of motion (ROM). Patients with severe reflex sympathetic dystrophy may have very limited motion, and surgery in these patients should be approached very cautiously because it can exacerbate this disorder. Patients with neuromuscular disorders, including those who have had a stroke, should also be approached with caution, because one cannot correct their underlying disorder. Patients with a history of knee sepsis may also have a stiff knee. Before considering arthroplasty, one must absolutely rule out low-grade sepsis.

PREOPERATIVE PLANNING

The pathologic anatomic conditions encountered in cases of stiffness of the knee may include shortening and tightness of the ligaments and muscles, fibrosis of the quadriceps muscle, intraarticular or extraarticular fibrosis, and intraarticular or extraarticular bony blocks from malalignment or new bone formation. The surgeon must be able to address any or all of these conditions.

Preoperative planning for arthroplasty of the stiff knee must include a thorough clinical and radiographic evaluation of the knee. The preoperative ROM of the knee must be documented, along with any contractures, scars, or angular deformity. The circulation and sensation in the limb, and its motor function, particularly with regard to the quadriceps muscle, must be assessed. In addition, as in the case of any surgery, the patient's overall condition must be evaluated preoperatively, including the patient's desire and ability to comply with postoperative therapy.

Radiographic evaluation must include anteroposterior (AP), lateral, and patellar views, with additional studies such as computed tomography (CT), bone scans, or scanogram added as needed. As in a revision situation, alignment, bone loss, and bone quality must also be assessed. Additionally, any hardware present around the knee and that which will have to be removed must be identified so appropriate instrumentation for accomplishing this will be available at the time of surgery.

Finally, the surgeon must decide which prosthesis to use. A wide variety of modular systems are available and can accommodate almost any situation, but occasionally a custom prosthesis must be fabricated for a very small or large knee or a knee with severe bone loss or malalignment. Careful consideration must be given to expected soft-tissue deficiencies. With severe deformity, the posterior cruciate ligament is usually abnormal and the prosthesis must substitute for it. Additionally, the collateral ligaments may be deficient or may become functionally deficient if extensive soft-tissue releases are required, and a constrained option must be available.

SURGERY

Once preoperative planning is complete and an appropriate prosthesis has been selected, the surgeon can proceed. In a laminar flow operating room, the patient is put in the supine position with a tourniquet on the thigh of the leg that will undergo surgery. The leg is draped free, and a Vi drape is used to isolate the operative field. We use epidural anesthesia in all knee replacements. This technique is very safe and effective, and it provides the additional benefit of permitting the patient to be maintained postoperatively on continuous infusion. This dramatically decreases the patient's postoperative pain and narcotic usage.

The patient's ROM and ligamentous stability should be assessed under anesthesia prior to incision (Figs. 12-1 and 12-2). If there is no previous incision, a straight midline or slightly paramedian incision should be used. Old incisions should be incorporated as much as possible into new ones, making sure to leave no avascular islands or narrow strips of skin.

A medial parapatellar arthrotomy is then performed along the junction of the quadriceps tendon and vastus medialis muscle (Fig. 12-3). If the patella is ankylosed, it may be osteotomized at this time. Any adhesions between the quadriceps and femur on either side of the patella and gutter are released, and the quadriceps is mobilized from the femur (Figs. 12-4 through 12-9). Flexion of the knee is now assessed. If the knee cannot be flexed more than 30 degrees to 40 degrees, we perform a quadriceps release rather than a V-Y turndown or tibial tubercle osteotomy. A V-Y turndown devascularizes the extensor mechanism, and adjusting the final length of the quadriceps mechanism is difficult. Small tubercle osteotomies may create problems with nonunion or loss of fixation, and large osteotomies require substantial fixation. In addition, any tubercle osteotomy can change the position of the patella, and the final adjustment of quadriceps tension is again somewhat problematic.

Quadriceps Release

With the knee in extension, the patella is everted and the patellofemoral ligaments are released with electrocautery. Next, we routinely perform a lateral retinacular release from the inside out (Fig. 12-10). If preservation of the superior genicular artery prevents an adequate release, we sacrifice the artery.

After this, a careful dissection is done, releasing the vastus medialis, medial capsule, and superficial medial collateral ligament (MCL) from the medial and anterior femur, as well as leaving the superior attachment of the deep MCL, thus forming a long sleeve subperiosteally (Fig. 12-11). The dissection of the MCL is done subperiosteally to about the midplane of the tibia. If the tibia and femur are ankylosed, an osteotomy is performed at the joint line; in other cases, scar tissue in the joint is excised with a scalpel and the cruciate ligaments and menisci are released (Fig. 12-12). If the knee cannot be flexed at least 30 degrees to 40 degrees because of a tight quadriceps mechanism, a controlled Z-lengthening is done of the rectus femoris and vastus intermedius muscles, using six to eight small incisions made with a no. 11 blade. The rectus is first separated from the vastus, and the knee is then flexed to keep tension on the tendon. With each Z, the flexion of the knee increases in a controlled fashion, until 70 degrees to 80 degrees of flexion is reached (Figs. 12-13 to 12-15).

Once this is accomplished, the knee is flexed with the patella everted, occasionally without dislocation, and the tibia is externally rotated to avoid avulsing the tendon from the tubercle (Fig. 12-16). The subperiosteal medial release is then continued as the knee is further flexed and the tibia externally rotated. The release is carried around medially and posteriorly to at least the midplane of the tibia (Figs. 12-17 to 12-19). The attachment of the MCL to the femur is not detached subperiosteally unless it interferes with the balance of the soft-tissue sleeve once the trial implant is in place. Any remnant of the medial meniscus is carefully released.

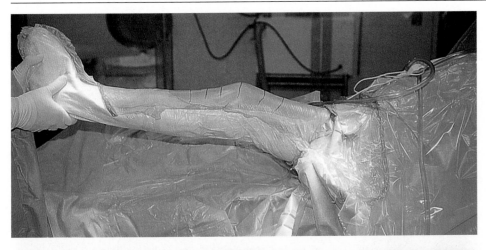

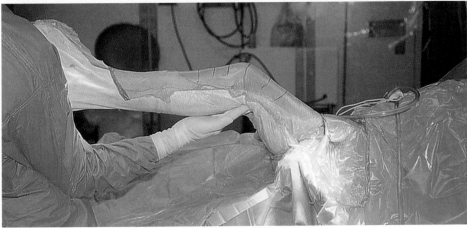

FIGURES 12-1 AND 12-2

Preoperative extension (−20 degrees) and flexion (50 degrees). Note that the leg is draped free.

Dissection is now done laterally with the knee flexed. The remaining patellofemoral ligaments are released (Figs. 12-20 and 12-21). The insertion of the iliotibial band is identified and preserved. The lateral capsular structures, including the popliteus and lateral collateral ligament, are released from the femur subperiosteally, using either a knife or an osteotome (Figs. 12-22 to 12-24). Lastly, if necessary, the iliotibial band is lengthened in a Z fashion. We then cut the proximal tibia, taking between 6 and 10 mm of bone and slightly more if a flexion contracture is present. The alignment of the cut is checked to be sure that it is neutral (0 degrees varus/valgus, 2 degrees to 3 degrees posterior slope) to the axis of the ankle (Figs. 12-25 and 12-26).

Intramedullary instrumentation is then placed in the femur and the distal femoral cut is made, removing 9 to 10 mm of bone from the lateral condyle to properly align the mechanical axis of the knee (Figs. 12-27 and 12-28). We generally make the femoral cut in 5 degrees of valgus, unless the patient had a severe valgus deformity. In this situation, we choose 3 degrees or even 0 degrees of valgus.

Thus, we create a rectangular gap approximately 20 mm in height, with medial and lateral soft-tissue sleeves.

The extension gap is checked using lamina spreaders or spacer blocks (Figs. 12-29 and 12-30). If the medial side is tight, the medial release is extended. In cases of severe valgus/flexion deformity, release of the lateral head of the gastrocnemius may occasionally be needed. If the knee lacks extension, the posterior capsule is released from the femur as needed. Occasionally, capsulotomy may be required.

After this, the anterior and posterior femoral cuts are made. The cutting blocks are placed to equalize the flexion gap medially and laterally and are then slightly externally rotated (Fig. 12-31). This helps keep the flexion gap equal as flexion increases and aids patellofemoral tracking.

(text continues on p. 154)

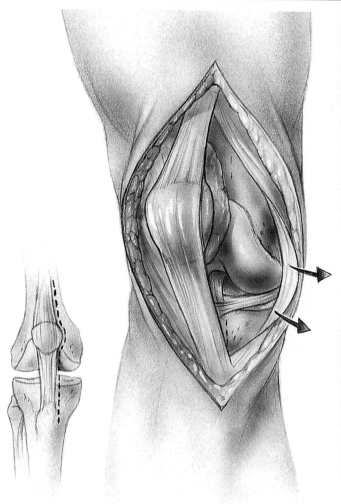

FIGURE 12-3
Initial incision and approach.

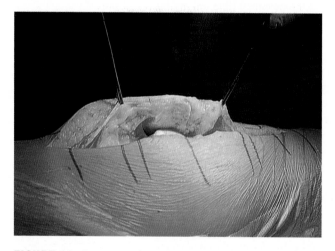

FIGURE 12-4
Lateral flap, with femur at left. Flap is full thickness, and a Kocher clamp is used to hold the edge.

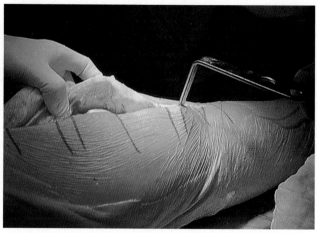

FIGURE 12-5
Early dissection of the lateral flap.

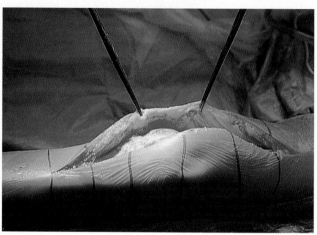

FIGURE 12-6
Medial flap. Note subperiosteal dissection of the tibia (*right*).

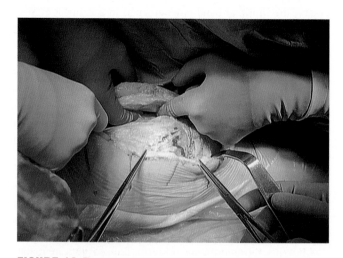

FIGURE 12-7
Lateral flap mobilization, femur at left. Adhesions in the gutter are released completely.

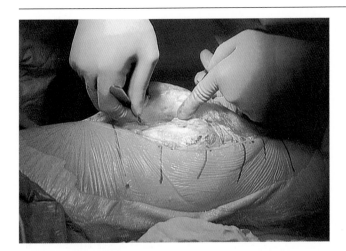

FIGURE 12-8
Lateral flap mobilization.

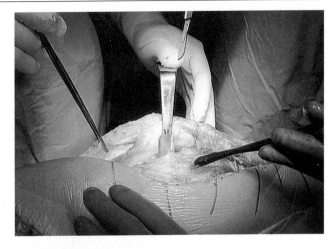

FIGURE 12-9
A small, angled Homan retractor is used for continued lateral mobilization.

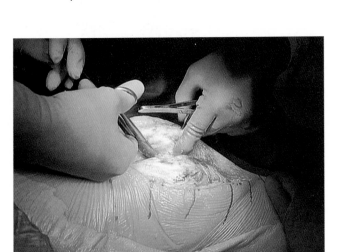

FIGURE 12-10
Beginning of lateral release, performed from the inside out. Complete retinacular release.

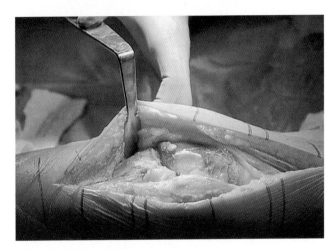

FIGURE 12-11
Beginning of deeper medial dissection, femur at left. An angled retractor is used.

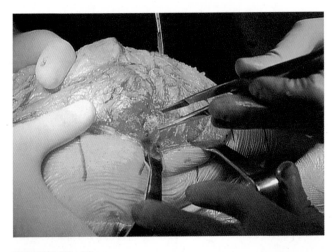

FIGURE 12-12
Excising scar tissue at medial joint line, femur to left.

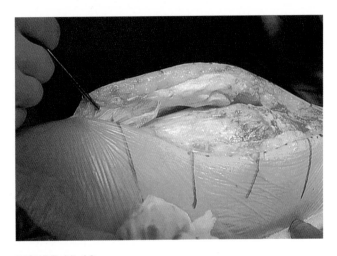

FIGURE 12-13
Beginning separation of rectus in preparation for Z-plasty. The easiest way to create this type of incision is with a scalpel.

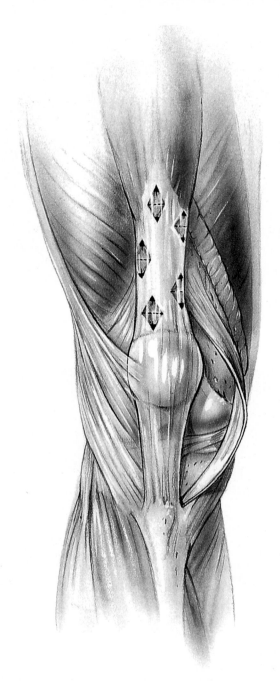

FIGURE 12-14
Anterior view of Z-lengthening.

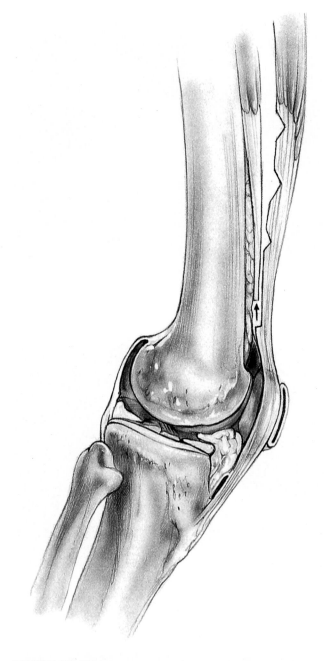

FIGURE 12-15
Lateral view of Z-lengthening. Note that the rectus is separated from the underlying vastus.

FIGURE 12-16
Tibia flexed up. Assistant externally rotates the foot to exert tension on the patellar tendon.

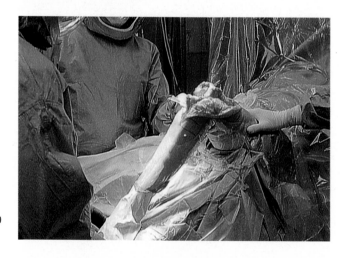

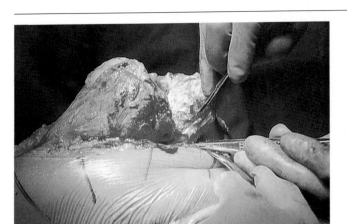
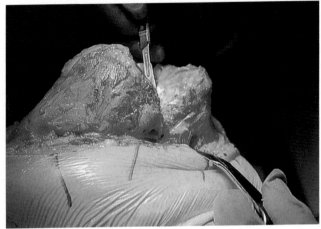

FIGURES 12-17 AND 12-18

Continuation of medial release. This subperiosteal dissection continues all the way to the posterior capsule.

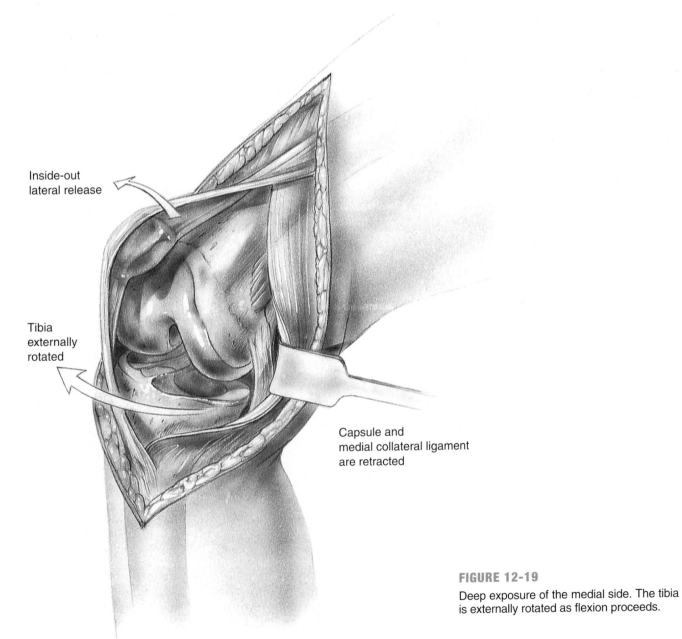

Inside-out lateral release

Tibia externally rotated

Capsule and medial collateral ligament are retracted

FIGURE 12-19

Deep exposure of the medial side. The tibia is externally rotated as flexion proceeds.

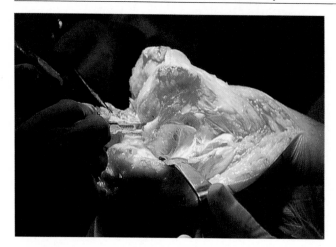

FIGURE 12-20

Lateral view of excision of lateral meniscus remnants.

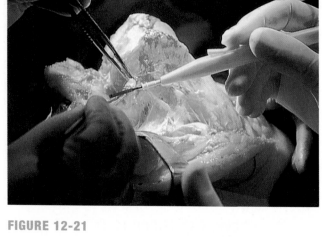

FIGURE 12-21

Final release of patellofemoral ligaments with cautery. This is an important and often overlooked step.

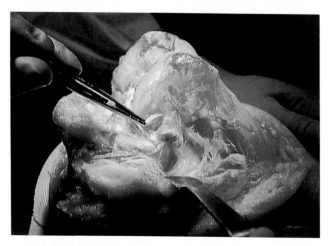

FIGURE 12-22

Lateral mobilization. Note external tibial rotation. If necessary, the subperiosteal dissection continues to or beyond the lower collateral ligament.

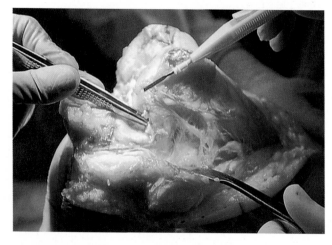

FIGURE 12-23

Lateral mobilization.

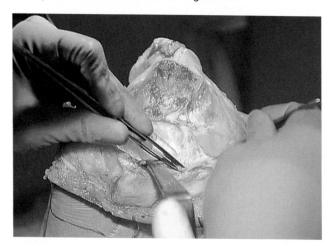

FIGURE 12-24

Extent of lateral mobilization.

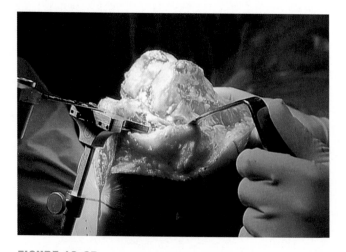

FIGURE 12-25

Cutting the tibia with an external alignment guide. Intramedullary guides may be used, but with attention to the possibility of bowed tibiae.

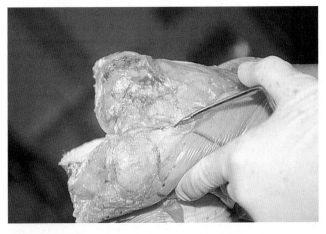

FIGURE 12-26

Lateral view after tibial resection. We typically resect the tibia first.

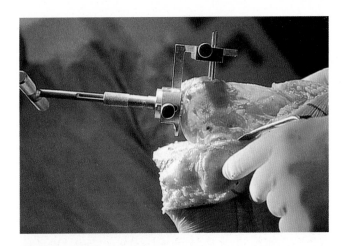

FIGURE 12-27

Femoral intramedullary instrumentation for distal resection. We enlarge the entry hole and irrigate and suction the femur to minimize the risk of fat embolization. The use of extramedullary guides for the tibia minimizes the chance of fat embolization from this bone.

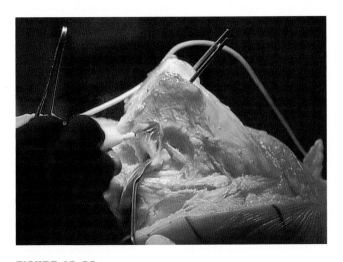

FIGURE 12-28

After resection. The pins are left in, should recutting prove necessary. Typically, patients with a flexion contracture will require more than a "standard" distal femoral resection. Leaving the pins in while checking the gap allows for easier replacement of the cutting guide.

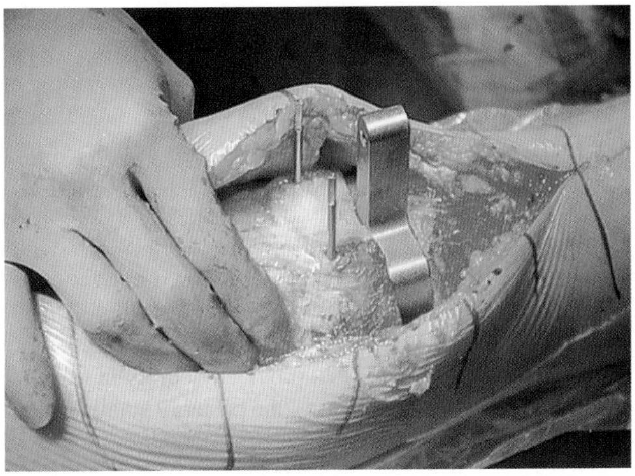

FIGURE 12-29

Spacer to check extension gap. We also use lamina spreaders, one applied medially and one applied laterally, to assess soft-tissue tension.

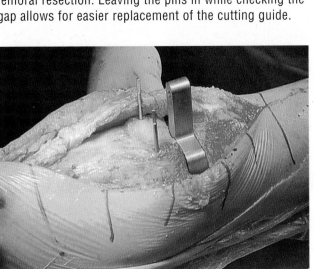

FIGURE 12-30

Valgus pressure to assess medial release and stability.

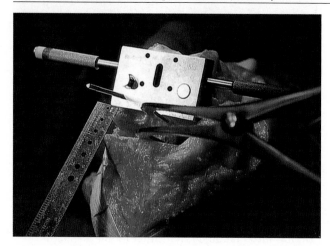

FIGURE 12-31

Anteroposterior cutting guide. The rectangular flexion gap is also checked with lamina spreaders.

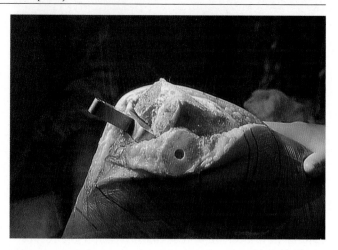

FIGURE 12-32

Spacer to check flexion gap.

If desired, spacer blocks can now be placed to assess the flexion and extension gaps. The intercondylar notch cut and chamfer cuts are made, and a femoral trial component is put in place (Figs. 12-32 and 12-33).

The tibial trial component is placed with the appropriate instrumentation. Care should be taken to ensure that the component is neutral or slightly externally rotated and aligned with the tubercle (Fig. 12-34). As determined either by measurement or by a spacer block, a tibial trial insert of the proper thickness is then placed, and the knee joint is reduced. A careful assessment of flexion and extension gaps, varus/valgus stability, and ROM must be made at this time. If the quadriceps mechanism is still tight and does not allow 30 degrees to 40 degrees of flexion with the implant in place, even with the tourniquet released, further controlled Z-lengthening is done (Fig. 12-35). It should be noted that in the stiff knee with a flexion contracture, there may be a disparity in the flexion and extension gaps, with the flexion gap the greater of the two. When this occurs, one must consider a constrained insert that provides stability in flexion while augmenting the function of the collateral ligament. In many cases, the posterior stabilized insert will allow appropriate stability.

If the trial components are satisfactory, they can be left in place while the permanent prosthesis is opened and the patella is cut. We always resurface the patella with an all-polyethylene tibial component, taking care not to increase the overall height of the patella (Figs. 12-36 and 12-37). Trial reduction of

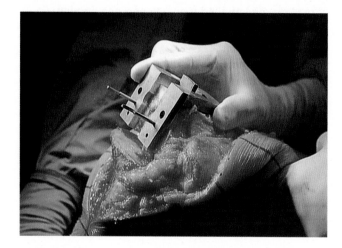

FIGURE 12-33

Notch guide placement. Proper placement of the guide is important, to leave sufficient bone medially and laterally so as not to weaken the condyles.

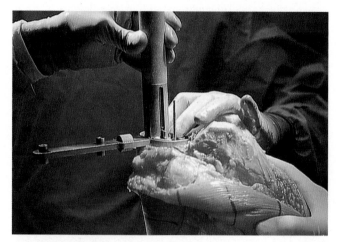

FIGURE 12-34

Tibial instrumentation. Care should be taken not to internally rotate the tibia relative to the tubercle.

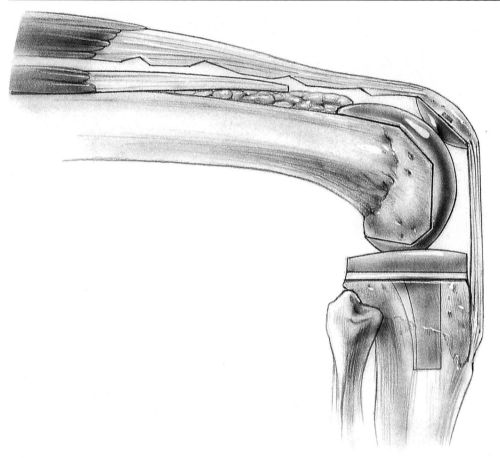

FIGURE 12-35

Lateral view with components in place. Note that if flexion is insufficient, further Z-lengthening of the rectus may be done.

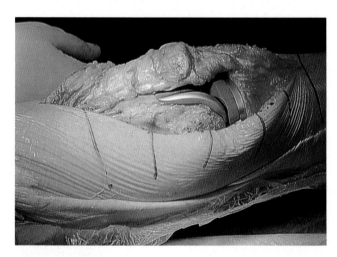

FIGURE 12-36

Trial reduction of femur and tibia. Flexion and extension should be checked.

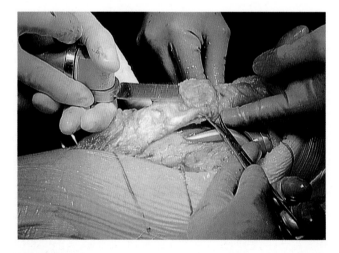

FIGURE 12-37

Cutting of the patella. A cutting guide may also be used. The patellar height should be measured before resection and after patellar trial placement to ensure that the height of the patella is not increased.

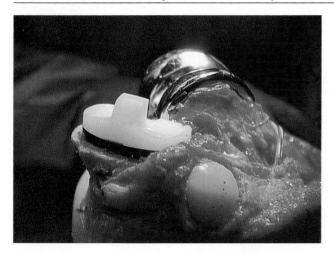

FIGURE 12-38

Placement of final components of prosthesis before reduction. The extensor mechanism should be protected by externally rotating the tibia. Care must be taken not to place the patella too far medially and to assess patellar tracking.

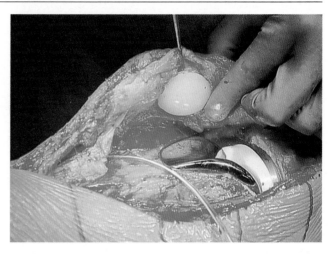

FIGURE 12-39

Extent of lateral release. The retinaculum is completely released, as is the insertion of the vastus lateralis.

all three components is done, and the knee is taken through a ROM. The patella should track easily, without tilting, using the "no thumb" technique.

Jet lavage is used to clean the bony beds of the patella, femur, and tibia, which are then carefully dried with a lap sponge. Once the cement is at a consistency of dough or toothpaste, it is finger pressured into the patella and femur. The patellar component of the prosthesis is held with a special clamp, and the femoral component is impacted using the appropriate tool. Any excess cement is removed with curettes. While this is occurring, an assistant mixes the second batch of cement for the tibia. Once this cement reaches the correct consistency, the tibial baseplate is cemented in position after finger pressurization of cement into the plateau. A trial polyethylene tibial component is placed, and the knee joint is reduced into extension. This "lever" action further pressurizes the cement, extruding some of it, which is removed with curettes. Once the cement has completely polymerized, the knee is flexed. Any excess cement is removed with osteotomes. The trial polyethylene tibial component is replaced with the real polyethylene insert, and the knee is reduced (Fig. 12-38). The knee is copiously irrigated with jet lavage.

At this point, we release the tourniquet and coagulate any bleeding vessels, paying particular attention to the area of the lateral release (Fig. 12-39). The limb is then re-exsanguinated with an

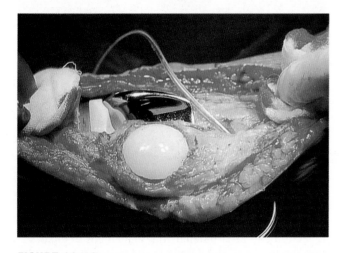

FIGURE 12-40

Drain placement. We pass a drain once from the inside out and leave the drain in the lateral gutter.

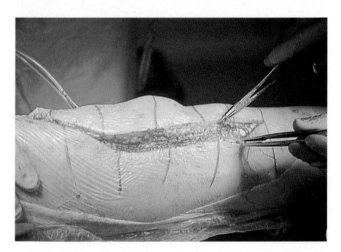

FIGURE 12-41

Arthrotomy closure with Tevdek and Vicryl sutures, spaced approximately 1 cm apart.

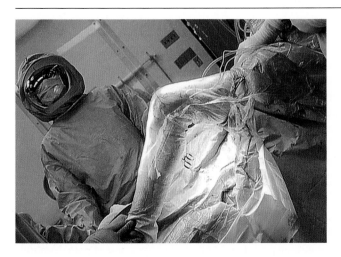

FIGURE 12-42

Note postoperative flexion of 80 degrees. The patient ultimately achieved 95 degrees of flexion by 6 months. Note that intraoperatively, the inflated tourniquet may "trap" the quadriceps. After closure, Betadine-soaked silk gauze, gauze sponges, and Webril are placed over the wound. Plaster splints are used to keep the knee in extension overnight unless the patient has a severe valgus or flexion deformity, in which case the knee is flexed approximately 15 degrees.

Esmarch bandage and the tourniquet is reinflated. More irrigation is performed. Two Constavac drains are placed. The arthrotomy is closed with no. 0 Tevdek and Vicryl sutures (Figs. 12-40 and 12-41). Subcutaneous tissues are closed in one layer with no. 0 Vicryl sutures and the skin is closed with a running 3-0 nylon suture. Several interrupted vertical mattress sutures are added. Subcutaneous closure with no. 0 and 3-0 Vicryl sutures followed by staples is preferred by some surgeons. Flexion and extension are again assessed (Fig. 12-42).

The wound is dressed with Betadine silk gauze, plain gauze, and soft padding. Two plaster splints are placed medially and laterally keeping the knee in extension, and an Ace bandage is placed. A radiograph is made in the recovery room. In cases of correction of valgus with flexion contracture, the knee is immobilized in 15 degrees of flexion to reduce the risk of peroneal nerve palsy.

POSTOPERATIVE MANAGEMENT

Drains and splints are removed on the first postoperative day and the patient is placed in a continuous passive motion (CPM) machine. Initially, this is set to a range from 0 degrees to 30 degrees, which is increased as tolerated, usually by about 10 degrees per day. If the patient had a preoperative flexion contracture or if the knee was tight in extension in the operating room, the patient is taken out of the CPM machine at night and must sleep with a knee immobilizer. On the afternoon of the first postoperative day or the morning of the second day, the patient, accompanied by a physical therapist, begins to ambulate with a walker. Ambulation is increased daily, and the patient is advanced to crutches or a cane as tolerated. The therapist also assists the patient with knee flexion exercises and straight leg raises.

The expectations of both the surgeon and the patient must be realistic. Even the most educated patient often hopes for a "normal" knee after arthroplasty, and the surgeon cannot paint too gloomy a picture. However, the surgeon must explain that the goal will be to improve the ROM and function of the knee, and not to make it normal or near normal. In patients with 50 degrees or less of knee motion preoperatively, 70 degrees to 80 degrees of motion without pain should be considered a successful outcome.

COMPLICATIONS

The following sections are devoted to major problems that may be encountered intraoperatively in arthroplasty of the stiff knee.

Avulsion of the Tibial Tubercle

This can be avoided with careful subperiosteal mobilization, with the tibia externally rotated, as the knee is flexed. This complication can usually be avoided. The emphasis is again on external rotation of the tibia along with flexion.

Unequal Flexion/Extension Gap

As mentioned, an unequal flexion-extension gap requires a constrained polyethylene insert and is associated with the correction of a flexion contracture or loss of condylar bone from previous surgery. We do not hesitate to release the MCL from the femur if this facilitates exposure and soft-tissue balance.

Bone of Ligament Loss

Compensation for loss of bone or ligament can usually be made with a modular knee system. Both kinds of loss must be considered preoperatively, and the surgeon should be prepared to deal with any possible loss. Remember, however, that the patient with limited motion has "aggressive fibroblasts" and will rarely end up with instability.

Other major problems encountered after arthroplasty of the stiff knee are as follows (excluding the usual concerns with deep vein thrombosis, infection, and others).

Loss of Range of Motion

Despite what the surgeon achieves in the operating room (i.e., 80 degrees to 90 degrees of flexion), the patient may have difficulty achieving motion postoperatively, usually because of pain. Continuous epidural anesthesia can diminish the pain, and appropriate physical therapy may help, but sometimes manipulation may be required. If the patient has not achieved 60 degrees of flexion by 6 weeks, we manipulate the knee under anesthesia.

Abnormalities in Wound Healing

Aside from the usual concerns, any knee that has had prior surgery, especially with multiple incisions, may be subject to drainage, or worse, to skin sloughing. Skin sloughing may often require a flap for reconstruction, and this possibility should always be considered preoperatively. Consultation with a plastic surgeon may prove helpful. We put patients who have persistent drainage on bedrest, with a clean sterilely applied compressive dressing. We allow no CPM or therapy until the drainage ceases.

Patient Expectations

Once having achieved an improved ROM, the patient may begin to expect that improvement will continue, resulting in a near-normal ROM. The patient must be reminded of preoperative goals and that the maximum benefit of the total knee replacement is only achieved by 8 to 10 months postoperatively.

RECOMMENDED READING

Aglietti P, Windsor RE, Buzzi R, et al. Arthroplasty for the stiff or ankylosed knee. *J Arthroplasty* 1989;41(1):1–5.

Kim J, Nelson CL, Lotke PA. Stiffness after TKA: Prevalence of the complication and outcomes after Revision. *J Bone Joint Surg* 2004;86:1479–1484.

Rand JA. Revision total knee arthroplasty: surgical technique. In: Rand JA, ed. *Total knee arthroplasty.* Baltimore, MD. Raven Press, 1993:155–176.

Scott RD. Revision total knee arthroplasty. *Clin Orthop* 1998;226:65–78.

Sculco TP, Faris PM. Total knee replacement in the stiff knee. *Techniques Orthop* 1988;3(2):5–8.

Vince K, Dorr LD. Total knee arthroplasty: principles and controversy. *Techniques Orthop* 1987;1(4):69–82.

Whiteside LA, Ohl MD. Tibial tubercle osteotomy for exposure of the difficult total knee arthroplasty. *Clin Orthop* 1990;260:6–9.

Windsor RE, Insall JN. Exposure in revision total knee arthroplasty: the femoral peel. *Techniques Orthop* 1988;3(2):1–4.

13 Simultaneous Total Knee Arthroplasty and Femoral Osteotomy

John M. Siliski

INDICATIONS/CONTRAINDICATIONS

Simultaneous femoral osteotomy and total knee arthroplasty (TKA) should be considered for the treatment of deformities of the femur that would compromise or complicate a TKA done for osteo- or posttraumatic arthritis. The deformities within the femur are most commonly the result of fracture malunion but may also be the result of metabolic conditions such as Paget's disease or rickets. Most patients have had prior surgical treatment of the femur and therefore may have significant prior surgical scars and retained hardware. The most common situation is a mid-to-distal femoral nonunion with a previous lateral subvastus approach and retained lateral plate (1–3).

The types of femoral deformities encountered include frontal plane angular (varus or valgus deformity), sagittal plane angular (flexion or extension deformity), and torsional (internal or external rotation deformity). Any combination of these deformities may be encountered.

Frontal plane angular deformities are the most common type that lead to an indication for simultaneous osteotomy and knee arthroplasty, because even 10 degrees of deformity in this plane, if left uncorrected, may have significant effects on bone cuts and collateral ligament balance. The location of the deformity along the femur can influence its impact on the distal femoral cut. Hip adduction or abduction can compensate for more proximal deformities so that when the distal femoral cut is made, there is little effect on collateral ligament balance. In the presence of a distal deformity, however, a femoral cut made perpendicular to the mechanical axis can have a much greater impact (Fig. 13-1). Although minor degrees of frontal plane angular deformity can be managed by asymmetric distal femoral bone cuts and ligament balancing, as the varus or valgus femoral deformity becomes greater, so does the asymmetry of the bone cuts and the collateral ligament imbalance (4). By the point at which the frontal plane deformity is 10 degrees or more, a TKA will present a difficult problem of collateral ligament balance in flexion but marked imbalance in extension. The choice may then be either to try to improve ligament balance in extension, which may then lead to imbalance in flexion, or to use a more constrained implant that substitutes for collateral ligament function. The option essentially uses an implant for a primary arthroplasty that is most commonly used to salvage difficult revision knee arthroplasties (5–7).

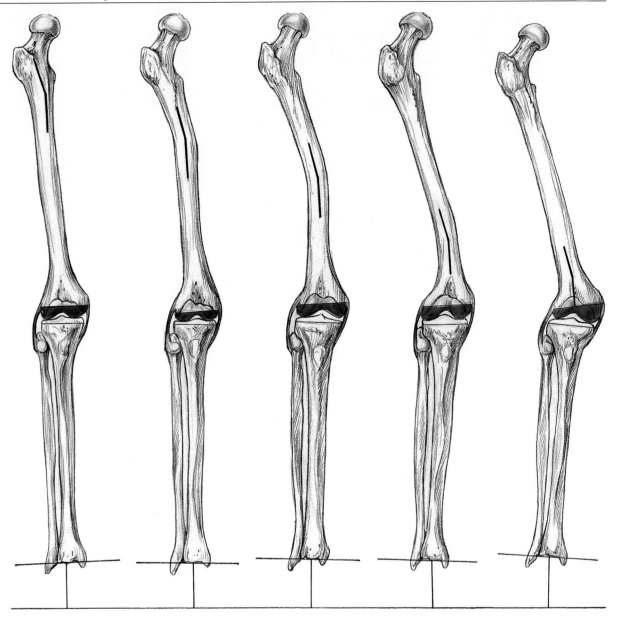

FIGURE 13-1

(A) Diagrams demonstrating the impact of a valgus femoral deformity at varying distances from the knee on the standard distal femoral resection made perpendicular to the mechanical axis. The collateral ligament origins and extension space geometry are more compromised as the deformities become more distal.

If left uncorrected, sagittal plane deformities create several potential problems. If the surgeon places the femoral implant in a normal position on the distal femur, the persisting femoral deformity will result in the joint line not being parallel to the ground, and the leg will have altered mechanics caused by the effective hyperextension or flexion from the periarticular deformity. If the femoral component is placed on the distal femur in a flexed or extended position in an attempt to correct the periarticular deformity, difficulties occur with either femoral notching or overresection of the posterior condyles. It also becomes difficult to maintain proper function of the posterior cruciate ligament and balancing of the flexion and extension gaps. Consequently, sagittal plane deformities above 10 to 20 degrees should be considered for simultaneous osteotomy at the time of knee arthroplasty.

Rotational deformities, if left uncorrected, will leave the knee and foot pointed out or in; this may be tolerable for smaller degrees of malrotation for less active patients. Unfortunately, rotational deformities are minimally correctable during knee arthroplasty because the rotational positioning of the femoral and tibial components must be guided by bony anatomy, patellofemoral tracking, tibiofemoral tracking, and balancing of the medial and lateral flexion gaps. For the active patient with a femoral rotational deformity greater than 20 degrees, a derotational osteotomy should be considered.

Contraindications to simultaneous femoral osteotomy and TKA include the following. Patients with knee pain but predicted future low demand for function, such as a nursing home patient who will permanently use a walker anyway, may best be treated without a corrective osteotomy. The knee arthroplasty may be performed with or without an attempt to correct the overall limb alignment. Patients who may have difficulty with the simultaneous rehabilitation of a healing osteotomy and a knee replacement should be considered for the alternative options. If there is any concern about residual infection in the femur, simultaneous osteotomy and knee arthroplasty should be avoided.

PREOPERATIVE PLANNING

Evaluation and Preparation

A standard orthopedic history should be obtained regarding the patient's past history of injury, treatment, and current symptoms. In most cases, there will be a remote history of a femoral fracture and the more recent development of significant knee pain as arthritic changes have developed. The evaluation must include all aspects of the old injury, any residual effects on the extremity, and the severity of the knee arthritis. The history, examination, and imaging studies must then be processed by the surgeon to decide on a detailed surgical plan that takes into account all aspects of the case: surgical approach, use of tourniquet for the entire procedure or for arthroplasty only, removal of retained hardware, level of the femoral osteotomy, fixation device for the osteotomy, type of knee implant, and type of femoral guide system to be used.

The patient must also be prepared for a combined procedure that requires a longer anesthesia time and greater blood loss. Preoperative autologous blood donations should be considered.

Examination and Imaging Studies

Physical examination should include all the standard aspects for a knee being prepared for arthroplasty, including a detailed knee examination as well as an examination of the hip, foot, and ankle and neurocirculatory function of the limb. In addition, there will be aspects of the examination that should focus on leg length discrepancy, femoral deformity, and pre-existing scars. Any pre-existing scars will need to be considered as part of the overall plan for the exposure for the simultaneous osteotomy and arthroplasty.

Imaging studies should include standard anteroposterior (AP) (standing), lateral, and skyline views to assess the arthritic changes in the knee and their contributions to frontal and sagittal plane deformities in the limb as a whole. A lateral view taken with the knee in maximal extension will help to define the presence or absence of a flexion contracture in the knee. A 3-foot AP view of the extremity will permit assessment of the limb's overall mechanical axis. AP and lateral views of the femur, based on the proximal segment, will permit assessment of the degree of frontal and sagittal plane angular deformities. An x-ray of the femur taken at the angle that maximizes the femoral angular deformity will permit measurement of the true maximal angular deformity, and in which plane it lies relative to the frontal and sagittal planes.

Instruments and Implants

Instruments for removing existing hardware and for placing the new internal fixation device (either a plate or intramedullary rod) will need to be available for the osteotomy. The surgeon may wish to have a C-arm image intensifier available to check the osteotomy, hardware placement, and mechanical axis. For the TKA, the surgeon needs to have available an extramedullary guide system if the internal fixation device will block use of an intramedullary guide. With the mechanical axis corrected with the osteotomy, a standard posterior cruciate ligament-retaining or substituting knee prosthesis should be all that is necessary for the arthroplasty unless there are additional complicating issues at the level of the knee.

SURGERY

Positioning

The patient is placed supine with a trochanteric roll. A radiolucent table may be chosen if use of image intensification is anticipated. If the limb is long and if the surgical incision will start at or below the midthigh, a tourniquet may be placed before preparation and draping. If a tourniquet will interfere with the exposure for the osteotomy, it may be better to perform the osteotomy without a tourniquet and then place a sterile tourniquet after the osteotomy part of the surgery is completed.

Exposure

The majority of these cases have used a previous lateral approach to the femur with placement of some type of plate (Figs. 13-2 and 13-3). The single surgical exposure that accommodates all aspects of the case is a lateral subvastus approach with tibial tubercle osteotomy. The old lateral incision is reopened and extended down along the lateral margin of the tibial tubercle. The vastus lateralis muscle is elevated off the intermuscular septum to expose the femoral shaft and the existing hardware (Fig. 13-4). Distally, the lateral capsule is incised, and a small portion of the anterior muscle compartment of the calf is elevated adjacent to the tibial tubercle. Osteotomy of the tibial tubercle is then performed (Figs. 13-5 and 13-6). The surgeon uses an osteotome to make a horizontal cut about 1 cm deep through the bone just proximal to the patellar tendon insertion. This cut leaves a "shelf," which will make the osteotomy more stable after the tubercle is reattached during closure. An oscillating saw can then be used to open the cortex along the lateral margin of the tubercle, curving anterior and out through the cortex. An osteotome is used to divide the cortex medial to the tubercle leaving most of the medial periosteum intact. An osteotome can be inserted through the lateral cortical incision to complete the osteotomy and elevate the tubercle in a medial direction. The medial soft tissues can be left intact and attached to the tubercle by using a scalpel and elevator to lift the soft tissue sleeve off the proximal medial tibia. Once the tibial tubercle and fat pad are freed up, the entire extensor mechanism can be mobilized medially for wide exposure of the distal femur and knee. The retained hardware is removed (8).

Femoral Osteotomy

The standard three-wire technique may be used on the distal femur for placement of a 95-degree angled blade plate for fixation of a supracondylar osteotomy. (Image intensification may be used as well.) One wire is placed over the distal femur, and a second wire is placed over the anterior trochlear surface. The third summation wire is drilled into the distal femur so that it is parallel to the distal and anterior surfaces (Fig. 13-7). The chisel for the blade plate is inserted parallel to the summation guide

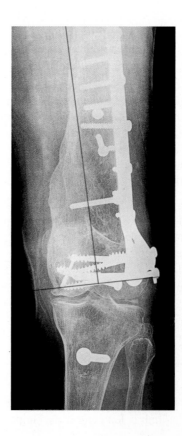
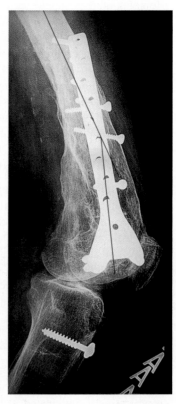

FIGURE 13-2

X-rays of a 78-year-old female who had sustained a left distal femoral fracture 18 years prior to knee replacement. There is a retained condylar buttress plate on the distal lateral femur. There is a 10-degree varus and 20-degree antecurvatum malunion of the old fracture. The knee has degenerative changes with varus malalignment. Templating for a total knee arthroplasty without a corrective femoral osteotomy indicated that a very asymmetric distal femoral resection would be necessary to correct the mechanical axis to neutral. The preoperative plan was for femoral osteotomy at the level of the malunion, with simultaneous total knee arthroplasty with a cruciate-retaining implant.

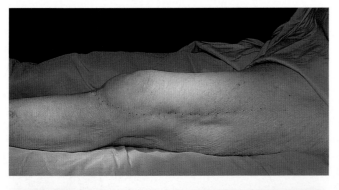

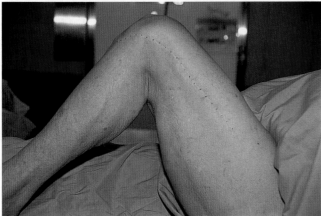

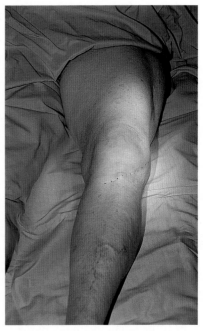

FIGURE 13-3

The preoperative clinical examination was notable for an old lateral surgical scar, motion 5 to 95 degrees, varus deformity at the level of the distal femoral shaft and the knee, and stable knee ligaments.

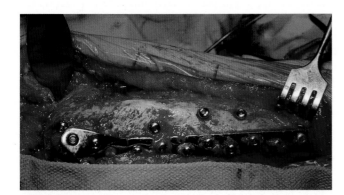

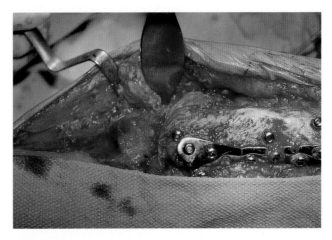

FIGURE 13-4

Under tourniquet control, a lateral subvastus approach to the distal femur has been performed, with exposure of the retained plate.

FIGURE 13-5

The lateral capsule has been opened, and osteotomy of the tibial tubercle has been performed. The entire extensor mechanism can be retracted medially for exposure of the distal femur and the knee joint.

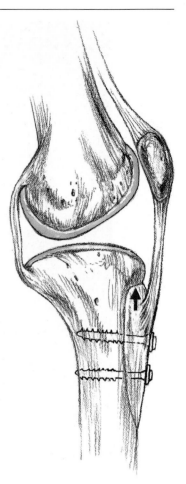

FIGURE 13-6

Diagram of the lateral view of the tibial tubercle osteotomy. The horizontal proximal cut just proximal to the patellar tendon insertion is done with an osteotome. The resulting shelf, upon fixation of the osteotomy, prevents proximal migration from tension provided by the extensor mechanism. The tubercle osteotomy should be about 1 cm deep, curving distally out the anterior cortex. A length of 7.5 cm provides a large surface area for internal fixation and healing. On the medial side of the tibial tubercle, a 0.25-inch osteotome can be placed through two or three small openings in the periosteum to cut through the medial cortex. The tubercle fragment can then be elevated out of its bed in a medial direction. A periosteal elevator is used to strip the soft tissues off the proximal medial tibia in continuity with the tubercle, thereby maintaining vascularity.

wire. It should be inserted sufficiently proximal to the distal articular surface so that the blade plate will not interfere with the pegs or central housing of the femoral component (Fig. 13-8). Instead of being 15 mm from the joint surface, as is recommended for fracture fixation, a distance of 25 mm is necessary to avoid contact with the prosthetic component. Once the tract for the blade has been created, the surgeon performs a femoral osteotomy with a power saw (Fig. 13-9). Most commonly, the osteotomy is at the level of the angular deformity, as was performed in this case. A small wedge of bone is resected from the lateral side for a varus deformity and from the medial side for a valgus deformity so that the osteotomy surfaces will be parallel when the realignment is performed. A 95-degree angled blade plate of appropriate length is inserted into the distal fragment. As the plate is brought into contact with the proximal fragment (femoral shaft), the femur is realigned. The plate is compressed, and the proximal screw holes are filled with cortical screws (Fig. 13-10). At this point in the surgery, the femoral anatomy has been restored to normal. Imaging studies may be performed to confirm hardware placement and alignment.

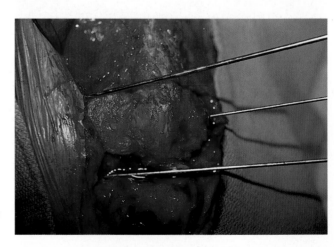

FIGURE 13-7

The three-wire technique is used on the distal femur to place a guide wire that is parallel to the joint surface.

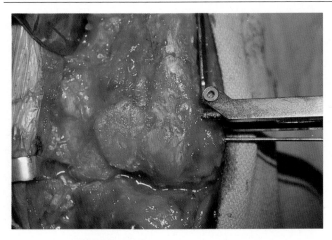

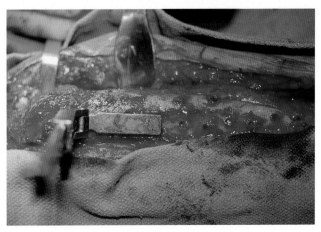

FIGURE 13-8

The chisel for the blade is inserted parallel to the guide wire. Because the femoral implant will extend into the femur, the chisel is placed somewhat more proximally (about 25 mm from the joint surface) than for fracture fixation.

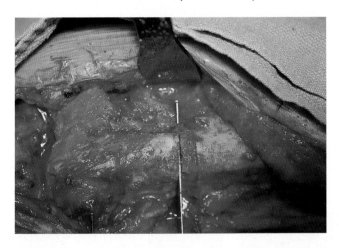

FIGURE 13-9

An osteotomy of the femur is performed, in this case, at the level of the angular malunion. A small lateral wedge is removed for a closing osteotomy.

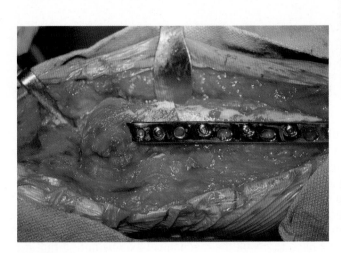

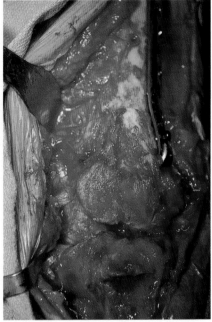

FIGURE 13-10

A 95-degree angled blade plate is then inserted into the chisel tract in the distal femur. The osteotomy is reduced and compressed as the plate is fixed to the femoral shaft.

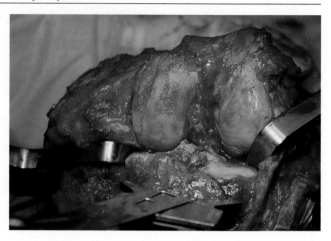

FIGURE 13-11

The proximal tibial resection is performed routinely with an extramedullary cutting guide.

An alternative fixation method is retrograde femoral nailing. The stem on a femoral component may not be sufficient fixation of the femoral osteotomy if used without supplemental plating.

TKA

The tibial resection is performed routinely (Fig. 13-11). On the femoral side, an intramedullary guide system cannot be used because of the hardware. An extramedullary guide system is used to make a proper cut on the distal femur (Figs. 13-12 and 13-13). Computer navigation is now readily

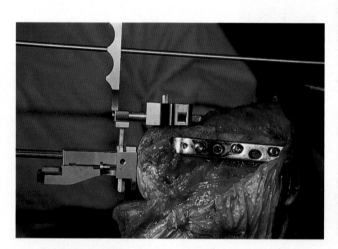

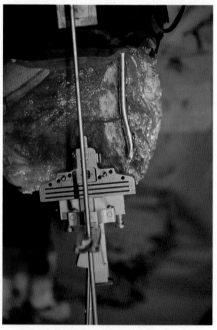

FIGURE 13-12

Because the blade part of the plate blocks placement of a long intramedullary femoral guide rod, an alternative method must be used for placing the distal femoral cutting jig. In this case, a guide is used that has a short post that fits into the distal femoral drill hole and which has an extramedullary rod that extends over the femur. With the femur exposed, the rod can be viewed from the lateral side to be sure the cutting jig will be at 90 degrees so the component will not be flexed or extended. The rod can be viewed from anterior to visually check for a 7-degree valgus alignment of the cutting jig on the distal femur. The rod can also be used to check the mechanical axis by noting that it projects over the center of the femoral head. This can be done with image intensification or by aligning the rod over a palpable marker placed preoperatively on the skin directly over the femoral head.

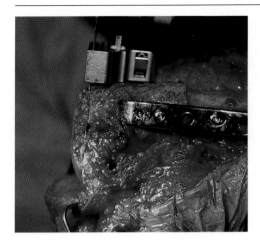

FIGURE 13-13

The distal femoral cut is made with an oscillating saw through the cutting jig.

available and presents a useful method for preparing the distal femur with appropriate coronal, sagittal, and axial alignment when hardware or deformity makes use of standard intramedullary instrumentation impossible. Thereafter, the remainder of the knee arthroplasty is performed in standard fashion. The femur is sized, and the additional femoral cuts are made in proper rotational alignment (Fig. 13-14). The trial implants are placed, and the knee is checked for alignment, motion, stability, and ligament balancing (Figs. 13-15 and 13-16). The prosthetic components are cemented in place (Fig. 13-17).

Closure

The surgeon reattaches the tibial tubercle fragment using two large fragment screws, placed just lateral to the stem of the tibial component (Fig. 13-18). The lateral capsule and quadriceps fascia are closed.

POSTOPERATIVE MANAGEMENT

Because the tibial tubercle osteotomy is securely fixed, early motion of the knee can be started. A continuous passive motion machine and active assisted motion are both used. Because of the femoral osteotomy, weight bearing is limited to touch down for the first 6 weeks until there are radiographic signs of early healing (Fig. 13-19).

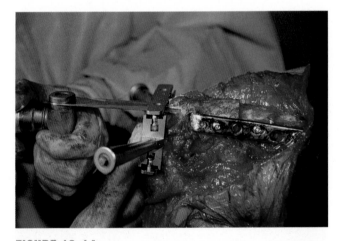

FIGURE 13-14

The additional femoral cuts are made with jig placed in proper rotational alignment.

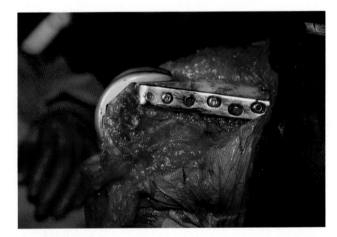

FIGURE 13-15

The trial femoral component is placed.

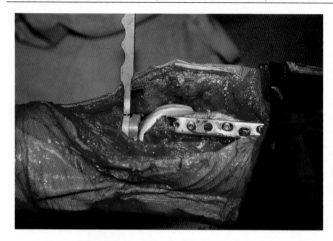
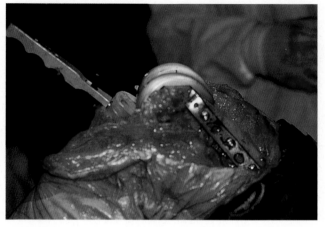

FIGURE 13-16

The knee is checked with trial components to assess extension, flexion, and ligament balancing.

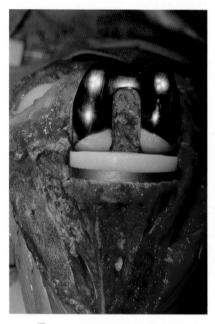
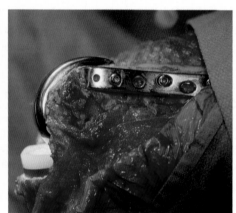
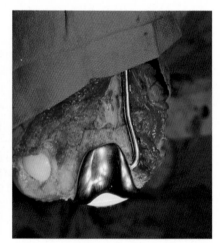

FIGURE 13-17

The implants are cemented into place.

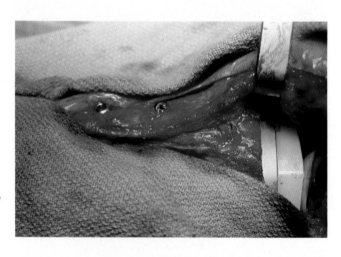

FIGURE 13-18

The tibial tubercle fragment is secured with two large fragment screws placed from anterior to posterior. Because the tubercle is lateral to the midline, it is usually easy to place these screws to the lateral side of the stem of the tibial component.

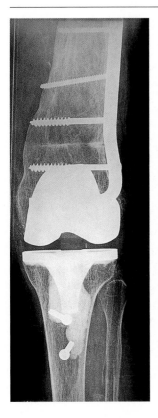
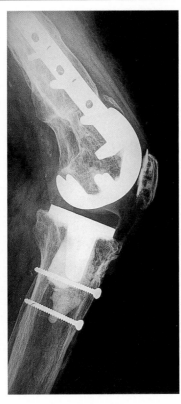

FIGURE 13-19

Post-operative x-rays at 8 weeks after surgery show healing femoral and tibial tubercle osteotomies, normal mechanical and anatomic axes, and a well-positioned and fixed total knee arthroplasty. At 6 months after surgery, the patient was pain-free and full weight bearing. The knee motion was 0 to 110 degrees. The knee had no instability, and quadriceps strength was equal to the opposite side.

COMPLICATIONS

The list of potential complications consists of those that can occur after femoral osteotomy, tibial tubercle osteotomy, and TKA: infection, deep vein thrombosis, nerve palsy, hemorrhage, loss of fixation, nonunion, and stiffness. Because of the exposure involving the quadriceps, there is an increased risk of adhesions and limited flexion. The knee should be followed closely in the early postoperative period for any difficulty with recovery of the expected flexion. It is better to do an early, gentle manipulation than a late, difficult manipulation that may put excessive stress on the tibial and femoral osteotomies.

REFERENCES

1. Austin KS, Siliski JM. Extensile exposure of the knee. In: Siliski JM, ed. *Traumatic Disorders of the Knee.* New York: Springer Verlag; 1994:69–82.
2. Lonner JH, Siliski JM, Lotke PA. Simultaneous femoral osteotomy and total knee arthroplasty for treatment of osteoarthritis associated with severe extra-articular deformity. *J Bone Joint Surg* 2000;82A:342–348.
3. Lonner JH, Pedlow FX, Siliski JM. Total knee arthroplasty for post-traumatic arthrosis. *J Arthroplasty* 1999;14:969–975.
4. Mann JW III, Insall JN, Scuderi GR. Total knee arthroplasty in patients with associated extra-articular deformity. *Orthop Trans* 1997;21:59.
5. Mast J. Nonunions and malunions about the knee. In: Siliski JM, ed. *Traumatic Disorders of the Knee.* New York: Springer Verlag; 1994:369–385.
6. Papdopoulos EC, Parvizi J, Lai CH, Lewallen DG. Total knee arthroplasty following prior distal femoral fracture. *Knee* 2002;9:267–274.
7. Vince KG, Berkowitz R, Spitzer A. Collateral Ligament Reconstruction in Difficult Primary and Revision Total Knee Arthroplasty. Read at the Scientific Meeting of the Knee Society, San Francisco, CA. February 16, 1997.
8. Wolff AM, Hungerford DS, Pepe CL. The effect of extraarticular varus and valgus deformity on total knee arthroplasty. *Clin Orthop* 1991;271:35–51.

14 Managing Patella Problems in Primary Total Knee Arthroplasty

Richard A. Hocking and Steven J. MacDonald

The incidence of postoperative problems and complications with the patella in primary knee replacement has fortunately been significantly reduced with a better understanding of the effects of component position and rotation on patellofemoral mechanics and in particular with the development of femoral components that have been designed to assist patella tracking. However, there remain several specific clinical scenarios in which the patella and/or the extensor mechanism present unique challenges to the reconstructive surgeon. These specific situations are the subject of this chapter.

Modern femoral components have an impact on patellar performance. They are side-specific and have a prominent anatomically designed trochlear groove, which proximally sweeps laterally to capture the patella in extension. The groove then sweeps medially to draw the patella between the medial and lateral condyles as the knee is flexed. Modern designs accommodate the morphology of both the native patella and a prosthetic patella whether the patellar prosthesis is an inlay or an onlay design.

The soft tissues also affect the tracking of the patellar tendon. The ability of the patella to track physiologically is determined by the balance of the forces exerted through the soft tissues around the knee. Manipulating these forces allows the surgeon to balance the patella. Extreme situations such as altered height of the patella, chronic dislocation of the patella, erosion of the patella, or absence of the patella have profound effects on these forces and are the subject of this chapter.

LATERALLY DISLOCATED PATELLA

Indications

On occasion, patients present with a laterally subluxed or chronically dislocated patella, which may be caused by congenital or acquired disorders of the patella. Congenital patella dislocations may occur in patients with Nail-patella syndrome in which there is a small, high patella. The majority of the patellae that present dislocated are acquired dislocations caused by secondary mechanical alignment changes of the limb (usually severe valgus) (Fig. 14-1) and erosions of the patella articular surface (more common in advanced rheumatoid arthritis) (Fig. 14-2A,B). The challenge in these situations is first to reduce the dislocations and then to achieve stability throughout the arc of motion.

Preoperative Preparation

Preoperative evaluation includes thorough history, examination, and radiological investigation. In the history, the nature of the onset and the duration of the dislocation should be sought. Symptoms

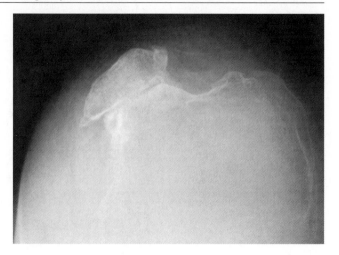

FIGURE 14-1

Sunrise radiograph showing a chronically subluxed patella in a valgus knee.

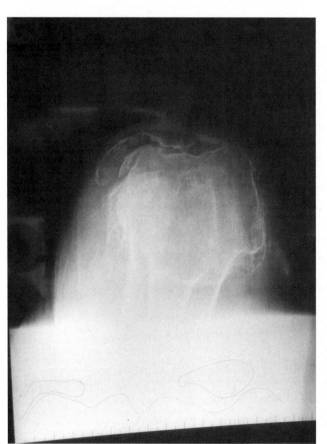

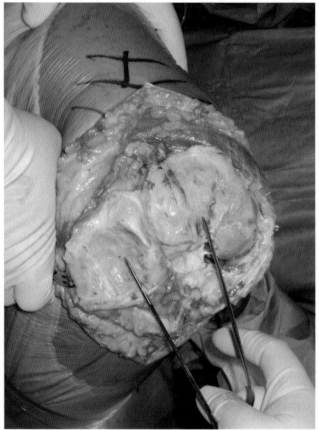

A

B

FIGURE 14-2

(A,B) Preoperative skyline radiograph demonstrates laterally dislocated and extremely thin patella. Clinically, the patient was noted to have less than a 10-mm thick patella with severe erosive changes. It was decided not to resurface the patella because resurfacing would have left the patella extremely thin and at risk for fracture or osteonecrosis. Peripheral osteophytes were removed, and the periphery of the patella was "neurotomized" with an electrocautery. Despite leaving an arthritic and erosive patella, the patient had very little patellofemoral pain after total knee arthroplasty.

of instability, particularly with single-leg weight bearing and loss of power in the affected knee are important to elucidate.

Physical examination should be directed at establishing the position of the patella in relation to varying positions of flexion. Is the patella always dislocated? Is it dislocated only in flexion (suggesting tight lateral structures and a contracted extensor mechanism), or does the patella reduce in deep flexion while being unstable in early flexion (suggesting either patella alta or a poorly formed trochlea)?

Imaging studies should include a standing 3-foot anteroposterior, lateral, and intercondylar views. A skyline view of the patellofemoral joint is also required. In these views, the anatomical and mechanical axes should be determined. The majority of cases with patella dislocation will be in knees with significant valgus deformity. The skyline view usually reveals a shallow or dome-shaped trochlea with a patella that has suffered erosion to conform to the dome-shaped trochlea (Fig. 14-2A). Although magnetic resonance imaging or computer tomography scans can be helpful for assessing the extent of bony erosions preoperatively, this additional information is generally unnecessary as long as the surgeon anticipates erosive changes and plans appropriately.

TECHNIQUE INCLUDING PEARLS AND PITFALLS

The surgeon approaches the knee via a midline incision and medial parapatellar arthrotomy. The medial release is initially kept to a minimum in keeping with the routine valgus knee exposure. An attempt is then made to evert the patella, which may or may not be successful at this stage. If successful, the surgeon continues with the preparation for implanting the tibial and femoral components, paying careful attention to the alignment and rotation of the components (information to follow). If the surgeon is unsuccessful in everting the patella, a decision needs to made as to whether the existing exposure is adequate to correctly orient the femoral and tibial components. If the existing exposure with lateral subluxation/dislocation of the patella without eversion is adequate, I continue with preparation for implantation. If the exposure is inadequate, the exposure needs to be improved by eversion of the patella.

Eversion of the patella may be achieved by performing a lateral release. My preference is to perform the release from inside the knee to outside. The patella is lifted anteriorly with one hand, and using a knife or electrocautery, the tight lateral retinaculum is divided. Initially, the retinaculum is divided immediately adjacent to the patella. An attempt at eversion is made, and if this is not successful, the retinaculum superior and inferior to the patella is palpated for tightness, and the release is extended accordingly. The release is continued until the patella is able to be everted.

The preparation of the proximal tibial and femoral surfaces is completed as outlined in Chapter 5, and coronal soft tissue balancing is addressed as outlined in Chapter 9, after which the patella is addressed. I prefer to resurface the patella with an inlay component (1). The thickness of the patella is determined with calipers. If the patella is less than 12 mm thick, the risk of a fracture either with intraoperative preparation or in the postoperative period is increased, and I will therefore leave that patella unresurfaced (2). I try to maximize the size of the patella button, and I center it on the patella bone to allow for the largest size patella. If the bone stock is adequate, I try to maximally medialize the patella button to enhance patella tracking, using the smallest patellar component possible so as not to compromise the lateral patellar facet if it is very thin and risks fracture. The patella is then reamed to a preset depth to allow seating of the implant inside a rim of bone. With the trial button in place, I remove excess bone using the oscillating saw such that there is a smooth transition from the prosthetic patella to the host patella surface. This creates a dome-shaped structure with the prosthetic patella at the center.

The knee is then put through a range of motion (ROM) with the trial components in place. The corrections to the coronal plane alignment are often all that is necessary to keep the patella balanced, particularly if a lateral release had been done during the approach. If the patella is not reduced at this stage, and a lateral release was not performed earlier, it is performed at this stage, after the tourniquet has been released and patellar tracking has been reassessed (Fig. 14-3) (3). The surgeon performs the release using a scalpel or electrocautery from inside the joint starting with the retinaculum immediately adjacent to the patella and then continuing the release proximally and distally as required. The knee is then put through a ROM, and the stability of the patella is assessed. It is important to distinguish between a patella that tends toward a tilt, versus those that are subluxing or dislocating. If the patella is simply tilting, one or two towel clips are used to approximate the medial arthrotomy closure, and patellar tracking is reassessed. In the vast majority of clinical scenarios, this simple move will resolve the tilt. Rarely, the patella may continue to dislocate as the knee goes into

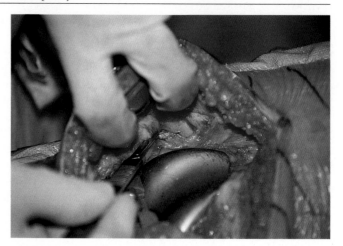

FIGURE 14-3

If the patella subluxes with the trial components in place, a lateral retinacular release is performed from the inside of the capsule, making an attempt to preserve the lateral geniculate vessels.

deeper flexion. The approach then is to tighten the medial side to see whether this will balance the forces across the patella (Fig. 14-4). Vastus medialis obliquus (VMO) advancement is simulated using two sharp towel clips to hold the VMO close to the lateral edge of the patella. The knee is then put through a ROM. This medial advancement should stabilize the patella. Further reinforcement to the medial structures can be achieved with recreation of the medial patellofemoral ligament with either autograft gracilis tendon or allograft tendon, although I have never needed to resort to this reconstruction to stabilize a dislocating patella. Additionally, although medialization of the tibial tubercle has been described for this scenario, I have not had to use that approach to centralize the patella, even in the most extreme cases (4–6).

The definitive components are now implanted. With the knee in extension, the medial parapatellar arthrotomy is closed with the VMO advanced to the position required for patella stability. I use interrupted no. 1 Vicryl sutures to close the quadriceps tendon and retinaculum superior and adjacent to the patella and a continuous suture from the inferior pole of the patella to the tubercle.

Having reduced the chronically dislocated patella, the ROM may be diminished compared with the preoperative range. I do not advocate lengthening the extensor mechanism to improve ROM, as I believe that it may lead to weakness in terminal extension and an extensor lag. I prefer to leave the patient with full power in extension, albeit with a reduced range of flexion, which may improve over time with appropriately aggressive physiotherapy.

POSTOPERATIVE MANAGEMENT

Postoperative management proceeds as per routine total knee replacement. If a lateral release has been performed, this area will be more tender and swollen than normally seen. Flexion is allowed as tolerated. It is important to document clearly the intraoperative flexion achieved to guide the therapist and the patient about what would be a reasonable goal for ultimate knee flexion. For reasons already discussed, these knees do have a tendency to have less flexion than a standard total knee replacement. The patients work with their physiotherapists to improve their flexion while maintaining full extension power through isometric quadriceps contractions. Patients treated with advancement of the VMO may be immobilized for 4 to 6 weeks to protect the repair; however, isometric exercises can be initiated immediately.

COMPLICATIONS

An early concern with any patient undergoing lateral retinacular release is the remote possibility of hematoma or prolonged wound drainage from bleeding from a lateral geniculate vessel. This risk can be reduced by deflating the tourniquet when a lateral release is performed and cauterizing the vessel if transected during the lateral release. A late complication is avascular necrosis of the patella and is identified postoperatively initially by sclerosis and later by fragmentation of the patella. This condition may or may not be symptomatic. Reconstruction may not be possible if the patella fragments and if the patella component loosens. If this should occur and the patient is symptomatic, the loose fragments may require excision, aiming toward retention of the largest remaining fragment, which will now remain unresurfaced within the balanced extensor mechanism.

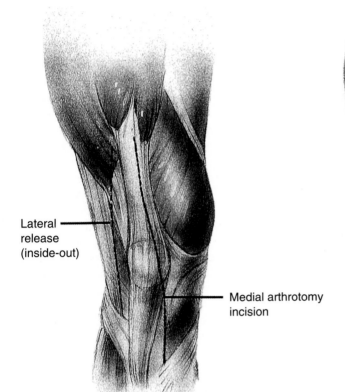

Lateral release (inside-out)

Medial arthrotomy incision

A

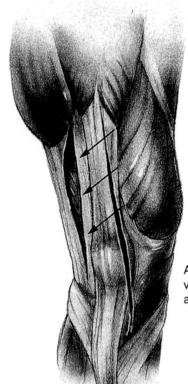

Arrows demonstrate vastus medialis advancement

B

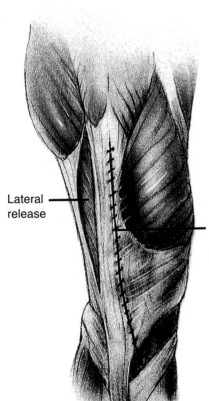

Lateral release

Medial imbrication over 50% to 75% of the width of the quadriceps tendon

C

FIGURE 14-4

(A) Proximal realignment for patellar maltracking. Shown are the medial parapatellar arthrotomy incision and the line of the inside-out lateral retinacular release (*dotted lines*). **(B)** Arthrotomy and lateral release have been performed. **(C)** Reefing of the medial retinaculum on the quadriceps tendon has been performed.

PATELLA BAJA

Indications

Patella baja is defined as an Insall-Salvati ratio (ratio of the patellar tendon length to the length of the patella) of less than 0.8. Patella baja can make exposure to the knee challenging, but the Insall-Salvati ratio neither helps determine how to proceed with surgery nor does it predict whether surgery will be successful in the long term. Many surgeons agree that component positioning has been shown to influence the long-term outcome of total knee replacement, but the absolute anatomic position of the patella is less critical with respect to outcomes, although it can influence function, particularly terminal flexion (7).

The etiology of the patella baja is likely to predict the effect the baja will have on the surgery. Patella baja may be congenital or acquired. In my experience, congenital baja is very rare and has not proved problematic from the perspective of surgical exposure, as these patellae are still often mobile and not scarred from previous surgery. The majority of cases of patella baja I confront are in association with postsurgical changes from either high tibial osteotomies (both lateral closing wedge and medial opening wedge) or tibial tubercle osteotomies performed historically for either patellofemoral instability or arthritis. A specific challenge in these cases is that the patellar tendon can become shortened with decreased mobility and can be quite scarred down and adherent to the anterior tibial surface. The patella tendon has shortened in relation to its previous length, which may lead to problems in exposure, particularly with everting the patella. Occasionally, the tibial tubercle has been moved distal to its original location, but the patella tendon retains its overall length (albeit with the patella in a lower-than- anatomic position), and in these scenarios, achieving adequate exposure to the knee is not usually as difficult.

TECHNIQUE INCLUDING PEARLS AND PITFALLS

I approach the knee with patella baja in the same way as all my primary total knee replacements. I perform a midline incision and a medial parapatellar arthrotomy. I next gain adequate exposure to the knee to allow accurate component positioning. I try to evert the patella in all of my cases. Routinely, I sharply dissect deep to the patella tendon to lift the capsular attachments and retropatellar bursa off the anterior tibia to the tibial tubercle. I perform the same maneuver in the knee with patella baja, gradually releasing scar tissue as required until my exposure allows patellar eversion. If following these soft tissue releases I still am unable to evert the patella, however, I will simply subluxate it laterally and perform the femoral and tibial cuts. Once these cuts are performed, the overall soft tissue tension in the knee is significantly reduced, and the patella should be able to be everted. If the surgeon is still struggling, a quadriceps snip could be performed to assist in exposure, but in my experience, that is not necessary unless one is insistent on everting the patella at the beginning of the case. If having performed the quadriceps snip I was still struggling for exposure, I would then perform a tibial tubercle osteotomy. Although this would be my plan, I have not encountered a case of patella baja in which I have needed to perform a tibial tubercle osteotomy because I was not able to gain adequate exposure to accurately implant the components of a primary total knee arthroplasty (TKA).

The next decision to make is how to deal with the patella itself. As previously stated, I resurface all patellae with adequate bone stock, so that is also my plan in cases of patella baja. If the patella is only moderately inferior in its location, then a routine resurfacing technique will suffice. With excessive baja, I will purposely use a smaller patellar button in a more superior location and an oscillating saw to remove the inferior portion of the patella that is impinging on the tibial tray. This can only be done if using an inlay patellar component, because it will have retained bone and cartilage distal to the patellar button. It is not feasible if an onlay patellar component is used, as the patellar resection typically is down to the level of attachment of the quadriceps or patellar tendons. Obviously, this technique allows you to only remove a few millimeters of bone, but I have found it a reproducible technique to gain a few extra degrees of flexion, before impingement between the patellar button and the tibial component (Fig. 14-5). Be careful not to jeopardize the attachment of the patellar tendon on the inferior pole of the patella.

Additionally, depending on which implant system you are using, some of the manufacturers now have high-flexion polyethylene options, which have a small recessed area anteriorly in the polyethylene to potentially allow greater flexion (Fig. 14-5). Although they may or may not actually achieve improved flexion, using those polyethylene options in the setting of patella baja creates more clearance anteriorly, once again minimizing the component to component impingement. Lastly, many times with

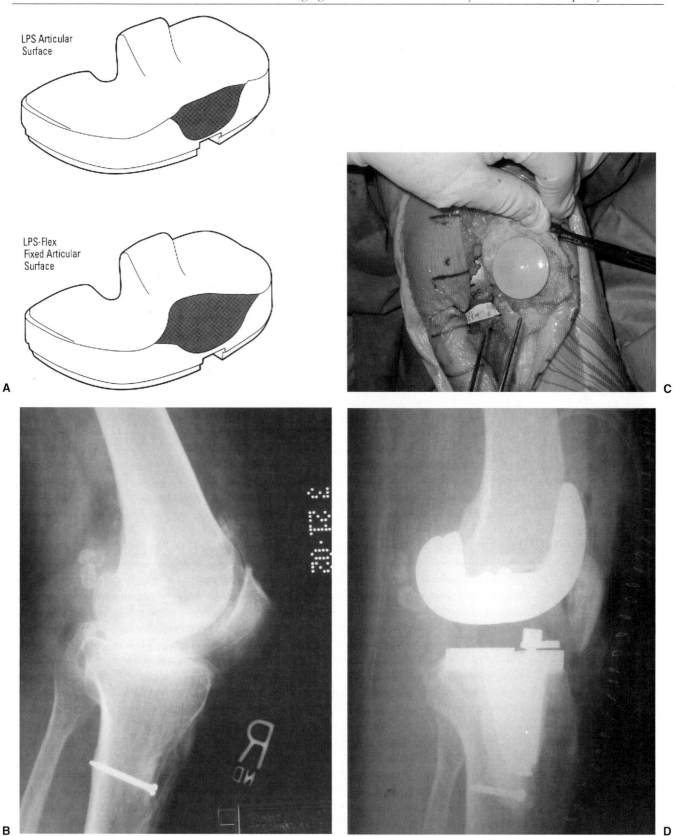

FIGURE 14-5

(A) Newer polyethylene inserts that accommodate high flexion are useful for patella baja because they have dished out anterior surfaces. **(B)** Preoperative radiograph demonstrates significant patella baja secondary to previous patellar realignment. **(C)** The patellar button is placed along the superior edge of the patella, and a dished-out polyethylene component is used. **(D)** Despite these efforts, there is still impingement of the patella on the polyethylene insert of the tibia, although the patient is asymptomatic.

baja, even after all of the techniques described have been performed, the surgeon will still see patellar-tibial component impingement in deep flexion. In my experience, these patients do not experience any pain in that location, and it is not a substantial clinical concern. For that reason, I would specifically not recommend doing anything more extensive, such as moving the extensor mechanism proximal with a tibial tubercle proximalization.

POSTOPERATIVE MANAGEMENT

There is no difference in the postoperative rehabilitation for patients with patella baja other than once again carefully documenting the intraoperative flexion you are able to achieve and communicating that to the therapist and the patient. If the patella component impinges on the polyethylene of the tibial component, it may be prudent to advise the patient to restrict excessive flexion.

Complications

In my experience, patients with patella baja are at no higher risk of complications than my routine total knee replacement patients. Care must be taken during the surgical exposure, however, to protect the patellar tendon attachment on the tibial tubercle, as it is at increased risk for avulsion.

Patellar Erosion

Patellar erosion is most common in patients with severe chronic erosive rheumatoid arthritis and chronic lateral patellar subluxation or dislocation. On radiographs, the patella is often subluxed or dislocated laterally (Fig. 14-2A,B). In patients with long-standing "burnt-out" rheumatoid arthritis, the patella may be elongated in the medial and lateral dimensions, with large flowing lateral osteophytes and apparent lateral subluxation. The patellar preparation is addressed as detailed in the section in this chapter on chronic patellar dislocation. Overaggressive preparation may put the patella at risk for fracture or potentially jeopardize the attachments of the quadriceps or patellar tendons. Therefore, I often opt to remove osteophytes and leave the patella unresurfaced if the bone is less than 12 mm thick. An alternative approach is to use a porous metal prosthesis that encourages bone ingrowth into the trabecular metal surface that is reamed into the deficient patellar bone and secured around the periphery with heavy suture (Fig. 14-6A–D). The polyethylene button is then cemented into the lug holes of the trabecular metal face. Early results have been encouraging with this technique (8).

POSTPATELLECTOMY TOTAL KNEE REPLACEMENT

It is not uncommon for patients who have had a patellectomy in the past to develop tibiofemoral arthrosis and ultimately require a TKA. The postpatellectomy knee will often present with either a fixed flexion contracture or an extensor lag. Noting the presence of these preoperative conditions is important for intraoperative choices and to direct postoperative rehabilitation.

Some authors have suggested techniques for recreating a patella in TKA postpatellectomy (9). This has not been my practice, and only short-term follow-up with a limited number of cases have been reported to date with those reconstructive techniques. My aims are no different in this clinical scenario than others—to perform a well-aligned, well-balanced knee arthroplasty but also paying particular attention to extensor mechanism tracking.

PREOPERATIVE PREPARATION

I choose to use posterior cruciate-substituting (PS) knees for all of my primary knee arthroplasties. Literature supports the use of PS knees when there has been a patellectomy. Thus, if you routinely use a cruciate-retaining knee for your primary total knee replacement, I recommend using a PS knee when confronted with a post-patellectomy knee. The extensor mechanism function, by virtue of the previous patellectomy, is compromised, and patients may already be experiencing symptoms of tibiofemoral instability. A PS replacement may aid in providing an additional restraint to instability.

TECHNIQUE INCLUDING PEARLS AND PITFALLS

I utilize the previous longitudinal incision that was used for the patellectomy. If the previous incision was horizontal, I traverse the scar with a standard longitudinal midline skin incision. I then perform

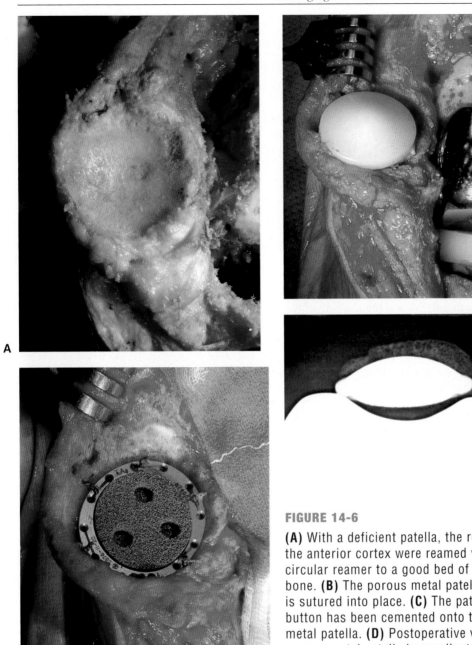

FIGURE 14-6

(A) With a deficient patella, the remnants of the anterior cortex were reamed with a circular reamer to a good bed of cortical bone. **(B)** The porous metal patellar button is sutured into place. **(C)** The patellar button has been cemented onto the porous metal patella. **(D)** Postoperative view of the porous metal patella in excellent position and stable at the 1-year follow-up. The patient has no anterior knee pain and remains comfortable.

my superficial dissection lifting the fat and loose connective tissue off the extensor mechanism. As previously described, using a sterile marking pen, I make a transverse mark at the distal extent of the VMO to assist with accurate closure. Next, I perform a medial-sided arthrotomy in the same fashion as if the patella had not been removed. Beginning proximally, the quadriceps tendon is divided longitudinally leaving a 0.5-cm cuff for later repair. At the VMO distal margin, the arthrotomy curves medially (concave laterally) as it would if the patella were still present such that there is a wide tendon remaining undivided in the femoral trochlea. The incision curves around medial to the medial edge of the patella tendon and continues toward the tibial tubercle. The proximal tibial soft tissue releases are performed in the usual fashion.

If an effort is not made to recreate a neopatella, the femoral component can be flexed slightly or marginally anteriorized to enhance the lever arm and improve the efficiency of the extensor mechanism (Fig. 14-7). Following femoral and tibial preparation, the trials are positioned, and the tracking of the extensor mechanism should be checked. The divided extensor mechanism may be

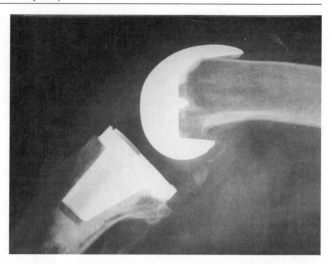

FIGURE 14-7

When performing a total knee arthroplasty after patellectomy, the femoral component can be flexed slightly to try to enhance the lever arm and improve the efficiency of the extensor mechanism.

approximated by either a sharp towel clip or a single figure-of-eight no. 1 Vicryl suture. The knee is passed through a ROM, and the tracking of the extensor mechanism is assessed. Implantation and closure occurs as for other primary total knee replacements. If a patient is noted preoperatively to have an extensor lag, however, I will attempt to tighten the extensor mechanism by intentionally malaligning the markings made on the tissues noted previously. Specifically, the extensor mechanism markings are reapproximated to an area more proximal on the medial arthrotomy tissue than the original marking location.

POSTOPERATIVE MANAGEMENT

Postoperatively, the physiotherapists are advised to work on maintaining full passive and active extension. Quadriceps-strengthening exercises are encouraged.

COMPLICATIONS

Extensor lag and terminal instability caused by quadriceps weakness are complications of the post-patellectomy total knee replacement.

RESULTS

Postoperative knee scores for patients who have had previous patellectomies are lower than seen in patients who have not had patellectomies. It should be emphasized, however, that both pain and function scores improve significantly compared to preoperative scores. Several investigators have compared PS to CR knees, and a consistent finding has been that PS knees have had more predictable results than CR knees. The number of years postpatellectomy has also been a factor found to positively predict results, with the longer time postpatellectomy predicting improved results (10–12).

CONCLUSION

This chapter has discussed the basic biomechanics of the patella and the extensor mechanism as it relates to TKA design and additionally to some of the unique challenges facing the arthroplasty reconstructive surgeon. Although I have discussed my preferred approach to the problems outlined, there are also other alternatives available. Regardless of the specific techniques used, adhering to the basic goals of total knee reconstruction—correct alignment and balancing—will provide consistent results, even in these very challenging cases.

REFERENCES

1. D'Lima DD, Chen PC, Kester MA, et al. Impact of patellofemoral design on patellofemoral forces and polyethylene stresses. *J Bone Joint Surg Am* 2003;85-A(suppl 4):85–93.
2. Burnett RS, Bourne RB. Indications for patellar resurfacing in total knee arthroplasty. *Instr Course Lect* 2004;53:167–186.

3. Benjamin J, Chilvers M. Correcting lateral patellar tilt at the time of total knee arthroplasty can result in overuse of lateral release. *J Arthroplasty* 2006;21:121–126.

4. Bullek DD, Scuderi GR, Insall JN. Management of the chronic irreducible patellar dislocation in total knee arthroplasty. *J Arthroplasty* 1996;11:339–345.

5. Hanssen A, Rand J. Management of the chronically dislocated patella during total knee arthroplasty. *Techniques Orthop* 1988;3:49–56.

6. Hudson J, Reddy VR, Krikler SJ. Total knee arthroplasty for neglected permanent post-traumatic patellar dislocation—case report. *Knee* 2003;10:207–212.

7. Meneghini RM, Ritter MA, Pierson JL, et al. The effect of the Insall-Salvati ratio on outcome after total knee arthroplasty. *J Arthroplasty* 2006;21:116–120.

8. Nelson CL, Lonner JH, Lahiji A, et al. Use of trabecular metal patella for marked patella bone loss during revision total knee arthroplasty. *J Arthrop* 2003;7(suppl):37–41.

9. Busfield BT, Ries MD. Whole patellar allograft for total knee arthroplasty after previous patellectomy. *Clin Orthop Relat Res* 2006;450:145–149.

10. Joshi AB, Lee CM, Markovic L, et al. Total knee arthroplasty after patellectomy. *J Bone Joint Surg Br* 1994;76:926–929.

11. Martin SD, Haas SB, Insall JN. Primary total knee arthroplasty after patellectomy. *J Bone Joint Surg Am* 1995;77:1323–1330.

12. Paletta GA, Laskin RS. Total knee arthroplasty after a previous patellectomy. *J Bone Joint Surg Am* 1995;77:1708–1721.

15 Use of a Varus-Valgus Constrained but Nonhinged Prosthesis for Ligament Insufficiency in Primary Total Knee Arthroplasty

Paul F. Lachiewicz

INDICATIONS

The prevention and management of instability after primary total knee arthroplasty (TKA) are important issues. Instability is a common mechanism of failure and need for revision after primary TKA. In one series of 440 revisions, 63% failed within 5 years, and instability was the reason for failure in 27% (1). In another study of 212 revisions, instability was the mechanism of failure in 21% of cases (2). Instability was the second most common mode of early failure and the third most common mode of late failure (2). Instability may be categorized as flexion instability, varus-valgus instability in extension, and global instability. Flexion instability may be a result of attenuation, rupture, or overrelease of the posterior cruciate ligament (PCL) with PCL-retaining prosthetic components (3). It may also occur with posterior cruciate substituting, rotating, bearing, and so-called deep-dish prostheses caused by improper gap balancing in flexion, undersizing of the femoral component, excessive posterolateral corner and lateral soft tissue releases, or poor design of the tibial spine (4).

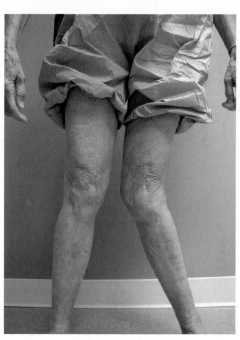

FIGURE 15-1

Preoperative photograph of the legs of an 86-year-old woman with instability of the left knee.

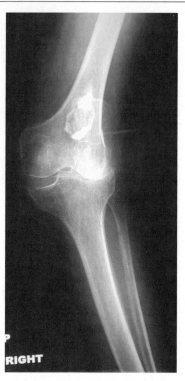

FIGURE 15-2

Preoperative radiograph measures 34 degrees of anatomical valgus alignment. There is medial gapping, suggesting incompetence of the medial collateral ligament.

There are numerous indications for the use of varus-valgus constrained (nonhinged) components in primary TKA. The most common indication is the arthritic knee, usually in an elderly, osteopenic female patient, with severe valgus deformity and attenuation or functional absence of the medial collateral ligament (MCL) (Fig. 15–1) (5). These knees usually have a valgus deformity of 20 degrees or greater (Fig. 15-2). In all patients with a preoperative valgus deformity, the author's primary goal is a balanced, stable knee in 4 to 6 degrees valgus alignment. In knees with fixed deformities, ligament balancing, with release of contracted structures on the concave side of the deformity, is performed (6). The author routinely uses a posterior cruciate substituting prosthesis for primary TKA. Spacer bars are used to check varus-valgus stability after bone resection and appropriate ligament release. The author implants the varus-valgus constrained components only if the MCL cannot be tensioned properly. The author has no experience with MCL advancement or grafting in primary TKA (7,8). The presence of a screw or staple at the origin or insertion of the MCL on preoperative radiographs should raise the surgeon's suspicion that this ligament may be incompetent once the bone resections are performed. Iatrogenic damage transection of the MCL or lateral collateral ligament can infrequently occur during primary TKA. The collateral ligaments may be especially vulnerable during proximal tibial or posterior femoral condylar resections. It has been reported that primary repair of the MCL can be successful in knees with retention of the PCL (9). The author, however, uses a varus-valgus constrained component in this clinical situation as, in his opinion, suture repair of the collateral ligament is unreliable and avoids the need for postoperative bracing. The other disorders and diagnoses for which a varus-valgus constrained component may be necessary are listed in Table 15-1 (Figs. 15-3 and 15-4).

In these clinical situations, the author initially attempts to perform a posterior cruciate-substituting prosthesis if at all possible. If one or both collateral ligaments appear incompetent, however, the author proceeds with the varus-valgus constrained components rather than prolonged postoperative immobilization or bracing.

TABLE 15-1. Possible Indications for Varus-Valgus Constrained Components

- Severe valgus deformity (incompetent medial collateral ligament)
- Posttraumatic arthritis
- Advanced rheumatoid arthritis
- Iatrogenic damage to medial collateral ligament
- Charcot and "pseudo-Charcot" arthropathy (Fig. 15-3)
- Paget's disease (Fig. 15-4)
- Poliomyelitis
- Hemophiliac arthropathy

CONTRAINDICATIONS

Varus-valgus constrained components should not be implanted if the MCL and lateral collateral ligaments are intact and the knee is able to be balanced in both flexion and extension. With certain implant systems, however, a posterior stabilized (rather than constrained) tibial polyethylene liner may be used if the constrained condylar components are deemed necessary because of bone deficiencies of the distal femur or proximal tibia. The major contraindication to the use of these components is complete absence of either collateral ligament or deficiency of the medial epicondyle or medial femoral condyle, such that even a constrained condylar component will not provide stability. In such cases, a hinged-linked prosthesis may be required (10,11). However, this situation should be very unusual in primary TKA.

TECHNIQUE

Patients with ligament insufficiency and a knee deformity that will require a varus-valgus constrained TKA are generally not candidates for a "mini-incision" approach. A thigh tourniquet set at 100 mm Hg above systolic blood pressure is routinely used. The author uses a 15- to 18-cm midline skin incision and a medial parapatellar capsular approach.

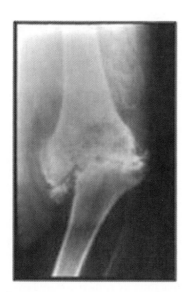

FIGURE 15-3

Patient with Charcot's arthropathy and severe bone loss and multiplanar instability.

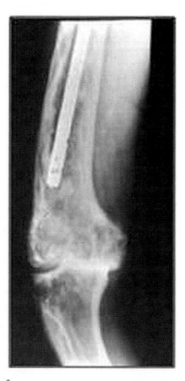

FIGURE 15-4

Patient with Paget's disease and medial collateral ligament incompetence.

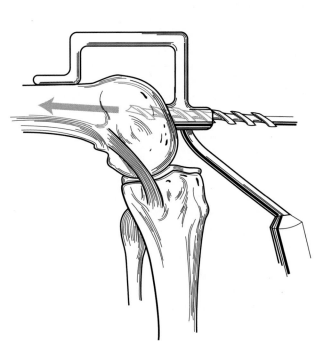

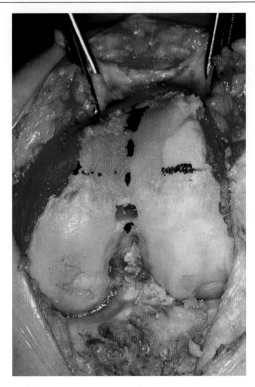

FIGURE 15-5

After exposure of the knee, the medullary canal of the distal femur is entered using an anterior referencing jig.

FIGURE 15-6

Line representing Whiteside's lines indicating the anteroposterior axis. The epicondylar axis of the distal femur is marked, and the initial anterior femoral resection is performed.

After exposure of the knee and removal of periarticular osteophytes, the surgeon drills the medullary canal of the distal femur using an anterior referencing jig (Fig. 15-5). Using the so-called Whiteside's line, the correct rotational alignment for the femoral component (epicondylar axis) is marked with methylene blue (Fig. 15-6) (12). Using a long intramedullary rod, the femoral jig is applied perpendicular to Whiteside's line (anteroposterior axis of the femur, from the low point of the trochlear groove to the high point of the intercondylar notch) or parallel to the epicondylar axis (a line from the medial epicondylar sulcus to the lateral epicondyles), and the initial anterior osteotomy is completed. The distal femur is resected at 6 degrees of valgus to match the angle of the stem housing of the constrained condylar femoral component (Fig. 15-7). The anterior to posterior size of the distal femur is measured using a sizing jig, and the surgeon selects the closest size component that will not overhang (Fig. 15-8). The next femoral jig is placed, and the posterior condylar and final anterior resections are performed (Fig. 15-9). The proximal tibia is then resected perpendicular to the long axis of the tibial shaft, using an extramedullary cutting jig. Balancing of the knee at 90 degrees of flexion and full extension is assisted by the use of spacer bars. In general, these knees with severe valgus deformity and ligament insufficiency will have tight lateral structures. A "pie-crusting" lateral ligament release is performed first, with cautery of the inferior lateral geniculate artery (6). Occasionally, additional release of the popliteus tendon and lateral collateral ligament from the lateral femoral condyle may be required (see Chapter 9).

If appropriate tensioning of the MCL cannot be achieved, the author proceeds with the constrained condylar components. The proximal tibia is prepared first using a cutting-drilling jig aligned with the medial border of the tibial tubercle, and a trial component is placed (Fig. 15-10A,B). For the distal femur preparation, the author first places a 10-mm reamer rod completely up the femoral medullary canal (Fig. 15-11). The first femoral intercondylar preparation jig is then centered over this rod. After the jig is pinned, the 10-mm rod is removed, and the distal femoral intercondylar region is reamed to 16 mm for the "housing" of the constrained condylar femoral component. The distal femoral medullary canal is sized for the appropriate diameter 100-mm femoral stem extension (5). The trial

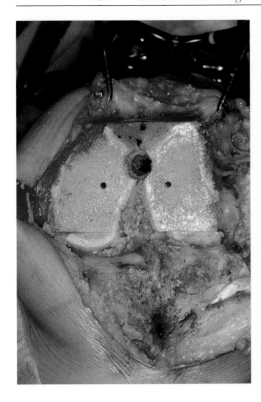

FIGURE 15-7

Distal femoral resection (6 degrees of valgus) is then performed.

stem extension is placed on the second femoral intercondylar jig, which is then placed into the distal femur and pinned anteriorly (Fig. 15-12). The intercondylar box resection and anterior/posterior chamfer resections are performed with a reciprocating saw (Fig. 15-13). (The second jig is then removed, and the trial femoral component with stem extension is inserted.) Trial reduction is performed using the appropriate tibial polyethylene thickness based on the spacer bar thickness. The knee should come into full extension and flex to at least 105 degrees. The flexion and extension gaps should be balanced. Preparation for the patella component and trial patellofemoral tracking is then performed using standard techniques.

The tibial component with its short (35 mm) stem extension and the femoral component with usually a 100-mm stem extension are put together on the back table with clean gloves. After standard bone preparation with pulsatile lavage, the entire tibial component is cemented first, followed by the

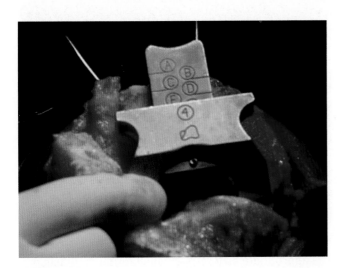

FIGURE 15-8

A sizing jig is used to measure the correct anterior-to-posterior dimension of the femoral component.

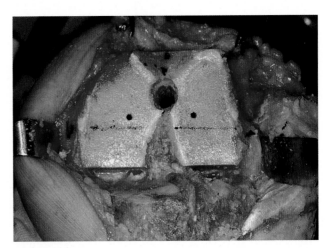

FIGURE 15-9

Posterior (first), then final anterior resections of distal femur are performed.

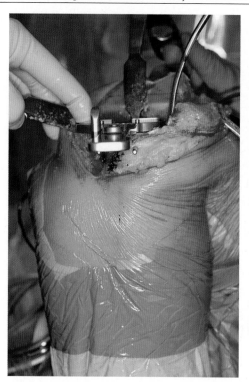
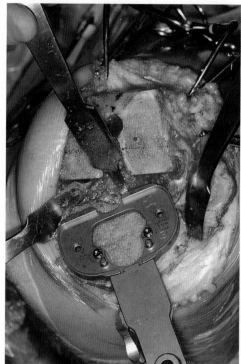

FIGURE 15-10

(A) For proper rotation, the trial plate for the tibial component is aligned with the medial border of the tibial tubercle. **(B)** The tibial plate is fixed with two pins.

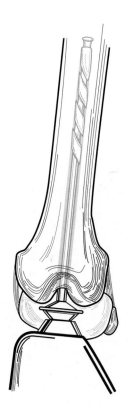

FIGURE 15-11

After the decision has been made to proceed to constrained condylar prosthesis, a 10-mm reamer rod is placed deeply into the femoral medullary canal.

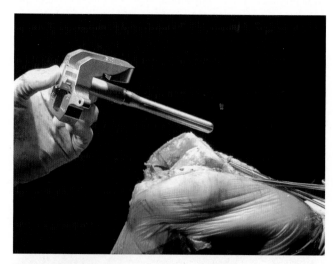

FIGURE 15-12

The appropriate size stem extension trial is attached to the intercondylar jig and placed into the distal femur. Generally, a 100-mm stem extension is used for the femoral component.

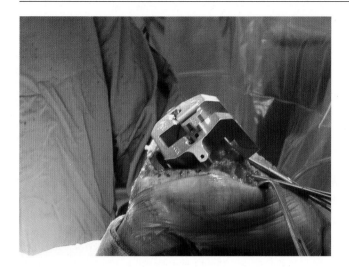

FIGURE 15-13

After two anterior fixation pins are placed in the femur, the stem extension trial is removed.

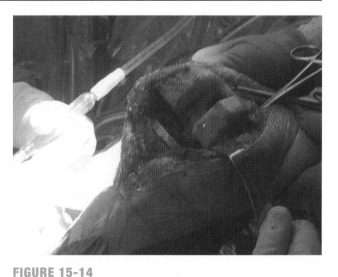

FIGURE 15-14

The distal femoral preparation is completed. The tibial plate trial with "stubby" stem extension has already been inserted. Reduction with trial components is then performed.

patella component and the femoral component. The stem extension of the femoral component is not routinely cemented unless there is deficiency of the medial or lateral femoral condyles (5). After cement polymerization, the tibial polyethylene is inserted into the tray, fixed with a locking screw using a torque wrench, and the knee is reduced (Fig. 15-14). A drain is placed, and capsular closure is performed with nonabsorbable sutures.

POSTOPERATIVE MANAGEMENT

A sterile compression dressing is used around the knee, with calf-length support hose and a rapid-inflation calf pneumatic compression device (Venaflow; DJO, Vista, CA). A hinged knee brace or knee immobilizer is not used unless there has been a serious injury to the extensor mechanism of the knee. A continuous passive motion machine, initially set at 0 to 40 degrees of flexion, is begun on the first postoperative day, for 1 hour three times daily. A physical therapist assists the patient with transfer activities and ambulation. The drain is removed at 24 to 48 hours. The dressing is changed on postoperative day 3 or 4, prior to discharge. Patients use a walker or crutches and progress to a cane at 4 weeks postoperatively. Knee manipulation is rarely necessary after a constrained condylar knee arthroplasty.

COMPLICATIONS

Tibial Postbreakage/Wear

Varus-valgus constrained components allow little (1 to 2 degrees) or no rotation with flexion-extension of the knee (13). Because of this, it is crucial to obtain the proper rotational alignment of both femoral and tibial components when using varus-valgus constrained components. The author has successfully used Whiteside's line for rotational alignment of the femoral components (12). There is some controversy about using a fixed anatomic structure for rotational alignment of the tibial component; however, the author has routinely aligned the rotation of the tibial component with the medial border of the tibial tubercle. After trial reduction of the knee, the lower leg and foot should not have excessive internal or external rotatory deformity, and the patella prosthesis should track without tilt or subluxation. If either of these are present, the rotational alignment of the components should be rechecked. If these are accurate, a lateral retinacular release is performed to centralize the patella.

Breakage of the tibial post of varus-valgus constrained components has been rarely reported (14). Most cases involve revision rather than primary arthroplasty. Tibial post-breakage could be more frequent in knees that are not properly balanced or are unstable with stress testing in extension. It has been suggested that tibial postwear debris may be responsible for osteolysis after TKA, but this may be more related to the tibial base plate design and polyethylene locking mechanism (13).

Dislocation

Varus-valgus constrained component could theoretically dislocate with a hyperflexion-valgus maneuver if the knee is not balanced (left excessively loose in flexion). This should be avoided by proper ligament balancing at 90 degrees of flexion.

Patella Problems

Because varus-valgus constrained components allow little or no rotation with flexion-extension of the knee (13), the patellofemoral joint and patella may also be subjected to greater shear forces than less constrained prostheses. With excessive lateral ligament releases, the patella could theoretically become devascularized with late fragmentation, from osteonecrosis or fracture (5). Patella subluxation, bony or soft tissue crepitus, or residual patella pain may occur with both posterior stabilized and varus-valgus constrained components (5). It may be related to femoral component design or residual unresected peripatellar soft tissue. Observation and palpation of the patellofemoral joint during the trial reduction is important to prevent this complication.

RESULTS

There are few recent published reports on the results of primary repair of disruption of the MCL or medial reconstructions for severe valgus deformity in primary TKA. In a series of 600 primary total knee arthroplasties at one center, there were 16 knees with intraoperative disruption of the MCL treated with primary repair (9). Twelve knees had PCL-retaining prostheses, and four had posterior-stabilized prostheses. All patients wore a hinged knee brace for 6 weeks. At a mean follow-up time of 45 months, there were no revisions, and all knees regained normal stability. In a series of eight patients with a mean preoperative valgus deformity of 22 degrees (range, 15 to 30 degrees), MCL advancement with a bone plug-suture technique was performed with a posterior cruciate- retaining prosthesis (7). Varus-valgus constrained prostheses were not available for use at that institution during that time. At a mean follow-up time of 6 years (range, 4 to 9 years), all knees were stable, and there were no revisions. A long leg brace for at least 6 weeks is mandatory with this reconstruction. Currently, this technique is recommended only for severe valgus knees in "younger, more active patients." To our knowledge, there are no published reports of this technique in such a patient population.

There are a wide variety of designs of varus-valgus constrained prostheses. At least 12 implant companies manufacture at least 22 different models of varus-valgus constrained (nonlinked) total knee prostheses. It is important to realize that the short- and longer-term results of these prostheses in primary TKA may be design specific. Most published series of these prostheses report the results of the nonmodular Total Condylar III prostheses (Depuy, Johnson & Johnson, Warsaw, IN) (15–19) or the modular constrained condylar Insall-Burstein II prosthesis (Zimmer; CCK, Warsaw, IN) (Figs. 15-15 and 15-16) (5,20). These studies are difficult to analyze because many include both primary and revision arthroplasties, and there is a relatively small number of patients with short-term follow-up. In one series of 17 patients treated with either a TC III or CCK prosthesis for multiplanar instability or severe bone loss in primary TKA, there were no revisions at a mean follow-up time of 5 years (17). Another study reported the results of 44 consecutive primary CCK prostheses in elderly patients with severe valgus deformities. There were no failures in 28 knees followed for a mean of 7.8 years (20). Finally, the author reported the 10-year survival rate of 54 consecutive TC III and CCK prostheses in primary TKA (5). With failure defined as revision for component loosening, the 10-year survival rate was 96% (confidence interval, 90.6% to 100%). There was no difference in the clinical or radiographic results between 37 knees in patients age 62 years or older and 17 knees in younger-age patients. There was no knee with a fractured tibial post at a mean follow-up time of 9 years (range, 5 to 16 years), and there was only one knee with osteolysis.

There are no clear advantages of either cemented or uncemented stem extensions for either the femoral or tibial component with varus-valgus constrained prostheses. The author generally uses a 35-mm cemented stem extension for the tibial component and a 100-mm uncemented stem extension for the femoral component (Fig. 15-17). The final choice, however, should be based on periarticular bone quality and the presence of condylar defects.

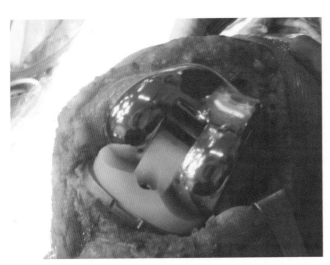

FIGURE 15-15

The components have been inserted, and the knee is reduced.

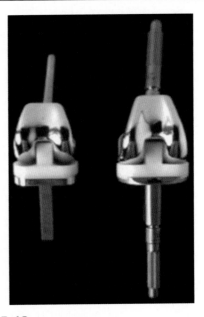

FIGURE 15-16

The nonmodular TCP III prosthesis is on the left, and the modular Insall-Burstein II CCK is on the right.

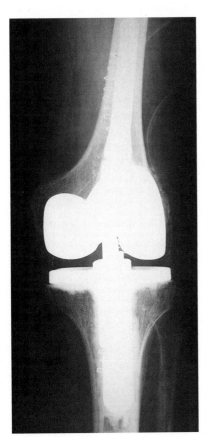

FIGURE 15-17

The postoperative radiograph measures 6 degrees of anatomical valgus alignment.

REFERENCES

1. Fehring TK, Odum S, Griffin WL, et al. Early failures in total knee arthroplasty. *Clin Orthop* 2001;392:315–318.
2. Sharkey PF, Hozack WJ, Rothman RH, et al. Why are total knee arthroplasties failing today? *Clin Orthop* 2002;404:7–13.
3. Waslewski GL, Marson BM, Benjamin JB. Early, incapacitating instability of posterior cruciate ligament-retaining total knee arthroplasty. *J Arthroplasty* 1998;13:763–767.
4. Pagnano MW, Hanssen AD, Lewallen DG, et al. Flexion instability after primary posterior cruciate retaining total knee arthroplasty. *Clin Orthop* 1998;356:39–46.
5. Lachiewicz PF, Soileau ES. Ten-year survival and clinical results of constrained components in primary total knee arthroplasty. *J Arthroplasty* 2006;21:803–808.
6. Mihalko WM, Krackow KA. Anatomic and biomechanical aspects of pie crusting posterolateral structures for valgus deformity correction in total knee arthroplasty: a cadaveric study. *Am J Orthop* 2000;15:347–353.
7. Healy WL, Iorio R, Lemos DW. Medial reconstruction during total knee arthroplasty for severe valgus deformity. *Clin Orthop* 1998;356:161–169.
8. Krackow KA, Madanagopal SG. Managing ligament loss. In: Lotke PA, Lonner JH, eds. *Knee Arthroplasty*, 2nd ed. Philadelphia: Lippincott Williams & Wilkins; 2003:167–193.
9. Leopold SS, McStay C, Klafeta K, et al. Primary repair of intraoperative disruption of the medial collateral ligament during total knee arthroplasty. *J Bone Joint Surg* 2001;83A:86–91.
10. Pour AE, Parvizi J, Slenker N, et al. Rotating hinged total knee replacement: use with caution. *J Bone Joint Surg Am* 2007;89:1735–1741.
11. Westrich GH, Mollano AV, Sculco TP, et al. Rotating hinge total knee arthroplasty in severely affected knees. *Clin Orthop* 2000;379:195–207.
12. Arima J, Whiteside LA, McCarthy DS, et al. Femoral rotational alignment, based on the anteroposterior axis, in total knee arthroplasty in a valgus knee. *J Bone Joint Surg* 1995;77-A:1331–1334.
13. Naudie DD, Rorabeck CH. Managing instability in total knee arthroplasty with constrained and linked implants. *Inst Course Lect* 2004;53:207–215.
14. McPherson EJ, Vince KG. Breakage of a total condylar III knee prosthesis. A case report. *J Arthroplasty* 1993;8:561–563.
15. Chotivichit AL, Cracchiolo A III, Chow GH, et al. Total knee arthroplasty using the total condylar III knee prosthesis. *J Arthroplasty* 1991;6:341–350.
16. Donaldson WF III, Sculco TP, Insall JN, et al. Total condylar III knee prosthesis. Long-term follow-up study. *Clin Orthop* 1988;226:21–28.
17. Hartford JM, Goodman SB, Schurman DJ, et al. Complex primary and revision total knee arthroplasty using the condylar constrained prosthesis: an average 5-year follow-up. *J Arthroplasty* 1998;13:380–387.
18. Lachiewicz PF, Falatyn SP. Clinical and radiographic results of the total condylar III and constrained condylar total knee arthroplasty. *J Arthroplasty* 1996;11:916–922.
19. Sculco TP. Total condylar III prosthesis in ligament instability. *Orthop Clin North Am* 1989;20:221–226.
20. Easley MD, Insall JN, Scuderi GR, et al. Primary constrained condylar knee arthroplasty for the arthritic valgus knee. *Clin Orthop* 2000;380:58–64.

16 Removal of a Well-Fixed Total Knee Arthroplasty

Daniel J. Berry

Removal of a well-fixed total knee arthroplasty component is required in many circumstances during revision total knee arthroplasty. Minimally traumatic removal of implants is essential to preserve critical ligamentous structures and as much good-quality bone as possible to facilitate the subsequent revision. Furthermore, efficient implant removal is essential to allow revision surgery to be performed in a timely manner. Finally, avoiding complications during the implant process removal is also important to optimize the outcome of the revision surgery (1–3).

Methods of implant removal have evolved over the past 3 decades. From a wide variety of techniques, a moderate number of methods have emerged, which most surgeons agree are most successful and efficient. Better instruments have also been developed, which make implant removal simultaneously simpler and more bone sparing.

INDICATIONS AND CONTRAINDICATIONS

Indications for removal of well-fixed total knee arthroplasty components include all circumstances in which an implant must be removed to optimize the results of the subsequent revision. As implant removal techniques have evolved and improved, surgeons have become more willing to remove well-fixed implants to optimize the subsequent reconstruction. That is, surgeons have become less fearful of the drawbacks of removing well-fixed implants and at the same time, have become more conscious of the value of starting with fresh implants that do not compromise options available for the subsequent reconstruction.

Indications for removal of well-fixed implants include the following:

1. Chronic infection in which a one- or two-stage procedure is being planned
2. Revision for implant malposition, in any plane including rotation
3. Revision for problematic implant sizing
4. Revision for knee instability for cases in which a high level of constraint is required
5. Selected cases of revision for bearing surface wear and for osteolysis when prosthetic retention is not desirable
6. Selected cases of periprosthetic fracture that cannot be treated with implant fixation
7. Removal of well-fixed implants to accommodate implants of new design when any other part of the arthroplasty is removed for implant failure of any reason, including loosening
8. Revision of well-fixed but fractured implants

Removal of well-fixed implants is relatively contraindicated when the implant can be preserved at revision surgery without compromising the reconstruction results. In some cases, a well-fixed, well-positioned tibial component that has parts compatible with modern femoral components may be preserved. A well-fixed femoral component may also be preserved in special circumstances; however, it is important to understand that preserving the well-fixed femoral component limits the surgeon's ability to adjust the position of the joint line, and therefore the flexion and extension balance. A well-fixed femoral component can be preserved less frequently than a well-fixed tibial component.

A well-fixed patellar component can often be preserved even when tibial and femoral revision are required. To be retained, the patellar component should not demonstrate severe polyethylene damage and should be reasonably compatible with the geometry of the trochlear groove of the planned new femoral component. Most dome-shaped patellar components articulate sufficiently well with the trochlear groove of most femoral implants to be considered compatible (4).

When the surgeon considers removing any implant, the risks and benefits of the decision must be weighed carefully. The surgeon must consider the following questions: How important is it to remove the implant for the subsequent reconstruction? How much bone is likely to be lost at the time of implant removal? If the anticipated amount of bone is lost, how much will this affect the subsequent revision options and success? What is the likelihood of more bone than expected being lost during implant removal? What is the likelihood of a catastrophic problem occurring during implant removal such as fracture of the major supportive portion of the bone? If major bone loss or a fracture occurs during implant removal, how much will this affect the results of the proposed reconstruction? How much time is implant removal likely to take, and what risk does the extra operative time pose to the individual patient? What benefits are likely to be realized by an implant removal? Are these benefits important enough to justify the risks previously mentioned?

TOOLS AND PREOPERATIVE PLANNING

The preoperative plan should take into account the diagnosis for which the patient is being revised and should include careful consideration of the specific interventions necessary to solve the existing problems with the knee arthroplasty. Before surgery, anticipate which implants will require removal to accomplish the surgical plan, and in turn, have appropriate tools available to accomplish the anticipated implant removal.

Before the surgery, make every effort to identify the specific implants already in place by manufacturer and design. Familiarize yourself with the design of the implants to be removed and methods of implant disassembly. Some implants can be removed much more easily if proper implant disassembly tools or implant-specific removal instruments are on hand, and in such cases, when possible, make arrangements in advance to have these instruments available.

Consider the tools needed for implant removal, including osteotomes, oscillating saws, punches, and universal tibial and femoral implant extraction devices. Also, have available specialized instruments such as high-speed metal cutting instruments and ultrasonic devices for cement removal. When necessary, have available specialized intramedullary cement column removal instruments when cemented stemmed implants must be removed.

As part of the preoperative plan, consider the order in which implants will be removed and have back-up plans available should the initial plan for implant removal fail. Also consider alternative plans if more bone loss than expected occurs during implant removal.

SURGICAL TECHNIQUE

Effective implant removal is based on using specific instruments for specific tasks. The following is a list of commonly used instruments with a discussion of strengths and weaknesses of each.

Hand Instruments

Osteotomes   Osteotomes can be used very effectively to divide the prosthesis-cement interfaces of cemented implants. Osteotomes can also be used effectively in some circumstances to cut uncemented implant-bone interfaces; thin flexible osteotomes are most useful in these cases. Stacked osteotomes can be used as wedges to lift implants out of bone.

Drawbacks of osteotomes include the fact that they can wander away from an implant-bone interface and cause bone destruction. When used as levering devices, osteotomes tend to crush bone, particularly when the bone is soft.

Punches   Good-quality punches are used to exert an axial force to accomplish implant removal. Punches should be used as a means of extracting the implant in most cases only after the implant interfaces have been disrupted. Good-quality punches can help extract well-fixed stems as well as the condylar portions of implants.

Gigli Saws   Gigli saws can be used to cut implants away from bone. These saws allow access to certain interfaces that are difficult to reach with other saws. The main drawback of Gigli saws, which has recently led to their less-frequent use, is their tendency to wander away from prosthesis interfaces and into good-quality bone, which leads to bone loss.

Power Instruments

Power Saws   Power saws efficiently cut both prosthesis-cement interfaces and prosthesis-bone interfaces. Certain saw blades, especially narrow blades and relatively short blades, are particularly helpful. Trying to stay close to the implant with the saw blade is an important aspect of safe and effective use of a power saw. Keep in mind that saw blades can wander away from implant interfaces, and relatively short passes with a saw blade from multiple sides of the implant reduce the risk of the blade wandering far from the implant. Saw blades become dull when used against metal implants and need to be exchanged frequently. "Past pointing" with saw blades can cause damage to soft tissue structures.

Ultrasonic Instruments   Ultrasonic instruments can melt and cut cement (5,6). As such, they are effective for dividing cemented implant-periprosthesis interfaces (7). Ultrasonic instruments can also be used to remove well-fixed intramedullary cement. Drawbacks of ultrasonic instruments include the fact that they create heat and can burn bone, particularly when a tourniquet is inflated, thus lavage should be used in conjunction with ultrasonic instruments (8). Ultrasonic instruments are more expensive than hand instruments, and in some cases, they are not as fast to use as hand instruments.

Metal Cutting Instruments   Metal cutting instruments are essential for certain specific tasks in implant removal. They can facilitate cutting away well-fixed portions of an implant to allow access to other interfaces. They are particularly useful for dividing the well-fixed pegs of an uncemented metal-back patellar component and for removing the condylar portion of the tibial or femoral implant to allow access to underlying well-fixed stems.

IMPLANT REMOVAL

Sequence of Implant Removal

Good exposure is essential for all aspects of revision knee arthroplasty including implant removal. Poor exposure during implant removal increases the risk of soft tissue structure damage and may lead to excessive bone loss. Therefore, establishing adequate exposure before attempted implant removal is important. On the other hand, the surgeon should understand that as implants are successively removed from the knee, more space is created, and exposure is simultaneously facilitated. Details of exposure techniques are discussed in Chapter 32.

In selected cases of partial knee revision, the sequence of implant removal is dictated by the specific implants being removed. In most cases, however, when a full knee revision is being planned, the following sequence of implant removal is most effective.

After knee exposure, remove the polyethylene insert of the tibia, which creates space in the knee and facilitates exposure. Next, remove the femoral component. Once the femoral component is removed, better access to the tibial component is facilitated. Remove the tibial component next, then cement from the canal of the femur or tibia. If necessary, remove the patellar component, usually as a last step. Removing the patellar component as the last step protects the patella—which has thin, easily damaged bone from retractors—during removal of the other components of the arthroplasty.

Removal of the Polyethylene Insert

In most cases, removal of a modular polyethylene insert is simple. Understand the locking mechanism involved. If locking screws, bolts, or pin-type devices are present, remove them, then extract the polyethylene insert. Most polyethylene inserts are removed by levering them out of the tibial tray from anteriorly to posteriorly (with an osteotome or implant-specific device). Some polyethylene inserts are designed to load from the side, however, and if the surgeon is aware of this, the implant can be slid out of the medial side of the tibia once adequate exposure is obtained.

When polyethylene is very difficult to remove from the tibial tray, either in the case of a nonmodular implant or a modular implant that does not disassemble easily, the polyethylene can be cut into pieces with an osteotome or saw and then removed in a piecemeal manner.

Removal of the Well-Fixed Femoral Component

After good exposure of the femoral component, begin by dividing the femoral prosthesis-cement interfaces (9). It is important that the exact metal-cement interface is identified to facilitate removal of the implant without excessive bone loss. Gain very good exposure of the interface itself by removing soft tissues with a small rongeur. Divide the implant-cement interface with an oscillating saw, osteotomes, or thin ultrasonic cutting device (Fig. 16–1A,B). In most cases, start by dividing the bone at the anterior flange, anterior chamfer, and distal cut. The posterior chamfers and posterior condylar portions of the implant may be divided carefully with a narrow osteotome: angled osteotomes are helpful for this particular part of the process, as these portions of the implant are difficult to access.

During the process of dividing interfaces, work from both the medial and lateral side of the implant to avoid having saws or osteotomes wander away from the prosthesis-cement interface. Once the implant interfaces have been divided, disimpact the implant from the femur with a punch against the anterior flange of the implant or with an implant-specific extractor that provides axial force (Fig. 16-2).

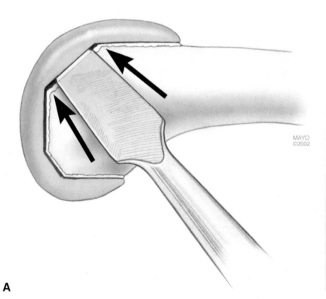

MAYO
©2002

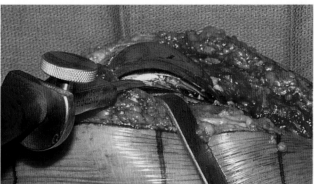

A   B

FIGURE 16-1

(A,B) An osteotome is used to divide/disrupt the prosthesis-cement interface of a well-fixed femoral component.

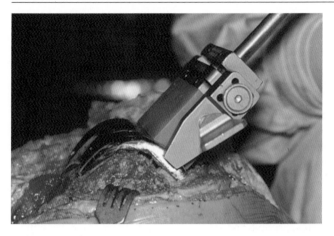

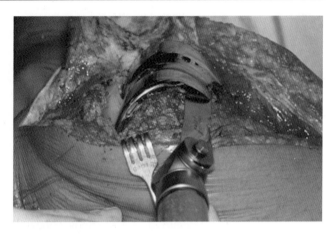

FIGURE 16-2

Disimpaction of a femoral component after division of implant-bone interfaces.

FIGURE 16-3

A saw is used to divide the prosthesis-bone interface.

Avoid excessive force during this process; the need for high forces suggests a portion of the implant remains well fixed, and very aggressive disimpaction may lead to notable bone loss during the implant extraction process.

Once the implant has been taken out, remove the cement from the bone interface with hand instruments or a high-speed burr. If there is any indication of an infection, strive to remove all cement. Be particularly conscientious to look for cement where previous lugs or drill holes may have existed in the femur.

When a posterior stabilized implant with a closed box is in place, recognize that the cemented interface of the box is not easily accessible (10). In most cases, once the remainder of the implant is freed from the cement, the box portion will disengage from the cement without excessive bone loss. Make sure the implant is extracted directly axially (as opposed to at an angle) to reduce the risk of femoral condyle fracture produced by impingement of the box during implant removal.

Removal of the Well-Fixed Uncemented Femoral Component

Many of the same principles of implant removal apply for the uncemented implant as a cemented implant. The uncemented prosthesis-bone interface is most easily divided with oscillating saws (Fig. 16-3). Interfaces that are difficult to access can often be divided with an osteotome. Particularly for bone-ingrown uncemented implants, it is important for the surgeon to make sure that all possible prosthesis-bone interfaces are divided before attempting implant extraction to avoid major bone loss.

Removal of the Cemented Tibial Component

Removal of the cemented tibial component begins by gaining good access to the anterior and medial aspects of the tibial component. Place particular emphasis on gaining good access to the posterior medial aspect of the tibial component by releasing sufficient tissue in this area (such as the postero-medial capsule and semimembranosus tendon) to externally rotate the tibia. As for the femoral component, excellent exposure of the prosthesis-cement interface is essential. Use saws or osteotomes to divide the implant-cement interface. In most cases, stems or pegs on the tibial component to some degree limit access to the posterior aspects of the tibia from instruments inserted from anterior to posterior. Therefore, once the anterior aspects of the interfaces have been divided, work from the posterior medial aspect of the tray, beneath the posterior extent of the tibial component to divide the remaining interfaces. It is important during this process to avoid damage to critical posterior soft tissue structures. Recognize there may be a small portion of the posterior lateral aspect of the tibia that is not always easily divided with instruments inserted from anterior to posterior or from medial to lateral. In most cases, the small remaining cement interface in this area of the implant nevertheless can be debonded safely during axial implant disimpaction.

Once the condylar portion of the tibia has been freed of some of its attachments to cement, the implant usually can be extracted successfully. This implies that the implant will be debonded from the prosthesis-cement interface along the tibial stem or pegs. In selected cases, when rough or porous coated stems are bonded very tightly to cement, debonding cannot be expected to occur. In these cases, alternate techniques may be considered (information to follow).

There are different methods of applying axial load to extract the tibial component, including implant-specific or universal tibial extraction devices. Stacked osteotomes may also be used, as they provide a wedge to lift the tibial component (Fig. 16-4A,B). Use the broadest osteotomes possible against the bone or the cement to avoid crushing tibial bone. Alternatively, a punch may be used to extract the tibial component. The punch can gain purchase against the anterior or medial aspect of the tibial tray. Alternatively, make a small hole in the tibia (either medial or lateral to the tubercle) to facilitate tibial disimpaction with a punch directed at the tibial tray (Fig. 16-5). As the tibial tray is extracted, concentrate on avoiding damage to the bone of the lateral femoral condyle. Hyperflexion of the knee at this stage allows the trajectory of the tibial component to be moved anterior to the femur during extraction, thereby protecting the femoral condyles. The more tibial cement that is left behind with the bone, the better, as this tends to protect the underlying bone. Once the implant is removed, cement removal under direct vision is simple and safe.

Removal of the Well-Fixed Uncemented Tibial Component

Removal of uncemented tibial components follows the same guidelines as removing cemented implants. Like removal of the femoral component, cutting of the uncemented tibial prosthesis-bone interface is most effectively performed with a saw. Difficult-to-access areas can be divided with an osteotome. Be aware that if there are uncemented porous-coated stems in place, disimpaction of stems can cause marked bone loss if bone adheres to the implant. If the stem is against only cancellous bone, in many cases, the implant can be removed with only modest central cancellous bone loss.

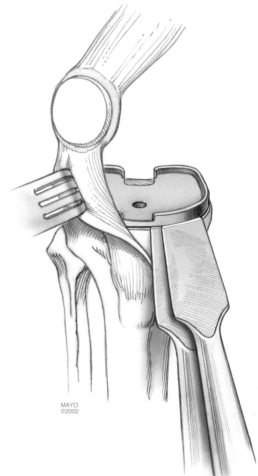

MAYO
©2002

A

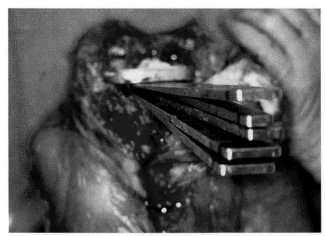

B

FIGURE 16-4

(A,B) Stacked osteotomes may be used to elevate a tibial component away from the bone. The broadest osteotome is used closest to the bone to avoid crushing tibial bone.

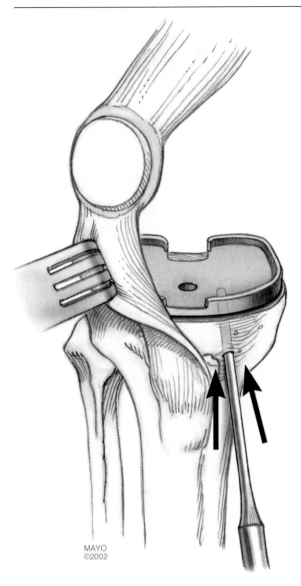

MAYO
©2002

FIGURE 16-5

A punch may be introduced through a small drill hole in the tibia to provide direct axial disimpaction force for tibial component removal.

If the well-fixed stem is against cortical bone and appears to be bone ingrown, however, exert great caution because vigorous disimpaction before all interfaces are divided can lead to removal of a large segmental portion of the tibia. In these cases, direct access to the stem to divide the stem-bone interfaces before stem extraction may be necessary (information to follow).

Removal of Patellar Component

The patella is a small bone, and very little bone loss can be tolerated before reconstruction becomes problematic. Removal of most well-fixed all-polyethylene patellar components is straightforward. Use a saw to divide the patellar polyethylene at the cement interface. Remove underlying cement with hand instruments or a high-speed burr. When a metal-backed patellar component is present, particularly if it is an uncemented implant, avoid the temptation to try to lever the prosthesis away from the bone. Rather, it is safest to use a high-speed diamond cutting wheel to cut the prosthesis away from the bone and away from the fixation pegs (Fig. 16-6) (11). Once the prosthesis has been removed, the fixation pegs may either be left in place (if they will not compromise the subsequent reconstruction) or removed by directly accessing the peg-bone interfaces with a very small high-speed cutting burr (Fig. 16-7).

Removal of Well-Fixed Stems and Well-Fixed Intramedullary Cement

Removal of well-fixed stems of the femoral or tibial component is among the most challenging elements of well-fixed implant removal.

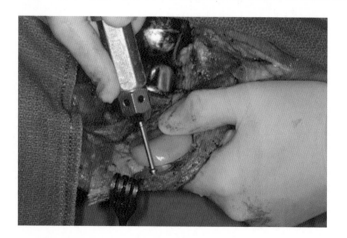

FIGURE 16-6

A diamond wheel may be used to divide the bone-prosthesis interface and fixation pegs of a metal patellar component.

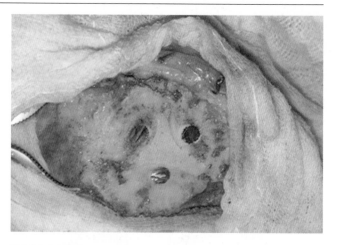

FIGURE 16-7

Metal fixation pegs remaining after the implant is cut away from the patella with a diamond wheel may be removed with a very small burr.

Some stems are designed not to bond to the cement or the bone and can be removed in a straightforward manner. In these cases, the condylar portions of the implant are separated from the bone, and then punches or implant-specific extraction instruments are used to disimpact the condylar part of the femur or tibia, and the stem comes out of the bone with the implant.

In some other cases, however, stems are present with a very rough surface finish, or geometric features such as kinks, slots, or expansions are present that preclude easy removal from cement. Also, in some cases, a porous-coated or rough surface finish uncemented stem may be fixed directly to the bone. When these conditions are present, consider alternate strategies for implant removal because very vigorous axial disimpaction may be unsuccessful or may lead to femoral or tibial fracture. Often, the best strategy for implant removal in such circumstances is to remove the condylar portion of the femoral or tibial component and then gain direct access to the stem. When specific disassembly instruments are available from the manufacturer, this process may be facilitated. If the condylar portion of the implant cannot be disengaged from the stem, consider using high-speed metal cutting instruments to cut the condylar portion of the implant away from the stem (Figs. 16-8 and 16-9).

After removal of the condylar portion of the implant, high-speed cutting instruments, ultrasonic instruments, and hand instruments can be used to divide interfaces along the stem. Once a sufficient amount of the stem has been accessed, the stem usually can be disimpacted. Manufacturer-specific devices that screw into a stem or lock onto a stem are quite helpful to facilitate firm axial disimpaction. Vise grip extractors can also be used to grip a stem, as may special metal cutting instruments and taps (12).

Uncommonly, well-fixed stems cannot be accessed satisfactorily because the condylar portions of the implant cannot be removed easily. In such cases, alternate methods that provide direct transosseous stem access by osteotomy may be considered. Extended tibial tubercle osteotomy can provide good access to the well-fixed tibial stem, but before using this method, consider the pros and cons of extended tibial tubercle osteotomy. A well-fixed femoral stem can be accessed by creating a window in the distal anterior femur by lifting a flap of bone. This technique is needed very rarely.

Once stems have been removed from the canals, well-fixed intramedullary cement may need to be removed. Methods of intramedullary cement removal are well established from revision hip surgery. Gain good visualization of the tibial or femoral canal. Remove cement in a sequential fashion, starting with cement closest to the joint, and work gradually away from the joint. Hand instruments and cement taps are very effective for this process. Ultrasonic cutting instruments can create longitudinal cuts in the cement to facilitate segmental extraction of cement. High-speed cutting burrs also can be used to remove cement, but avoid blindly using high-speed cutting instruments that can perforate femoral or tibial bone. Ultrasonic instruments (plug-pulling devices) and taps can be very helpful to remove cement plugs. Fluoroscopy can guide cement removal but is not necessary in most cases. Remove remaining intramedullary cement and membrane with back-biting hand instruments before beginning intramedullary reaming for the knee reconstruction.

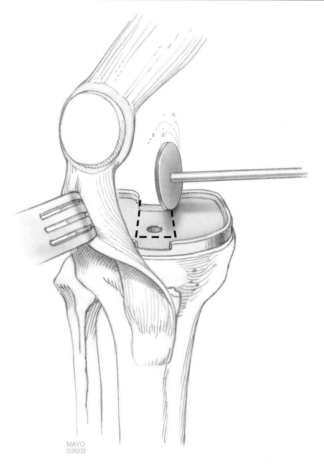

FIGURE 16-8

Access to a well-fixed tibial stem may be gained by cutting the metal tray from the stem. After the stem is removed, direct access to the interface along the stem is obtained.

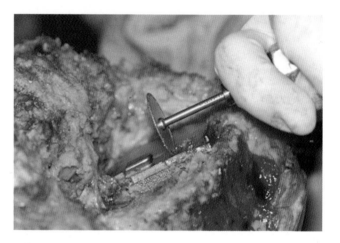

FIGURE 16-9

A diamond wheel is used to cut away the condylar portion of a tibial component to gain direct access to the very well-fixed stem.

COMPLICATIONS

Complications associated with removal of a well-fixed knee replacement can arise from inadequate exposure or hasty implant extraction. Avulsion of the patellar tendon or medial collateral ligament injury are vulnerable during the exposure for revision knee arthroplasty and can be avoided by taking care to use some of the extensile surgical exposures outlined in Chapters 1 and 4. Additionally, fracture may occur, or a large condylar fragment may come off during implant removal if care is not taken to develop the interfaces between implant and cement or bone.

REFERENCES

1. Berry DJ. Component removal during revision total knee arthroplasty. In: Lotke PA, Garino JP, eds. *Revision Total Knee Arthroplasty*. Philadelphia: Lippincott-Raven Publishers; 1999:187–196.
2. Mason JB, Fehring TK. Removing well-fixed total knee arthroplasty implants. *Clin Orthop* 2006;446:76–82.
3. Masri BA, Mitchell PA, Duncan CP. Removal of solidly fixed implants during revision hip and knee arthroplasty. *J Am Acad Orthop Surg* 2005;13:18–27.
4. Lonner JH, Mont MA, Sharkey P, et al. Fate of the unrevised all-polyethylene patellar component in revision total knee arthroplasty. *J Bone Joint Surg* 2003;85A:56–59.
5. Klapper RC, Caillouette JT. The use of ultrasonic tools in revision arthroplasty procedures. *Contemp Orthop* 1990;20:273–278.
6. Klapper RC, Caillouette JT, Callaghan JJ, et al. Ultrasonic technology in revision joint arthroplasty. *Clin Orthop* 1992;285:147–154.
7. Caillouette JT, Gorab RS, Klapper RC, et al. Revision arthroplasty facilitated by ultrasonic tool cement removal. *Orthop Rev* 1991;20:353–440.

8. Brooks AT, Nelson CL, Stewart CL, et al. Effect of an ultrasonic device on temperatures generated in bone and on bone-cement structure. *J Arthroplasty* 1993;8:413–418.

9. Firestone TP, Krackow KA. Removal of femoral components during revision knee arthroplasty. *J Bone Joint Surg* 1991;73B(3):514.

10. Alpert SW, Stuchin SA, Lubliner JA. Technique for removal of femoral components with intercondylar articulation in total knee arthroplasty. *Bull Hosp Joint Dis* 1995;53:48–49.

11. Dennis DA. Removal of well-fixed cementless metal-backed patellar components. *J Arthroplasty* 1992;7:217–220.

12. Harris WH, White RE Jr, Mitchell S, et al. Removal of broken stems of total joint components by a new method: drilling, undercutting and extracting without damage to bone. In: Salvati EA, ed. *The Hip*. St. Louis: C. V. Mosby; 1981:37.

17 Implanting the Revision Total Knee Arthroplasty

Kelly G. Vince and Martin Bedard

ORIGIN OF THE TECHNIQUE

Although there is more than one way to revise the failed total knee arthroplasty (TKA), the technique proposed here applies to most implant systems and all causes of failure. This technique has been practiced and refined since first devised in 1989 and published in 1993 (1). It is based on classic principles of balancing flexion and extension gaps.

KEYS TO REVISION TKA

Although this chapter deals specifically with the technical aspects of implanting the revision TKA, some concepts are integral to the technique. First, revision knee arthroplasty is distinctly different from primary surgery. Most attempts to render a revision as a "primary" are ill fated. Second, the simple keys to revision knee arthroplasty are:

1. The flexion gap is primarily a function of femoral component size and rotation (and to a lesser extent, position).
2. The extension gap is a function of femoral component proximal distal position. It follows that the tibial component, because it is part of both the flexion and extension gaps is not useful to selectively control either of them.

Indications

The indication for revision knee arthroplasty is in general: function sufficiently compromised by pain, instability, or stiffness that the promise of gain to the patient is worth the risk of surgery. Symptoms should be distinguished from diagnoses. Therefore, "pain" is not a diagnosis and "instability" is an incomplete diagnosis. Considering instability as an example:

1. Does the patient describe "buckling and instability" because the extensor mechanism is dislocating?
2. Is the knee collapsing into valgus because of malalignment and ligamentous instability?
3. Is the tibia dislocating posteriorly in flexion?

A worksheet approach (Table 17-1) is helpful to ensure that the cause of failure is understood completely, that the revision is indicated, and that the surgery is likely to succeed.

Contraindications

In general, the contraindications to revision knee arthroplasty may be described as (a) insufficient data to explain the etiology of pain or failure and establish a diagnosis, (b) very low probability of success, (c) unreconstructable extensor mechanism, (d) active infection, and (e) severe medical

TABLE 17-1. Worksheet for Failed Revision Total Knee Arthroplasty

	Diagnoses	Patient:				Implant Type:		Y/N
1	Infection	Clinical Drainage: Erythema: Swelling:	ESR ( ) CRP ( )	Asp. WBC(<2500) Asp. Diff(<50%) % PMN	C&S subcult.			
2	Extensor Mech. Rupt.	Extensor lag:	PalpDefect	InsallSalvati	Avulsed	PatFract	QuadsRupt.	
3	Stiff	ext-flexion	ipsi-hip OK?	CT Tibia	CT Femur	tibial slope: femoral size: fem flex/ext: pat thick:		
4	Tibial-femoral instability	Clinical VarusValgus arc: AP (in flexion): Recurvatum:		CT Tibia	CT Femur	Loose Y/N Breakage Y/N Mech axis: deg. Var/Val		
5	Fracture	XR tib:		XR fem:				
6	Loose	Subside?	Radioluc.?	BoneScan	Fluoro	Mech axis: deg. Var/Val CT-osteolysis		
7	Patella & malrotation	Maltrack Y/N	Tilt degrees	Displacement	Pat. Comp	CT Femur	CT Femur	
8	Breakage	Instab: Y/N		X-Ray: Y/N				
9	No diagnosis	AP pelvis	LS-Spine	BoneScan	RSD	Pre TKA XR		

impairment. Revision knee arthroplasty must not be performed until the patient's symptoms are understood, the cause of failure identified, and a plan formulated to specifically correct that cause. Revision knee arthroplasty is contraindicated until the status of the spine and ipsilateral hip joint have been defined (and recorded in the medical record) and until the possible role of internal rotation of the tibial and/or femoral components has been considered. Surgery is contraindicated until the possibility of active infection has been eliminated.

The ultimate contraindication to revision surgery is persistent or recurrent infection. Most other mechanical problems (bone loss, extensor rupture, etc.) can be overcome. The results of a second, two-stage reimplantation protocol for a failed two-stage reimplantation are discouraging (2). This situation may be anticipated in the patient who is a "poor host" and unable to mount the necessary resistance to infection (3). The combination of sepsis and either bone or extensor mechanism deficits are relative contraindications for even a two-stage revision because of the challenge posed by foreign material, both allograft and large implants, in an environment that was at one time dominated by microbes. Despite some success with massive structural allografts (4) (including the extensor mechanism) after infection, the predilection of microbes for avascular tissue cannot be ignored (Table 17-2).

TABLE 17-2. Relative Contraindications to Revision Total Knee Arthroplasty

Relative Contraindications		
Sepsis	and	Failed two-stage reimplantation
Sepsis	and	Poor host
Sepsis	and	Massive bone loss
Sepsis	and	Extensor mechanism rupture

Preoperative Preparation

Although comprehensive history taking and physical examination represent the standard of care, the preoperative evaluation should be disciplined, repetitive, and focused, if not streamlined. The history should establish if the knee is the source of the pain or if symptoms have been referred from the hip or spine. Delayed wound healing, drainage, or any other experiences that raise the suspicion of infection are extremely important. Whether the arthritic symptoms were ever relieved by the original arthroplasty, or if a previously successful reconstruction has recently become problematic is important. The exact meaning of the patient's description of instability, as discussed previously, should be probed.

Physical examination must evaluate the status of the ipsilateral hip, in particular how far it rotates internally and whether this movement produces pain. Does the knee look infected? Motion and stability of the problem knee arthroplasty must be quantified. Gait evaluation should record scoliosis, hip abductor dysfunction, antalgic features, limb alignment, and dynamic instability.

After the history and physical examination, a reliable differential diagnosis will have been established. Necessary laboratory investigations include a complete blood count, erythrocyte sedimentation rate determination, and a C-reactive protein test to evaluate sepsis. Any abnormality mandates an aspiration of the arthroplasty (with the patient off of antibiotic therapy for at least 10 days if not longer) at which time, synovial fluid must be evaluated for cell count, differential, and culture. Three radiographs of the knee joint, anteroposterior (AP), lateral, and patellofemoral, represent the minimum evaluation. The AP yields more information if performed with the patient standing on the affected leg only as the so-called single-leg weight bearing view. A lateral view will be more instructive if the patient is standing on one limb alone, when flexion contracture and recurvatum can now be quantified (Fig. 17-1).

Revision surgery for instability or loosening can be planned more easily if a full-length radiograph is obtained that shows the hip, knee, and ankle joint for evaluation of limb alignment. This study will also reveal hip pathology and extra-articular deformity. Without it, an AP radiograph of the pelvis is an important way to identify ipsilateral hip pathology, one of the contraindications to revision.

Computerized tomography (CT) can quantify rotational positioning of both the femoral and tibial components (5). This plays an important etiological role in patellar complications, instability, and stiffness. CT scans reveal bone loss from osteolysis much more accurately than plain radiography (6). Radioisotope studies are rarely helpful, except if they are "normal" in the mysterious, problem TKA, which suggests that further surgery should be avoided.

A–D

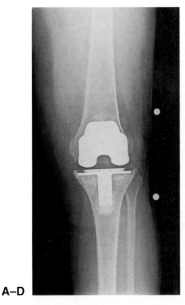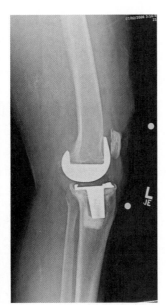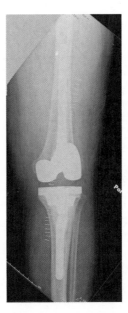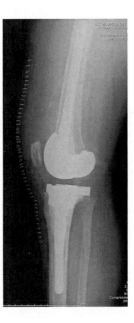

FIGURE 17-1

Radiographs. **(A)** Pre-revision anteroposterior and lateral view of failed Insall-Burstein II prostheses, modular posterior stabilized arthroplasty at 17 years postprimary secondary to wear, osteolysis, and loosening. **(B)** Postrevision with posterior stabilized articular, offset press-fit stem extensions on the tibia and femur with porous, metal cone augment on the tibia to enhance fixation. The three-step technique described later was used.

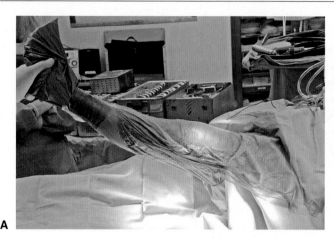
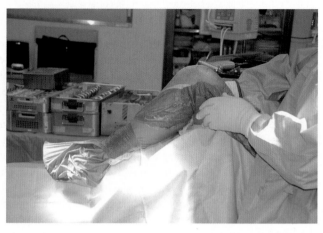

A
B

FIGURE 17-2

Intraoperative examination I. **(A)** A disciplined approach to revision knee arthroplasty includes examining the knee fully under anesthesia for stability and motion, with particular attention to flexion contractures and recurvatum deformities. These have implications for surgical technique. **(B)** Flexion is quantified by allowing the knee to fall freely.

SURGICAL TECHNIQUE

A disciplined approach to revision knee arthroplasty includes examining the knee fully, under anesthesia for stability and motion. Particular attention is paid to flexion contractures and recurvatum deformities, which have implications for surgical technique. Flexion is quantified, by allowing the knee to fall freely (Fig. 17-2A,B). The surgical approach to the knee is methodical and performed in a routine stepwise fashion, using the principles discussed in Chapters 1 and 4. Two scalpels, attached side by side with Steri-Strips, enable the surgeon to excise preexisting scar, assuming that there is enough supple skin remaining for closure. This technique produces a superior cosmetic result, respects the principle that preexisting incisions should be used, and eliminates very narrow (millimeters wide or smaller) strips of skin that may lie between two incisions, strips that must not have very good vascularization (Fig. 17-3A,B). A straight arthrotomy, extending from the medial base of the tibial tubercle to the medial aspect of the quadriceps tendon will transect fewer longitudinal fibers than a medial parapatellar arthrotomy. No more than about 1 cm of tissue will be removed from the top of the patella (Fig. 17-4).

Careful dissection, initiated with a scalpel and completed with a periosteal elevator will preserve this layer of tissue intact. The danger of multiple, longitudinal strokes of the blade will be to convert a single essential layer into useless strips that compromise closure and invite drainage (Fig. 17-5).

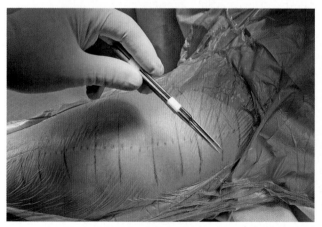
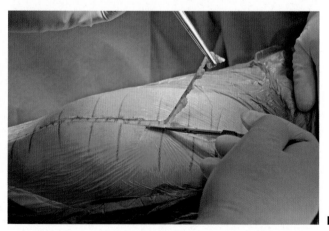

A
B

FIGURE 17-3

Scar excision. **(A)** Two scalpels secured with Steri-Strips enable the surgeon to excise the preexisting scar, assuming that there is enough supple skin remaining for closure. **(B)** This technique produces a superior cosmetic result, respects the principle that preexisting incisions should be used, and eliminates very narrow (millimeters wide or less) strips of skin that may lie between two incisions, strips that must not have very good vascularization.

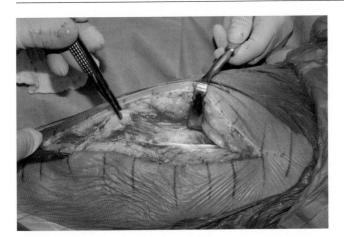

FIGURE 17-4

Arthrotomy. A straight arthrotomy, extending from the medial base of the tibial tubercle to the medial aspect of the quadriceps tendon will transect fewer longitudinal fibers than a medial parapatellar arthrotomy. No more than about 1 cm of tissue will be removed from the top of the patella.

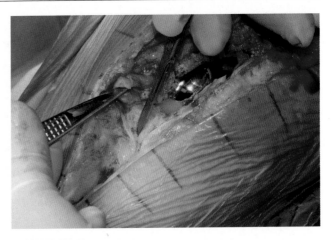

FIGURE 17-5

Elevation of the medial capsule. Careful dissection, initiated with a scalpel and completed with a periosteal elevator will preserve this layer of tissue intact. The danger of multiple, longitudinal strokes of the blade will be to convert a single essential layer into useless strips that compromise closure and invite drainage.

The synovial layer is invariably thickened at revision surgery. This scarred layer may be grasped by several Kocher clamps without concern of crushing the tissue. By contrast, sharp clamps are applied to the patient's own tissue, causing less damage. The interval is easily developed with cutting cautery. On the medial side, the thickened synovial layer may be separated with an index finger. A thick layer can be removed. In this case of loosening and osteolysis, the removed scar will contain a large volume of polyethylene wear debris. Removing this layer facilitates the exposure without recourse to more aggressive maneuvers such as tibial tubercle osteotomy or quadriceps turndown (Fig. 17-6). The lateral synovectomy layer is more difficult to develop. Cautery will be required and care must be taken not to impair the quadriceps tendon (Fig. 17-7). Both sides of the femur are usually scarred to the extensor mechanism. Cautery and blunt division restores this interval facilitating exposure, increasing quadriceps excursion and knee flexion (Fig. 17-8A,B). Scar around the patella should be removed. Note the wear of the patellar component (Fig. 17-9). The patellar tendon is held with sharp clamps and the scar on its deep surface with Kocher clamps. Removing this layer restores the tendon's ability to "twist" aiding exposure and flexion. It will sometimes improve patella baja modestly (Fig. 17-10). The very long-handled Mayo scissors may be introduced, "open" into the space above the anterior femur to release scars that tether the extensor. This step should be followed by a gentle manipulation before any components are removed and will be particularly helpful in revision of the stiff knee (Fig. 17-11).

The examination continues once the arthroplasty is open. Varus and valgus stability must be evaluated, remembering that instability is more often the result of wear, loosening, or component position than it is of ligament failure. Varus and valgus stability must be evaluated not only in full extension where the effect of the posterior structures may be misleading but also with the knee flexed to 30 degrees (Fig. 17-12A). The dimension of the flexion gap is best quantified by distraction, as shown here, giving the surgeon a quantitative idea of how large the mismatch is between flexion and extension gaps (Fig. 17-12B). With the patient's foot off the edge of the operating table, the surgeon may apply pressure with his or her thigh to flex the patient's knee and externally rotate the tibia. External rotation moves the tibial tubercle laterally, decreases the force on the extensor mechanism, and will eventually bring the tibia forward, out from under the femoral component (Fig. 17-13A). Cautery can be used to detach the medial capsule, and if a medial release is required, to balance the knee, as the tibia is externally rotated. This step decreases the need for more aggressive exposure maneuvers (Fig. 17-13B).

After the surgical approach has been completed, every revision arthroplasty, no matter the cause of the original failure, can be performed in a sequence of three steps:

1. Reestablish tibial platform.
2. Stabilize the knee in flexion.
3. Extend the knee to stabilize the knee in extension.

(text continues on p. 210)

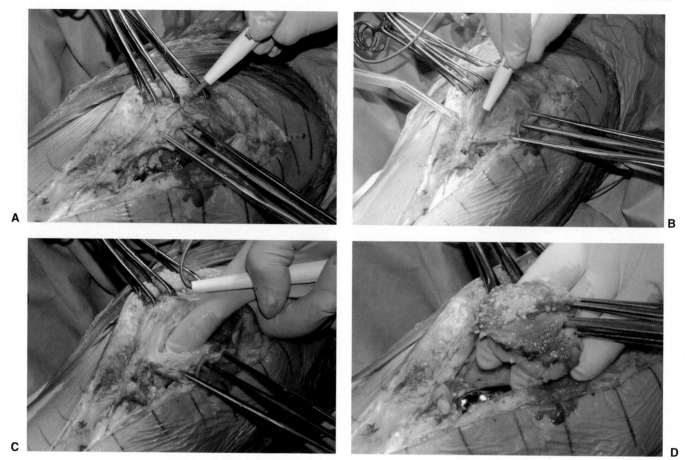

FIGURE 17-6

Medial synovectomy. **(A)** The synovial layer is invariably thickened at revision surgery. This scarred layer may be grasped by several Kocher clamps without concern for crushing the tissue. By contrast, sharp clamps are applied to the patient's own tissue, causing less damage. **(B)** The interval is easily developed with cutting cautery. **(C)** On the medial side, the thickened synovial layer may be separated with an index finger. **(D)** A thick layer can be removed. In this case of loosening and osteolysis, the removed scar will contain a large volume of polyethylene wear debris. Removing this layer facilitates the exposure without recourse to more aggressive maneuvers such as tibial tubercle osteotomy or quadriceps turndown.

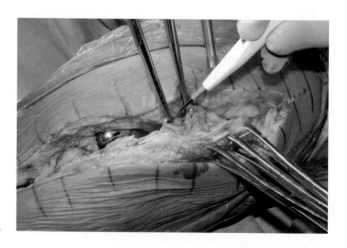

FIGURE 17-7

Lateral synovectomy. The lateral synovectomy layer is more difficult to develop. Cautery will be required and care must be taken not to impair the quadriceps tendon.

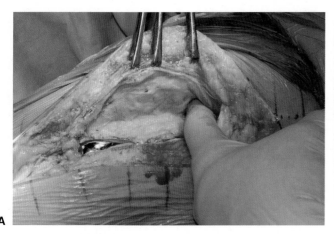

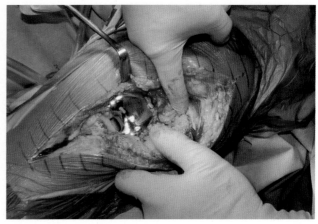

A   B

FIGURE 17-8

Reestablish "gutters." **(A,B)** Both sides of the femur are usually scarred to the extensor mechanism. Cautery and blunt division restores this interval facilitating exposure, increasing quadriceps excursion, and knee flexion.

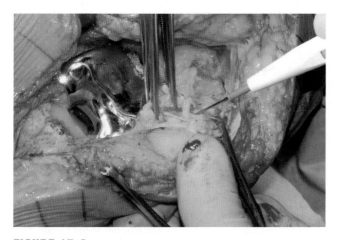

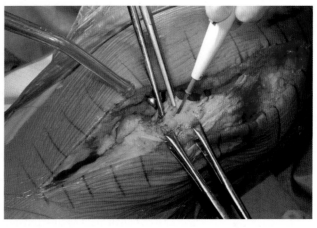

FIGURE 17-9

Peripatellar scar. Scar around the patella should be removed. Note the wear of the patellar component.

FIGURE 17-10

Scar on the deep surface of the patellar tendon: The patellar tendon is held with sharp clamps and the scar on its deep surface with Kocher clamps. Removal of this layer restores the ability of the tendon to twist, aiding exposure and flexion. It will sometimes improve patella baja modestly.

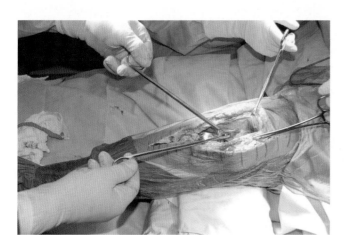

FIGURE 17-11

Liberation of quadriceps. The very long-handled Mayo scissors may be introduced, open into the space above the anterior femur to release scars that tether the extensor. This step should be followed by a gentle manipulation before any components are removed and will be particularly helpful in revision of the stiff knee.

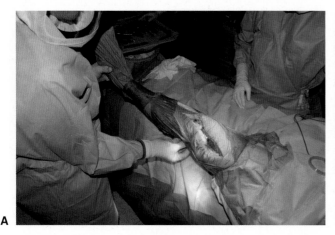

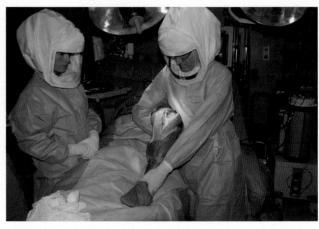

FIGURE 17-12

Intraoperative examination II. **(A)** The examination continues once the arthroplasty is open. Varus and valgus stability must be evaluated, remembering that instability is more often the result of wear, loosening, or component position than it is of ligament failure. Varus and valgus stability must be evaluated not only in full extension where the effect of the posterior structures may be misleading but also with the knee flexed to 30 degrees. **(B)** The dimension of the flexion gap is best quantified by distraction, as shown here. This gives the surgeon a quantitative idea of how large the mismatch is between the flexion and extension gaps.

The specific problems that must be solved at each step in this sequence will vary by the cause of failure. For example, if the patella had been dislocating, then the major problem to be corrected in step 1 will be tibial component rotation and in step 2, femoral component rotation (Fig. 17-14). By contrast, if loosening and osteolysis have been the problem, then reconstruction of bone defects will be necessary in all three steps accompanied by reduction of varus mechanical alignment when placing the femoral component.

Although component removal is discussed elsewhere in this text, recognizing that there is a "budget" of time for the surgery, I prefer to saw off the components, which is the most expeditious method. A narrow reciprocating blade works well on the femoral interface and can be introduced in all interfaces except the posterior condyle where a curved 0.25-inch osteotome works well. A blow of the mallet on a large punch, held against the most proximal edge of the femoral flange and parallel to the femur, will

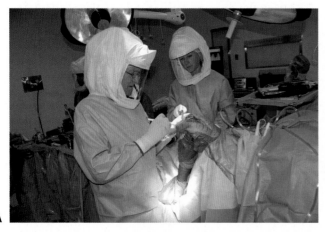

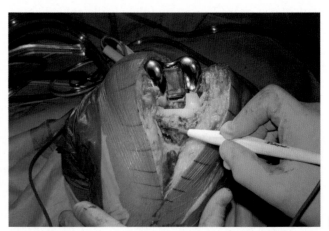

FIGURE 17-13

Exposure. Externally the rotate tibia. **(A)** With the patient's foot off the edge of the operating table, the surgeon may apply pressure with his or her thigh to flex the patient's knee and externally rotate the tibia. External rotation moves the tibial tubercle laterally, decreases the force on the extensor mechanism, and will eventually bring the tibia forward, out from under the femoral component. **(B)** Cautery can be used to detach the medial capsule and if a medial release is required, to balance the knee, as the tibia is externally rotated. This step decreases the need for more aggressive exposure maneuvers.

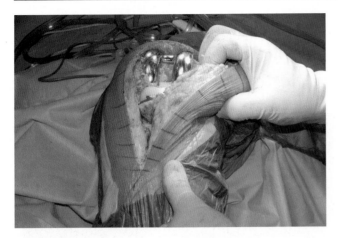

FIGURE 17-14

Intraoperative examination III. Rotational positioning of tibial and femoral components is most easily quantified by prerevision computerized tomography. The discipline of examining the knee continues, however. The tibial component should line up with the tibial tubercle, as seen here. The surgeon's lower thumb is on the tibial crest, corresponding to the extensor attachment. The position of the femoral component on computed tomography scan should be compared with the position intraoperatively, to plan the position of the revision implant.

rapidly and safely remove the component. Ignore residual cement that is well fixed to bone unless sepsis is present (Fig. 17-15). Obsession with its removal at this stage will waste time and perhaps bone. Any femoral cement that does not belong will come off in steps 2 and 3, with saw cuts.

The tibial component is similarly removed with a saw: initially, a wide blade to disrupt most of the fixation interface, preferably between the bone and the cement. Later, a reciprocating saw will

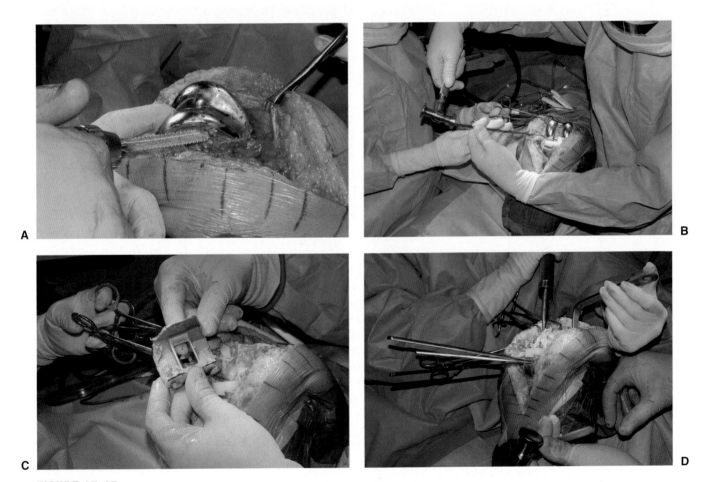

FIGURE 17-15

Component removal. **(A)** A reciprocating saw can be easily admitted into the bone-cement interface at 45 degrees as seen here, to prevent the saw mechanism from simply banging against the knee if admitted straight on. **(B)** The posterior condyles are not easily accessible to the saw but may be reached with narrow (0.25-inch) curved osteotomes. **(C)** With the interface disrupted, the femoral component can be removed and bone preserved. **(D)** After sawing through the tibial interface, the component is extricated from the bone with stacked osteotomes.

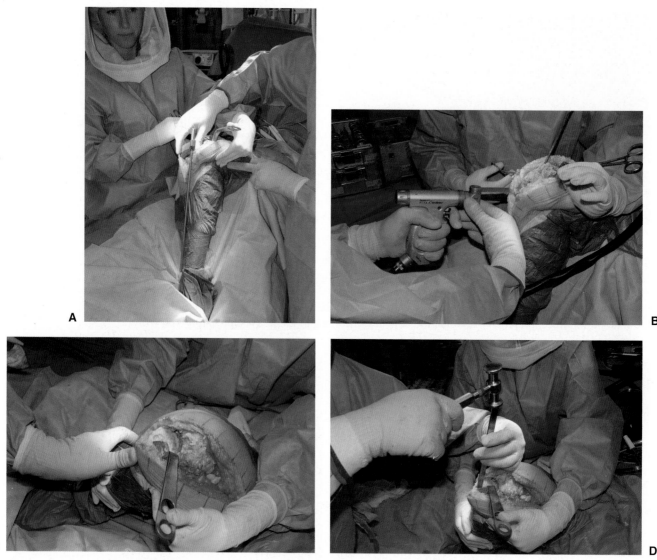

FIGURE 17-16

Tibial orientation. **(A)** Even a rudimentary extramedullary alignment guide will give useful information. Here, the spacer block and alignment rod are used. This provides a rough idea of the angulation and slope of the proximal tibia with the component removed. It is premature to try and achieve the "perfect cut" at this time, as this may result in excess removal of bone. **(B)** A tibial cut may be performed freehand or with instruments; keep in mind, however, that most instruments devised for primary surgeries will not sit easily at the new level of tibial resection and that most attempts to make a primary-type cut will sacrifice inordinate amounts of bone. Further, the position of the component will be determined by the stem extensions engaging the endosteum rather than the cut. **(C)** Rotational orientation of the tibial component should be with the tibial tubercle to enhance patellar tracking. Here, the position is confirmed, as the previous component also had the desired orientation. **(D)** A rectangular-shaped access to the canal is created with an osteotome. This provides access to old bone cement and commits visually and structurally to the desired rotational orientation of the revision implant.

reach corners of the plateau. The postero-lateral corner is problematic, and an offset chisel or osteotome will work well.

A good approximation of a neutral tibial cut can be achieved freehand when the component is removed. Remember that most tibial cutting guides will not necessarily fit the revision tibia very well, particularly when there is scarring of the infrapatellar tendon. A simple extramedullary spacer block or trial tray and an extension rod works well to evaluate the orientation of the cut (Fig. 17-16). Accordingly, the precise cut, which by itself determines alignment in the primary is not required here, as an asymmetric press fit stem and contact of the tibial component with a large percentage of the host bone will suffice. Attempts to create the "perfect" tibial cut tend to sacrifice bone and place the component at a level where the funnel shape of the tibia has a reduced diameter and further diminished strength.

RATIONALE FOR THE SEQUENCE

The general rationale for this sequence starts with the phrase "tibial platform," which I carefully selected when first describing this technique, to indicate a foundation on which to build the knee. This is neither the joint line nor the tibial articular surface. It is the location of a tibial trial component, held by modular, press-fit stem extensions. The rationale for establishing the tibial component first lies in the fact that it is common to both the flexion and extension gaps and accordingly cannot be used to manipulate the relative dimensions of either gap.

The subsequent rationale for then proceeding to the flexion gap has been described (7) but can be reduced to the argument that the idea of a two- dimensional "joint line" should be replaced by the fact that the joint line is three- dimensional and corresponds to the complex shape of the femoral component, from its distal surface to the most posterior articulation. In addition, if the femoral component determines the flexion gap, and if we can usually go up or down one component size, which affords an adjustment of about 8 mm. By contrast, the extension gap can be manipulated up or down as much as 30 mm in challenging cases. It then makes sense to commit to the more limiting flexion gap that can then be more easily matched by the more variable extension gap.

Step 1: Reestablish Tibial Platform

The tibial platform is easily reestablished with a minimal bone cut and solid press fit of an asymmetric stem extension inside the asymmetric tibial bone. The center of the tibial diaphysis is, on average, 4 mm medial to the center of the articular surface (8). This means that if a straight press-fit stem is used, one of three situations will ensue:

1. The stem fits and lies in valgus, often more valgus than the surgeon intended. This is not distressing if revising a knee that has failed in varus (i.e., varus overload leading to medial wear, osteolysis, and loosening) but can be problematic when treating valgus instability.
2. The stem fits and is parallel to the mechanical axis, but the tibial component is no longer centered on the tibia so that it must be either undersized or allowed to overhang medially.
3. An undersized tibial stem extension is aligned parallel to the tibial bone and allowed to dangle in the medullary canal.

The only strategy for retaining the desired size of component that does not overhang, respecting neutral alignment and also filling the medullary canal of the diaphysis to enhance fixation, is to implant some type of asymmetric or offset stem, although a short thin cemented stem is an alternative.

The entry point for the reamer should stand on the tibial plateau, over the diaphyseal point where the stem tip will eventually reside. Rather than drilling this starting point, it works well to note the tibial tubercle as a landmark for rotation and then remove a rectangle of bone with a 0.5-inch osteotome. This gives good access to the canal and forces the surgeon to actively select the rotational position of the tibial component. The tibial crest is a reliable and easily palpable landmark for both rotation, varus-valgus alignment, and the destination of the reamers.

Unlike reaming for fracture fixation, in which the surgeon tends to look down the canal, it is advantageous to hold the reamer at arm's length and keep the alignment in view (Fig. 17-17). Although it is called a reamer, the instrument (whether powered or driven by hand), should only be used to measure the diameter of the medullary canal. The path of the reamer will be the position of the stem extension and in turn, the alignment of the component. As progressively larger-diameter reamers are applied, the instrument will, at some point, "jump" out of alignment, following the curve of the canal. The last diameter reamer that sat parallel to the mechanical axis (i.e., still pointed at the center of the talus) should be the size of stem that is selected.

A trial tibial component and offset stem are then selected and positioned (Fig. 17-18). Despite the many suggestions regarding how to exploit the offset of some medullary stems, I believe the stem should be placed medially and the component laterally in virtually every case, to accommodate tibial anatomy, achieve neutral alignment, fill the canal, and avoid component overhang.

Bone defects should be noted by clearing osteolytic membrane but are ignored at this point (Fig. 17-19). The position of the trial component will define the defects clearly, and they can be dealt

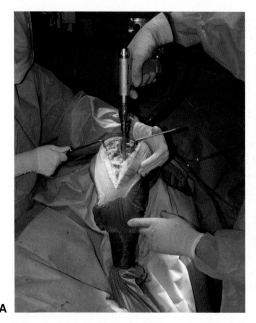
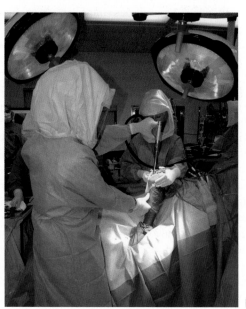

A

B

FIGURE 17-17

Reaming the tibia. **(A)** The tibial crest, as an indicator of the diaphysis, is a reliable target. **(B)** Unlike reaming for fractures, the surgeon should stand back and visualize the orientation of the reamer, as this will be the alignment of the component. Very little bone should be removed with reaming.

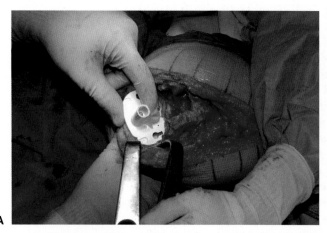
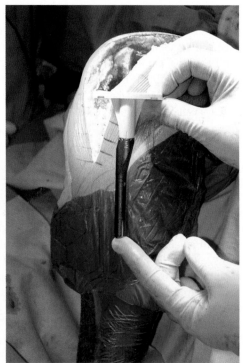

A

B

FIGURE 17-18

Place the tibial trial. **(A)** A quick way to size the tibial trial is to place one, upside down, on the cut surface of the tibia. This dispenses with an entire set of templates. **(B)** In the vast majority of cases, corresponding to the anatomy of the tibia, the offset of the stem should be used to place the stem medial and the prosthesis lateral. *(continued)*

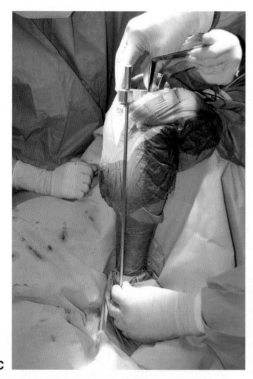

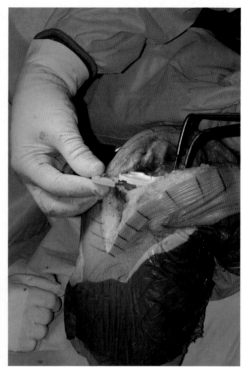

C

D

FIGURE 17-18 *(Continued)*

(C) Once the trial is in place, the alignment should be confirmed with an extramedullary guide. Here again, the simple spacer and rod. Remember to orient the rod over the tubercle. **(D)** If the fixation is solid with the trial, and if the alignment is satisfactory, there may not be perfect contact of the component with all of the host bone. These defects now define the role of augments.

with later. For the moment, we are interested in the big picture: alignment, stability, and component size and position.

Step 2: The Flexion Gap

This second phase of the procedure accomplishes the most important work of the revision. It can be divided into three phases:

1. Determine and commit to the desired femoral component rotation.
2. Select the size of the femoral component that stabilizes the knee in flexion.
3. Assess the level of the joint line relative to the patella, with a modular polyethylene insert in place that stabilizes the arthroplasty in flexion.

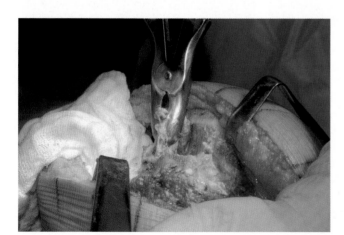

FIGURE 17-19

Osteolytic membrane. Abundant amounts of osteolytic membrane must be removed from cases that have failed from wear and loosening to expose healthy bone for fixation.

Step 2A: Establish Correct Rotational Position of the Femoral Component

The femoral component should ideally be oriented rotationally, parallel to the transepicondylar axis. This anatomic landmark, often difficult to locate in a primary, may be tougher to find in a revision (Fig. 17-20). The other guides to rotational positioning: the trochlear groove (Whiteside's line) (9,10) and the posterior articular surfaces (11) simply do not exist at revision. Rotational positioning is best determined in the revision arthroplasty by:

1. Pre-revision CT scan
2. The amount of residual posterior condyle
3. Patellar tracking

The CT scan is helpful for virtually every revision surgery. The surgeon who orders and studies the preoperative CT scan will better understand the failed arthroplasty. The internally rotated femoral component can be marked and corrected with a posterolateral femoral augment. Alternately, the surgeon can palpate the residual posterior condylar bone, where an internally rotated femoral component will

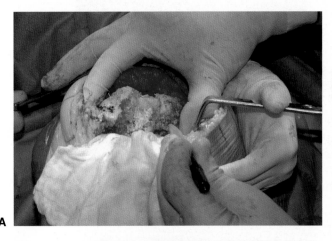
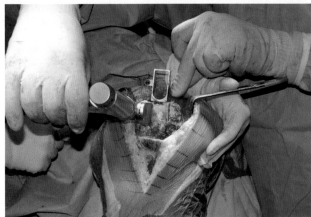
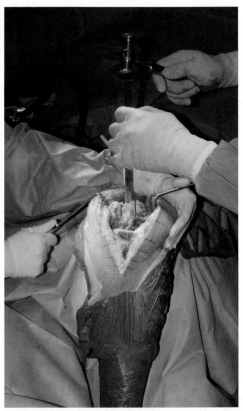

FIGURE 17-20

Step 2A: femoral component rotation. **(A)** The transepicondylar axis is identified and marked. The sulcus between the attachments of the medial superficial and deep ligaments is reliable, as is the single prominence to which the lateral collateral attaches. There are few other landmarks for rotation in the revision knee. **(B)** A physical commitment to rotational position can be established by cutting the intercondylar notch at this point. For many implant systems, the dimensions of the notch will be very similar for the range of possible sizes. Here, the modular "box" is used to verify the width of the cut. Alternately, the canal may be opened with a drill, but this destroys an otherwise useful block of bone. **(C)** The depth of the intercondylar notch will not be known until step 3 when the extension gap is established. A relatively shallow amount of bone may be resected with the osteotome at this stage.

have left more posterior bone on the medial side. Ultimately, if the trial patellar does not track centrally, additional external rotation of the femoral and tibial components should be considered.

The surgeon can commit to the desired femoral component rotational position consciously and visually by sawing the intercondylar notch, either by using a modular version of the intercondylar box or freehand. The depth of this cut will not yet be determined until step 3.

Step 2B: Stabilize the Knee in Flexion

In Step 2B, we put our first "key to revision surgery" into action: the flexion gap is controlled by the size (and position) of the femoral component. In virtually all revisions, the only consistently reliable anatomic landmark will be the intramedullary canal. As such, diaphyseal-length press-fit stems can be implantable instruments. Even if surgeons ultimately prefer a fully cemented narrow stem, using larger-diameter press-fit stems at this stage will establish component size and position and which augments are necessary to maintain that position. With these augments applied, component position will be ensured even if the stem diameter is reduced.

Reaming technique influences stem position. As in the tibia, the surgeon should not use the reamer to remove much bone but rather to guide component position and measure the diameter of the canal. There is a general tendency, probably because of the reamer's weight and working hand posture, for the surgeon to unconsciously lower the handpiece and establish a flexed trajectory for the instrument and then the implant (Fig. 17-21). Holding the reamer up, against the anterior endosteum will favor a position parallel to the bone. In the medial-lateral plane, a diaphyseal engaging stem can be placed in more valgus (for the knee that has failed from loosening and varus alignment) if the reamer is pulled toward the lateral endosteum. This would normally create lateral overhang of the femoral component that can be avoided with an offset stem: the prosthesis sitting medially, and the stem in the bone sits laterally. Conversely, (remembering that the proximal tip of the reamer/the stem is immobilized in the diaphysis) reaming against the medial cortex will provide several more degrees of varus, with the offset used to centralize the component by moving it laterally to correct, for example, the knee that has failed with valgus instability (12).

Femoral component size influences soft tissue tension in flexion (Fig. 17-22). Simply replicating "normal" osseous anatomy with the component may lead to trouble. In effect, the soft tissues have often changed irrevocably at revision surgery, when previously perfect choices of sizing are no

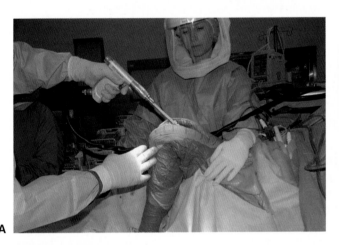
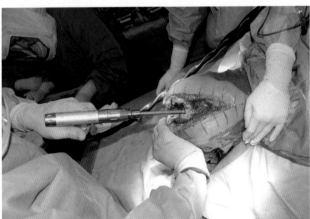

A   **B**

FIGURE 17-21

Femoral canal reaming. **(A)** There is a tendency to drop the hand holding the reamer, and so the instrument takes a "flexed" position relative to the femoral canal, as will the stem extension and ultimately the femoral component. This limits the size of stem extension that may be used. The surgeon should keep the hand up while reaming. This also clarifies the need for an anterior augment in most cases. **(B)** Greater varus or valgus alignment may be obtained by the medial or lateral position of the reamer. Here, to reduce varus alignment and medial loading in a case that failed from wear and osteolysis, the reamer is pulled toward the lateral endosteum for more valgus alignment. The tip of the stem will be centralized in the diaphysis of the femur, and the component will be centralized by the medial position of the offset stem.

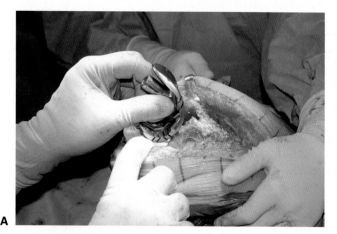

A

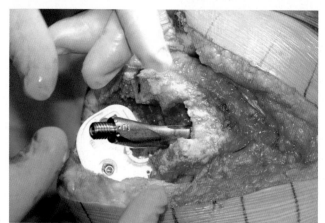

B

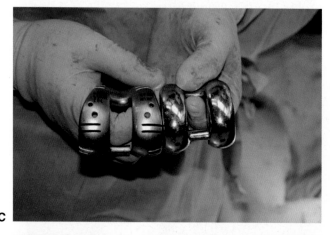

C

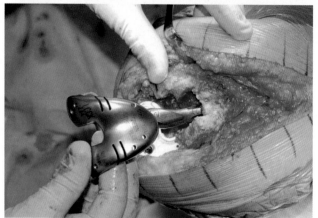

D

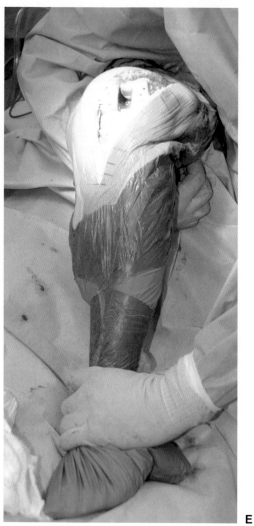

E

FIGURE 17-22

Step 2B: femoral component size and anteroposterior position.
(A) A quick indication of the largest femoral component that can be used comes from placing the articular surface of the component up against the distal femur. The one that extends from medial to lateral cortex will be the upper limit, as we would not want a component to overhang. The actual component that best serves this reconstruction will be this one or something smaller. It would be bigger if we are revising a case of instability and smaller if we are revising a case of stiffness. **(B)** Additional valgus alignment comes from reaming up against the lateral endosteum; a centralization of the component comes from the offset stem. Here, reaming laterally for valgus and the offset medial to centralize. **(C)** In this case, a femoral component larger than what had been removed was necessary to stabilize the flexion gap. **(D)** Alignment and centralization have been achieved. **(E).** Test stability of the flexion gap by distracting the knee in 90 degrees of flexion.

longer effective. For example, the revision of a knee that has instability in flexion must either decrease the size of the flexion gap (larger femoral component) or increase the size of the extension gap (resect additional distal femoral bone and raise the joint line). The stiff knee, by contrast (in addition to rectifying rotational problems), usually requires a more spacious flexion gap, which can be achieved with a smaller femoral component or by decreasing the extension gap with distal femoral augmentation. It will be the condition of the soft tissues, scarring and contracture or stretching and plastic deformation, which determines appropriate sizing. In the event that soft tissues have simply failed, constraint may be necessary.

The advice to select a revision femoral component based on the size of the removed component, the dimension from the prearthroplasty radiograph, or the radiograph of the unoperated contralateral side, should be taken with caution. The soft tissues at the time of the revision should guide the choice of size. Accordingly, as an initial rough guide to sizing during the revision, we may determine the largest feasible size by placing the articular surface of a trial component up against the distal femoral bone. Clearly, the one that overhangs medial to lateral will be too big, and so we will have defined the largest possible for the case. If this is a case of instability, that largest size may be perfect. If the case is one of limited flexion, something smaller will be required. At this stage, the majority of femurs will have an anterior defect that responds well to an augment.

Step 2C: Evaluation of Joint Line

With the tibial platform established and a potential femoral component in position, the modular tibial insert that will stabilize the knee in flexion is selected (Fig. 17-23). The thickness of this

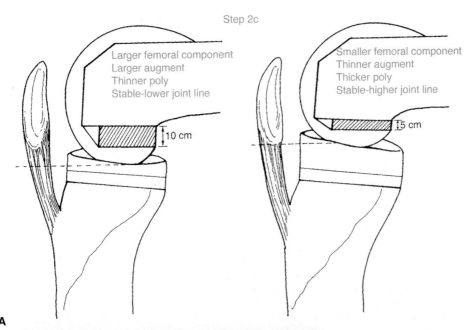

Step 2c

Larger femoral component
Larger augment
Thinner poly
Stable-lower joint line

10 cm

Smaller femoral component
Thinner augment
Thicker poly
Stable-higher joint line

5 cm

A

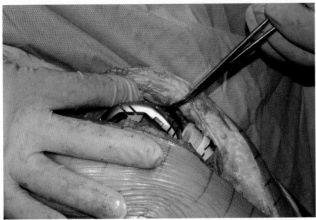

B

FIGURE 17-23

Step 2C: joint line height. **(A)** The trial femoral component and trial tibial insert were selected in Figure 17-21, and the stability in flexion was verified. However, the flexion gap could also be stabilized with the combination of a smaller femoral component and a thicker tibial polyethylene insert or even a larger femoral component and a thinner insert. Although all three combinations would be stable, the difference would be the height of the joint line in flexion. This height relative to the patella would be replicated in extension. **(B)** Here, the position of the inferior pole of the patella (with a normal patellar tendon) is compared to the joint line.

insert has implications for how high the joint line will be lifted in flexion. Although numerous methods have been suggested for evaluating the joint line, I use the relationship of the articulation (in flexion) relative to the inferior pole of the patella, assuming there is a relatively normal patellar tendon length.

Accordingly, a larger femoral component requires a thinner polyethylene with a resultant lower joint line relative to the patella. A smaller femoral component will require a thicker tibial insert for flexion stability, which will drive the joint line higher. I do not believe that the joint line should "chase" a pathologically low patella (patella infera/baja) from patellar tendon contracture or that any surgery should be attempted to lengthen a scarred patellar tendon.

Step 3: Stabilize the Knee in Extension

By now, the tibia has been reconstructed and the knee stabilized in flexion. The femoral component size and AP position have been established. The only remaining problems to address are the proximal-distal position of the femoral component with the requisite distal femoral augmentations and whether the patient's collateral ligaments can be expected to provide stability without mechanical constraint. This is the third step—stabilizing the knee in extension (Fig. 17-24).

Most of the difficult work in the knee has been accomplished already. In this third step, the knee is brought into full extension with all components temporarily secured with stem extensions. To accommodate the tibial polyethylene that has stabilized the knee in flexion, the femoral component will be pushed into the femur as the knee reaches extension. The limb should neither be allowed to remain in residual flexion nor should it permitted to reach recurvatum. In full extension, the femoral component position is noted and secured with pins if the system allows, indicating to what extent distal augmentation will be required. Usually, small amounts of irregular, residual distal femoral bone must be resected to accommodate an augment. Cutting slots in some trial femoral components facilitate this step. The proximal-distal position has been finalized, and so the requisite depth of the intercondylar cut has been determined.

Indications for Constraint

There are two specific indications for constraint, both resulting from plastic deformation of supporting soft tissues, that can be evaluated during these steps:

1. flexion gap larger than the extension gap, to the point that even the largest femoral component with a thick polyethylene does not provide stability, and
2. varus-valgus instability in extension (or enough flexion to relax the posterior structures) caused by collateral ligament failure.

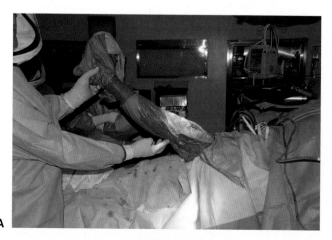
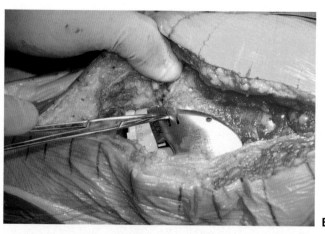

A

B

FIGURE 17-24

Step 3: extension. **(A)** All components are in place, and the knee is extended fully with neither recurvatum nor residual flexion. This will force the femoral component into the desired position for a balanced extension gap. **(B)** Cutting slots in the trial components of several systems then guide the surgeon as to precisely how much bone to resect to accommodate with augments.

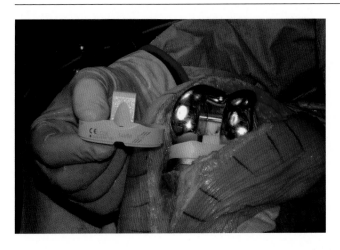

FIGURE 17-25

Need for constraint. With the final tibial and femoral components installed, both the flexion gap and the extension gap are stable with a posterior stabilized tibial insert. Accordingly, we see the actual (white) polyethylene insert implanted. At this stage, however, the option of a nonlinked constrained insert was feasible to eliminate instability from collateral ligament insufficiency.

The majority of these cases can be successfully stabilized with a nonlinked constrained implant. The specific conditions that necessitate a linked constrained or hinged device are debated. The mechanical strategy for overcoming recurvatum secondary to extensor mechanism paralysis has not been established. Hinges will not eliminate quadriceps buckling, and any hyperextension stop in the implant is mechanically demanding (Fig. 17-25).

PEARLS

Femoral Augments: Kinematic Implications

From the first attempts at revising a failed knee arthroplasty, surgeons have been faced with the often-dramatic challenge of reconstituting lost bone (Table 17-3). This is of course exacerbated by multiple surgeries, osteolysis, and surgical treatment of infection. Metal modular augments were originally developed as simple bone substitutes. Each of them has more significant kinematic implications—the ability to alter the position of components and accordingly to influence forces on the knee, fixation, and the relationship between stability and mobility. For example, distal femoral augments do more than replace missing distal femoral bone. On the medial side, they increase valgus alignment and on the lateral, varus alignment. When combined with a distal lateral augment, the femoral component is positioned more distally, decreasing the size of the extension gap, resolving nonneurological recurvatum, and balancing instability where the flexion gap is small. The joint line will also be lowered in extension by medial and lateral distal femoral augments (Fig. 17-26).

Posterior femoral augments have a different effect on rotation, depending on which side is used. Posterolateral augments are used most frequently to correct the internal rotation associated with

TABLE 17-3. Augments				
Component	**Location**	**Primary Effect**	**Secondary Effect**	**Commonly Used to Treat**
Femur	Anterior	Femur out of flexion	Increase femoral stem fill	All modes of failure
	Distal-lateral	Increase varus	Decrease valgus destructive force	Valgus instability (common)
	Distal-medial	Increase valgus	Decrease varus overload	Loosening caused by medial wear and osteolysis
	Posterolateral	External rotation	Enhance patellar tracking	Malrotation and patellar complications
	Posteromedial	Internal rotation	Rarely required	Loosening and osteolysis
	Posteromedial and lateral	Increase femoral component size	Decrease size flexion gap	Flexion instability
Tibia	Medial	Increase valgus	Decrease varus overload	Loosening and osteolysis
	Lateral	Increase varus	Rarely required	Prior high tibial osteotomy (uncommon)
	Medial and lateral	Brings tibial component and stem extension up, out of tibia	Enhances fit of offset stem extension. Decreases flexion and extension gaps	Bone loss after 1. Infection 2. Osteolysis 3. Multiple revisions 4. Instability

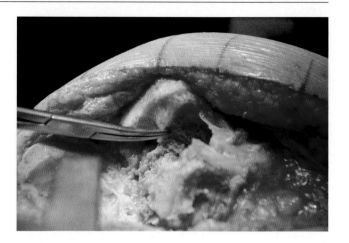

FIGURE 17-26

Femoral bone defects. Conventional block augments have been added to the distal and posterior femoral component as the result of steps 1 through 3, providing a solid fit between implant and host bone. The residual femur has some cancellous bone available for cement intrusions, and a decision is made against porous metal augmentation.

patellar tracking problems. Posteromedial augments are rarely used alone but are more commonly combined with a postero-lateral augment to permit a larger femoral component, thus decreasing the size of the flexion gap, which is a common problem in flexion instability.

Cementing Femur

When modular uncemented stems were first introduced, cement was restricted to the cut surface of either the tibia or femur. Loosening still complicated revision knee arthroplasty. Accordingly, the current recommended technique is to place cement on the cut bone surface, introduce the uncemented stem into the femur (or tibia) to about 10 cm short of seating (to occlude the canal), and then to fill the metaphyseal area with cement using a gun (Fig. 17-27A). The component is gradually seated as the cement is introduced. Once the posterior condyles contact the host bone, so that a closed space has been created, additional cement can be introduced to ensure that all defects are filled (Fig. 17-27B). The posterior augments are selected to determine femoral component size, rotation, and impact stability in flexion. The distal femoral augment thickness is selected to normalize the joint line and ensure that the polyethylene tibial insert that had been chosen to stabilize the knee in flexion is also the correct one to balance the knee in extension (Fig. 17-27C).

Anterior Femoral Augments: Fixation

Anterior femoral augments bring the femoral component up out of the anterior defect and eliminate the flexed position of a femoral component (Fig. 17-28). This brings any stem extension parallel to the medullary canal where the maximum diameter can be accommodated without being limited by impingement on the anterior endosteum. This enhances fixation with press-fit stem extensions. Eliminating the femoral component flexed position also prevents relative hyperextension of the components when the knee is fully extended and the resultant, damaging tibial spine impingement.

Tibial Augments: Stem Fit

Even asymmetric tibial stem extensions may not fit the anatomic tibial canal, especially if there has been considerable loss of proximal tibial bone. Typically, the lateral aspect of the tibial stem extension will abut on the endosteum of the tibial canal, pushing the component medially or into varus. If both medial and lateral block augments are added, the tibial component is lifted up out of the canal slightly where this contact is avoided (Fig. 17-29). These augments will have the additional benefit of decreasing both the flexion and extension gaps, so that in the face of instability or bone loss, the surgeon will not be forced to the limits of the polyethylene thickness inventory.

Patellar Osteotomy

There are many strategies for dealing with patellar bone loss in revision arthroplasty. If bone loss has left little more than the anterior shell, resulting in a residual scaphoid shape that hugs the lateral femoral condyle and tracks laterally, a simple split of the patella from top to bottom, followed by cracking the medial and lateral halves anteriorly will create a shape that fits more easily in the femoral groove and tracks well. These two pieces generally consolidate with time (13).

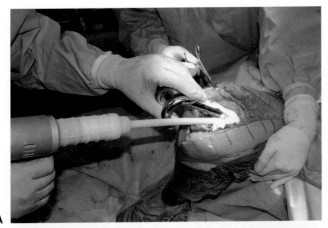

A

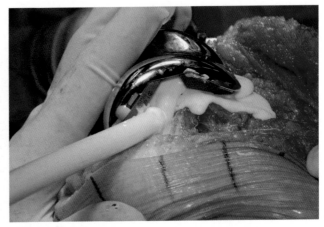

B

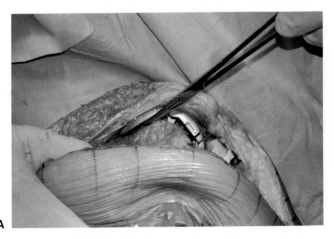

C

FIGURE 17-27

Cementing femur. **(A)** When modular uncemented stems were first introduced, cement was restricted to the cut surface of either the tibia or femur. Loosening still complicated revision knee arthroplasty. Accordingly, the current recommended technique is to place cement on the cut bone surface, introduce the uncemented stem into the femur (or tibia) to about 10 cm short of seating (to occlude the canal), and to fill the metaphyseal area with cement using a gun. **(B)** The component is gradually seated as the cement is introduced. Once the posterior condyles contact the host bone, so that a closed space has been created, additional cement can be introduced to ensure that all defects are filled. **(C)** The actual femoral component has been implanted. The posterolateral augment seen here allowed a sufficiently large femoral component to be implanted to ensure stability in flexion. The distal femoral augment thickness was determined in step 3 by trimming a small amount of irregular distal femur through the cutting slots to ensure that the polyethylene tibial insert that had been chosen to stabilize the knee in flexion is also the correct one to balance the knee in extension.

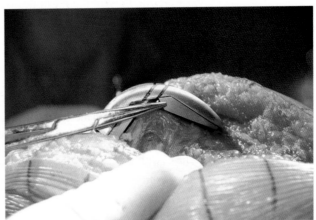

A

B

FIGURE 17-28

Anterior augment. **(A)** Medial view of anterior defect. This defect was defined by reaming the canal, with the handpiece held up, parallel to the medullary canal and using a diaphyseal-filling stem. **(B)** Lateral view of anterior defect with anterior augment in place. This ensures parallel position of the stem in the canal.

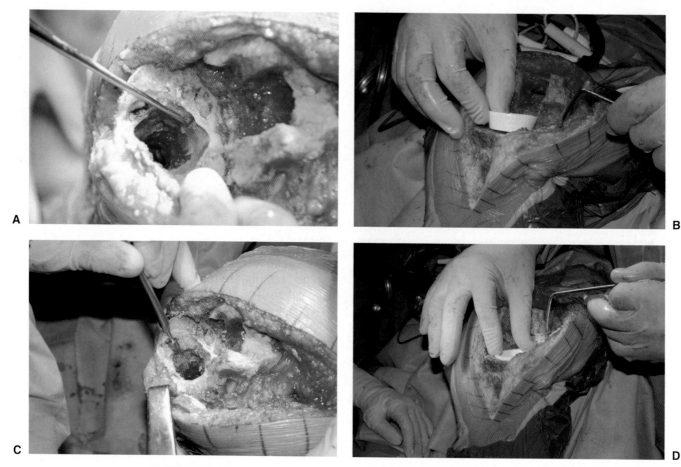

FIGURE 17-29

Tibial defects and the role of porous metal augments. **(A)** Contained tibial defect after failure from wear, osteolysis, and loosening. The defect is not large and could be filled with bone graft or cement. The bone surface quality, however, is poor for cement fixation. **(B)** Porous metal augments may be used to enhance fixation. If the revision bone grows into the porous metal, and then the component is cemented into the porous metal, a solid transition of interfaces will have been created. Here, a trial plastic conical augment is positioned. **(C)** A judgment is made to remove a small amount of sclerotic bone to accommodate the conical augment rather than place the cement up against the smooth, sclerotic host bone. **(D)** The trial cone is seated flush. *(continued)*

PEARLS

1. Establish a diagnosis. As with every field of medicine, an articulate diagnosis must guide therapy. Although there are different approaches to diagnosis, a strong argument can be made that the following eight causes of failure embrace all the indications for revision: loosening/wear, infection, tibiofemoral instability, stiffness, patella maltracking and tibial/femoral component malrotation, extensor mechanism rupture, fracture, and implant breakage (14). Surgery for unexplained pain cannot be justified (Table 17-1).
2. Revise the failed arthroplasty, do not simply perform a repeat surgery. Once the failure has been explained, the revision strategy should address the cause. For example, valgus instability should be corrected by reducing valgus alignment and restoring stability (15) and patellar tracking problems must address rotational positioning of tibial and femoral components (16), etc.
3. Use revision implant systems. The revision is not a primary arthroplasty, and primary implants cannot be expected to address issues of fixation to compromised bone, augmentation of structural deficiency, or constraint for ligamentous instability. Results are superior with revision systems (17).

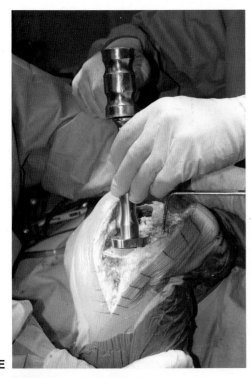

E

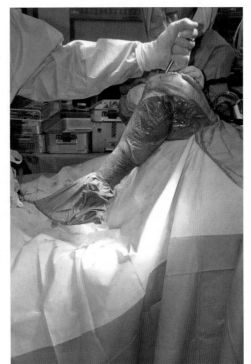

G

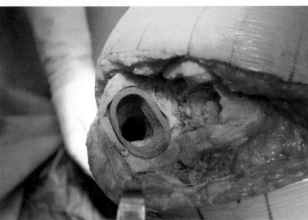

F

FIGURE 17-29 *(Continued)*

(E) Actual porous cone is impacted. **(F)** The rotational position of the cone is immaterial, as long as it does not compromise the correct position of the actual implant. Gaps between the cone and host are filled with bone graft to prevent intrusion of methacrylate cement.
(G) The interference fit of the porous cone is sufficiently solid that a bone hook placed inside of it is able to lift the tibia without dislodging the conical augment.

4. Do a complete revision arthroplasty. The insistence on leaving well-fixed components, while understandable, has been demonstrated empirically to yield poor results, except in select cases (18–22). There are explanations for this. If only the tibia is revised, exposure is difficult, and the collaterals may be stretched. Yet the flexion and extension gaps may be difficult to balance unless the femur is also revised. If only one component is revised, malrotation (typically internal rotation) of a well-fixed and unrevised tibial or femoral component may be overlooked. Finally, constraint will not be an option if it is necessary.

5. Couple the tibia to the femur, accepting what has become of the soft tissues as a result of the failed arthroplasty. This is the essence of the three-step technique described here (23). Insistence upon restoration of normal anatomy (i.e., joint lines in the revision) fails to acknowledge that the soft tissues have been substantially and unpredictably altered by the failed arthroplasty.

PITFALLS

Excess Valgus Femur and Tibia

Many revision knee arthroplasties end up with the femoral (and sometimes the tibial) components in more valgus than the surgeon intended. This may not be problematic unless the knee has been revised for valgus instability. It is difficult to be certain why this happens on the femur, except that most surgeons operate from the same side of the table as the joint and tend to "pull" reamers, trials, and implants toward themselves (i.e., into valgus). The lateral femoral condyle is generally smaller and certainly less strong than the medial. This is difficult to appreciate in a revision where there are so few landmarks. This tendency can be avoided if press-fit stems are large enough to engage the endosteum and long enough to bypass the very funnel shape of the distal femur. In addition, given the anatomy of the distal femur, where the center of the medullary canal lies medial to the distal femur, an offset stem with the component placed laterally and the stem medially will decrease valgus.

Internal Rotation Tibia

There is a tendency to replicate the position of components that are removed, even if this position contributed to the failure, hence the advice to perform a revision, not a repeat arthroplasty. This is best avoided with conscious appreciation of what the rotation was—something that a CT scan and an intraoperative examination provide. I believe that the tibial component needs to be rotated over the tibial tubercle and the extensor mechanism. The tendency to internal rotation will be exacerbated by large amounts of proximal tibial bone loss, especially when this extends to the tip of the fibular head. Once the tibial bone that was above the fibula is lost, the only way to achieve coverage is to internally rotate the component, with adverse effects on patellar function. Even if the surgeon is aware of the risk of internal rotation and plans the ideal position, the posterolateral part of the component may encroach on the femoral bone if the knee is tight or on the femoral component if a partial revision is done. This will force the component to rotate internally.

Accepting Excess Tibial Bone Loss—Small-Diameter Tibia—All Cortical Bone

There is a temptation to accept large amounts of proximal tibia bone loss and simply augment the defect with metal blocks. These cannot have the same fixation to the residual sclerotic cortical bone as is enjoyed in the primary, against cancellous bone. In addition, the size of the tibial component will be small, corresponding to the diameter of the tibial centimeters distal to the original joint. This means that the tibial component is unnaturally small. Despite some interchangeability in most systems between femoral and tibial components, it may not be possible to mate the ideally sized femur with the smaller tibia and will be even more difficult if constraint is needed. Accordingly, the undesirably smaller femoral component will leave the patient with a larger flexion gap of a resection of distal femoral bone, a very thick polyethylene insert, and a markedly elevated joint line. The solution will be the more challenging, proximal tibial allograft.

POSTOPERATIVE MANAGEMENT

The postoperative management of a revision total knee depends on the quality of bone support, integrity of the soft tissues, and stability of the components of the prosthesis. For a routine revision, with an intact medial collateral ligament and only moderate bone loss, where the flexion-extension balance has been reestablished and the joint line reconstructed, the postoperative management duplicates that of a primary total knee.

On the other hand, as structural and ligamentous losses become more complex, the rehabilitation program is slowed proportionately. It is suggested that the revised soft tissue sleeve be allowed to consolidate before applying excessive stress. In the more complex revisions, gentle range of motion is allowed immediately after surgery, but undue force on the knee is avoided, and the impulse to aggressively rebuild muscle strength by means other than isometrics is tempered. Physical therapy should focus on gait training and range of motion for the initial 4 to 6 weeks after revision arthroplasty; quadriceps strengthening can begin after extensor mechanism healing. If a tibial tubercle osteotomy has been used, range of motion, weight bearing, and strengthening may be protected until healing progresses, but it depends on the tubercle's stability of fixation. In addition, weight bearing is started immediately after surgery but protected for longer periods of time compared to primary knee arthroplasty with a walker or crutches. If structural bone grafting has been performed, weight bearing is protected for a longer period of time until consolidation occurs. The postoperative management of the patient after extensor mechanism allografting is discussed in detail in Chapter 31.

Alterations in the typical rehabilitation course should be discussed in detail with the patient, physical therapists, and other personnel involved in the patient's care.

COMPLICATIONS

The single greatest complications related to revision knee replacement surgery are the intraoperative technical problems that can profoundly compromise the outcomes. The most common of these include avulsion or peeling of the patellar tendon from the tibial tubercle, failure to reestablish the joint line, flexion-extension imbalance, patellar maltracking, fracture or loss of bone during implant removal, fracturing of a patella which is too thin, avulsion or transection of the medial collateral ligament, and component malposition. In addition, there are the same potential problems that affect a primary total knee but with an increased risk of occurrence. These problems may include stiffness, delayed wound healing, hematoma, infection, neurapraxia, and others.

REFERENCES

1. Vince KG. Revision knee arthroplasty technique. *Instr Course Lect* 1993;42:325–339.
2. Hanssen AD, Trousdale RT, Osmon DR. Patient outcome with reinfection following reimplantation for the infected total knee arthroplasty. *Clin Orthop Relat Res* 1995;321:55–67.
3. Cierny G 3rd, DiPasquale D. Periprosthetic total joint infections: staging, treatment, and outcomes. *Clin Orthop Relat Res* 2002;403:23–28.
4. Clatworthy MG, Ballance J, Brick CW, et al. The use of structural allograft for uncontained defects in revision total knee arthroplasty. A minimum five-year review. *J Bone Joint Surg Am* 2001;83-A:404–411.
5. Berger RA, Crossett LS, Jacobs JJ, et al. Malrotation causing patellofemoral complications after total knee arthroplasty. *Clin Orthop Relat Res* 1998;356:144–153.
6. Reish TG, Clarke HD, Scuderi GR, et al. Use of multi-detector computed tomography for the detection of periprosthetic osteolysis in total knee arthroplasty. *J Knee Surg* 2006;19:259–264.
7. Vince KG, Droll KP, Chivas D. Your next revision total knee arthroplasty: why start in flexion? *Orthopedics* 2007;30:791–792.
8. Nakasone CK, Abdeen A, Khachatourians AG, et al. Component alignment in revision total knee arthroplasty using diaphyseal engaging modular offset press-fit stems. *J Arthroplasty* 2007 Dec 10 [Epub ahead of print].
9. Whiteside LA, Arima J. The anteroposterior axis for femoral rotational alignment in valgus total knee arthroplasty. *Clin Orthop Relat Res* 1995;321:168–172.
10. Arima J, Whiteside LA, McCarthy DS, et al. Femoral rotational alignment, based on the anteroposterior axis, in total knee arthroplasty in a valgus knee. A technical note. *J Bone Joint Surg Am* 1995;77:331–334.
11. Griffin FM, Math K, Scuderi GR, et al. Anatomy of the epicondyles of the distal femur: MRI analysis of normal knees. *J Arthroplasty* 2000;15:354–359.
12. Vince KG, Abdeen A. Revision TKA: four cases that taught me new things. *Orthopedics* 2006;29:853–855.
13. Vince K, Roidis N, Blackburn D. Gullwing sagittal patellar osteotomy in total knee arthroplasty. *Techniques in Knee Surgery* 2002;1:106–112.
14. Vince KG. Why knees fail. *J Arthroplasty* 2003;18(3 Suppl 1):39–44.
15. Vince KG, Abdeen A, Sugimori T. The unstable total knee arthroplasty: causes and cures. *J Arthroplasty* 2006;21(4 Suppl 1):44–49.
16. Malo M, Vince KG. The unstable patella after total knee arthroplasty: etiology, prevention, and management. *J Am Acad Orthop Surg* 2003;11:364–371.
17. Bugbee WD, Ammeen DJ, Engh GA. Does implant selection affect outcome of revision knee arthroplasty? *J Arthroplasty* 2001;16:581–585.
18. Babis GC, Trousdale RT, Morrey BF. The effectiveness of isolated tibial insert exchange in revision total knee arthroplasty. *J Bone Joint Surg Am* 2002;84-A:64–68.
19. Babis GC, Trousdale RT, Pagnano MW, et al. Poor outcomes of isolated tibial insert exchange and arthrolysis for the management of stiffness following total knee arthroplasty. *J Bone Joint Surg Am* 2001;83-A:1534–1536.
20. Fehring TK, Odum S, Griffin WL, et al. Outcome comparison of partial and full component revision TKA. *Clin Orthop Relat Res* 2005;440:131–134.
21. Mackay DC, Siddique MS. The results of revision knee arthroplasty with and without retention of secure cemented femoral components. *J Bone Joint Surg Br* 2003;85:517–520.
22. Knutson K, Lewold S, Robertsson O, et al. The Swedish knee arthroplasty register. A nation-wide study of 30,003 knees 1976-1992. *Acta Orthop Scand* 1994;65:375–386.
23. Vince KG. A step-wise approach to revision TKA. *Orthopedics* 2005;28:999–1001.

18 Managing Medial Collateral Ligament Deficiency with Soft Tissue Reconstruction

Kenneth A. Krackow

INDICATIONS/CONTRAINDICATIONS

Loss of ligament stability in total knee replacement, both in primary and revision situations, is commonly addressed by increasing the prostheses' constraint (1–5). But use of constrained prostheses, particularly rotating hinges, as well as constrained intercondylar prostheses (CIPs), may not be an optimal solution. This is particularly true in younger active patients, as shown by numerous studies (1–5). Furthermore, major reliance on the constrained prosthesis alone may not lead to success if the prosthesis is used without adequate soft tissue balance.

There are special situations in primary total knee replacement in which ligament loss or incompetence is encountered, either preoperatively or intraoperatively, and our preferred techniques for managing these situations are described herein. This ligament advancement or reconstruction approach is used at the time of knee arthroplasty to adjust major soft tissue sleeve imbalance caused by ligament loss or incompetence. It is not used as a technique for managing unstable total knee arthroplasty at a second separate procedure. Also, this chapter deals with ligament incompetence situations, not soft tissue balance techniques in general, which usually involve releasing tight structures on the concave side of a deformity and which are covered in Chapter 9.

Ligament imbalance in a primary total knee can be managed by different methods:

- Soft tissue balancing (generally done by releasing tight structures on the concave side of the deformity)
- Ligament reconstruction (which may include proximal and distal advancement of ligaments or ligament substitution or augmentation)
- Constrained prostheses (which may range from total stabilizing to a hinged prosthesis)
- A combination of any two or more

We use the term *CIP* to indicate total knee components with intra-articular "peg" mechanisms that provide medial lateral and posterior stability. This term has been adopted to provide a generic alternative to the cumbersome attempts at not favoring a particular brand by simultaneously always mentioning two or three, for example, constrained condylar knee, total condylar III, superstabilizer, and others.

We define ligament loss or incompetence as a situation in which the ligament is either stretched and attenuated or injured and in discontinuity. In these situations, releasing the opposite side to balance the soft tissue sleeve may not be an ideal solution. It may likely be impractical to expect to lengthen the now relatively tight side enough to balance out to an abnormally lengthened position assumed on the damaged side. Also, neither the original damaged side nor the released surgically lengthened side will possess normal ligament strength. Therefore, ligament reconstruction or the use of a more constrained prosthesis or a combination of both may be necessary to achieve adequate stability.

CIPs have been shown to have encouraging results in the intermediate-term follow-up in elderly patients with low physical demand (3). In individuals who are younger and more active, however, the constrained knee may transfer stress to the implant–cement–bone fixation interface and may lead to early failure. Therefore, to avoid excessive prosthesis constraint in patients who are not elderly, ligament reconstruction can be a workable alternative. Key features of the indications for soft tissue advancement or reconstruction as described in this chapter relate to a strong desire to avoid the use of a CIP.

It should also be clear that we are dealing with a situation that by definition is not amenable to a solution by use of posterior-substituting components alone. Most posterior-stabilized components provide no collateral stability; they provide posterior stability and some medial lateral translation stability.

PREOPERATIVE LIGAMENT LOSS

Preoperative ligament loss can be the result of traumatic ligament injury or stretching, or as part of these a priori primary deformities.

Valgus Deformity

Valgus deformity in an arthritic knee may be classified as type I, type II, or type III (Fig. 18-1A–C) (6,7). The type II valgus knee is found in a small subgroup of patients with greater bony deformity with two specific soft tissue problems: lateral soft tissue contracture and medial soft tissue attenuation. Medial ligament reconstruction procedures are considered in those cases in which adequate medial stability has not or cannot be achieved, despite essentially maximum soft tissue release. Such release would include posterior cruciate ligament release or recession and extensive release of lateral collateral structures.

While considering special deformity situations that may be addressed by ligament reconstruction technique, it may also be appropriate to consider and discuss type III valgus deformity. An example of this is a severely overcorrected closing wedge-style proximal tibial osteotomy as a result of malunion, late collapse, wear in the lateral compartment, or overcorrection at the time of surgery. This situation is not exactly an example of ligament damage or incompetence, but its management is unusual and fits in with other techniques discussed in this chapter.

In this situation, in addition to the grossly abnormal valgus-oriented proximal tibia, there is an asymmetry of the soft tissue sleeve, which is different from the average valgus knee. The dissection at the lateral aspect of the knee and soft tissue handling of the iliotibial band and lateral collateral ligament during the previous proximal tibial osteotomy together can make the standard lateral soft tissue release more difficult. Achieving sufficient lateral release in any of these examples to achieve simultaneous balance of collateral ligaments and the normal 6 degrees of valgus tibiofemoral angle may simply be impossible (8,9). Therefore, medial ligament reconstruction may be considered to achieve adequate balance, particularly in younger active individuals in whom we want to avoid excessive constraint. Furthermore, in our experience, the tibial osteotomy is done in the younger age group, and the truly overcorrected example becomes a major problem within 18 months to 2 years after osteotomy. Therefore, patients with type III valgus presenting for treatment are relatively young patients in whom the surgeon would like to avoid the use of a CIP.

Today, type III valgus knees may also be managed by simultaneous tibial osteotomy during arthroplasty, with fixation using press-fit intramedullary stems. The complex ligament reconstruction procedure was developed before such implants became available (8). Other options, such as

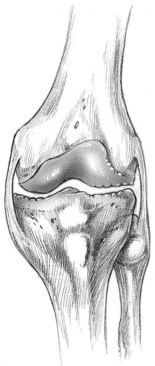
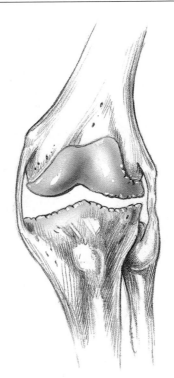
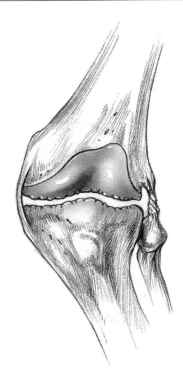

A–C

FIGURE 18-1

Classification of valgus deformity for total knee arthroplasty. **(A)** Type I valgus deformity has mild-to-moderate deformity with medial capsular ligamentous soft tissues intact—that is, without excessive attenuation. **(B)** Type II valgus deformity is more severe than type I and has an attenuation of the medial capsular ligamentous sleeve. **(C)** Type III valgus deformity occurs when significant overcorrection is present after valgus proximal tibial osteotomy or conceivably tibial plateau fracture, resulting in the same configuration. Valgus-oriented tibial joint surface in combination with relatively varus-oriented distal femoral situation. Deformity is by definition significant, and soft tissue structures to both the medial and the lateral side are usually intact.

corrective osteotomy alone could even be considered for some cases. TKA should be offered only when the patient is, in general terms, considered an arthroplasty candidate because of significant intra-articular degeneration requiring joint resurfacing.

Procedures

The following procedures are indicated for preoperative ligament loss, depending on the nature of the injury. Medial collateral ligament (MCL) reconstruction is indicated for preoperative traumatic MCL injury and type II and type III valgus deformity.

INTRAOPERATIVE LIGAMENT LOSS

MCL

The MCL is probably the most common collateral ligament injured intraoperatively. The exact incidence of this complication is not known. In our personal experience, it is less than 1%. There are reports of an incidence rate as high as 8% in a selected group of morbidly obese individuals (10). Whatever the incidence may be, intraoperative disruption of MCL injury could cause significant soft tissue imbalance and late postoperative medial instability with valgus deformity.

Situations in which there is a high risk of injuring the MCL intraoperatively are as follows:

- Markedly obese individuals with difficult exposures
- Tight varus knees, typically with overhanging medial femoral and tibial osteophytes
- Surgical inexperience

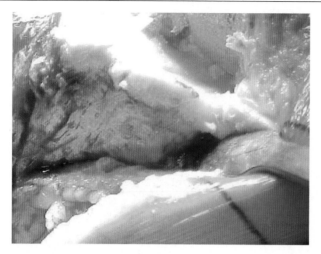

FIGURE 18-2

Subperiosteal dissection of the medial tibial condyle and placement of the retractor under the medial collateral ligament.

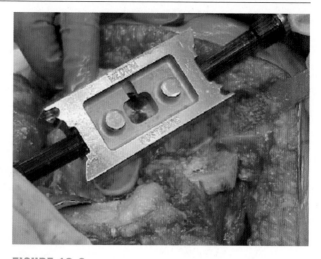

FIGURE 18-3

Protecting the collateral ligaments by placing the retractors at the same level as the saw blade while doing bone preparation.

Intraoperative MCL injury occurs when the surgeon fails to remain close enough to the bone and dissect under the MCL at the medial tibia, just below the osteophyte. In certain cases, the superficial MCL remains closely apposed to the bone here. The surgeon or the assistant who does not appreciate this fact may lacerate the MCL if it is not adequately retracted during sharp dissection when attempting to uncover the osteophyte, during sawing the tibial or posterior femoral cut, or while excising the medial meniscus without proper tension or exposure.

Clearly, the best practice is to avoid injury. Surgical tips to avoid injuring the MCL include the following:

- Medial tibial condyle dissection must be subperiosteal and therefore deep to the MCL.
- Placement of an elevator or retractor must clearly be under the MCL (Fig. 18-2) on bare bone.
- The collateral ligaments should be protected by placing appropriate retractors while performing the bony preparation (Fig. 18-3) and making certain that the retractors are at the same level as the saw blade.
- Release the mid and posterior midmedial capsular margin and deep MCL before cutting the medial tibia (Fig. 18-4) so that it is possible to perform adequate protecting retraction.

Recognizing the MCL injury is one of the key elements in its management. Most of the time, the MCL injury is masked in full extension caused by secondary supporting structures at the posterior and posteromedial corner of the knee. The increased instability becomes evident only in flexion. The injury can be confirmed by doing further dissection or by palpating the ligament directly.

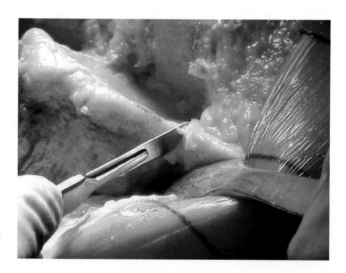

FIGURE 18-4

The medial capsular margin and the deep medial collateral ligament are being released before cutting the medial tibial condyle.

Sometimes, a major clue can be sudden ease of delivering the tibia forward, together with an apparent external rotation while working in flexion.

Once injury is recognized, the next course of action is still debatable. It is well known that an unstable total knee does not do well. For this reason, we stress the importance of being confident that the soft tissues are not left with inappropriate imbalance (11–15). It seems logical to repair the injured ligament to maintain such soft tissue balance (16). In the presence of direct injury, repair would be the surgeon's immediate thought. Direct repair may be very feasible and the option of choice, particularly in the case of a partial laceration.

In other cases of complete laceration, the surgeon must also examine the setting to see if direct repair is practical. In the case of a tight varus deformity that requires medial release, reapplication of the ends with direct repair may be impractical. This basic consideration is the main rationale for our use of a semitendinosus augmentation technique.

A technique we have been using to address MCL injury at TKA may be considered. Despite the limited experience, it adheres to general orthopedic principles and may extricate the surgeon from a difficult situation if the available structure and surfaces are proper and intact. The method involves semitendinosus tendon augmentation, left attached to its tibial insertion and fixed at (or somewhere proximal to) the epicenter of medial femoral rotation. This technique is only feasible if (a) the distal semitendinosus insertion remains intact, (b) host bone at the medial femoral condyle is adequate, and (c) stable fixation of the tendon graft to the femoral bone is possible.

PREOPERATIVE PLANNING

If ligament reconstruction is favored, preoperative workup should include the following:

- Assessment of the deformity's severity and the instability
- Availability of workable tissues such as semitendinosus tendon
- Prosthetic availability (if adequate stability cannot be achieved at the time of surgery with ligament reconstruction, the option of increasing the constraint in the prosthesis should be available)

SURGERY

Surgery for Preoperative MCL Attenuation

Techniques have been refined for both proximal and distal advancement of soft tissue capsular ligamentous elements on the medial aspect of the knee. Clearly, they are intended to address medial attenuation in valgus deformity. We generally restrict the technique to proximal advancement on the femur for several reasons. On the medial side, the ligamentous complex has a delta or deltoid configuration, spanning from an epicenter at the femur to broad attachment at the tibia. Adequately cinching up the medial side by distal advancement requires elevation of the entire distal medial sleeve from the tibia—including the superficial MCL, posteromedial capsule, and posterior oblique ligament—after such elevation. The entire sleeve needs to reattach distally to the tibia. The dissection is large, the technical requirements are greater, and the possibility for disruption (and alternatively protection) of the reconstruction seems less favorable.

With this background, it was considered that proximal advancement would be easier, safer, and overall more successful. It is important to appreciate that proximal advancement is performed with the goal of establishing the final reattachment point at the presumed epicenter of rotation to which the original end of the ligament extends.

MCL Reconstruction

The technique described is more simple than one might imagine. For valgus deformity, the medial capsular ligamentous flap is elevated from the epicondylar origin, creating a trapezoid flap of tissue, which remains distally attached (Fig. 18-5A). The elevated tissue has substantial thickness and will hold sutures well. Our preference is not to start with a bone flap or bone island, because this practice may weaken the residual future attachment site (Fig. 18-6). We also focus attention on achieving the major security of the advancement tissue at the more proximal location, not at the center of rotation, most likely closer to the original point of elevation. But we still want to achieve attachment at an area that might be removed (i.e., the center of rotation) if we take off a bony surface (Fig. 18-5B).

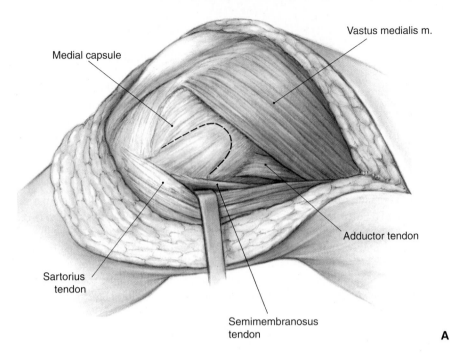

Medial capsule

Vastus medialis m.

Sartorius
tendon

Semimembranosus
tendon

Adductor tendon

A

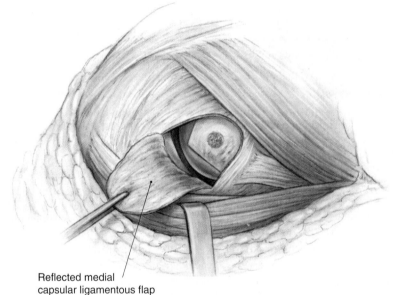

Reflected medial
capsular ligamentous flap

B

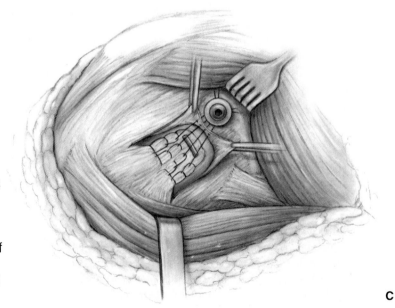

FIGURE 18-5

Proximal advancement of the medial collateral
ligament. **(A)** The medial capsular ligamentous
flap is elevated from the epicondylar origin,
creating a trapezoidal flap of tissue that remains
attached distally. **(B)** The center of rotation is
determined to be beneath this reflected
ligamentous flap. **(C)** The flap is advanced
proximally and secured proximal to the center of
rotation. One or two locking loop ligament
sutures are placed into the ligamentous flap and
secured proximally.

C

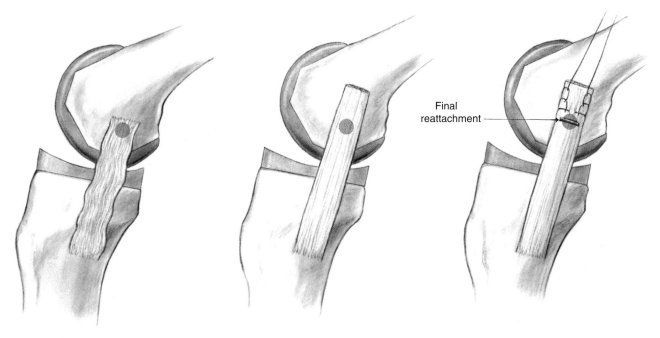

FIGURE 18-6

Proximal attachment of the medial collateral ligament requires elevation of the proximal ligament. However, the final reattachment point on the femur is at the presumed epicenter of rotation for the femoral condyle and not the new proximal end of the ligament.

It is imperative at the first stage of tissue elevation that this is accomplished completely so that the flap of tissue being handled is disconnected entirely from the femur. Pulling on it directly should be resisted only by attachments at the tibia.

The surgeon places one or two locking loop ligament sutures using suitably stout material (such as no. 5 Ethibond) (Fig. 18-5C) (17,18). The epicenter of the femoral condylar geometry is generally estimated by visual inspection. The flap is manipulated anteroproximally, straight proximally, or possibly proximal posteriorly to find the best-fitting arrangement. This position is usually cephalad and anterior (Fig. 18-7A,B). The soft tissue is reapplied to the femur at the epicenter with a soft tissue staple or a screw–ligament–washer combination.

The "tails" of the sutures are tied more proximally to a "post." We generally use a long screw with a washer. The screw, if possible, should be long enough to reach the far lateral cortex. Also, it is aimed obliquely, rather than straight medial laterally.

Oblique orientation of the proximal fixation screw is used because a more transversely directed screw undergoes a larger moment created by a distally originating force. It seems that a transversely oriented screw has less stability to resist the force than a similar but longer type of screw directed more obliquely and closer in line with distraction force (Fig. 18-8).

The working side, originally the convex side of the deformity, may be quite soft (from disuse osteoporosis) because it has been underloaded. For this reason, pay special attention to the soft tissue fixation methods because the soft bone does not typically provide strong staple fixation.

The suture fixation to this proximal screw is the real strength of the reattachment. The point of reattachment of the ligament to bone, however, is at the epicenter where the soft tissue is applied by the first-mentioned staple or ligament–screw–washer combination.

The surgeon performs reconstruction after final placement of the actual components, and assuming that a proper center of rotation reattachment point has been selected, tension is set at approximately 25 to 30 degrees of flexion.

This technique would quite possibly be employed with the use of a stemmed femoral component and possibly one that has an intercondylar box associated with a posterior-substituting design, so the orientation of the fixation devices (screw or staple) must be planned carefully to "dodge" these metallic elements of the femoral component. We do not use this technique in combination with the CIP type of prosthesis and use an imbrication technique in those situations.

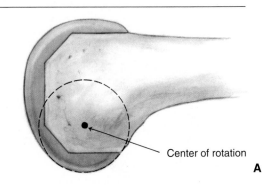

Center of rotation

A

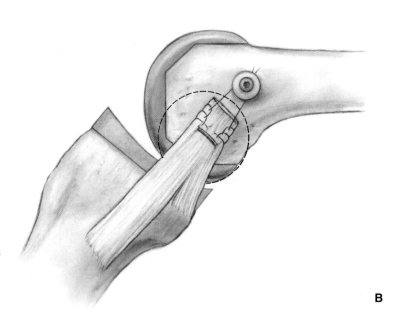

B

FIGURE 18-7

(A) Determination of the epicenter. The epicenter is determined according to the outline of the femoral joint surface. **(B)** Technique of reattachment. The flap is manipulated anteriorly and proximally to re-establish the epicenter with a soft tissue center or screw–ligament–washer combination. The tails of the suture are tied more proximal to a screw post.

Passing the suture tails through separate drill holes to the far cortex and tying the sutures over that cortex is an alternative if the proximal screw washer seems not to be possible (Fig. 18-9).

The added requisite exposure to perform this proximal advancement is really not as great as may be imagined. The exposure plus the advancement is more often less surgery than one might undertake for accomplishment of the alternative rather gigantic concave side release, which would be necessary in a greater attempt to achieve collateral balance. Also, this latter attempt may be inadequate because of the inherent limitation of concave release.

FIGURE 18-8

(A,B) The bone on the unloaded knee condyle is frequently soft, and good fixation is important. We prefer to use an obliquely directed screw because it will resist distraction of forces, offering more resistance to distraction forces.

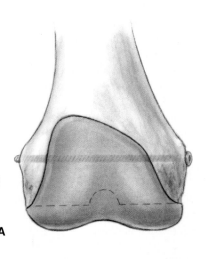

A

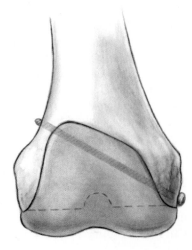

B

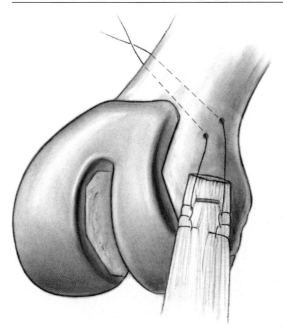

FIGURE 18-9

An alternative to proximal screw fixation is making separate drill holes through the proximal cortex and securing the sutures through them. This step is useful if the bone is very soft, but it may be difficult with a stemmed component.

Semitendinosus Augmentation for MCL Disruption

The semitendinosus tendon is accessed by reflecting the cephalad margin of the pes anserinus group peripherally and distal posteromedially (Fig. 18-10A). The tendon is identified, looped, and pulled up into view with a curved clamp (Fig. 18-10B). Scissors dissection is used to free the tendon from the surrounding sheath and attached soft tissue and muscle (Fig. 18-10C). The surgery at this point is essentially identical to what the surgeon would perform for harvesting a semitendinosus piece for anterior cruciate ligament reconstruction work. Deep narrow retractors, long scissors, a tendon stripper, and a remote tendon cutter are all helpful.

After the tendon is freed and released proximally, the femoral attachment point is selected with a trial or final femoral component in place. If there is no attached MCL tissue, the center-of-rotation attachment point can be selected without consideration for plans to imbricate the MCL.

If the femoral origin of the MCL remains and seems to be at the proper epicenter of rotation, clearly, the semitendinosus tendon used as a ligament augmentation device will need to be attached elsewhere.

Considering the requirement of maintaining essentially equal flexion-extension gaps, a 45-degree line drawn distal posterior to proximal anterior going through the equal ligament length or flexion-extension gap situations for the tibia at 0 and 90 degrees. Positioning on this line proximal and anterior to the epicenter of rotation, which itself is isometric at 0 degrees, will be relatively tight at angles in between. This can be seen geometrically and has been shown in cadaver experiments by Martin and Whiteside (19). Attachment points selected distal and posterior to the epicondylar region will similarly have isometry at 0 and 90 degrees but laxity at points in between (Fig. 18-11A–D).

The surgeon must then examine the tibiofemoral gapping situation to determine if the gapping in flexion seems to be greater, equal to, or less than in extension and adjust the placement point accordingly. Attachment above the 45-degree line leads to relative tightness in flexion, whereas attachment below leads to relative laxity in flexion and relative tightness in extension.

Attachment of the semitendinosus augmentation is via a through-and-through drill hole directed from the chosen medial entry point, directed laterally and exiting generally slightly proximal and anterior to the respective entry point. The hole should be drilled at a diameter equal to or very slightly smaller (by 1 to 2 mm) than the estimated diameter of the semitendinosus tendon (Fig. 18-10D).

Passage of this equal-sized or oversized tendon is accomplished by using what we refer to as a homemade Chinese fingertrap (Fig. 18-12) (20). To ensure permanence of the Chinese fingertrap device's grip, the surgeon places a single suture as indicated to resist initial slippage and to activate or invoke the constricting behavior, which is the essence of the grasping function provided by the trap (Fig. 18-13) (20). With careful construction of the trap, it is possible to pull a tendon easily through a rather snug drill hole.

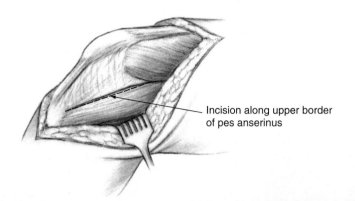

Incision along upper border of pes anserinus

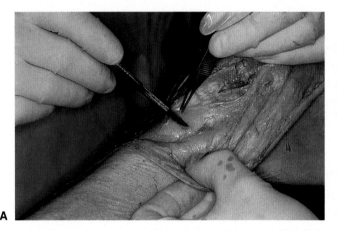

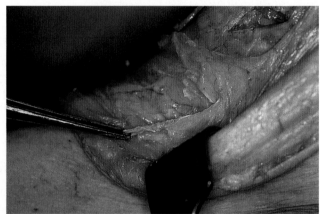

A

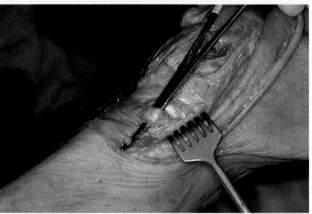

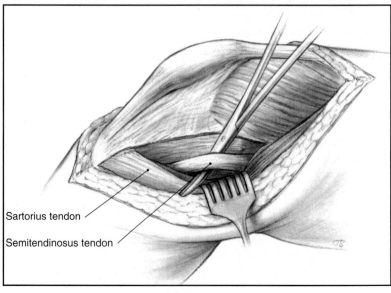

Sartorius tendon

Semitendinosus tendon

B

FIGURE 18-10

Semitendinosus augmentation for deficiency in the medial collateral ligament. **(A)** The pes anserinus group is identified by palpation and with a longitudinal incision just anterior to the group. **(B)** The tendon is identified, looped, and pulled into view with a curved clamp. *(continued)*

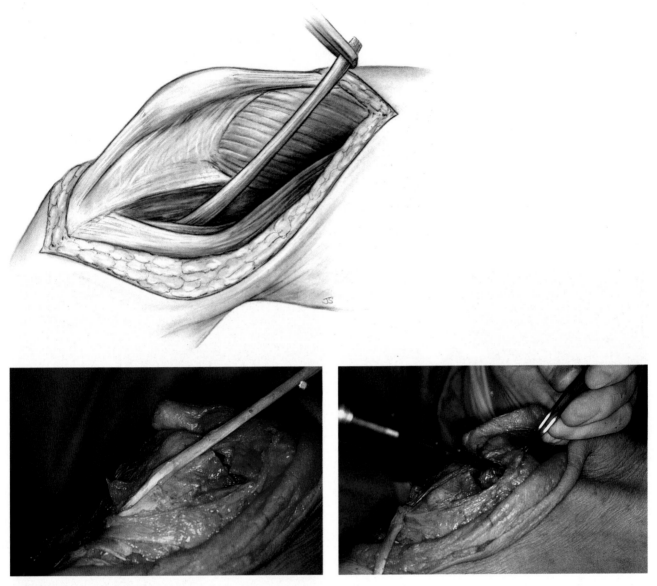

FIGURE 18-10 *(Continued)*

(C) The tendon is freed from the surrounding sheath detached at the muscular tendinous junction. *(continued)*

The four suture tails are passed through to the far side of the tunnel. The semitendinosus tendon is pulled into the tunnel. Depending on the length of the tendon, it either will be through and exiting at the lateral cortex or have its endpoint situated within femoral bone.

Stabilization of the tendon will primarily be achieved by tethering of the suture tails from the fingertrap. This fixation may be accomplished by tying over a screw, washer, or staple (Fig. 18-14). In addition to securing the tails, when the tendon is long enough to exit the lateral femoral cortex, a soft tissue staple may be added, approximating the tendinous tissue to the cortex in the exit region. The tails of the homemade Chinese fingertrap, however, are still secured in a somewhat remote region.

One might use a Mitec or other suture anchor as well, although we have not used those types of sutures. This equipment is perhaps more expensive and may be less secure compared with a ligament staple or screws when used in relatively osteoporotic bone, which is present in older patients requiring these techniques.

As with techniques previously described, final positioning and tensioning of the semitendinosus, and whatever imbrication is performed on residual medical collateral tissue, are performed after final components are in place.

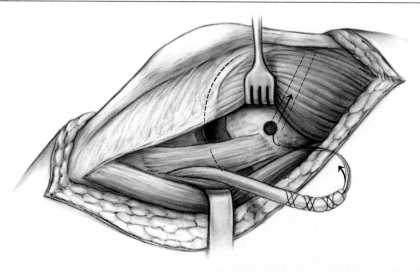

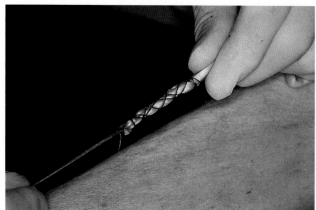

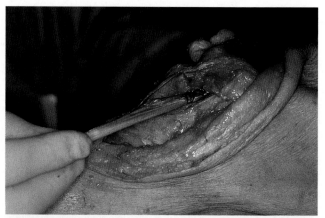

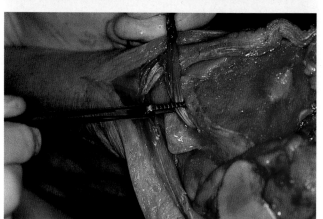

FIGURE 18-10 (Continued)

(D) A homemade Chinese fingertrap is wrapped around the proximal portion of the semitendinosus tendon. The semitendinosus tendon is pulled into the tunnel at the proper epicenter of rotation. The tendon may be stabilized by the suture anchor or by the screw over the staple on the lateral cortex.

POSTOPERATIVE MANAGEMENT

Preoperative Ligament Loss

The situation after proper performance of ligament repair should look quite stable, but the surgeon must not be overconfident and undertake a program of minimal attention or protection, which is suboptimal. Appreciation of the possibility of failure is, we believe, appropriate and most essential. We seek a postoperative regimen that permits range-of-motion (ROM) exercise, however, protection and caution are in order.

The two most vulnerable times would seem to be very early in the postoperative course from time 0 through 3 to 5 days, during which, the patient may be relatively unable to call into play his or her own active muscular protective mechanisms, secondary to pain and analgesic sedation. Unprotected movement of the extremity by nursing or physical therapy staff could be disruptive.

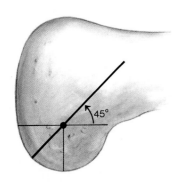

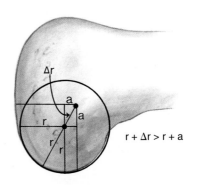

$r + \Delta r > r + a$

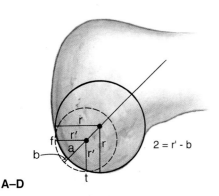

$2 = r' - b$

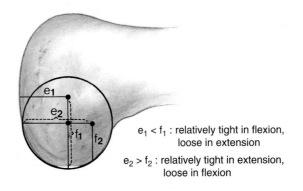

$e_1 < f_1$: relatively tight in flexion, loose in extension

$e_2 > f_2$: relatively tight in extension, loose in flexion

A–D

FIGURE 18-11

Determining the proper epicenter of rotation on the medial femoral condyle. **(A)** A line drawn 45 degrees to the distal posterior femoral cortex and going through the femoral epicondylar area will maintain equal flexion and extension gaps. **(B)** Positioning of the line proximal and anterior to the epicenter of rotation, which itself is isometric at 0 and 90 degrees, will be relatively tight at angles in between. **(C)** Attachment points selected distally and posteriorly at the condylar region will similarly have isometry at 0 and 90 degrees but laxity at points in between. **(D)** In a revision situation, the surgeon may have to move a more proximal reattachment. The surgeon must carefully examine the tibial femoral gapping situation to determine which position is best.

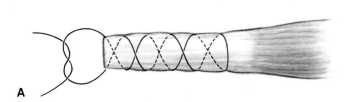

A

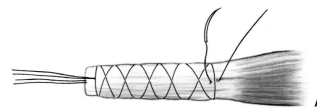

A

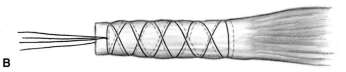

B

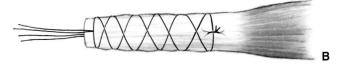

B

FIGURE 18-12

(A,B) The homemade tendon Chinese fingertrap can stabilize the free tendon edge. The suture material is wrapped around the distal end of the tendon and tied to prevent loosening of the trap.

FIGURE 18-13

(A,B) To ensure permanence of the grip of the Chinese fingertrap device, a single suture is placed, as indicated, to activate or invoke the constricting behavior, which is the essence of the grasping function provided by the trap.

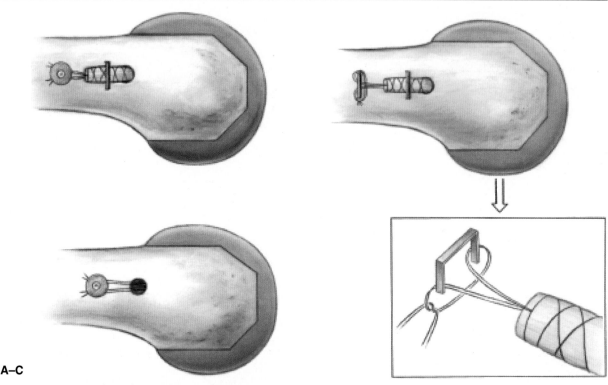

A–C

FIGURE 18-14

Securing the semitendinosus tendon on the lateral cortex. **(A)** If the tendon is long enough to come out of the lateral cortex hole, it can be secured with a staple while the suture tails are secured over a screw. **(B)** The suture tails may also be secured under and about a stale placed more proximally. **(C)** If the tendon is too short, it can be secured with a suture anchor in the bone, and the tails can be stabilized around a screw on the lateral cortex.

Similarly, as the patient gets past the second or third week and has good ROM with substantially less pain and generally less protective attention to the knee, the possibility of untoward movement and stress seems significant—these are times at which extra caution is in order.

Continuous passive motion (CPM) is avoided in the earliest stage (0 to 5 postoperative days). The patients are braced near full extension for the first 3 to 4 weeks, removing the brace frequently for specific active and active-assisted ROM exercise. The splint is replaced to protect against unconscious untoward movement and force. Continuous passive motion could possibly be used to a degree, but we have not specifically done this. At 3 to 4 weeks, the long leg splint or knee immobilizer may be changed to a hinged device. Similarly, this latter type of brace is removed for specific ROM sessions and then is replaced. It is worn at night as well. At 6 weeks, a relatively simple, hinged knee brace is used while the patient is awake and up and for about the next 6 weeks to 3 months.

RESULTS

The techniques described in this chapter have been effective at restoring knee stability and achieving success despite MCL deficiency noted preoperatively or occuring intraoperatively. One study by Healy et al (12), reported on the results of eight knees with type II valgus deformity treated with proximal MCL advancement and bone plug recession. In that series, the mean patient age was 75 years, and the mean preoperative tibiofemoral alignment was 22 degrees of valgus (range, 15 to 30 degrees valgus). Posterior cruciate-retaining implant designs were used in seven knees; one had a posterior-stabilized implant. No additional implant constraint was necessary. Unrestricted motion was allowed in a hinged knee brace for 6 weeks. At most recent follow-up, 100% of patients were satisfied, there were no knees with coronal laxity, and the mean knee ROM improved from 87 degrees preoperatively to 113 degrees postoperatively.

REFERENCES

1. Chotivichit AL, Cracchiolo A III, Chow GH, et al. Total knee arthroplasty using the total condylar III knee prosthesis. *J Arthroplasty* 1991;6(4):341–350.
2. Donaldson WF III, Sculco TP, Insall JN, et al. Total condylar III knee prosthesis. Long-term follow-up study. *Clin Orthop* 1988;226:21–28.
3. Easley ME, Insall JN, Scuderi GR, et al. Primary constrained condylar knee arthroplasty for the arthritic valgus knee. *Clin Orthop* 2000;380:58–64.
4. Rand JA. Revision total knee arthroplasty using the total condylar III prosthesis. *J Arthroplasty* 1991;6(3):279–284.
5. Sculco TP. Total condylar III prosthesis in ligament instability. *Orthop Clin North Am* 1989;20(2):221–226.
6. Krackow KA. *The Technique of Total Knee Arthroplasty.* St. Louis: C.V. Mosby; 1990.
7. Krackow KA, Jones MM, Teeny SM, et al. Primary total knee arthroplasty in patients with fixed valgus deformity. *Clin Orthop* 1991;273:9–18.
8. Krackow KA, Holtgrewe JL. Experience with a new technique for managing severely overcorrected valgus high tibial osteotomy at total knee arthroplasty. *Clin Orthop* 1990;258:213–224.
9. Mont MA, Alexander N, Krackow KA, et al. Total knee arthroplasty after failed high tibial osteotomy. *Orthop Clin North Am* 1994;25(3):515–525.
10. Winiarsky R, Barth P, Lotke P. Total knee arthroplasty in morbidly obese patients. *J Bone Joint Surg* 1998;80:1770–1774.
11. Griffin FM, Insall JN, Scuderi GR. Accuracy of soft tissue balancing in total knee arthroplasty. *J Arthroplasty* 2000;15(8):970–973.
12. Healy WL, Iorio R, Lemos DW. Medial reconstruction during total knee arthroplasty for severe valgus deformity. *Clin Orthop* 1998;356:161–169.
13. Krackow KA, Miller CD, Mihalko WM, et al. Thinking about deformity and alignment in TKA. *Orthopedics* 1997;20(9):825–826.
14. Takahashi T, Wada Y, Yamamoto H. Soft-tissue balancing with pressure distribution during total knee arthroplasty. *J Bone Joint Surg Br* 1997;79(2):235–239.
15. Whiteside LA, Saeki K, Mihalko WM. Functional medial ligament balancing in total knee arthroplasty. *Clin Orthop* 2000;380:45–57.
16. Leopold SS, McStay C, Klafeta K, et al. Primary repair of intraoperative disruption of the medical collateral ligament during total knee arthroplasty. *J Bone Joint Surg Am* 2001;83(1):86–91.
17. Krackow KA, Thomas SC, Jones LC. A new stitch for ligament-tendon fixation [Brief note]. *J Bone Joint Surg Am* 1986;68(5):764–766.
18. Krackow KA, Thomas SC, Jones LC. Ligament-tendon fixation: analysis of a new stitch and comparison with standard techniques. *Orthopedics* 1988;11(6):909–917.
19. Martin JW, Whiteside LA. The influence of joint line position on knee stability after condylar knee arthroplasty. *Clin Orthop* 1990;259(6):909–917.
20. Krackow KA, Cohn BT. A new technique for passing tendon through bone [Brief note]. *J Bone Joint Surg Am* 1987;69(6):922–924.

19 Managing Bone Loss with Metal Augments

Henry D. Clarke and Arlen D. Hanssen

INDICATIONS

Primary total knee arthroplasty (TKA) has proven reliable, yet failures do occur (1,2). Contemporary causes of failure include aseptic loosening, infection, and osteolysis caused by particulate wear debris (3,4). Each of these etiologies can result in significant bone loss that must be managed at the time of revision TKA.

The management of this bone loss in revision TKA is based on the size and type of defects that are encountered during the procedure. Numerous options exist and in many circumstances, alternative reconstructive techniques may be considered, including:

- Cement
- Particulate and structural bone grafts
- Metal augments
- Allograft prosthetic composites
- Segmental replacement prostheses

The strategy used by each surgeon may be influenced by factors including availability of the required items, surgeon experience, operative time, cost, and age and activity level of the patient. As for many surgeons, our preferred choice primarily depends on the size of the defect.

Numerous classification systems have been previously described to aid in both pre-operative planning and intraoperative management of bone loss in revision TKA. We favor the use of the Anderson Orthopaedic Research Institute (AORI) classification, which is relatively simple and has been validated (Table 19-1) (5,6).

Practical guidelines have been published, based on the AORI classification, to aid the surgeon in managing the bone loss encountered in revision TKA (5,7). With the introduction of larger standard and trabecular metal augments, the spectrum of defects that can be managed with this technique has increased and represents our primary choice in most circumstances. Based on the size of the lesion, our preferred techniques are as follows:

- AORI type 1 defects of the femur and tibia, including small, contained defects less than or equal to 5 mm in depth can be managed with cement or traditional metal augments.
- AORI type 2 defects, whether unicondylar or bicondylar, including uncontained defects up to 20 mm in depth can usually be addressed with conventional metal or trabecular-metal augments.
- AORI type 3 defects have historically been managed with structural allograft bone, allograft prosthetic composites, or megaprostheses. However, the introduction of very large trabecular metal augments, which can be used with a variety of prosthesis systems, has largely replaced our use of structural allografts.

TABLE 19-1. AORI Classification of Bone Defects in Total Knee Arthroplasty

Type 1	Intact metaphyseal bone	Good cancellous bone at or near the normal joint line
Type 2	Damaged metaphyseal bone	Loss of cancellous bone that requires reconstruction to restore joint line
Type 3	Deficient metaphyseal bone	Deficient bone compromises major portion of either condyle or plateau.
Femoral and tibial defects are classified independently	A = One condyle or hemiplateau B = Both condyles or entire plateau	

Adapted and reprinted with permission from Engh GA, Ammeen DJ. Bone loss with revision total knee arthroplasty: defect classification and alternatives for reconstruction. *AAOS Instructional Course Lectures* 1999;48:167–175.

Standard metal augments are augments that regardless of size, attach directly to the body of the prosthesis with cement, snap, taper fit, or screw fixation. They may be composed of titanium, cobalt chrome, or tantalum. These augments are system specific and are available in a variety of sizes and styles. Femoral augments, typically blocks 5- to 20-mm thick, attach to the distal or posterior condyles of the prosthesis (Fig. 19-1A). Tibial augments include blocks and partial or full wedges that attach to undersurface of the tibial tray (Fig.19-1A,B). These tibial augments also replace up to 15 to 20 mm of bone loss. In addition, sleeve augments are available in some systems for the tibia and femur. These sleeve augments insert over the stem of a revision component and are designed to fill metaphyseal defects.

Very large trabecular metal cone augments do not attach to the prosthesis but instead are impacted directly into large areas of femoral or tibial metaphyseal bone loss (Fig. 19-2). These trabecular metal cone augments allow the restoration of a stable foundation upon which the prosthesis with or without additional standard augments can be supported. This ability to use these augments independently of the prosthesis as a structural bone graft substitute differentiates trabecular metal cone augments from other porous-coated metaphyseal filling metal augments. Currently

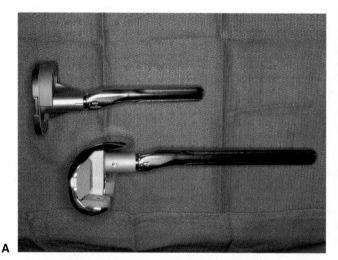
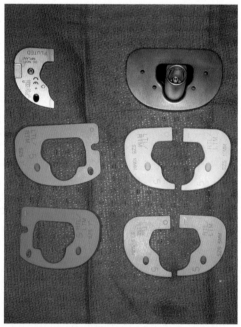

A   B

FIGURE 19-1

(A) Femoral and tibial components demonstrating a variety of metal augments in different thicknesses and composition. The femoral augments are composed of tantalum trabecular metal and are attached via screw fixation, whereas the conventional metal tibial augment is cemented to the tray. **(B)** In each knee system, a variety of trial tibial augments are available, including blocks and wedges of varying thicknesses.

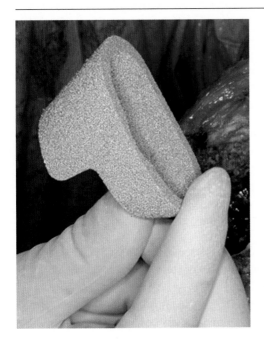

FIGURE 19-2

Trabecular metal cone augments are used independently of the prosthesis to reconstruct metaphyseal bone loss in the tibia or femur. A stepped tibial cone is shown before implantation.

available trabecular metal cone augments are all manufactured by a single company (Zimmer, Warsaw, IN) from commercially pure tantalum. This material is formed into a porous trabecular geometry that approximates the structure of cancellous bone (8,9). Trabecular metal has two to three times the porosity of conventional porous metal coatings, which helps maximize the potential for bone ingrowth (8,9). In addition, because of its inherent strength, it may be used without the need for conventional metal backing to create structural augments. Widespread use in many areas of orthopedic reconstruction has shown the rapid manner in which osseous ingrowth into this tantalum substrate occurs (8). Potential advantages of the trabecular metal cone augments versus structural bone graft include:

- Availability of a wide variety of prefabricated shapes and sizes of augments
- Quick and easy use
- Ability to contour to obtain a custom fit
- Immediate load bearing
- Rapid bone ingrowth with stable long-term fixation

In distinction, although structural grafts and impaction grafting techniques have been reported to have acceptable results in complex revision hip and knee arthroplasty cases, reservations persist (10–13). Potential problems with large bone grafts include:

- Limited availability
- Risk of bacterial and viral disease transmission
- Increased intraoperative time
- Prolonged weight-bearing restrictions until graft incorporation has occurred
- Graft resorption in 5% to 20% of cases (10,12).

As a result of these ongoing concerns with the use of structural bone grafts, coupled with the increasing availability of the large cone augments and good early results in the revision TKA setting, we have increased our use of trabecular metal cones in AORI type 2 and 3 bone defects, where we would have previously used bone graft material.

CONTRAINDICATIONS

Absolute contraindications for the use of standard and very large trabecular metal cone augments include typical contraindications for TKA, such as infection. Relative contraindications for the use of all metal augments regardless of size and composition include absence of host bone support. In cases in which massive bicondylar bone loss exists with absence of any rim of cortical bone, allograft prosthetic composites or segmental replacement prostheses should be considered.

PREOPERATIVE PREPARATION

Accurate preoperative assessment and classification of bone loss is important to ensure that appropriate augments or bone graft material are available. Because of the potential for iatrogenic bone loss during component removal, however, the final classification of the bone defects must be based on the intraoperative findings after prosthesis removal and debridement. Therefore, in revision TKA, the surgeon must be prepared for several contingencies.

Although not definitive, preoperative studies can provide helpful information about the type of defects that may be encountered intraoperatively.

- Knee radiographs are low cost but may fail to allow accurate assessment of the number and size of lesions, especially in the setting of osteolysis (14,15).
- Computed tomography (CT) is a more sensitive tool. In a recent study comparing radiographs to multidetector CT, the radiographs only identified 17% of the osteolytic lesions identified on the CT scans (14).
- Metal suppression protocol, magnetic resonance imaging also appears to provide superior data to radiographs for evaluating osteolysis (15). This capability may not be routinely available in all centers, however.

Therefore, although radiographs remain an important tool for evaluating limb alignment and component positioning in the coronal and sagittal planes, additional studies should be considered for evaluating bone loss, especially when osteolysis is suspected.

Evaluation of radiographs and CT or magnetic resonance imaging scans pre-operatively is especially important if revision surgery is performed in centers where a complete array of standard and very large trabecular metal cone augments and revision knee prostheses are not immediately available. This allows the surgeon to procure the prosthetic and augment options that may be required.

SURGICAL TECHNIQUE

In this section, we address in a stepwise manner the use of both standard metal and trabecular metal cone augments for managing AORI type 2 and 3 defects.

Evaluation of Bone Loss

- After obtaining adequate exposure, the original components are removed.
- Loose cement and bone is debrided.
- Classification of femoral and tibial bone loss is performed according to the previously described AORI system.
- A tentative reconstructive plan is formulated.
- The tibial surface is freshened with a saw to create a flat surface.
- The femoral and tibial canals must be opened up and reamed to size the appropriate stem extensions.
- When conical metaphyseal-diaphyseal defects exist, preparation for trabecular metal cone augments is best performed at this stage, before prosthesis sizing. A significant advantage of the cone augments is that they are not fixed directly to the prosthesis but are independently sized and impacted to create a foundation for the prosthesis. Therefore, they may be used with a wide variety of prostheses systems, and the decision to use these augments is independent of prosthesis choice.

Preparation for Trabecular Metal Cone Augments

- In some cases, only a tibial or femoral cone augment is required; however, when both the femur and tibial have large bone defects that require reconstruction, start with reconstruction of the tibia.
- A variety of full femoral and tibial trabecular metal cones as well as asymmetric stepped tibial designs are available (Fig. 19-3A,B).
- A trial augment is used to size the defect. The trial augment that best fits the bone defect and produces the optimal peripheral contact with the remaining host bone is selected (Fig. 19-4A–D).
- In most cases, the bone defect does not exactly match one of the available sizes; a high-speed burr can be used to the contour the host bone or augment itself (Fig. 19-5).

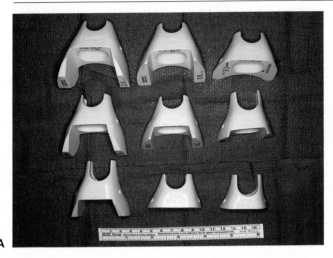
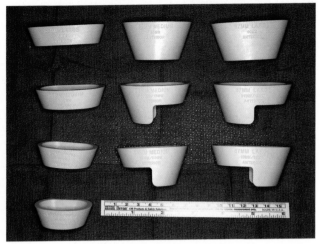

FIGURE 19-3

Trial large trabecular metal cone augments for the femur **(A)** and tibia **(B)** are available in a number of different shapes and sizes.

- Once the tibial trial has a good press fit with maximal peripheral contact, the real cone augment can be selected and impacted in place (Fig. 19-6A–D).
- The femur can be prepared in a similar manner if required (Fig. 19-7A,B).
- Selection of the trial prosthetic components begins after the tibial and femoral cone bone defects have been addressed.

Restoration of Flexion and Extension Gaps

Prosthesis sizing and positioning is used to recreate balanced flexion and extension gaps. At this stage, appropriate component rotation and alignment must be set, and component sizes, stem extensions, and

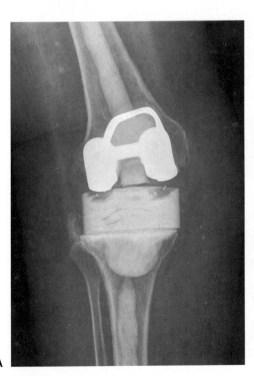
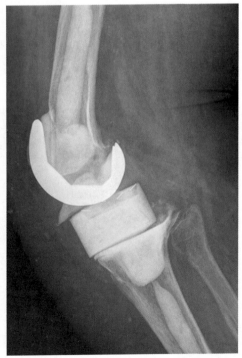

FIGURE 19-4

(A) Preoperative anteroposterior x-ray of a patient with an articulating cement spacer for deep prosthetic infection. Conical bone loss is anticipated in the tibial metaphysis.
(B Preoperative lateral x-ray of the same patient. *(continued)*

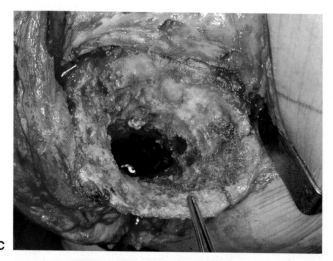

C

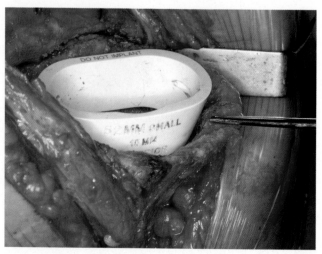

D

FIGURE 19-4 *(Continued)*

(C) Intraoperative photo of the same patient demonstrating a conical defect of the tibial metaphysis after cement spacer removal. **(D)** The trial tibial cone augment that most closely matches the conical defect is selected. However, it sits proud because of impingement on the host bone.

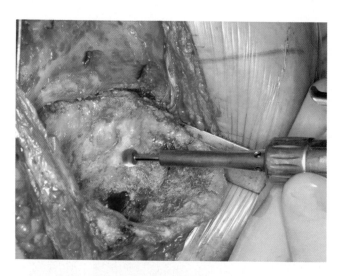

FIGURE 19-5

A high-speed burr is used to contour the host bone to accommodate the trial cone augment with maximal peripheral contact possible.

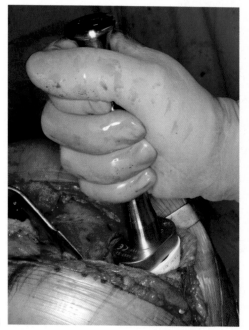

A

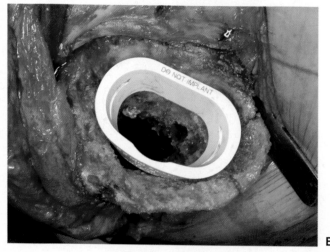

B

FIGURE 19-6

(A) The trial is gently impacted to assess fit and stability. **(B)** The cone trial after press-fit shows acceptable peripheral contact. *(continued)*

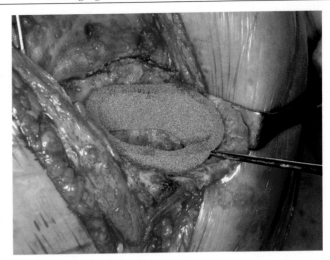

C   **D**

FIGURE 19-6 *(Continued)*

(C) The real trabecular metal cone augment is selected. **(D)** The real cone after impaction. The remaining peripheral voids will be filled with bone graft or bone matrix putty to prevent cement intrusion before implanting the real components.

conventional modular augments must be selected and assembled. In most cases in which cone augments have been used, standard metal or trabecular metal block augments are also required for addressing distal or posterior femoral bone loss, especially if isolated to one condyle.

Prosthesis Selection

● Beginning on the tibial side, the trial component that adequately covers the proximal surface is selected, and the appropriate rotation is set.

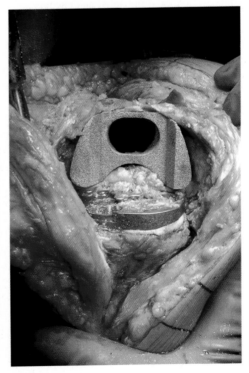

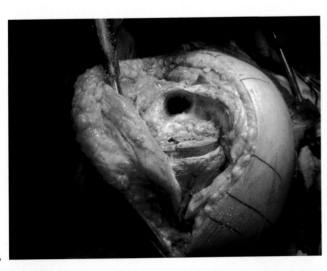

A   **B**

FIGURE 19-7

(A) Intraoperative photo demonstrating femoral bone loss. **(B)** Intraoperative photo with a trabecular metal cone augment impacted into the femoral defect.

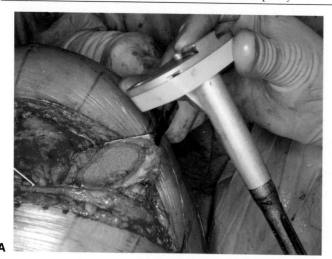

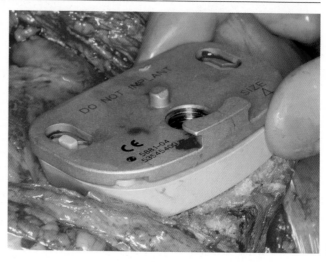

A

B

FIGURE 19-8

(A) Conventional augments on the tibial trials may be required in addition to the cone augments. **(B)** The trial is then impacted through the trabecular metal cone, and correct is rotation set.

- The appropriate-diameter stem extension, sized earlier in the case, is selected and attached to the trial. To optimize alignment initially, the longest available stem extension is selected. When the cone augment has been placed asymmetrically because of the location of bone loss, an offset stem may be required.
- The trial component with the appropriate diameter and length stem extension is then impacted through the trial cone augment (Fig. 19-8A,B).
- Axial alignment is then verified with a drop rod, and adjustments are made as required.
- Once alignment has been optimized, the extent of any remaining bone defects are assessed, and block or wedge augments are selected. The trial is removed, and the augments are attached and then reimpacted and checked.
- Femur preparation begins by identifying the transepicondylar axis.
- The femoral component size and stem are then selected. As with the tibia, long diaphyseal engaging stem trials are used initially to optimize alignment.
- The surgeon then performs the box cut by inserting the jig attached to the previously determined stem extension. Rotation is set along the epicondylar axis, the jig is pinned in place, and the cut is performed.
- The trial femoral component is assembled with distal augments to set the preliminary distal joint line approximately 25 to 30 mm distal to the epicondyles (Fig. 19-9). It is impacted, and distal and posterior bone gaps are evaluated.

FIGURE 19-9

A trial femoral component is impacted with conventional augments to provisionally restore distal joint line position 25 to 30 mm distal to the epicondyles.

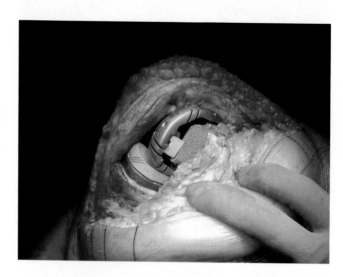

- The trial is removed, and standard augments distally and posteriorly are optimized.
- A tibial polyethylene trial is then inserted that tensions the flexion gap.
- The knee is extended, and the extension gap is evaluated.
- If the knee has a residual flexion contracture, the distal augments are reduced, and the femoral component is moved more proximally. Alternatively, the next larger femoral component can be selected to better fill the flexion gap, if it can be accommodated by the medial-lateral dimension of the femur. This will allow a thinner polyethylene insert to be used.
- If the knee hyperextends, additional distal augments are added onto the distal femur, which better fills the extension gap.
- When either the medial or lateral collateral ligament is nonfunctional, or in cases in which a gross mismatch exists between the flexion and extension gap that cannot be managed by adjusting the position or size of the femoral component, a more constrained condylar prosthesis or hinged device must be used.
- The trial components are removed, and the final stem selections are determined based on whether cemented or uncemented stems are to be used. The trials with the final stem trials are reinserted to ensure that component alignment and position is not affected.
- An x-ray may be obtained to verify appropriate sizing and alignment of the components before final insertion.

Insertion of the Femoral and Tibial Components

- The real modular components are assembled with the appropriate stem extensions and standard metal augments (Fig. 19-10).
- Any remaining small gaps between the trabecular cone augments that have been previously impacted and the host are filled with either morcelized cancellous bone graft or demineralized bone matrix putty (Fig. 19-11). This minimizes cement intrusion between the augment and host bone and furthermore may promote bone ingrowth around the entire periphery of the trabecular metal augment.
- Finally, the real prosthetic components are cemented through the trabecular metal augments (Fig. 19-12A–C).

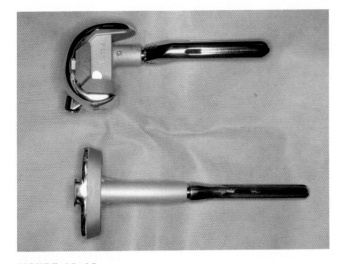

FIGURE 19-10

The real components with appropriate augments are assembled.

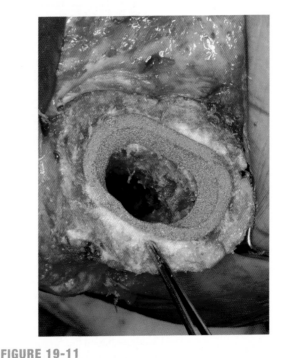

FIGURE 19-11

The real trabecular metal cone has been impacted, and the small cone-host bone gaps are packed with demineralized bone matrix putty.

FIGURE 19-12

(A) Final tibial construct cemented in place.
(B) Postoperative anteroposterior x-ray of the same patient demonstrating the tibial trabecular metal cone augment. **(C)** Post-operative lateral x-ray of the same patient.

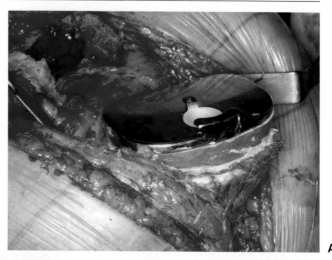

A

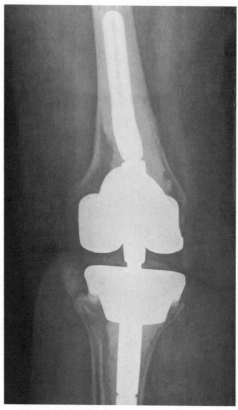

B

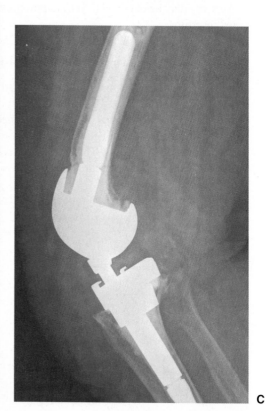

C

PEARLS AND PITFALLS

- When preparing conical femoral or tibial bone defects with the high-speed burr to accept trabecular metal cone trials, unnecessary bone removal should be avoided. Even with the plastic trial augments, however, rigorous impaction can produce a fracture in the bone. Therefore, the preparation process is a precision technique, and the trials should be used frequently to assess fit. Although a snug fit is desirable, avoid excessive force during impaction of the trials or final augments.

- In most cases, the authors avoid using complete or partial wedges because of the shear stress on the interface between the augment and the cement mantle. Instead, we recommend converting a wedge-shaped defect to a step configuration to allow use of a block augment. This preparation can be performed either freehand, using the trial tray and block to mark the bone that must be removed, or with the use of an intramedullary cutting jig.

- The debate regarding cemented and uncemented stem extensions in revision TKA persists, but we favor the use of cemented stem extensions in most circumstances requiring the use of the trabecular cone augments (16–19). However, unless preoperative x-rays have shown a significant extra-articular deformity, during the early trial stages, the longest stem trials (180- to 220-mm combined length) help to optimize alignment by engaging the diaphysis. In most cases, it is not necessary to cement a stem of this length, and therefore, before opening the real components, selection of a shorter, wider stem is appropriate. A stem that gives a combined length of 80 to 150 mm is usually adequate. Especially on the femoral side, it is helpful to mark the trial component position circumferentially with methylene blue before and after selecting the final stem to ensure that unintended changes in medial-lateral or distal positioning do not occur.

- When cementing both femoral and tibial stems, it is preferable to cement the tibia first. To prevent malrotation during the cementing process, the tibial cement should be allowed to cure before proceeding with cementation of the femoral component. Use of a canal plug, cement gun, and pressurization for the tibia and femur helps achieve an optimal cement mantle. Antibiotic-impregnated cement is used in every revision case.

POSTOPERATIVE MANAGEMENT

When a stable construct has been created with the use of a trabecular metal cone in conjunction with a cemented stem extension and cement about the core implant, the patient is allowed to weight bear as tolerated on the operated extremity. Most patients require the use of a walker or crutches for approximately 3 weeks and may then progress to a cane. The authors do not currently use continuous passive motion machines with most revision knee arthroplasties but do allow the majority of patients to participate in range of motion exercises in physical therapy. A brace or knee immobilizer is used when ambulating if a tibial tubercle osteotomy was performed.

COMPLICATIONS

In revision TKA, use of trabecular metal cone augments may be associated with all the usual complications that can occur in these difficult cases. These problems include mechanical failure of the prosthesis, instability, infection, and aseptic loosening. Specific concerns regarding the augments include the potential for failure caused by inadequate bone in-growth or failure because of mechanical overload when the augments are used in uncontained defects in which there is no potential for load sharing with surrounding host bone. At short-term follow-up in two small series of patients, a deep infection rate of about 10% has been the major cause of early failure (1 of 10 and 2 of 15 patients, respectively) (9,20). In each of these cases complicated by deep infection, the tibial cones demonstrated stable bone ingrowth. In these two series, there was one additional failure caused by a loosening of the femoral component; however again, in this case, the tibial cone showed stable bone ingrowth (20).

RESULTS

Successful midterm results following revision total knee replacement have been reported using conventional block and wedge augments in cases with AORI type 2 defects (21,22). In distinction, few published results exist regarding the use of very large trabecular metal augments in revision TKA. In numerous other applications including primary and revision hip arthroplasty, however, tantalum trabecular metal has shown reliable and rapid osseous ingrowth with stable long-term fixation. Two small series have reported encouraging early results in revision TKA. Radney and Scuderi reported good very short-term follow-up at a mean of 10 months (range, 5 to 14 months) for both femoral and tibial trabecular metal cones (9). In 10 revision cases performed in nine patients, a total of 10 tibial and two femoral trabecular metal cone augments were used. The core components had been cemented in every case, and either a press-fit or cemented stem extension was used for additional fixation (9). Results at this very early point were favorable with nine of 10 ten knees functioning well and a mean range of motion of 103 degrees (9). Review of the radiograph for each case revealed incorporation of the tibial and femoral cones into the adjacent bone without evidence of subsidence or change in position (9). In a second report, Meneghini et al presented results with trabecular metal tibial cone augments in 15 patients with AORI type 2B or type 3 tibial defects (20). In this series in which all patients were reviewed at 24 to 38 months follow-up, all tibial cone augments showed bone ingrowth without evidence of loosening or migration (20).

At the present time, the very large trabecular metal cone augments are manufactured by one manufacturer from tantalum. Because of the potential advantages of these augments versus allograft, research into alternative trabecular metal augments and prostheses from other elements, including titanium, is currently ongoing. It is anticipated that alternative trabecular metal technology will be commercially available in the next 5 years. Further studies will be required with these new products to verify similar promising results.

REFERENCES

1. Kelly MA, Clarke HD. Long-term results of posterior cruciate-substituting total knee arthroplasty. *Clin Orthop* 2002;404:51–57.
2. Sierra RJ, Cooney WP IV, Pagnano MW, et al. Reoperations after 3200 revision TKAs: rates, etiology, and lessons learned. *Clin Orthop* 2004;425:200–206.
3. Fehring TK, Odum S, Griffin WL, et al. Early failures in total knee arthroplasty. *Clin Orthop* 2001;392:315–318.
4. Sharkey PF, Hozack WJ, Rothman RH. Why are total knee arthroplasties failing today? *Clin Orthop* 2002;404:7–13.
5. Engh GA, Ammeen DJ. Bone loss with revision total knee arthroplasty: Defect classification and alternatives for reconstruction. AAOS Instructional Course Lectures 1999;48:167–175.
6. Mulhall KJ, Ghomrawi HM, Engh GA, et al. Radiographic predictions of intraoperative bone loss in knee arthroplasty revision. *Clin Orthop* 2006;446:51–58.
7. Lucey SD, Scuderi GR, Kelly MA, et al. A practical approach to dealing with bone loss in total knee arthroplasty. *Orthopedics* 2000;23:1036–1041.
8. Bobyn JD, Poggie RA, Krygier JJ, et al. Clinical validation of a structural porous tantalum biomaterial for adult reconstruction. *J Bone Joint Surg Am* 2004;86(Supp 2):123–129.
9. Radnay CS, Scuderi GR. Management of bone loss: augments, cones, offset stems. *Clin Orthop* 2006;446:83–92.
10. Backstein D, Safir O, Gross A. Management of bone loss: structural grafts in revision total knee arthroplasty. *Clin Orthop* 2006;446:104–112.
11. Engh G, Herzwurm PJ, Parks NL. Treatment of major defects of bone with bulk allografts and stemmed components during total knee arthroplasty. *J Bone Joint Surg Am* 1997;79:1030–1039.
12. Haddad FS, Spangehl MJ, Masri BA, et al. Circumferential allograft replacement of the proximal femur: a critical analysis. *Clin Orthop* 2000;371:98–107.
13. Lotke PA, Carolan GF, Puri N. Impaction grafting for bone defects in revision total knee arthroplasty. *Clin Orthop* 2006;446:99–103.
14. Reish TG, Clarke HD, Scuderi GR, et al. Use of multi-detector computed tomography for the detection of periprosthetic osteolysis in total knee arthroplasty. *J Knee Surg* 2006;19:259–264.
15. Vessely MB, Frick MA, Oakes D et al. Magnetic resonance imaging with metal suppression for evaluation of periprosthetic osteolysis after total knee arthroplasty. *J Arthroplasty* 2006;21:826–831.
16. Fehring TK, Odum S, Olekson C, et al. Stem fixation in revision total knee arthroplasty: a comparative analysis. *Clin Orthop* 2003;416:217–224.
17. Haas SB, Insall JN, Montgomery W III, et al. Revision total knee arthroplasty with use of modular components with stems inserted without cement. *J Bone Joint Surg Am* 1995;77:1700–1707.
18. Shannon BD, Klassen JF, Rand JA, et al. Revision total knee arthroplasty with cemented components and uncemented intramedullary stems. *J Arthroplasty* 2003;(7 Suppl 1):27–32.
19. Whaley AL, Trousdale RT, Rand JA. Cemented long-stem revision total knee arthroplasty. *J Arthroplasty* 2003;18:592–599.
20. Meneghini RM, Lewallen DG, Hanssen AD. Treatment of Severe Tibial Bone Loss Using Porous Tantalum Metaphyseal Cones in Revision TKR. Presented at the American Academy of Orthopedic Surgeons Annual Meeting, Chicago, Illinois, March 24, 2006. Available online at: http://www3.aaos.org/education/anmeet/anmt2006/podium/podium.cfm?Pevent=405. Accessed September 2, 2008.
21. Pagnano MW, Trousdale RT, Rand JA. Tibial wedge augmentation for bone deficiency in total knee arthroplasty: a follow-up study. *Clin Orthop* 1995;321:151–155.
22. Patel JV, Masonis JL, Guerin J, et al. The fate of augments to treat type-2 bone defects in revision knee arthroplasty. *J Bone Joint Surg Br* 2004;86:195–199.

20 Managing Bone Loss with Bulk Allograft

Gerard A. Engh

INDICATIONS

Bone loss is a complication encountered quite frequently at the time of revision total knee arthroplasty (TKA). The bone loss can be caused by progressive bone destruction secondary to debris-generated osteolysis or can be caused by implant loosening, breakage, and migration that occurred over time (Fig. 20-1). Also, bone loss can result from multiple revision procedures in which additional bone was removed with each surgery to obtain a satisfactory fixation interface for new components.

As a rule, implant augments can be used in the femur or tibia to manage defects that extend 10 to 15 mm into the metaphyseal bone. If the depth of the bone loss in the metaphyseal segment is greater than 15 mm, the only reasonable options for repairing such a defect would be to replace the lost bone with a large structural allograft (femoral head), impaction allografting, or use of a trabecular metal cone (an augment that is not integral to the component itself). In such cases, restoration/reconstruction of bone stock is beneficial to achieve satisfactory fixation for the revision component.

PREOPERATIVE CLASSIFICATION OF BONE DEFICIENCY

A useful tool in the planning for revision surgery is classifying the bone defect from preoperative radiographs (Fig. 20-2). According to the Anderson Orthopedic Research Institute (AORI) Bone Defect Classification (1), a type 3 defect has bone too deficient to support an implant. Type 3 bone defects are best managed with large structural allografts. Structural allografts provide additional support for the implant and an interface that rapidly heals to host bone. Impaction grafting also works relatively well to manage type 3 defects if the bone defect is contained in the metaphyseal region such that adequate cortical bone support is available to avoid implant subsidence or if wire mesh is added to provide additional support for an uncontained tibial defect (2,3).

CONTRAINDICATIONS

The contraindications for structural allografts in revision surgery are active infection, and in rare instances, severe bone loss such that the metaphyseal region is not adequate to contain a femoral head allograft. In other words, a structural femoral head allograft would be contraindicated in a knee with an absent metaphyseal segment. The more appropriate alternative for this type of extensive bone defect is either the combination of a segmental allograft and a long-stemmed revision component or a tumor prosthesis.

It is important to bypass an area of repaired bone damage to offload stress from an allograft. A diaphyseal filling stem provides long-term component stability and protects an allograft from stress overload. On rare occasions, a diaphyseal deformity may prohibit the use of a long-stemmed component.

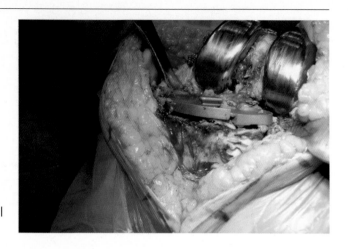

FIGURE 20-1

Broken titanium tibial tray over an area of tibial osteolysis.

PREOPERATIVE PREPARATION

An allograft bone segment can be obtained from a variety of sources. The American Society of Tissue Banks provides guidelines and requirements to ensure the safety of allograft bone. Such bone is readily available from the American Red Cross or other reputable tissue banks. Allograft bone must be maintained in a bone freezer at $-70°C$ or delivered on the day before surgery and kept frozen with dry ice. The most viable source of large structural allografts is femoral heads retrieved at the time of primary total hip arthroplasty. The diameter of the bone segment is available with the packaged allograft. An allograft that is larger than the anticipated size of the bone defect is essential.

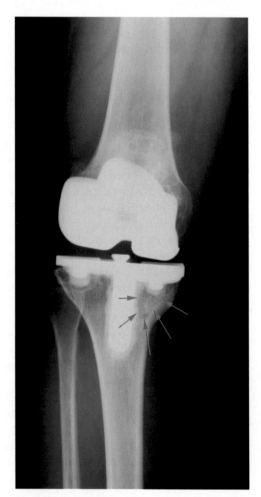

FIGURE 20-2

A large osteolytic lesion in the medial tibial plateau (*arrows*) is evident on this preoperative radiograph. A smaller lesion (*arrow*) is also noted in the lateral plateau.

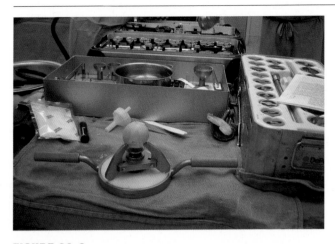

FIGURE 20-3

A femoral head allograft mounted in an Allogrip device before preparation for use.

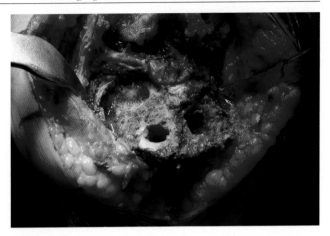

FIGURE 20-4

A broken titanium tibial tray that rested on an area of tibial osteolysis was removed and the defect classified (AORI type 3 tibial defect).

It is also essential to have the appropriate instrumentation for allograft preparation. The Allogrip (DePuy, Warsaw, IN) bone-holding device is best for preparing femoral head allografts (Fig. 20-3). The femoral head is anchored in the device for decortication and preparation. If the allograft is damaged or contaminated during preparation, it is important to have a back-up allograft available. The surgeon should always plan for the worst- case scenario to avoid the situation in which there is inadequate material to repair the bone deficiency.

ALLOGRAFTING TECHNIQUE

Preparation of Host Bone

The surgical technique used to repair a major bone defect (AORI type 3 defect [1]) with an allograft begins with creating a host bed that will provide stability for the allograft and viability for rapid union between the allograft and the host bone. The base of the bone defect is generally filled with a combination of fibrous tissue, osteolytic membrane, and sclerotic underlying bone (Fig. 20-4). The membranous tissue must be vigorously débrided, and the sclerotic and dead cancellous bone is removed until encountering viable cancellous host bone at the base of the defect that can heal rapidly to an allograft. Often, a high-speed burr is needed to remove irregularly shaped sclerotic bone prior to using the hemispheric male-type reamer (Fig. 20-5) to create a hemispherical shape for the femoral head allograft. It is important to avoid creating an uncontained defect by removing additional cortical margins of the host bone during allograft preparation. However, it is necessary to ream deep enough such that the resulting bone defect is semicontained and viable bone is exposed for allograft union.

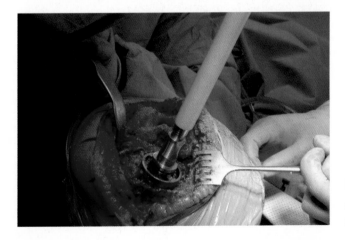

FIGURE 20-5

A male-type reamer was used to prepare the tibial bone defect secondary to osteolysis.

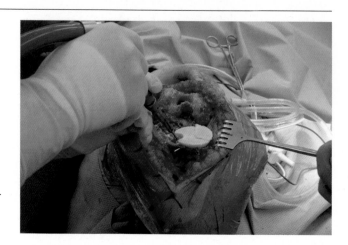

FIGURE 20-6

Opening the intramedullary canal with a high-speed burr after a femoral head allograft is placed in the medial tibial defect.

Preparation of the Allograft

The allograft should be prepared to the same size or one size larger than the hemispherical bone defect in the host bone. An allograft holding device is used to stabilize the femoral head allograft while it is prepared on a back table of the operating room. Using hemispherical female-type reamers, the allograft is decorticated through the subchondral plate to an area of uniformly cancellous bone. All the marrow elements are flushed from the cancellous bone with a power-washing device and saline material.

Insertion of the Allograft and Preparation for a Stemmed Component

The allograft is either impacted into place when the defect is fully contained or positioned in the defect and held with tenaculums while Kirschner (K-wires) are inserted that temporarily secure the allograft to the host bone. The position of the K-wires must not interfere with the central canal for the stem of the revision component. Once the allograft is seated and held in place with K-wires, a rough cut can be performed to remove the obvious excess allograft bone. After the rough cut, a high-speed burr is used to initially open the intramedullary canal (Fig. 20-6). Rigid intramedullary reamers are then used to re-establish a central canal for the stem of the revision component. As a rule, stems that engage the diaphyseal segment work best with revision cases that require allograft bone defect repair. These stems should reach into the diaphyseal segment of the adjacent host bone.

After the intramedullary canal is prepared, the long-stemmed trial implant is inserted. The excess bone is trimmed from the allograft until the implant is adequately seated on the allograft and host bone. In some instances, both of the distal femoral condyles or both proximal tibial plateaus can be repaired with two femoral head allografts (Fig. 20-7). In such cases, it may not be possible to seat the implant onto any viable host bone (Fig. 20-8). One goal of this allograft repair is joint line

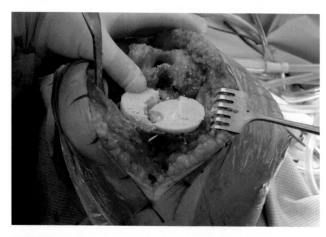

FIGURE 20-7

A portion of a second femoral head allograft is placed in the lateral tibial defect.

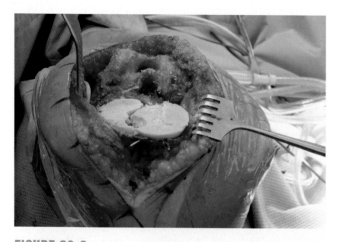

FIGURE 20-8

The two femoral head allografts will provide support for the revision implant.

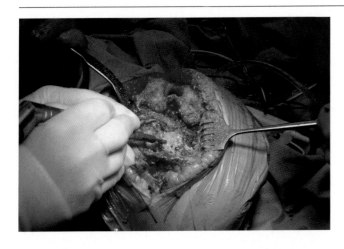

FIGURE 20-9

Sclerotic bone is removed at the base of the defect with a high-speed burr.

restoration. Trim the excess bone from the allograft until an appropriately sized implant can be seated at an appropriate joint line level.

Trial components are used to assess ligamentous stability in both flexion and extension. It is best to use the trial device with the least constraint necessary to evaluate knee stability. This will determine the appropriate amount of constraint needed for adequate knee stability with the final components.

Implanting the Final Components

The surgeon cements the final component into place with antibiotic-impregnated bone cement. The bone cement is finger-packed both into the allograft and any viable adjacent cancellous host bone. It is important to avoid cement penetrating the host-graft junction. The metaphyseal segment of the implant is cemented, but cement should not be used in the diaphyseal region or onto the extended stem of the component. Using an uncemented stem permits axial loading across the host-graft junction and the transfer of stress through the allograft as well, as the stem encourages graft union. Some surgeons prefer to use cemented stems, but there are no clear data to support either cemented or cementless stem fixation.

The K-wires holding the allograft in place are removed once the cement is cured. The allograft is captured between the component itself and the adjacent viable host bone. The cement bond between the implant and the allograft further stabilizes the graft (Fig. 20-9).

STEP-BY-STEP TECHNIQUE FOR STRUCTURAL FEMORAL HEAD ALLOGRAFTING

The following steps can be used to repair either a contained or uncontained metaphyseal bone defect with a structural femoral head allograft:

1. Remove the implant (Fig. 20-4) and débride all nonviable host tissue.
2. Use a high-speed burr (Fig. 20-9) to remove any sclerotic nonviable bone.
3. If necessary, create a central recess at the base of the bone defect (Fig. 20-8) to capture or contain a male-type reamer.
4. Ream the metaphyseal bone defect to a hemispheric shape (Fig. 20-5).
5. Ream to viable cancellous bone without creating an uncontained defect.
6. Prepare the allograft in an Allogrip holding device (Fig. 20-3).
   - Use a female-type reamer (Fig. 20-11) either the same size or one size larger than the male-type reamer used to prepare the host bone defect. After decortication (Fig. 20-12), power wash the allograft to remove marrow elements.
7. Impact the graft and secure with K-wires.
   - Avoid placing the K-wires where they would interfere with the stem of the component (Fig. 20-13).
8. Make a rough cut to remove excess allograft bone (Fig. 20-14).
9. Using a high-speed burr and rigid reamers, re-establish the central canal for a stemmed component (Fig. 20-6).
10. If any adjacent bone defects are present, repair the remaining defects with a separate allograft or a component augment (Fig. 20-7).

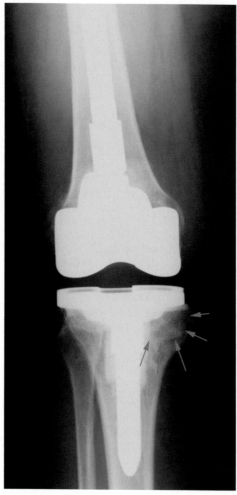

FIGURE 20-10

The type 3 defect in the medial tibial plateau was reconstructed with a femoral head allograft (*arrows*).

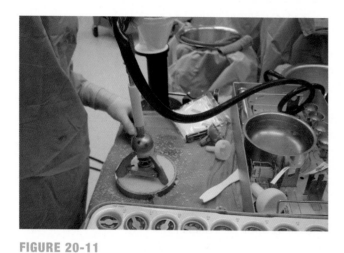

FIGURE 20-11

The femoral head allograft is prepared with a hemispheric female-type reamer to remove cortical bone from the surface.

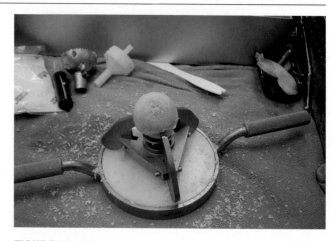

FIGURE 20-12

A prepared allograft with a fully uncovered cancellous surface.

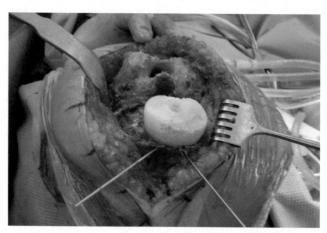

FIGURE 20-13

The allograft is held in place with Kirschner wires.

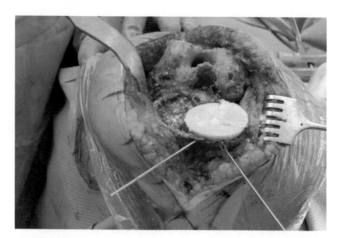

FIGURE 20-14

A rough cut of the femoral head allograft in the medial tibial defect.

11. Place a stemmed trial component into the prepared intramedullary canal and seat the component onto the surface of the allograft. Continue to resect excess bone until the component is fully seated on a combination of host and allograft bone.
12. After all bone preparation is complete, use antibiotic-impregnated cement to secure the component.
13. Remove the K-wires.

COMPLICATIONS AND PITFALLS WITH FEMORAL HEAD ALLOGRAFT PROCEDURES

1. Allograft is too small.
   - Select allografts that are large enough to fill any bone defects that may be encountered. Remember that the defects usually are larger than anticipated from radiographs.
2. Inadequate reaming.
   - Ream the defect until reaching cancellous, bleeding bone at the base of the bone defect to ensure allograft-host bone union.
3. Inadequate union of allograft.
   - If available, place autogenous, cancellous bone at the base of the prepared bone defect to enhance bone union.
4. Fracture of the allograft.
   - If the component has fins or pegs, prepare the allograft bone and adjacent host bone for the fins or pegs of the component with an oscillating saw, high-speed burr, or drill to avoid fractures with the use of punches designed for bone preparation for the implant's fins or pegs.
5. Damage of the allograft.
   - Always have an extra allograft reserved in case the graft becomes contaminated or damaged during preparation.
6. Bacterial or viral infection.
   - The risk of bacterial infection is concerning when structural allograft is utilized. The use of antibiotic-impregnated cement may reduce the risk of bacterial infection in this setting. Viral transmission, such as hepatitis and human immunodeficiency virus has been reduced with contemporary screening techniques, but grafts should be procured from reputable companies.
7. Graft resorption.
   - This can occur over time as the graft goes through a process of revascularization during the healing process that typically occurs between 5 and 7 years after implantation.

POSTOPERATIVE MANAGEMENT

As a rule, full weight bearing is encouraged after a revision TKA using a large structural allograft. The stem of the component should be of adequate length and diameter to offload the graft and satisfactorily protect the allograft until union occurs. If there is a precarious situation, particularly in cases in which the allograft is largely uncontained and unprotected, then protected weight bearing is essential until host allograft union is accomplished. This usually takes approximately 3 to 6 months.

RESULTS

One published series reviewed the results of 46 revision TKAs in which structural allografting was performed to treat severe tibial bone loss. At a mean of 97 months after surgery (minimum of 5 years) there were no instances of graft collapse or aseptic loosening associated with the graft. Two failures occurred as a result of deep infection; an additional two failures occurred as a result of femoral osteolysis, instability, or arthrofibrosis. At the time of additional surgeries, the grafts tended to appear stable, and histological evaluation of two autopsy specimens performed within 5 years of revision arthroplasty showed union between the host bone and allograft (4).

CONCLUSIONS

Nonunion of the allograft is more likely to occur with poorly contained defects and with fully cemented stems. Graft union to host bone is rapid, whereas graft resorption appears to be a very slow process and seems to occur only from the adjacent periosteum. Large contained allografts appear to remain structurally intact well beyond 10 years (4). Because the allograft remains as dead bone indefinitely, a healing response within the graft is not possible. Unlike large structural allografts that have had a high failure rate when used to repair large acetabular bone defects, the low failure rate with revision TKA seems to rely on the use of a long-stemmed component. A revision knee component with a large canal-filling stem protects the allograft from overload and microfracture.

REFERENCES

1. Engh GA. Bone defect classification. In: Engh GA, Rorabeck CH, eds. *Revision Total Knee Arthroplasty.* Baltimore: Williams & Wilkins; 1997:63–120.
2. Lotke PA, Carolan GF, Puri N. Impaction grafting for bone defects in revision total knee arthroplasty. *Clin Orthop Rel Res* 2006;446:99–103.
3. Lonner JH, Lotke PA, Kim J, Nelson C. Impaction grafting and wire mesh for uncontained defects in revision knee arthroplasty. *Clin Orthop Rel Res* 2002;404:145–151.
4. Engh GA, Ammeen DJ. Use of structural allograft in revision total knee arthroplasty in knees with severe tibial bone loss. *J Bone Joint Surg* 2007;89A:2640–2647.

21 Impaction Bone Grafting for Large Bone Defects

Paul A. Lotke and Jess H. Lonner

INDICATIONS

Large bone defects are frequently encountered during revision surgery for total knee arthroplasty. These are usually caused by osteolysis secondary to polyethylene wear or particulate debris. Large bone defects are also noted after removal of a prior prosthesis, however, especially if large femoral and tibial stems were present or after staged procedures for sepsis. The defects are frequently irregular in contour. This irregularity makes it difficult to use preformed spacers or augments without sacrificing additional bone (1). The impacted bone-grafting technique offers the ability to fill the irregular defects, as well as the opportunity to reconstitute bone. It has had long-term success in total hip arthroplasty and more recently for revision total knee surgery.

The combination of a long stem, cemented and imbedded within impacted bone graft creates a rigid, structurally sound support for large defects in the femoral or tibial metaphyses. Uncontained defects, in either of these metaphyseal areas, can be enclosed with wire mesh (2). Therefore, impacted bone grafting is clinically versatile and can be used in a wide variety of clinical situations.

CONTRAINDICATIONS

There are few absolute contraindications for use of impacted bone graft other than the presence of sepsis. It is time consuming, especially with uncontained defects requiring wire mesh enclosure. However, the ability to reconstruct bone and fill irregular defects can balance the time expended in using this technique.

ALTERNATIVES

Alternative methods of biological reconstruction include bulk allografts, however, they are technically difficult to fit and never incorporated into the host. Non-biologic materials, such as metallic augments and metaphyseal cones are also available, especially with the porous ingrowth metals. The ability to ultimately reconstruct bone makes impaction grafting a particularly advantageous alternative, however, especially in younger patients.

The alternative treatments include re-enforcing cement, metallic augments, metaphyseal porous metal cones, and structural allografts.

PREOPERATIVE PREPARATION

Standard anterior, posterior, lateral, and patellar radiographs should be used to evaluate all painful total knee arthroplasties (Fig. 21-1A,B). It is well recognized, however, that the standard

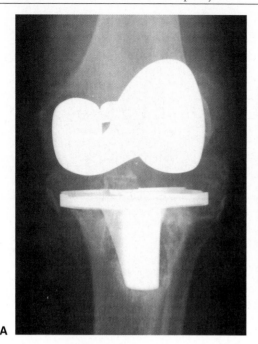

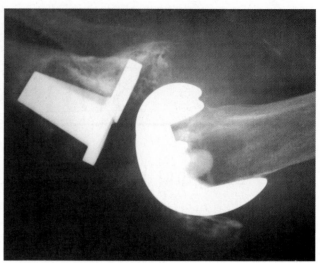

A   B

FIGURE 21-1

(A,B) Anteroposterior and lateral x-rays show a large bone defect in the tibial metaphyseal from a failing knee replacement. In addition, there is suggestion of lysis in the central portion of the femoral component.

radiographs routinely underestimate the extent of osteolysis that occurs in metaphyseal bone and behind the prostheses. Special sequence magnetic resonance imaging scans and computed tomography can be helpful for determining bone defects but depend on the imaging techniques and can be misleading as well. As with all preoperative preparations for revision total knee surgery, care should be taken to rule out the possibility of infection. If infection is suspected, multiple aspirations of the knee should be done, sedimentation rate and C-reactive protein laboratory studies obtained before surgery, and frozen pathology sections should be requested at the time of surgery.

SURGICAL TECHNIQUE

The patient is positioned, prepped, and draped in the usual manner. A cross-table foot post may be used to help stabilize the knee in the fully flexed position.

The exposure should generally utilize the prior skin incision and excise the widened stretched scar. Given the complexity of many revision total knee arthroplasties, in the presence of massive bone loss, a medial parapatellar arthrotomy is extensile and recommended. When extending the incision proximally, care should be taken to remain within the quadriceps tendon, so that a quadriceps snip across the tendon to obtain better exposure can be readily repaired. Care should be taken to avoid crossing the quadriceps tendon too distally or entering into the medialis muscle, as it makes repairing the quadriceps snip more problematic. Care should also be taken to protect the patella tendon attachment from peeling off the tibial tubercle. The patella should be subluxed, and rarely if ever, everted. In many of the knees with massive osteolysis, the tibial tubercle bone or the bones under the femoral condyles may be so thin that fracture is possible. Special care should be taken to avoid losing the integrity of these structures.

After reasonable exposure has been carefully obtained, we recommend a complete synovectomy to obtain full exposure and relaxation of the remaining soft tissue sleeve. As noted in Figures 21-2 through 21-4, the synovium can be removed sharply with its surrounding capsule. First, we remove the synovium from the suprapatellar pouch and then the medial and lateral extensions. When the synovium has been removed, it relaxes the medial and lateral soft tissue sleeves, making the knee more mobile and exposes the prosthetic interfaces. The remainder of the posterior synovium can be resected after the prosthesis has been removed.

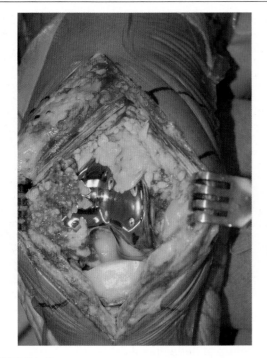

FIGURE 21-2

Exposure of the knee demonstrating marked synovial proliferation surrounding the prosthetic component and obscuring vision.

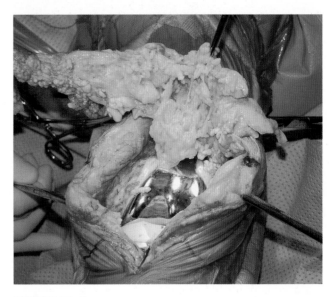

FIGURE 21-3

Removal of synovium by sharp dissection. The combined synovium and capsule are first removed from the suprapatellar pouch and medial-lateral extensions.

The prosthesis can be removed by standard techniques depending on its fixation, remaining bone stock, and style of prosthesis. Flexible osteotomes, thin saw blades, and osteotomes are standard requirements for removing the prothesis with the least amount of additional bone loss. It is best to remember not to insert a primary prosthesis that cannot be readily removed. Porous stems, notches imbedded within cement mantles, and rough textured surfaces make it extremely difficult to remove prostheses from the femur and tibia and should be avoided if possible.

In preparation for impacted bone grafting, the osteolytic, necrotic debris should be carefully curetted and cleaned from the intact bone surfaces. As shown in Figures 21-5 through 21-7, a

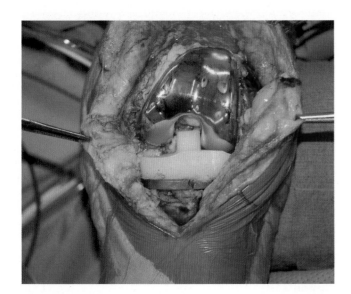

FIGURE 21-4

After synovectomy, exposure is readily obtained with good relaxation of the medial and lateral tissue sleeves.

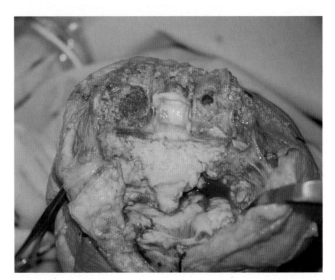

FIGURE 21-5

The prosthesis is removed. The debris behind the prosthesis can be extensive and hide large defects.

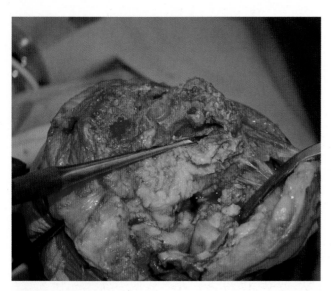

FIGURE 21-6

The bone is carefully curetted from the bone and removed with the aid of a rongeur.

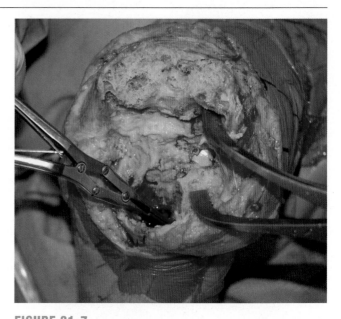

FIGURE 21-7

The surgeon carefully cleans the bone from the soft tissue debris to define the defects.

curette is carefully used to remove the debris down to healthy bone. Occasionally (Fig. 21-8), a high-speed burr can be used to remove small pockets of necrotic bone or fibrous debris. We think it is important to get back to healthy bone, not only to achieve a bleeding ingrowth but also to define the remaining bone support. After the bone has been débrided, a trial prosthesis can be inserted to determine the stem length and component size that will be required for reconstructing the prosthesis (Fig. 21-9).

The surgeon begins the impacted bone-grafting process by inserting a free stem, 2 to 3 mm wider than the anticipated stem, into the shaft of the femur. It should be held by a few pieces of impacted bone-grafting material to determine if the position of the stem is perfectly placed. It is very important that the temporary stem be placed in the exact location of the final prosthetic stem. Oversizing by a few millimeters allows some degree of compensation.

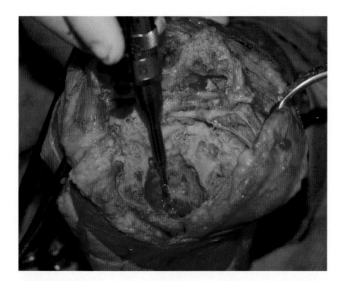

FIGURE 21-8

A high-speed burr can be used to remove pieces of cement, debris, or hidden areas of soft tissue pockets.

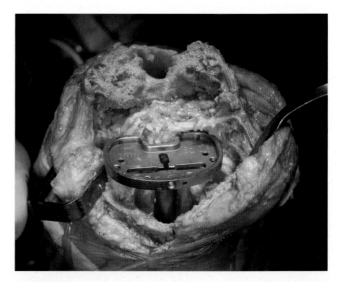

FIGURE 21-9

A trial prosthesis is inserted to find the defects in the tibia.

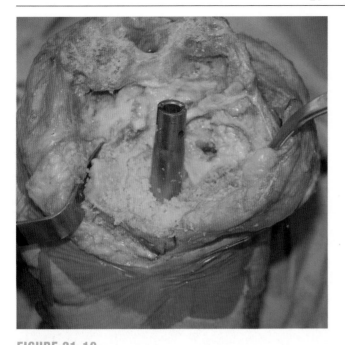

FIGURE 21-10

A temporary stem is placed in the central portion of the tibial shaft around which cancellous chips are carefully impacted.

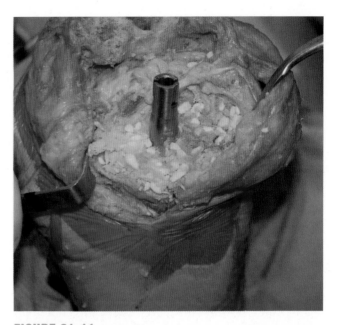

FIGURE 21-11

Some cortical chips are added to the cancellous morsels and raised above the cortical margins.

The bone graft is prepared from cancellous fragments. If the defect is exceptionally large, cortical bone can be added to give some additional structure to the bone graft; however, it does not mold well to the smaller defects. The chips should be irrigated and soaked in antibiotic solution before insertion. Either fresh-frozen morselized cancellous bone or freeze-dried cancellous morsels can be used for this process.

After the bone graft material has been prepared and the stem placed in the exact position for the final prosthesis, the bone graft morsels are progressively impacted around the side of the stem (Figs. 21-10 and 21-11). This is done in stages with an impactor and building layers of the impacted bone graft around the stem. Be careful that the stem is located in the correct position. At the top edge of the impacted graft, we may find loss of containment. In general, we can pack slightly above the contained level. If the cortical defect is more than 1.5 cm, however, a wire mesh should be considered to contain the impacted graft. The impacted graft is continued proximally until the entire defect has been filled.

The prosthesis is then cemented into place by carefully removing the temporary stem and by carefully placing cement and the prosthetic stem into the channel left for the stem (Fig. 21-12). Before the prosthesis is inserted, a thin smear of cement may be placed around the edge of the impacted bone to hold the fragments in place.

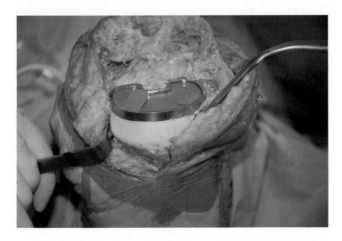

FIGURE 21-12

The temporary stem has been removed, and the prosthesis has been cemented into the central portion of the tibial shaft. A smear of cement has been placed over the uncontained defects.

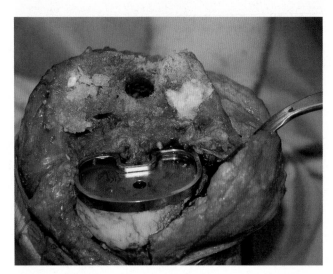

FIGURE 21-13

Smaller defects in the femoral canal are filled with impacted bone graft material.

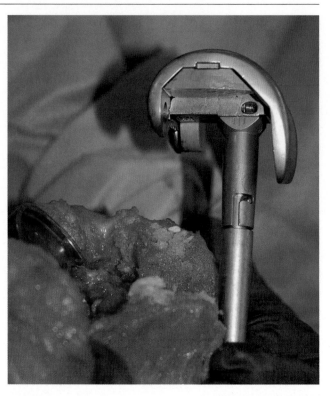

FIGURE 21-14

Final positioning of the reconstructed prosthesis with balancing of the flexion and extension spaces.

The tibial component is always placed first because it will be used to determine the transverse the long axis of the tibia and becomes the fixed reference onto which the flexion-extension gaps will be balanced (see principles of revision surgery).

On the femoral side of the knee (Figs. 21-13 to 21-18), it is particularly recommended to use impacted bone graft in defects that underlie thin cortical metaphyseal zones into which the medial and lateral collateral ligaments insert. These could fracture over cement or other metallic augments. The ability to reconstruct bone under the thin cortical remnants of the collateral ligaments is an important advantage of using impacted bone graft. On the femoral side, there is a tendency for the morsels of bone to disassociate on the surface. A thin coating of cement can be applied to the exposed surfaces of the cancellous bone to keep the morselized fragments in place (Fig. 21-18B).

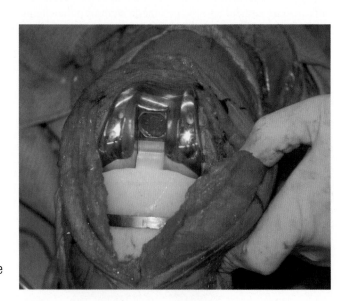

FIGURE 21-15

The prosthesis is in place. Thin cement on the anterior tibia coats the graft and prevents loosening of the bone morsels.

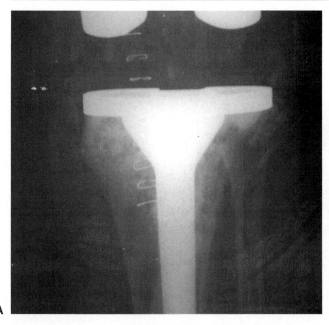

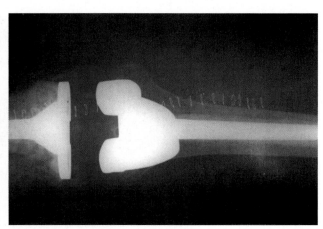

A

B

FIGURE 21-16

(A,B) Postoperative radiographs showing the impacted bone graft imbedded into the proximal tibia and the long tapered stems used for the fixation of the components.

UNCONTAINED DEFECTS

Uncontained defects in the proximal, tibial, or posterior femur can be treated with wire mesh attached to intact cortices with unicortical screws. The alternative is to rely on a soft tissue sleeve or a thin smear of cement over the bone surfaces. If wire mesh is used, a sheet of mesh can be cut the appropriate size and held in place with relatively few screws (Fig. 21-18).

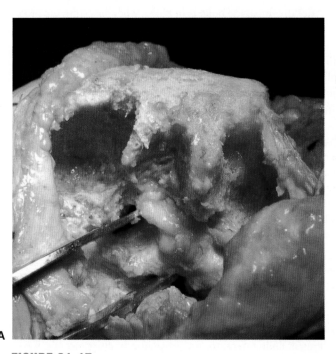

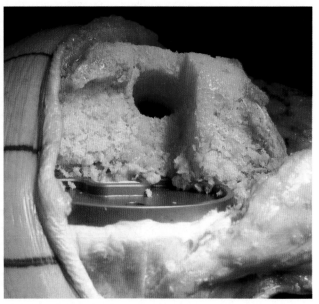

A

B

FIGURE 21-17

(A,B) Large defects in the femur are filed with impacted cancellous chips.

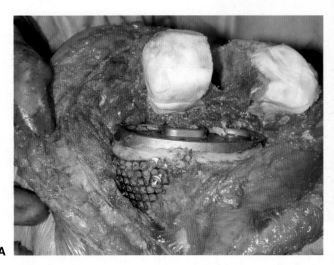

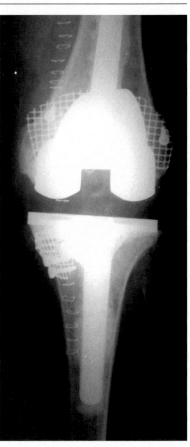

A

FIGURE 21-18

(A,B) Wire mesh has been used to contain the graft in a large defect in the proximal medial tibia. A thin coating of cement has been placed over the bone graft in the distal femur.

B

PEARLS AND PITFALLS

The perils of this technique involve impacting of the bone into the irregular bone defects. Smaller defects can be managed with cancellous bone. Cortical chips do not mold well to small defects and should be reserved for larger bone loss. After the impacted bone is in place, when inserting the prosthesis, care should be taken to avoid displacing the bone graft down into the hole where the temporary prosthetic stem was removed. This must be done carefully.

The principal pitfall with this technique is the amount of time it takes to adequately impact the bone graft. In addition, if the stem is placed in the wrong position, it will not allow proper positioning of the femur or tibial components in relationship with each other. Therefore, a trial reduction and accurate position of the stems before impacting bone graft is important.

POSTOPERATIVE MANAGEMENT

The postoperative course is similar to any revision total knee replacement. Generally, patients start protected weight bearing with a walker immediately after surgery. Progressive activity depends on other defects that are encountered in the total knee. If impacted bone is the only defect, patients should be managed the same as any other postoperative revision total knee patient. In general, patients are out of bed the next morning and walking with protected weight bearing with a walker. Because of the impacted bone graft, we may continue protected weight bearing with a walker or crutches, for as long as 6 weeks and then start the patient on a cane.

COMPLICATIONS

Complications can occur in all types of revision knee replacement surgery but have been reported with relatively limited frequency. Problems include infection, periprosthetic fracture, aseptic loosening, collapse of the bone graft, failure to incorporate, and junctional nonunion. The impacted bone-grafted procedure has shown itself to be relatively free of unusual complications.

RESULTS

The authors reported on 40 knees, including 12 uncontained defects requiring wire mesh. The knee score improved from 57 to 90 points, and the functional scores went from 52 to 80 points. At the mean of 3.8 years after surgery, there were no failures of prosthetic component loosening.There were two postoperative infections that were treated successfully and two late periprosthetic fractures caused by direct trauma. There were no mechanical failures, and the radiographs continued to show incorporation of the bone graft (1,2).

REFERENCES

1. Lotke PA, Carolan GF. Impaction grafting for bone defects and revision knee arthroplasties *Clin Orthop* 2006;446:99–103.
2. Lonner JH, Lotke PA, Kim J, et al. Impaction, grafting and wire mesh for uncontained defects in revision knee arthroplasties. *Clin Orthop* 2002;404:145–151.

22 Staged Revision of the Infected Total Knee Arthroplasty

Jess H. Lonner and Javad Parvizi

INDICATIONS/CONTRAINDICATIONS

Despite all attempts for prevention, periprosthetic joint infection continues to pose a great clinical problem, and its incidence may be on the rise (1–3). In fact, periprosthetic infection may now be the main cause of failure of total knee arthroplasty (TKA). The challenges of treating this complication relate to difficulty in diagnosis in some patients and selection of the most appropriate treatment modality. The main objective of the treatment is to eradicate infection and provide a functioning and pain-free joint for affected patients. The latter, however, can be difficult to accomplish in some cases.

We use a simple classification scheme that helps define an appropriate treatment algorithm for the infected TKA. Simplistically, this scheme distinguishes between acute and late infections. Acute perioperative infections generally occur within 3 weeks of surgery and can occasionally be treated effectively with thorough open debridement and lavage with retention of the implants, depending on the organism. Success with irrigation and debridement ranges from 8% to 56%, however, depending on whether the infectious organism is *Staphylococcus aureus* or *S. epidermidis* (4). Late infections, occurring more 3 to 4 weeks after index surgery, are either latent infections that arose from contamination during initial arthroplasty or hematogenous infections. Late infections that developed as indolent low-grade sepsis are often more difficult to eradicate than those arising more acutely from a hematogenous source. A late infection of a well-fixed TKA with acute onset of symptoms for less than 1 or 2 weeks may sometimes be treated effectively with arthrotomy, polyethylene exchange, thorough synovectomy, and soft tissue debridement with a 6-week course of parenteral antibiotics. This type of treatment is particularly effective with highly sensitive organisms of low virulence in immunocompetent patients (4). However, chronic low-grade infections tend to be more difficult to eradicate by debridement and implant retention. Other options such as serial aspirations, arthroscopic debridement, and chronic antibiotic suppression, alone, are often ineffective and therefore not recommended for treating late infections. We recommend two-stage exchange arthroplasty for chronic or late infections, acute infections by resistant organisms, infection in an immunocompromised or malnourished host, or patients with soft tissue deficiency (5–13).

Patients in whom an attempt at staged reimplantation has failed are candidates for salvage procedures including resection arthroplasty, knee fusion, and above-the-knee amputation. Patients with extensive medical comorbidities who are unable to tolerate multiple surgical procedures may be best suited to treatment with implant resection and debridement without use of intervening antibiotic spacers. These patients may go on to spontaneous autofusion if treated in a cast. Those with persistent ongoing infection despite multiple attempted staged revision arthroplasties and those with nonhealing sinus tract problems, a compromised soft tissue envelope, or extensor mechanism incompetence are also not suitable for reimplantation. If incompetence of the extensor mechanism is observed at the time of implant extraction and debridement, we usually plan for staged fusion.

Whether planning eventual reimplantation, resection arthroplasty, or fusion, an initial meticulous soft tissue and bone debridement, as well as complete removal of polymethylmethacrylate is paramount.

DIAGNOSING DEEP INFECTION

Establishing a diagnosis of deep infection after TKA may be a considerable challenge but is of utmost importance so that appropriate treatment can be initiated (1,14–16). Purulent drainage, sinus tract formation, fevers, and chills are uncommon in deep knee infection. A methodical application of available diagnostic tests is advisable, but reflexive overutilization of studies is often unnecessary and wasteful of time and resources (14). A careful history regarding the onset of symptoms and a meticulous physical examination will often give important clues as to the source of failure. Radiographs rarely distinguish between septic and aseptic failure, but select serologic studies are very useful for diagnosis (Figs. 22-1 and 22-2). A peripheral white blood cell count is rarely elevated, but a preponderance of polymorphonuclear cells may suggest infection. Used in concert, the sedimentation rate and C-reactive protein (CRP) are more accurate serologic studies, particularly for late infections (14,17–19). Knee aspiration is the most effective method for identifying a deep knee infection after TKA (17,20–22). The knee is an easy joint to aspirate and serial aspirations, with the patient off antibiotics for 3 or 4 weeks, may significantly enhance the diagnostic yield. If a patient with chronic insidious symptoms had been put on antibiotics empirically by another physician without having first aspirated and cultured the synovial fluid, then we tend to discontinue antibiotics for 4 weeks (provided symptoms or signs of bacteremia do not develop) and then re-aspirate the knee. Recent studies suggest that a white blood cell count of greater than as little as 2500 to 3120 cells/μL and neutrophil differential >60% to 65% in the knee aspirate carries over 95% accuracy in diagnosing periprosthetic joint infection (17,21,22). Serial aspirations have been shown to increase diagnostic yield of cultured fluid, so in cases of heightened clinical suspicion, serial aspirations are performed (23). Gram stains of the aspirate are often not helpful, but occasionally, bacteria may be seen. We rarely use nuclear studies such as labeled white blood cell scans, although total body technetium scans may be useful in ruling out metachronous infection in a patient with multiple painful prosthetic joints, when one joint implant is infected (24,25). We believe that intraoperative frozen-section histoanalysis can be very useful in identifying occult infection, but it is extremely sensitive

FIGURE 22-1

(A,B) Anteroposterior and lateral radiographs of a total knee arthroplasty that had been performed 3 months prior to presentation. Persistent unremitting pain prompted referral, and aspiration confirmed coagulase-negative staphylococcus infection. Note that despite the femoral notching, there is no evidence of loosening or other radiographic changes that would suggest infection. This patient was considered to have a chronic infection despite only 3 months of symptoms.

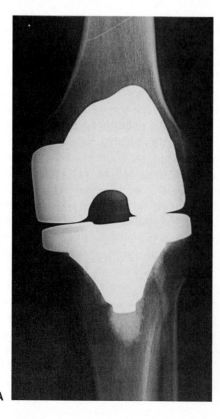

A

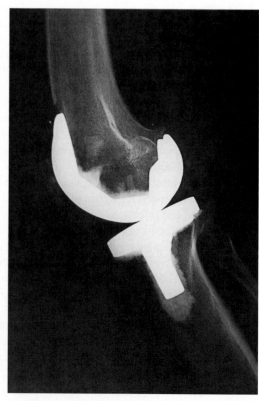

B

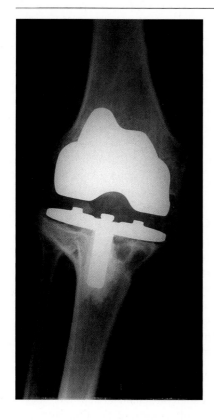

FIGURE 22-2

In contradistinction to the earlier radiographs, this radiograph shows marked radiographic changes in a chronically infected knee with cystic changes, gross loosening of the implant, and periosteal reaction.

to errors in tissue sampling and depends on the expertise of the histopathologist examining the tissues (26–28). Thus, institutions with available expertise can benefit from the use of frozen section in select cases. To improve yield and accuracy of frozen-section and intraoperative culture, representative multiple tissue samples from affected regions of the joint must be obtained. Interface tissue between the prosthesis and bone is mostly preferred, but inflamed synovial tissue or granulation tissue can also be useful. Fibrous or fibrin-rich tissue is difficult to interpret and should not be sent. At least two tissue samples should be sent from each knee, and the five most cellular fields should be analyzed under high-power magnification. The presence of more than 10 polymorphonuclear leukocytes per high-power field in five or more fields is almost uniformly consistent with deep periprosthetic infection. Between five and nine polymorphonuclear leukocytes per high-power field may suggest infection but should be considered in concert with other preoperative diagnostic tests.

Intraoperative cultures, although considered the most reliable determinant of infection, may be negative in 5% to 8% of acute and as many as 20% of chronic or indolent infections (16). When there is a strong clinical suspicion for infection despite negative intraoperative cultures, the knee should be treated as infected. We use a number of important strategies that improve the accuracy of intraoperative cultures. First, to increase the likelihood of organism isolation, preoperative antibiotics are withheld from patients with suspected infection in whom the infecting organism is not identified. (This is different from how antibiotics are given when infection is not suspected, in which case preoperative antibiotics are given within 30 to 60 minutes of tourniquet inflation.) Second, we usually send between four to five tissue samples from various affected regions of the knee. The tissue samples intended for culture are obtained with the use of clean and unused instruments and are transferred into containers without allowing them to come into contact with the gloves or drapes. Once multiple samples from different affected areas are obtained, the culture samples are sent to microbiology labs immediately. The latter strategy is effective in reducing the false-positive rate of infection. The tissues are sent for aerobic and anaerobic culture, which increases the likelihood of identifying not only indolent infection but also polymicrobial infection. Fungal or microbacterial testing is not routinely done, except in unusual cases. After cultures are taken, antibiotics may be administered with deflation of the tourniquet. The choice of antibiotic is based on the results of preoperative aspiration culture. If the infecting organism is not known, a broad-spectrum antibiotic such as vancomycin is administered. Culturing of draining wounds or sinus tracts is not recommended because of the likelihood of false-positive cultures from contamination.

SURGICAL TECHNIQUE

Surgical Exposure

The basic tenets of the surgical approach to the infected knee undergoing arthroplasty are similar to those for all revisions. In the knee with multiple surgical scars, the most lateral incision through which a standard arthrotomy can be performed is most often used. Small skin bridges should be avoided to minimize the risk of soft tissue hypoperfusion and potential for tissue necrosis. Sinus tracts within the margins of the skin incision are elliptically excised down to and through the capsule. Sinus tracts in other areas away from the surgical incision are also excised to minimize the risk of further contamination. An atrophic skin envelope, a multiply scarred knee, or a knee with large sinus tracts should prompt preoperative consultation with a plastic surgeon. In some cases, muscle flap and skin graft coverage may be required during the initial resection arthroplasty. Adequate soft tissue coverage helps promote healing and is critical for eradicating infection.

The surgical procedure proceeds in a systematic and organized manner that enables the surgeon to resect all infected tissues. At the time of arthrotomy, cultures are taken both of synovial fluid and inflamed soft tissues (Fig. 22-3). Remnants of all unabsorbed sutures are removed. Thorough synovectomy is performed before flexing the knee. The synovectomy is started from one area of the knee and performed in a stepwise fashion until healthy-appearing tissue is exposed. Lateral capsular tension is applied with the use of two Kocher clamps (Fig. 22-4). The surgeon also débrides the medial gutter and suprapatellar pouch in a similar fashion until healthy and viable tissue remains (Fig. 22-5). Often, extensive synovectomy provides ample exposure to allow flexion of the knee. Occasionally, however, undue tension is placed on the distal insertion of the patellar tendon, and the tibial insert may be removed at the outset to reduce the risk of patellar tendon avulsion (Fig. 22-6). A subperiosteal release of the deep medial collateral ligament, capsular sleeve, and semimembranosus insertion may facilitate anterolateral subluxation of the tibia and also relieve stress on the patellar tendon. The surgeon inserts a towel clamp or 1/8-inch pin through the patellar tendon insertion to further reduce the risk of avulsion (Fig. 22-7). At times, ancillary

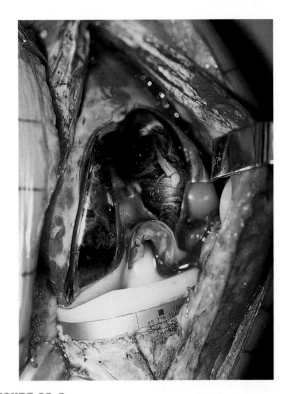

FIGURE 22-3

There is acute and diffuse inflammation of periarticular soft tissues.

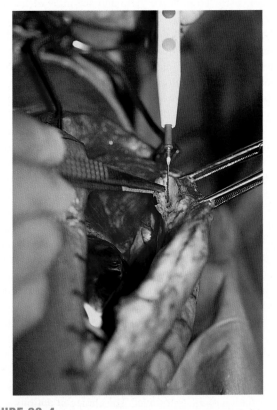

FIGURE 22-4

Synovectomy of the lateral soft tissues and gutter can be performed with the knee in extension.

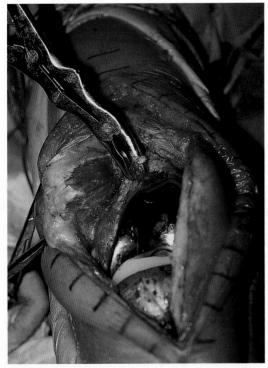

FIGURE 22-5

A rongeur may be used to débride the inflamed periprosthetic tissues, and a medial synovectomy may be performed with the knee extended.

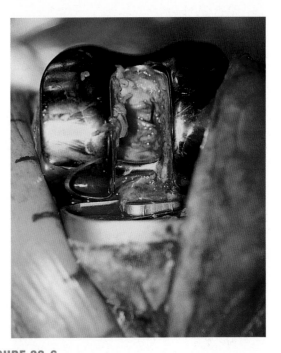

FIGURE 22-6

The polyethylene insert may be removed to facilitate flexion of the knee and exposure of the posterior aspect of the joint.

extensile approaches are necessary to achieve adequate exposure. Our preference is an inverted V-plasty of the proximal quadriceps tendon. A short oblique incision measuring 1 to 2 cm is directed laterally and distally from the proximal extent of the medial parapatellar incision at an angle of approximately 45 degrees (Fig. 22-8). This approach is safe and generally does not devascularize the proximal edge of the quadriceps tendon, because unlike a formal Coonse-Adams turndown, the superolateral geniculate vessels may be preserved. This approach, coupled with a lateral retinacular release from the inside out, with preservation of the superolateral geniculate vessels, provides ample exposure (Fig. 22-9). Quadriceps advancement is generally not performed. Other proximal releases may be performed, including the Insall snip, although for particularly tight knees, this approach may not be adequate. A tibial tubercle osteotomy, although potentially useful at the time of reimplantation, should be avoided at the time of implant extraction because of the risk of infected nonunion of the tibial tubercle, and the presence of hardware may compromise the ability to completely eradicate the infection.

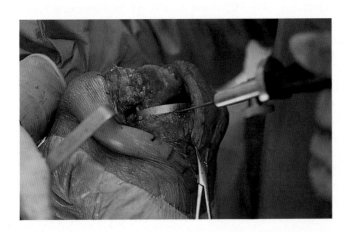

FIGURE 22-7

A thin, flexible osteotome may be used to define the interface of the undersurface of the tibial component and prepare it for removal. Note that a towel clamp is used to help provisionally reinforce the patellar tendon insertion and protect it from avulsion during the surgical procedure.

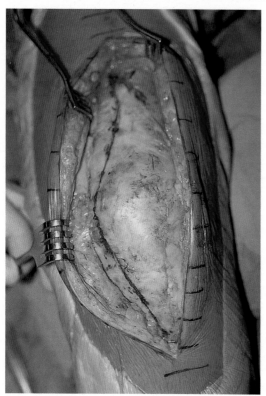

FIGURE 22-8

The planned arthrotomy incision is marked and includes a small lateral limb that may be used if an extensive approach is necessary for exposure.

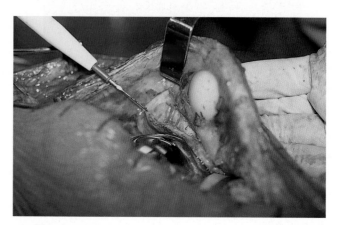

FIGURE 22-9

To facilitate exposure, a lateral retinacular release may be performed, preserving the superolateral geniculate vessels if possible, which are evident in this photograph.

IMPLANT REMOVAL

Once adequate exposure is obtained, removal of components begins. Removing well-fixed implants may be arduous, but uninfected bone stock and collateral ligament attachments need to be preserved with care. Attempts at component extraction are withheld until the interfaces are meticulously cleared and freed from underlying bone to minimize the risk of inadvertent bone removal. The interface edges beneath the components are demarcated with either a rongeur or small curette. We prefer to remove the femoral component first, as this often facilitates exposure of the tibia and avoids deposition of cement fragments and other debris into the medullary canal of the tibia. The femoral component can be removed with a combination of flexible and rigid osteotomes or a Gigli saw (Figs. 22-10 and 22-11). If applicable, all cement and necrotic tissue must be removed from the exposed bone surfaces and lug holes (Fig. 22-12). The tibial and patellar components are removed with a combination of small saw blades and osteotomes (Figs. 22-7 and 22-13). All of the cement is removed with a saw, osteotome, and burr (Fig. 22-14). When all implants are removed, synovectomy of the posterior aspect of the joint is performed.

Debridement of necrotic or infected bone is critical. Although preservation of ligamentous attachments and bone stock is important, thorough debridement of infected or devitalized tissue takes precedence to clear the infection. It is plausible that a high percentage of recurrent infections are caused by inadequate debridement of infected bone. Suspicious bone should be cultured and histologically analyzed to rule out osteomyelitis. Occasionally, further surgery is necessary to more thoroughly address foci of osteomyelitis.

After removing all cement and necrotic tissue, the knee is irrigated copiously with 6 to 9 liters of pulsatile lavage using solution that contains bacitracin and/or polymixin (Fig. 22-15). Before implanting the antibiotic spacers, the extent of bone loss and the integrity of the collateral ligaments should be assessed in an effort to prepare preliminarily for eventual reimplantation.

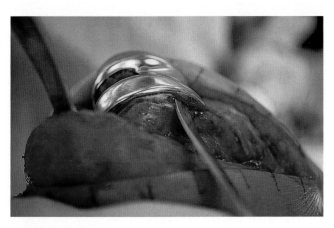

FIGURE 22-10
After the prosthetic interfaces are cleared and the interface edges demarcated, the femoral component is removed with an osteotome.

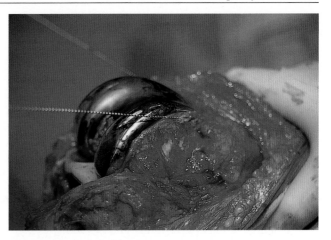

FIGURE 22-11
Alternatively, a Gigli saw may be used to remove the femoral component.

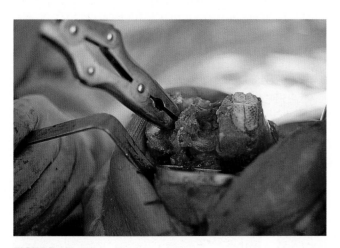

FIGURE 22-12
After femoral prosthesis extraction, cement and fibrous tissue are removed from the distal femur. Additionally, necrotic bone and inflamed tissue should be removed at this stage.

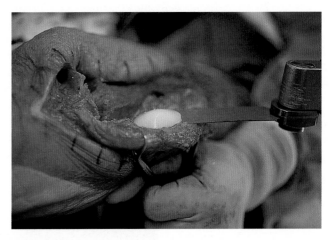

FIGURE 22-13
The patella is removed with an oscillating saw, and all underlying cement is removed from the lug holes using a high-speed burr, osteotome, or saw.

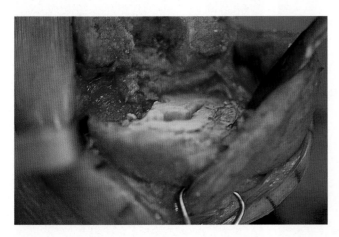

FIGURE 22-14
After prosthesis removal, tibial bone stock should be assessed and any further cement removed.

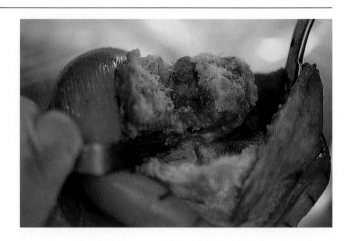

FIGURE 22-15

After thorough debridement, pulsatile irrigation can be used to clear debris from the bone surfaces and identify any further tissue in need of debridement.

INTERVAL ANTIBIOTIC SPACERS

We prefer two-stage revision with an interval period of antibiotic-impregnated cement spacers for most late infections (5,6,12). Antibiotic-loaded cement provides a vehicle for local delivery of relatively high concentrations of local antibiotics (which are eluted up to 6 weeks), confers mechanical stability of the knee during ambulation, and limits contracture of the soft tissue envelope, which simplifies exposure of the joint during subsequent reimplantation. Several types of antibiotic spacers can be considered. Our preferences are either an articulating spacer or two contoured, static cement spacers, one capping the femur and the other the tibia. (Figs. 22-16 and 22-17). Unlike standard spacer blocks that do not allow motion, articulating spacers allow partial weight bearing, enhance short-term limb function, and enable immediate range of motion, which reduces scarring and ultimately facilitates surgical exposure at reimplantation (5,7,10,29). We do not use a monoblock spacer in most cases, as it can be difficult to extract at secondary reimplantation.

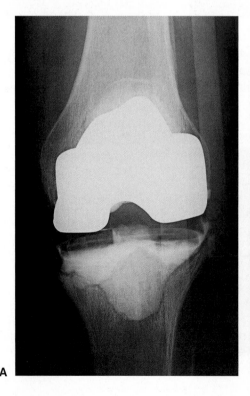
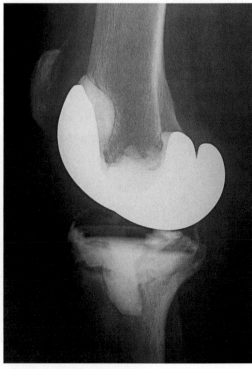

FIGURE 22-16

(A,B) Radiographs of a dynamic articulating spacer.

A

B

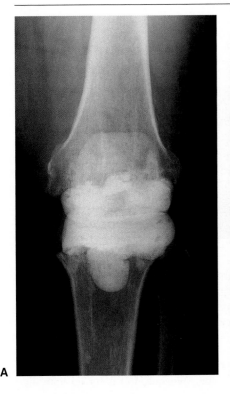
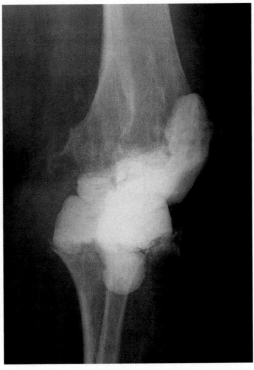

A

B

FIGURE 22-17

(A,B) Radiographs of a static spacer.

TECHNIQUE OF CEMENT SPACER INSERTION

For infections with sensitive organisms, acute onset, and good soft tissues, we prefer to use a dynamic articulating spacer. In this technique, all adherent cement is cleared off the backside of the extracted femoral component, which is then sterilized for 20 minutes in the autoclave (Figs. 22-18 to 22-20). A fresh polyethylene insert appropriately mated to the femoral component is used as the articulating countersurface, selecting a thickness that will allow reasonable balancing of the flexion and extension spaces (Figs. 22-21 and 22-22). Because the articulating spacer will be in for a relatively short time, wear per se is not a concern; therefore, there can be a manufacturer mismatch between the sterilized

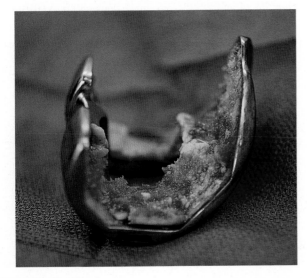

FIGURE 22-18

The undersurface of the femoral component after removal shows adherent cement.

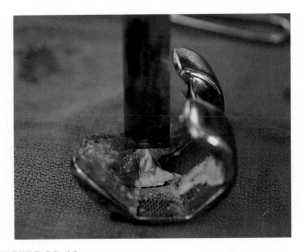

FIGURE 22-19

If an articulating spacer is to be used, all cement is removed from the femoral component using an osteotome.

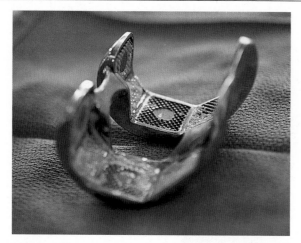

FIGURE 22-20

Photograph of the femoral component after cement had been removed and the prosthesis sterilized in the autoclave for 20 minutes.

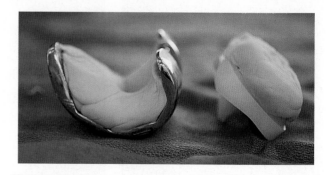

FIGURE 22-21

The underlying surfaces of the femoral component and a fresh polyethylene tibial insert are coated with a mixture of Palacos cement and high concentrations of tobramycin and vancomycin.

femoral component that had been removed and the newly opened polyethylene insert without concern regarding adverse consequences. Palacos cement (Zimmer, Inc., Warsaw, IN) is mixed with high concentrations of antibiotics (3 g of vancomycin mixed with either 3.6 g of tobramycin or 240 mg of gentamycin per 40 g of methylmethacrylate) to provide a high localized dose of broad-spectrum antibiotics. The cement is hand mixed as presence of bubbles in the cement improves antibiotic elusion. We prefer Palacos cement at this stage because of its superior antibiotic elution kinetics. For most cases, two or three packets of cement are adequate. The cement-antibiotic mixture is applied to the undersurfaces of the sterilized femoral component and polyethylene tibial insert in a doughy stage (Fig. 22-21). An appropriately sized polyethylene tibial component is implanted first, with caution not to pressurize the cement into the trabeculae of the metaphyseal bone. The doughy cement is laid gently onto the bony surface, irrigated with water, and backed off periodically to avoid interdigitation of the cement and cancellous bone (Fig. 22-22). The same technique is used for the femoral component with the knee flexed 90 degrees, leaving the cement mantle several millimeters thick (Fig. 22-23).

As the cement cures, the knee is brought through an arc of motion several times to ensure preservation of appropriate soft tissue tension (Figs. 22-24 and 22-25). We make sure not to overdistend

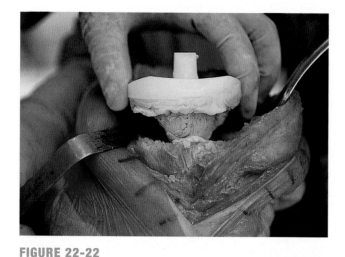

FIGURE 22-22

In the doughy stage, the cement of the tibial spacer is inserted into the keel defect and the surface of the proximal tibia, avoiding pressurization of cement within the trabecular bone.

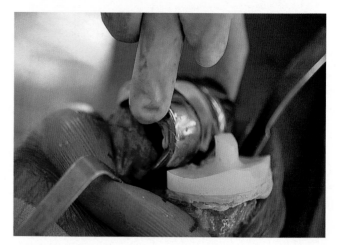

FIGURE 22-23

The femoral component is inserted similarly.

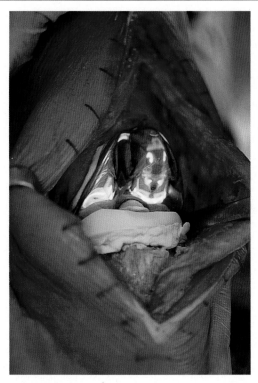

FIGURE 22-24

The stability of the articulating spacer is assessed, in part, in extension. Note the liberal cement mantle, which ensures that the cement is not pressurized into the exposed trabecular bone.

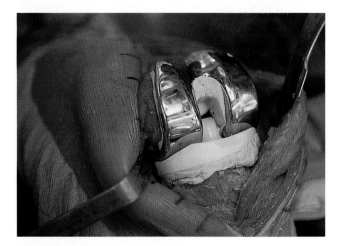

FIGURE 22-25

The stability of the articulating spacer is also assessed in flexion.

the extension space, as this may put the collateral ligaments on stretch and potentially render them incompetent at the time of revision arthroplasty. Alternatively, undertensioning may cause subluxation or dislocation of the polyethylene insert (Fig. 22-26). The latter problem can be avoided by using an all-polyethylene insert with a central keel as the tibial bearing.

An alternative to dynamic articulating spacers is standard antibiotic spacer blocks alone, with similar concentrations of antibiotics per unit of polymethylmethacrylate as in articulating spacers. The tibia is first capped with a disc of cement with a small central knob that extends into the debrided metaphyseal defect in which the previous tibial keel and cement resided (Fig. 22-27). Appropriate sizing of the tibial disc is important. It must be thick enough to provide a stable base, narrow enough to allow capsular closure, but have enough underlying cancellous and cortical support to minimize subsidence and protect trabecular bone stock. The femoral spacer contour and size are equally important. It should be no more than approximately 1 cm thick anteriorly, and the anterior flange should taper proximally to facilitate capsular closure (Fig. 22-28). The femoral spacer is curved distally and posteriorly around the distal femoral condyles.

Antibiotic-impregnated cement dowels are inserted into the medullary canals when revising stemmed implants (Fig. 22-29). It is important to ensure that the dowels are thinner than the inner canal dimensions to avoid incarceration in the femoral or tibial canals. It is also prudent to check the "fit" of the dowels during the cement polymerization process. We prefer cement dowels to beads on a metal wire or heavy suture because the latter can become entrapped by abundant fibrous tissue or organized clot that eventually fill the canals.

A closed suction drain is not used because it has been shown to reduce the effective dose of local antibiotics. The knee is then sutured in layers. A no. 1 monofilament, nonbraided suture is used for capsular closure, as this may be less of a nidus for infection than braided suture. Subcutaneous closure is performed with a 2.0 monofilament suture, and the skin is generally stapled unless the surgeon is concerned about the skin tissue's integrity, in which case nylon sutures are used to close in an interrupted fashion, sometimes using retention sutures. As mentioned earlier, a muscle flap should be considered if the closure is compromised.

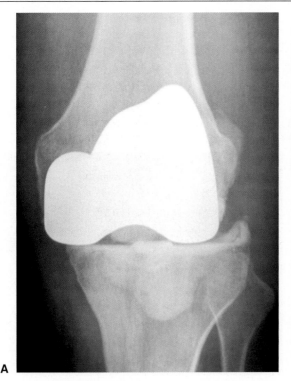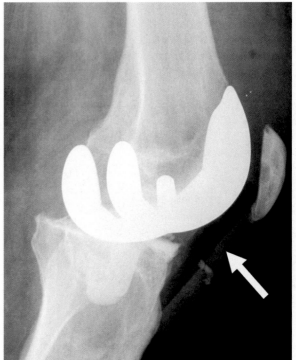

A

B

FIGURE 22-26

(A,B) Anteroposterior radiograph of an articulating spacer shows apparent loss of the "clear space" that should be occupied by the polyethylene insert. The lateral radiograph shows that the insert has dissociated from the underlying cement and displaced into the anterior aspect of the knee. This could result in laceration of the extensor mechanism or collateral ligaments.

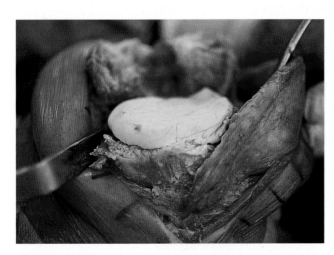

FIGURE 22-27

If nonarticulating cement spacers are used, the tibial spacer is fashioned to fit on the cut and prepared surface of the proximal tibia. The margins of the spacer should not extend beyond the margins of the cut metaphyseal surface.

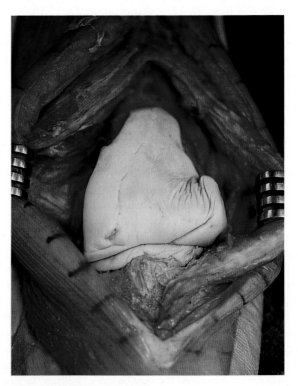

FIGURE 22-28

The femoral and tibial static spacers with the knee in full extension.

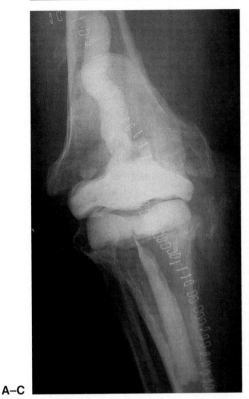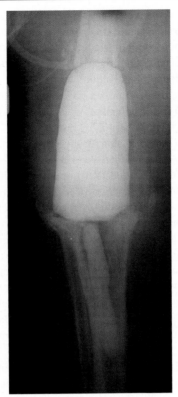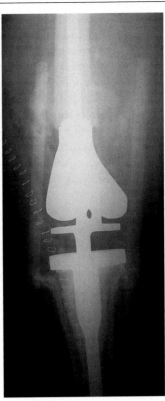

A–C

FIGURE 22-29

(A–C) Anteroposterior radiograph of a knee after implantation of spacers, including dowels, after removal of an infected revision style total knee arthroplasty. Note periosteal reaction of the medial and lateral metaphyseal flares of the distal femur. Intraoperative biopsies of these bony sites showed chronic osteomyelitis. A distal femoral resection was necessary to eradicate the extensive osteomyelitis of the distal femur and eventually, a hinged knee arthroplasty with distal femoral modular augments was necessary.

ROLE OF INTERVAL DEBRIDEMENT BEFORE IMPLANTATION

On occasion, a secondary interval debridement is performed. We perform an additional debridement before eventual reimplantation in patients in whom there is concern of inadequate initial debridement (such as cases performed elsewhere); when the initial cultures confirm osteomyelitis; when CRP is not normalizing despite a 6-week course of antibiotics; when the knee remains markedly inflamed; or when cultures of a repeat knee aspirate performed 4 weeks after discontinuing antibiotics are positive. Secondary debridement provides an opportunity to reculture the bone and soft tissues to determine therapeutic response. Occasionally, chronic recalcitrant osteomyelitis requires such aggressive osseous resection that treatment with a rotating hinge arthroplasty with bulk modules is necessary (Fig. 22-29).

POSTOPERATIVE MANAGEMENT WITH SPACER BLOCKS

Patients are maintained on 6 weeks of parenteral antibiotics specific for organisms cultured on preoperative aspirates, with modification of antibiotics made as necessary depending on the results of intraoperative cultures. If intraoperative cultures are negative, but frozen and permanent sections of analyzed tissues suggest infection, then antibiotics are administered empirically with the assumption that there is an infection with a fastidious organism. A peripherally inserted central catheter is inserted for a minimum of 6 weeks and perhaps longer if additional debridement is necessary before staged reimplantation.

In the initial acute postoperative period, the wound is assessed carefully. Persistent drainage is treated aggressively with early debridement. Wound necrosis is treated with debridement, and a local gastrocnemius muscle flap is used to gain wound coverage and enhance the vascularity of the local environment.

Isometric exercises are initiated immediately to promote quadriceps rehabilitation and to reduce the formation of retropatellar adhesions. If an articulating spacer is used, a continuous passive motion machine is employed while the patient is hospitalized, unless immobilization is prudent to protect the surgical wound. Flexion is usually restricted to 90 degrees. Partial weight bearing with a knee immobilizer is allowed while ambulating.

If a nonarticulating spacer is used, we prefer to use a knee immobilizer, rather than a long leg cast, so that the surgical incision and knee may be evaluated during the postoperative period.

TIMING OF REIMPLANTATION

Reimplantation is performed when four important prerequisites are satisfied (30). First, and perhaps the most important, is that the CRP needs to return to normal and stay normal despite discontinuation of antibiotics, and the erythrocyte sedimentation rate should be normal or trending toward normal. Second, the underlying cause of infection (if identified) is adequately addressed. Patients with recurrent urinary tract infection, cellulitis, poor dentition, or skin ulceration need to be investigated, and all strategies for treatment and prevention of subsequent recurrence are implemented. Third, immunocompromised, malnourished, and medically unwell patients need to be fully optimized before reimplantation surgery. Finally, the soft tissues around the knee need to be fully healed and ready for another incision. The latter includes careful assessment of the vascular status of the limb to ensure that the likelihood of wound breakdown is minimized following reimplantation. Some of these patients, as alluded to previously, may require evaluation by plastic surgeons for possible coverage.

We prefer not to reflexively reimplant the knee upon completion of the antibiotic course, but rather to wait an additional 2 to 6 weeks after termination of antibiotics to allow for persistent infection to declare itself during the antibiotic-free period. During this period, the serology markers are checked on a weekly basis to ensure that they remain normal. Before reimplantation and at a minimum of 2 to 4 weeks after completion of the antibiotic course, we aspirate every knee. Aspiration while on antibiotics or within a short period of completing the course may provide false assurance for eradication of infection as organisms are being suppressed (2,18,31).

We find it useful to follow the trending patterns of the erythrocyte sedimentation rate and CRP to help guide us in determining the appropriateness of reimplantation. The sedimentation rate may remain elevated for 6 months after surgery, but CRP levels should generally normalize by 4 weeks postoperatively; therefore, if the CRP has normalized and the sedimentation rate trends toward normal, we would proceed with reimplantation. If an appropriate trend is not observed, however, we opt for further debridement, without reimplantation (18,30).

Occasionally, if we are concerned about the possibility of extensive osteomyelitis, we may obtain a bone scan to help determine the extent of infection and the need for further osseous debridement; however, we otherwise rarely obtain nuclear scans before reimplantation (25).

Once in the operating room, there are several important parameters that we use to guide us with appropriate decision making. An important part of reimplantation surgery is further debridement of the soft tissues and bone as needed. If during debridement, foci of infection are noted, or if the frozen section sent for examination shows signs of acute inflammation, we tend to abort reimplantation and place another antibiotic spacer (32). We reserve the frozen-section examination to cases in which there is concern regarding potential ongoing infection. We base our decision to reimplant a knee prosthesis on the results of intraoperative tissue analysis, but we use five (rather than 10) polymorphonuclear leukocytes per high-power field as the index of infection. Changing the histological threshold for infection reduces the risk of implanting a prosthesis into a persistently infected bed but potentially increases the tendency to withhold reimplantation when it may be appropriate.

SURGICAL TECHNIQUE OF TKA REIMPLANTATION

Once the surgeon has decided to proceed with reimplantation, the appropriate selection of surgical incisions and principles of exposure are paramount. Rotational muscle flaps (if present) are carefully elevated, without compromising their vascular pedicles. If the knee has an articulating spacer in place, relatively little scarring of the suprapatellar pouch and medial and lateral gutters facilitates surgical exposure (Fig. 22-30). After arthrotomy, synovectomy and excision of scar tissue and pseudocapsule are performed (Fig. 22-31). A lateral retinacular release may enhance exposure and allow subluxation

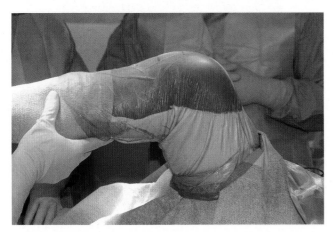

FIGURE 22-30

At the time of reimplantation, this knee, which has an articulating spacer, has 80 degrees of flexion.

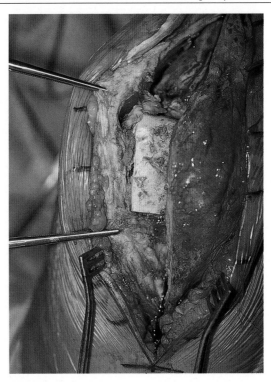

FIGURE 22-31

At the time of reimplantation, a standard arthrotomy is performed, and cultures of the synovial fluid are obtained. The gross appearance of the synovial fluid should be noted.

of the patella; patellar eversion is not absolutely necessary in most revision TKAs. Subperiosteal dissection along the medial edge and posteromedial corner of the tibia allows anterolateral subluxation of the tibia, optimizing exposure of the tibial surface and relieving tension on the patellar tendon insertion. If necessary, the surgeon performs a proximal inverted V-plasty of the quadriceps tendon, a quadriceps snip, or a tibial tubercle osteotomy. Our preference, once again, is to use a proximal ancillary exposure rather than a tibial tubercle osteotomy because of the inherent risk of tubercle nonunion, particularly if bone stock is compromised.

Synovial fluid and select tissue samples are sent for culture in all patients, and frozen- and permanent-section histoanalysis of interface tissues or synovium are performed if there is concern regarding ongoing infection. As stated, ongoing acute inflammatory response with more than five polymorphonuclear leukocytes per high-power field will prompt further debridement, implantation of interval antibiotic spacers, and delay of reimplantation.

The spacer blocks are removed, and further soft tissue and osseous debridement is performed (Figs. 22-32 and 22-33). Long-handled reverse curettes are used to clear fibrous tissue from the intramedullary canals (usually after failed stemmed revisions) (Fig. 22-34). The cut tibial, femoral, and patellar surfaces are cleared of adherent soft tissues. Posterior capsular scar tissue is carefully freed from the posterior femoral condylar surfaces using an elevator (Fig. 22-35). Pulsatile lavage of the knee is performed to define further the extent of bone loss and margins of nonviable soft tissues.

We prefer modular knee revision systems that provide the option of using stems and metallic augments of varying lengths and sizes, respectively, to provide the latitude and adaptability to fill bone defects and achieve stability, while restoring the joint line and normalizing component alignment. The decision regarding implant constraint is made primarily based on the integrity of the collateral ligaments and extent of bone stock compromise. We treat all reimplantations with stemmed implants and a posterior cruciate ligament-substituting device. An unlinked, but constrained prosthesis is selected if residual soft tissue instability exists after attempting to balance the soft tissues with the trials in place. In the event that complete incompetence of one or both collateral ligaments exists, a

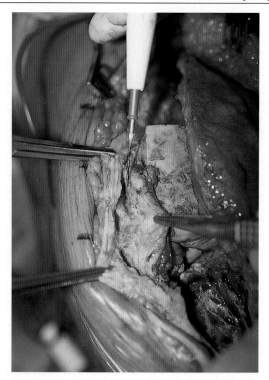

FIGURE 22-32

Synovectomy and excision of pseudocapsule is performed initially with the knee in extension.

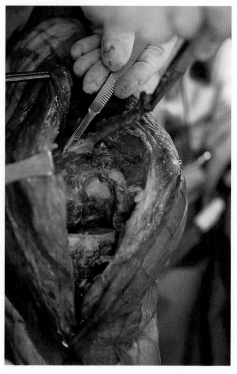

FIGURE 22-33

After removal of the articulating spacers, necrotic tissue, granulation tissue, and fibrous tissue can be observed on the cut surfaces of the femur and tibia. These should be entirely removed.

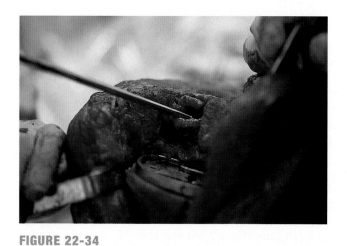

FIGURE 22-34

After capping the proximal tibia with the trial component to avoid deposition of debris within the prepared tibia, a variety of curettes may be used to remove fibrous tissue from within the femoral canal if a stemmed implant had been used.

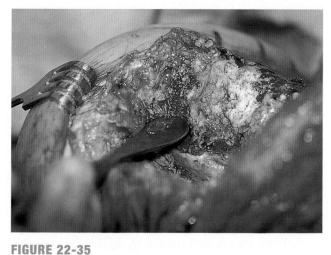

FIGURE 22-35

With the knee in flexion, scar tissue adherent to the posterior femoral condyles is freed using a periosteal elevator.

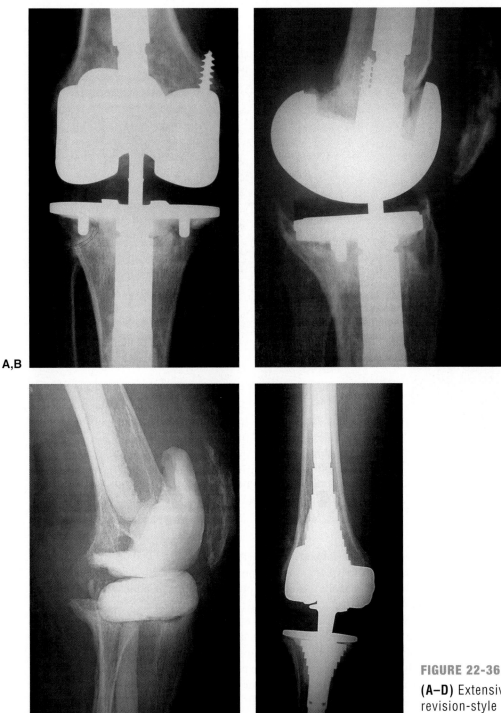

A,B

C,D

FIGURE 22-36

(A–D) Extensive osseous infection after revision-style implant required eventual revision total knee arthroplasty using a linked modular hinge.

rotating hinge prosthesis may be selected (Fig. 22-36). If extensive resection of the distal femur or proximal tibia is necessary for chronic osteomyelitis, a rotating hinge prosthesis with distal femoral or proximal tibial bulk augments is used (see Fig. 22-29).

Restoring the joint line and appropriate implantation of components in proper rotational and axial alignment are critical to optimize performance, restore appropriate kinematics, and enhance patellar tracking. We generally use metal augments, not allograft, for addressing bone loss in revisions for septic failure because of a concern that allograft may be more likely to become infected in the presence of persistent infection.

We proceed with the reimplantation in a stepwise fashion, addressing the tibia first to establish a stable platform from which we can determine femoral component rotation and gap balance.

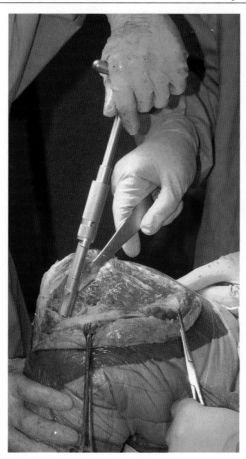

FIGURE 22-37

After adequate tissue debridement of the exposed metaphyseal surfaces, the tibia is prepared.

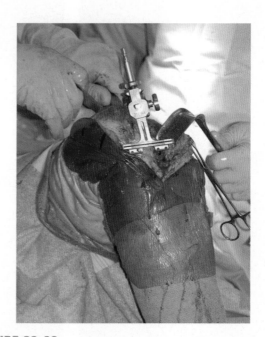

FIGURE 22-38

A proximal skim cut of tibia is performed, removing a minimal amount of bone to achieve a stable platform for the implant. In this case, an oblique slotted cutting block is pinned in place, anterior to the patellar tendon. The saw cut would have to be made from the medial-most edge of the guide to avoid damaging the patellar tendon. It is often easier to freehand the cut.

Referencing from the endosteal surfaces of both the tibial and femoral diaphysis is, in our hands, the most reproducible and accurate method of preparing the proximal tibia and distal femur (Fig. 22-37). Intramedullary reamers are used to size the canals for a press-fit stem; a tight press fit is not necessary. The tibial canal is easily accessible. Reaming of the intramedullary canal with sequentially increasing reamers allows engagement of the endosteum within the diaphysis. Reaming by hand or with a power reamer using low velocity affords better tactile sense, superior control of the reamers, and reduced risk of inadvertent cortical perforation, compared to aggressive powered reaming. The reamer, or an appropriately sized trial stem, engages the tibial endosteum and acts as a guide upon which a tibial cutting block is mounted so that the tibial metaphysis can be resected. Often, the skim cut is made at a right angle to the axis of the tibial shaft; however, occasionally, an oblique cut is made to accommodate an oblique deformity. Most often, we prefer to freshen the surface of the proximal tibia with a freehand cut because it is difficult to slide the cutting instrument under the scarred patellar tendon. The alternative is to pin the guide superficial to the patellar tendon and cut around it, but the stability of the guide is weakened, and there may be a certain amount of error by this technique or risk to the patellar tendon (Fig. 22-38). The surgeon aligns the block with the medial third of the tibial tubercle to avoid erroneously cutting the tibia in varus or valgus. This cut is usually quite conservative, but adequate osseous support is important. Metal augments or reinforced cement are used to fill uncontained bone defects of the proximal tibia.

After the tibial cut surface has been prepared, alignment is confirmed with an extramedullary rod (Fig. 22-39). The trial tray and stem are assembled; a component with offset may be helpful to maximize coverage and avoid overhang of the tibial tray (Fig. 22-40). Once the appropriate trial is set up and the need for offset established, a keel punch or burr is used if any bone needs to be cleared to orient the tray so that its center is aligned with the medial third of the tibial tubercle. The trial is left in place during femoral preparation.

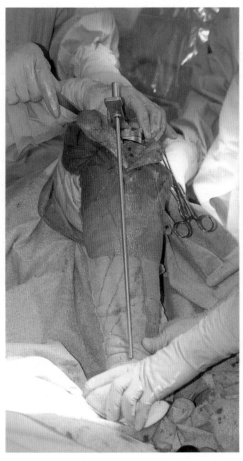

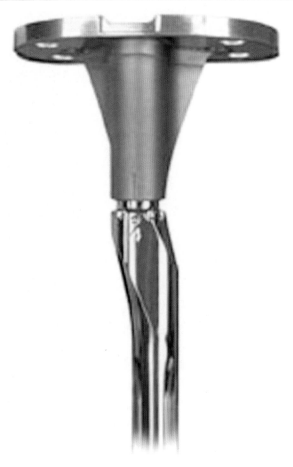

FIGURE 22-39

An extramedullary alignment rod attached to a trial tibial tray with a medial augment is used to confirm accuracy of the proximal tibial cut.

FIGURE 22-40

An offset tibial keel may be necessary to optimize tibial coverage and avoid component overhang.

Sequential reaming of the femoral canal is performed until the diaphyseal endosteum is engaged (Fig. 22-41). Usually, only a skim cut of the distal femur is necessary to freshen the bone ends. The orientation of the distal femur can be determined by mounting a cutting guide at the appropriate fixed angle (often between 5 and 7 degrees) on the reamer or trial stem, which is inserted in the femoral canal. A decision is made regarding the need for distal condylar augments, based on an assessment of the amount of bone loss relative to where the joint line should be (Fig. 22-42A,B). The joint line should be restored to 20 to 25 mm from the medial femoral epicondyle. If one considers that the femoral implant is approximately 9 mm thick, then any further condylar deficiency should be

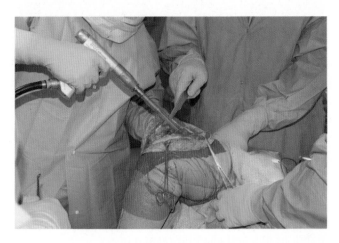

FIGURE 22-41

Femoral reaming is performed until endosteal contact is achieved.

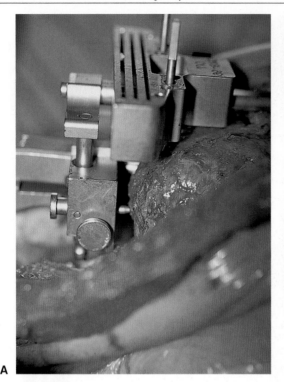
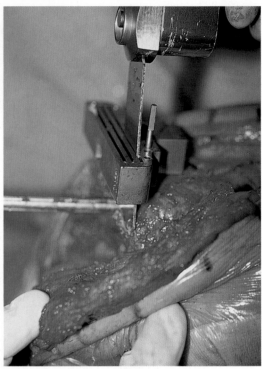

A   B

FIGURE 22-42

(A,B) A distal femoral cutting guide is applied to a trial stem or the reamer to resect the distal femur, generally at an angle of 5 to 7 degrees of valgus. The distal femoral condyles may be cut at different depths depending on the extent of bone loss.

restored with appropriately sized augments (Fig. 22-43). The size of the femoral component is selected to equalize the flexion and extension gaps after restoring the joint line with appropriate distal augments. The femoral size options are limited, in part, by the preselected size of the tibial component. Anteroposterior, chamfer, and box-cutting guides are mounted on the intramedullary reamer or trial stem with provisional distal augments applied to ensure that the depth of the box resection is appropriate and the chamfer cuts are appropriate (usually, the latter are "air balls") (Fig. 22-44).

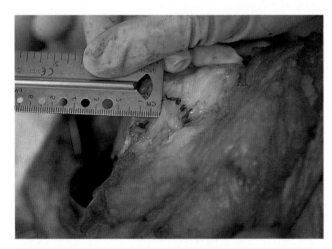

FIGURE 22-43

Measurements should be made to estimate the position of the joint line, which is approximately 20 to 25 mm from the medial epicondyle.

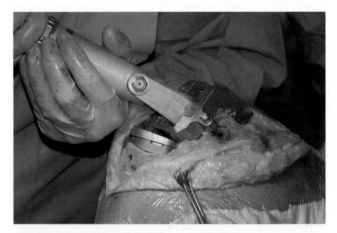

FIGURE 22-44

An appropriately sized chamfer and box-cutting block is secured to the distal femur parallel to the transepicondylar axis, mounted on a stem that engages the endosteum of the diaphysis to ensure appropriate coronal alignment of the instrument. Using augments, if necessary, ensures appropriate depth of box and chamfer resection.

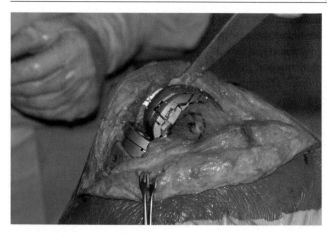

FIGURE 22-45

The trial components, with augments, are inserted. The joint line, measured from the medial epicondyle to the distal surface of the femoral component, is appropriately restored between 20 and 25 mm.

With the knee flexed 90 degrees, the guide is externally rotated, referencing it off of the cut tibial surface, manually tensioning the ligaments to re-establish a rectangular flexion space. The transverse axis of the cutting block should be parallel to the transepicondylar axis. Femoral offset options may improve position of the femoral component and normalize the flexion gap and patellofemoral space.

The decision to resurface the patella depends on the quality and thickness of residual bone. Pseudomeniscus and fibrous tissue are debrided from the surface and periphery of the patella. The patella is resurfaced if viable bone stock measures 10 to 15 mm; however, the remnant is left as a bony shell if it is too thin or has evidence of osteonecrosis. Leaving a bony shell may predispose to a moderate incidence of anterior knee discomfort; however, resurfacing of an excessively thin or osteonecrotic patella can result in fracture or disassociation of the patellar component. The introduction of trabecular metal patella components has allowed resurfacing of patellae that would be considered too thin. We usually use trabecular metal patella components if bone thickness is between 4 to 10 mm.

The trial components are assembled with the appropriate augments, and limb alignment, joint line position, stability, and patellar tracking are assessed (Figs. 22-45 and 22-46). Stability is checked both in full extension, midflexion, and 90 degrees of flexion. Initially, trialing is performed with a posterior stabilized insert, and additional constraint is used if necessary. If significant collateral imbalance persists, despite efforts of balancing and use of an unlinked constrained knee arthroplasty, a rotating hinge prosthesis is selected.

If an extensive release of the quadriceps tendon or tibial tubercle osteotomy were performed, patellar tracking is assessed with the osteotomy or quadriceps provisionally repaired. The evaluation of any patellar maltracking should include an assessment of soft tissue balancing, component rotation, patellar composite thickness, and tibial and femoral positioning. "Overstuffing" of the patellofemoral articulation with either an anteriorized femoral component, internally rotated femoral component, or excessively large patellar composite will predispose to subluxation. Malaligned

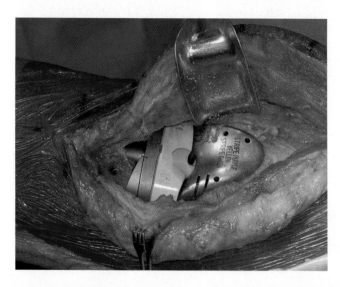

FIGURE 22-46

Appearance of trials in full extension.

implants should be reinserted correctly and tissue imbalance addressed. If satisfactory trialing has been achieved, the bony surfaces are then prepared for implantation.

We prefer to cement the condylar surfaces of the tibial and femoral components, including the tibial keel, but to use cementless, press-fit stems, unless bone is severely osteoporotic and canals are capacious, in which case the stems are cemented. There is no proven difference in the incidence of recurrent infection whether or not stems are cemented, but if reinfection develops, press-fit stems are easier to remove. We use antibiotic-impregnated Simplex Methyl methacrylate premixed with tobramycin (1.2 g tobramycin per 40 g of cement) in all revision surgeries, as this has been shown to significantly reduce the risk of recurrent infection without compromising the mechanical strength of cement. If an antibiotic is being added at the time of surgery instead of using the premixed cement, the antibiotic powder should be mixed with the powder of the cement polymer before adding the liquid monomer. When press-fitting the stems, it is useful to apply the cement directly to the undersurface of each component in a doughy stage, to avoid deposition into the medullary canals (Fig. 22-47A,B). The medullary trabecular surfaces are also coated with cement, leaving a space for passage of the stem.

Adequate balancing and tissue tension are confirmed with the trial tibial insert, and the final tibial polyethylene insert is impacted onto the clean and dry base plate. Once again, the knee is assessed for stability, range of motion, and patella tracking (Figs. 22-48A,B and 22-49A,B).

WOUND CLOSURE

The tourniquet is deflated, and hemostasis is achieved before wound closure. The wound is copiously irrigated with pulsatile lavage to evacuate debris. A midsized closed suction drain is inserted into the lateral gutter. Closure of the medial capsular arthrotomy and the lateral limb of an inverted V-plasty is performed with interrupted absorbable monofilament suture. We generally do not

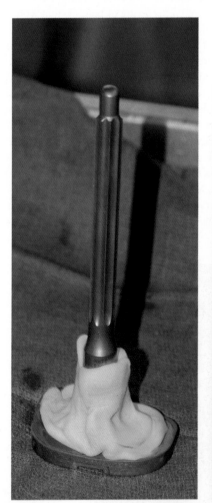
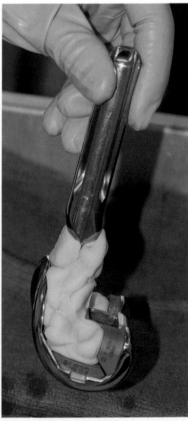

FIGURE 22-47

(A,B) When using press-fit stems, the cement/antibiotic mixture should be applied directly to the metaphyseal segment of the implant to ensure that cement does not extend into the canals.

A,B

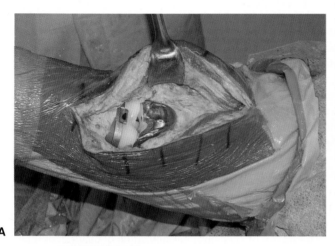

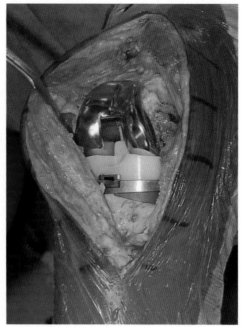

A

B

FIGURE 22-48

(A,B) Intraoperative photograph of the implanted components, with the knee in extension and flexion. The knee was stable and balanced without the need for constraint.

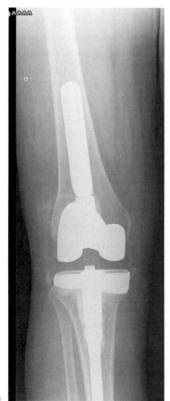

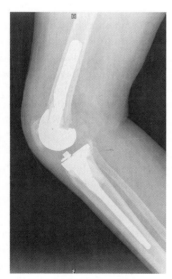

A,B

FIGURE 22-49

(A,B) Postoperative radiographs of the revision total knee arthroplasty showing a well-aligned implant. The thin patella was left as a bony shell.

perform V-Y quadriceps advancements because this increases the risk of an extensor lag. Once the capsule and arthrotomy are closed, passive motion against gravity is assessed to determine the quality of the capsular closure and to set limits for postoperative therapy. If the integrity of the skin is in question, coverage with a gastrocnemius flap should once again be considered.

POSTOPERATIVE MANAGEMENT

Antibiotics are continued empirically until the definitive culture results return, in 3 to 5 days. If intraoperative cultures are unexpectedly positive, consultation with an infectious diseases specialist is sought, and continuation of antibiotics for at least 6 weeks is considered unless deemed a contaminant. Although bacteria that grow on a solid medium are often appropriately considered true infections, it is not appropriate to reflexively dismiss as contaminants those bacteria that grow only in thioglycolate broth but not on a solid medium. In fact, about 50% of infections are so indolent that they may grow only in broth. In these cases, comparison to the results of histological analyses of harvested tissues can be invaluable. Occasionally, an additional debridement is performed, and long-term oral suppression is used in select cases.

The surgical wound is assessed on postoperative day one. If it appears viable and drainage is minimal, then continuous passive motion and physical therapy can commence. In general, when the lateral limb of an inverted V-plasty is no more than 2 to 3 cm in length, there is no alteration in our recommendations for range of motion or strengthening of the quadriceps, although patients are protected with a knee immobilizer and a walker or cane until normalization of quadriceps tone. For more extensile quadricepsplasties, or in the rare case of a V-Y advancement, strengthening exercises are restricted to isometrics, and flexion is limited to that achieved intraoperatively.

If wound drainage persists after initiating therapy or continuous passive motion, the knee is once again immediately immobilized. In the majority of cases, drainage will stop after 24 to 48 hours of immobilization. If, however, drainage persists despite immobilization, the patient is returned to the operating room for debridement of the deep knee wound and joint exploration. Closure is then once again performed in layers. Wound healing takes precedence over motion.

RESULTS

Two-stage revision TKA for late or chronic infection is successful in eradicating most infections in 80% to 90% of knees (5–10,12,13,29,33). When considering the treatment of the infection as the endpoint, there is no clear difference in the outcomes whether an articulating spacer or static spacer is used (5,7,10,29). However, the reduced periarticular scarring that is common to articulating spacers makes it easier to expose the knee during the reimplantation. Additionally, knees treated with an intervening articulating spacer block may ultimately have better function after reimplantation than those treated with a static spacer block, although pain scores may be similar (29).

As many as 30% to 55% of recurrent infections involve organisms different from those which grew during the initial debridement and implant removal. Some of these bacteria represent a new infection, whereas others are an expression of a previously present but unrecognized organism in a polymicrobial infection that was inadequately treated (8,9,12). The possibility that a relatively high percentage of recurrent infections may be from polymicrobial infections that were only partially treated should alert us to the practice of taking multiple fluid and tissue cultures at the time of resection arthroplasty and prompt us to consider other methods for determining whether there is ongoing infection before second-stage reimplantation.

The use of antibiotic-loaded cement at the time of reimplantation may be one of the most effective measures to reduce the risk of recurrent infection. It is inconclusive how other factors such as duration of antibiotics, interval to reimplantation, comorbidities, organism virulence, or the use of antibiotic-impregnated spacer blocks affect the reinfection rate (8).

S. aureus or *S. epidermidis* cause the majority of recurrent infections. Although *S. epidermidis* is often considered a low-virulent microorganism, it can be one of the more difficult bacteria to eradicate because of its tenacious glycocalyx, which can confer protection for bacteria from antibiotics and often adhere to retained tissues despite debridement. We recommend that aggressive and occasionally staged debridements be performed in the setting of *S. epidermidis* infection to reduce the risk of recurrent or persistent infection with these bacteria. The concerning spike in the incidence of antibiotic-resistant organisms, such as methicillin-resistant *S. aureus* or *S. epidermidis* has been associated with a recurrent infection rate that may be as high as 24% (13).

SUMMARY

In conclusion, although two-stage revision arthroplasty is the preferred method for treating most late and chronic prosthetic infections, a 10% to 20% recurrent infection rate may be unavoidable in the hands of many surgeons, despite thorough tissue debridement, appropriate and specific parenteral antibiotic therapy, and the use of antibiotic-impregnated cement. Unfortunately the success rate of treating infection may decline further with the rise of methicillin-resistant organisms. It is anticipated that a large number of periprosthetic infection cases over the coming decade will be caused by methicillin-resistant *S. aureus* and methicillin-resistant S. *epidermidis* species.

The treatment goals remain the successful eradication of infection and the restoration of limb function, and this is most likely to be achieved by diagnosing the infection quickly, identifying the infectious organisms, initiating surgical treatment without delay, and ensuring reasonable wound coverage. In the setting of infection, the balance between preservation of bone stock and adequacy of debridement is a challenge that must be addressed individually for each joint. Retaining foci of osteomyelitis is very likely an underappreciated source of recurrent infections. When we are comfortable that the infection has been treated, then it is paramount to follow the critical tenets of revision surgery, including selecting appropriate incisions, protecting the extensor mechanism, ensuring proper axial and rotational implant alignment, restoring the joint line, and monitoring postoperative rehabilitation.

REFERENCES

1. Ip D, Yam SK, Chen CK. Implications of the changing pattern of bacterial infections following total joint replacements. *J Orthop Surg (Hong Kong)* 2005;13:125–130.
2. Mohanty SS, Kay PR. Infection in total joint replacements. Why we screen MRSA when MRSE is the problem? *J Bone Joint Surg Br* 2004;86:266–268.
3. Phillips JE, Crane TP, Noy M, et al. The incidence of deep prosthetic infections in a specialist orthopaedic hospital: a 15-year prospective survey. *J Bone Joint Surg Br* 2006;88:943–948.
4. Deirmengian C, Greenbaum J, Stern J, et al. Open debridement of acute gram-positive infections after total knee arthroplasty. *Clin Orthop* 2003;416:129–134.
5. Fehring TK, Odum S, Calton TF, Mason JB. Articulating versus static spacers in revision total knee arthroplasty for sepsis. The Ranawat Award. *Clin Orthop* 2000;380:9–16.
6. Goldman RT, Scuderi GR, Insall JN. 2-stage reimplantation for infected total knee replacement. *Clin Orthop Relat Res* 1996;118–124.
7. Haddad FS, Masri BA, Campbell D, et al. The PROSTALAC functional spacer in two-stage revision for infected knee replacements. Prosthesis of antibiotic-loaded acrylic cement. *J Bone Joint Surg Br* 2000;82:807–812.
8. Hanssen AD, Rand JA, Osmon DR. Treatment of the infected total knee arthroplasty with insertion of another prosthesis. The effect of antibiotic-impregnated bone cement. *Clin Orthop Relat Res* 1994;44–55.
9. Hirakawa K, Stulberg BN, Wilde AH, et al. Results of 2-stage reimplantation for infected total knee arthroplasty. *J Arthrop* 1998;13:22–28.
10. Hofmann AA, Kane KR, Tkach TK, et al. Treatment of infected total knee arthroplasty using an articulating spacer. *Clin Orthop Relat Res* 1995;45–54.
11. Kilgus DJ, Howe DJ, Strang A. Results of periprosthetic hip and knee infections caused by resistant bacteria. *Clin Orthop Relat Res* 2002;116–124.
12. Lonner JH, Beck TD, Jr, Rees H, et al. Results of two-stage revision of the infected total knee arthroplasty. *Am J Knee Surg* 2001;14:65–67.
13. Mittal Y, Fehring TK, Hanssen A, et al. Two-stage reimplantation for periprosthetic knee infection involving resistant organisms. *J Bone Joint Surg Am* 2007; 89A:1227–1231.
14. Austin MS, Ghanem E, Joshi A, et al. A simple, cost-effective screening protocol to rule out periprosthetic infection. *J Arthrop* 2008;23:65–68.
15. Barrack RL, Aggarwal A, Burnett RS, et al. The fate of the unexpected positive intraoperative cultures after revision total knee arthroplasty. *J Arthrop* 2007;22(suppl):94–99.
16. Parvizi J, Ghanem E, Menashe S, et al. Periprosthetic infection: what are the diagnostic challenges? *J Bone Joint Surg Am* 2006;88(suppl) 4:138–147.
17. Della Valle CJ, Sporer SM, Jacobs JJ, et al. Preoperative testing for sepsis before revision total knee arthroplasty. *J Arthrop* 2007; 22(suppl):90–93.
18. Greidanus NV, Masri BA, Garbuz DS, et al. Use of erythrocyte sedimentation rate and C-reactive protein level to diagnose infection before revision total knee arthroplasty. A prospective evaluation. *J Bone Joint Surg Am* 2007;89A:1409–1416.
19. Niskanen RO, Korkala O, Pammo H. Serum C-reactive protein levels after total hip and knee arthroplasty. *J Bone Joint Surg Br* 1996;78:431–433.
20. Duff GP, Lachiewicz PF, Kelley SS. Aspiration of the knee joint before revision arthroplasty. *Clin Orthop Relat Res* 1996;132–139.
21. Mason JB, Fehring TK, Odum SM, et al. The value of white blood cell counts before revision total knee arthroplasty. *J Arthrop* 2003;18:1038–1043.

22. Trampuz A, Hanssen AD, Osmon DR, et al. Synovial fluid leukocyte count and differential for the diagnosis of prosthetic knee infection. *Am J Med* 2004;117:556–562.
23. Barrack RL, Jennings RW, Wolfe MW, Bertot AJ. The Coventry Award. The value of preoperative aspiration before total knee revision. *Clin Orthop Relat Res* 1997;8–16.
24. Levitsky KA, Hozack WJ, Balderston RA, et al. Evaluation of the painful prosthetic joint. Relative value of bone scan, sedimentation rate, and joint aspiration. *J Arthrop* 1991;6:237–244.
25. Scher DM, Pak K, Lonner JH, et al. The predictive value of indium-111 leukocyte scans in the diagnosis of infected total hip, knee, or resection arthroplasties. *J Arthrop* 2000;15:295–300.
26. Athanasou NA, Pandey R, de Steiger R, et al. Diagnosis of infection by frozen section during revision arthroplasty. *J Bone Joint Surg Br* 1995;77:28–33.
27. Feldman DS, Lonner JH, Desai P, Zuckerman JD. The role of intraoperative frozen sections in revision total joint arthroplasty. *J Bone Joint Surg Am* 1995;77:1807–1813.
28. Lonner JH, Desai P, Dicesare PE, et al. The reliability of analysis of intraoperative frozen sections for identifying active infection during revision hip or knee arthroplasty. *J Bone Joint Surg Am* 1996;78:1553–1558.
29. Freeman MG, Fehring TK, Odum SM, et al. Functional advantage of articulating versus static spacers in 2-stage revision for total knee arthroplasty infection. *J Arthrop* 2007;22:1116–1121.
30. Lonner JH. Identifying ongoing infection after resection arthroplasty and before second-stage reimplantation. *Am J Knee Surg* 2001;14:68–71.
31. Lonner JH, Siliski JM, Della VC, et al. Role of knee aspiration after resection of the infected total knee arthroplasty. *Am J Orthop* 2001;30:305–309.
32. Della Valle CJ, Bogner E, Desai P, et al. Analysis of frozen sections of intraoperative specimens obtained at the time of reoperation after hip or knee resection arthroplasty for the treatment of infection. *J Bone Joint Surg Am* 1999;81:684–689.
33. Haleem AA, Berry DJ, Hanssen AD. Mid-term to long-term followup of two-stage reimplantation for infected total knee arthroplasty. *Clin Orthop* 2004;428:35–39.

23 Rotating Hinge for Revision Total Knee Arthroplasty

Richard E. Jones

M ost patients who require revision total knee arthroplasty (TKA) can be managed adequately with posterior stabilized or varus-valgus constrained prostheses. However, if there is massive loss of bone or substantial compromise of soft tissue support and stability, a rotating hinge prosthesis may be necessary.

Walldius (1) described the initial use of a hinge for TKA, and it was used in primary and occasionally, in revision circumstances. Early hinge designs had unidirectional sagittal plane motion, metal-to-metal articulations, a paucity of sizes, and flat trochlear grooves, resulting in high rates of implant failure and complications (2,3).

Hinged TKA designs evolved, with dual articulations with built-in rotation introduced, when it was recognized that rotation is necessary to preserve some degree of gait kinematics and to ensure reasonable midterm implant survivorship. Newer designs had broad articulation surfaces to decrease deleterious stresses and better distribute load. Also, greater availability of implant sizes and manufacturing techniques produced more reliable clinical outcomes with contemporary rotating hinge TKA (4–6).

INDICATIONS

The goals of revision TKA surgery include bone preservation, restoration of symmetrical soft tissue support, establishment of the joint line, and alignment and balance of the knee. In principle, the extent of implant constraint should be consistent with the clinical situation. This chapter describes the surgical indications and technique for one particular system, the S-ROM rotating hinge (DePuy, Warsaw, IN), when maximum constraint is necessary during revision TKA.

The indications for a rotating hinge knee arthroplasty for revision TKA include (a) loss of the medial and/or lateral collateral ligaments, (b) extensive bone loss of Engh type II (metaphyseal loss with cortical shell intact) or Engh type III (loss of metaphyseal and cortical shell, including collateral insertions), (c) severe flexion-gap imbalance necessitating a linked system, and (d) sagittal instability with non-reconstructible extensor mechanism loss (Table 23-1).

In primary TKA, the rotating hinge option has provided positive outcomes for patients with neuromuscular diseases and conditions (e.g., poliomyelitis) that result in a flail or back-knee deformity from quadriceps weakness. The hinge axle-yoke mechanism of several rotating hinge knee arthroplasty systems provides for 5 degrees of hyperextension with a positive stop. This allows knee stabilization and an acceptable gait pattern for such patients. Patients undergoing TKA for traumatic arthrosis or take-down of a prior arthrodesis may have large flexion gaps at reconstruction, which may require use of a rotating hinge TKA.

TABLE 23-1. Bone and Soft Tissue Defect Classification Implant Selection

		SOFT TISSUE DEFECT →			
		All Intact	PCL Absent	LCL Absent	MCL Absent	All Absent
B O N E	T_1/F_1	Non stabilized, or stabilized	Stabilized insert	Stabilized or VVC	Hinge	Hinge
D E F E C T	T_2/F_2	VVC	VVC	VVC or hinge	Hinge	Hinge
	T_3/F_3	Hinge	Hinge	Hinge	Hinge	Hinge

LCL, lateral collateral ligament; MCL, medial collateral ligament; PCL, posterior cruciate ligament; VVC, varus-valgus constrained (unlinked) implant.

SURGICAL TECHNIQUE

Appropriate preoperative assessment is essential, and good planning is the hallmark of successful surgical outcomes. The use of a hinge is often a backup contingency, because many patients will require less constraint than anticipated at the time of reconstruction. Nonetheless, when ultimate constraint is needed, a rotating hinge is a practical option (Figs. 23-1 and 23-2).

The revision knee is evaluated under anesthesia for alignment, stability, and length. Selection of a skin incision in a knee with multiple previous incisions is dictated by the cutaneous vascular anatomy predominantly coursing from the medial side. Typically, the most lateral incision should be selected and excised upon approach. Thick fasciocutaneous flaps maintain the best blood supply. After arthrotomy, complete debridement of the often-thickened synovial scar removes debris and pathologic tissue and helps mobilize the extensor mechanism for retraction and exposure.

The author's favored approach is midvastus parapatellar arthrotomy, extending 5 to 7 mm distal, along the medial tibia to elevate a continuous sleeve of soft tissue. This allows patella subluxation without eversion, and external tibial rotation and forward subluxation expose the lateral tibial plateau. This exposure precludes the need for rectus snip, tibial tubercle osteotomy, or other quadricepsplasty techniques and is stable upon closure. It has been the author's surgical approach technique in more than 300 consecutive revision TKAs.

The revision TKA sequence begins with establishment of a stable tibial base. Careful removal of the tibial component is best accomplished by interrupting the interface with a small oscillating saw blade (Fig. 23-3). Cement chisels, punches, mallet, and extraction devices can be used to remove the tibial component (Fig. 23-4). Cement, wear debris, and interface tissues are completely excised with a combination of saws, burrs, curettes, and rongeurs. Jet lavage is essential to expose a clean, vascular bone bed.

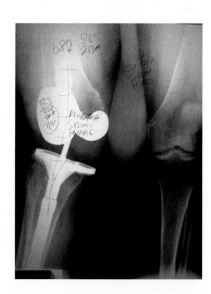

FIGURE 23-1

Preoperative anteroposterior radiograph of a 68-year-old female after revision total knee arthroplasty, with a varus-valgus constrained but unhinged implant with medial collateral deficiency.

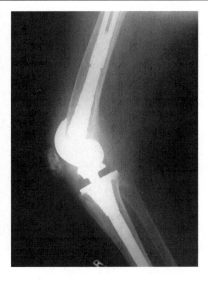

A,B

FIGURE 23-2

(A,B) Postoperative anteroposterior and lateral radiographs 48 months after S-ROM Rotating Hinge revision total knee arthroplasty.

This author prefers an intramedullary mounted instrument system, which requires progressive reaming of the tibia to achieve a cortical diaphyseal fill, anchoring the stem in good bone, followed by use of a tapered metaphyseal sleeve (Figs. 23-5 and 23-6). Larger metaphyseal defects may require the 150-mm stem, rather than the standard 100-mm stem, to provide the most stable construct.

Intramedullary pilot stems sized to the reaming diameter are mounted on metaphyseal sleeve broaches, and the tibial metaphysis is broached. Broach sizes are progressively increased until rotational stability is achieved and metaphyseal filling occurs (Fig. 23-7). Bone is trimmed using the top of the sleeve as a guide, and an appropriately sized tibial base plate is applied (Fig. 23-8). The tibial tray size is selected to maximize tibial coverage without overhanging into the soft tissues (Fig. 23-9). The provisional trial is assembled, with the metaphyseal sleeve size selected to match the final broach size and oriented appropriately to both fill the metaphyseal defect and ensure appropriate tibial tray alignment (Fig. 23-10).

The same combination of small saw blades and instruments will enable femoral component removal and bone preservation (Fig. 23-11). Posterior synovial scar is completely removed. Again, detritus and cement are débrided to expose live bone. The femur is reamed to achieve cortical intramedullary fill (Fig. 23-12). For larger defects, a more stable construct can be achieved with a curved 150-mm stem, which may be preferable to a straight 100-mm stem. For the 150-mm stem,

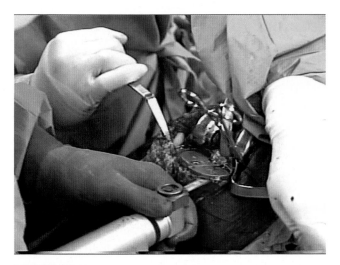

FIGURE 23-3

Small saw blade to interrupt tibial tray-bone interface.

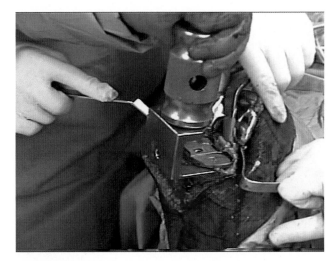

FIGURE 23-4

Removal of tibial component.

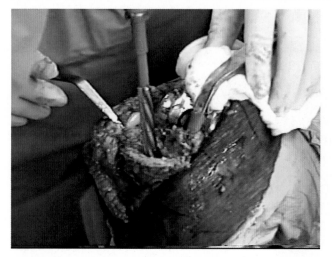

FIGURE 23-5
Ream tibial diaphysis.

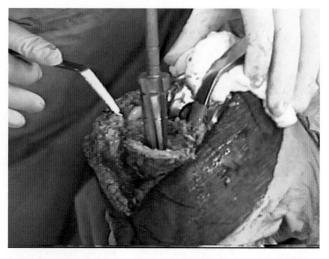

FIGURE 23-6
Twenty-millimeter pilot ream, tibia.

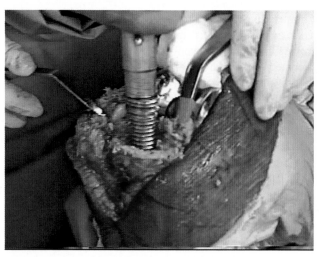

FIGURE 23-7
Broach seating, tibia.

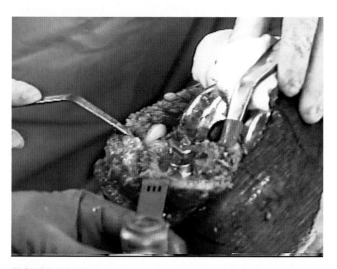

FIGURE 23-8
Trim bone using top of sleeve broach as a guide.

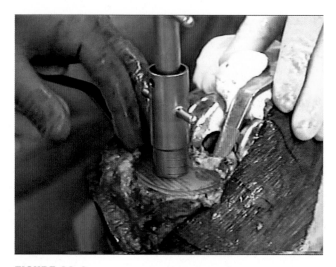

FIGURE 23-9
Size tibial base plate.

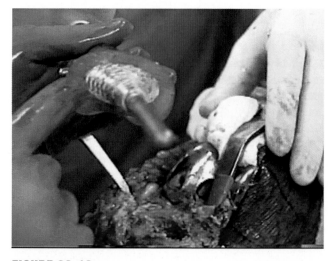

FIGURE 23-10
Rotation set on the tibial base plate and sleeve.

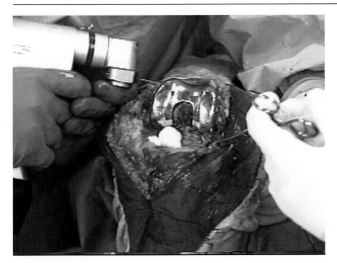

FIGURE 23-11

Small saw blade to interrupt interface femur.

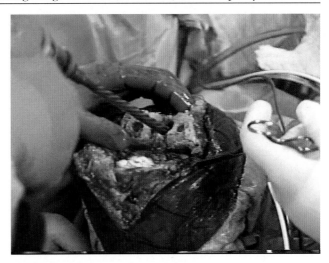

FIGURE 23-12

Ream femoral diaphysis.

flexible intramedullary reaming is performed to 1 to 1.5 mm above the straight ream diameter to accommodate the femur's anterior bow.

Metaphyseal broaches are attached to the appropriate size stem pilot and progressively engaged until rotationally stable (Fig. 23-13). Bone cuts are guided by stem-sleeve aligned intramedullary mounted instruments. Using the guide, distal cuts can be made in 0-, 5-, and 10-mm increments can adjust the joint line and determine the need for augments (Fig. 23-14). Even with a linked articulation, proper joint line position provides better joint kinematics (7). This is approximately 20 to 25 mm from the medial epicondyle. Proper establishment of femoral component rotation is essential. The transepicondylar axis, an effective guide for femoral rotation, is often not available in these complex revisions (Fig. 23-15). The greater trochanter is in line with the lateral epicondyle and can be used as a rotational guide. With the knee tensioned at 90 degrees of flexion, a rectangular flexion gap should be sought, provided the collateral ligaments are intact.

The trial components are assembled and mounted in the bone (Figs. 23-16 and 23-17). The appropriate polyethylene insert is selected to enable achievement of full extension, with an attempt to restore reasonable limb length (Fig. 23-18). With the axle-yolk bolt in place, accurate alignment and sagittal and coronal plane stability should be demonstrated (Fig. 23-19). Flex the knee to 90 degrees with the extensor mechanism subluxed laterally to evaluate flexion stability.

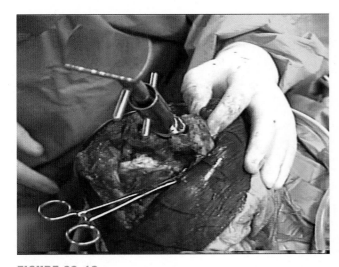

FIGURE 23-13

Seat femoral broach with pilot.

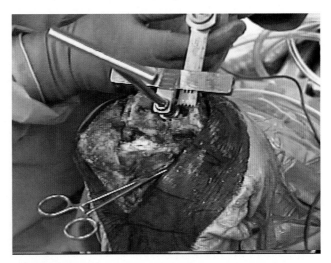

FIGURE 23-14

Distal femur trimmed for 5-mm augment.

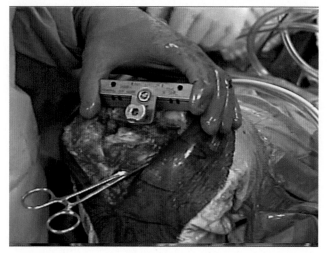

FIGURE 23-15
Set transepicondylar axis for oblique cuts.

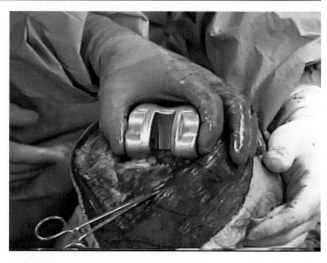

FIGURE 23-16
Seat femoral construct.

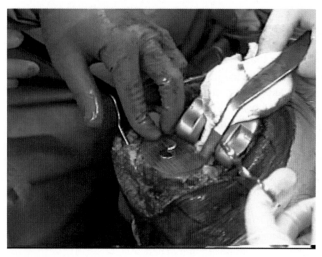

FIGURE 23-17
Seat tibial construct.

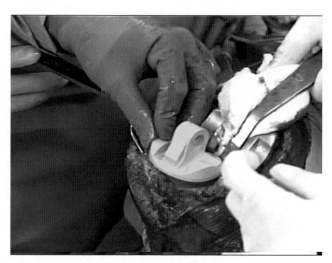

FIGURE 23-18
Poly-bearing dual articulation.

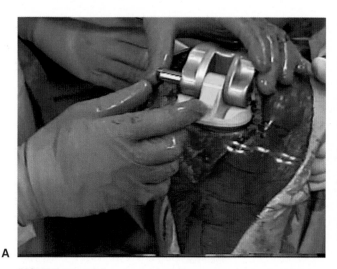

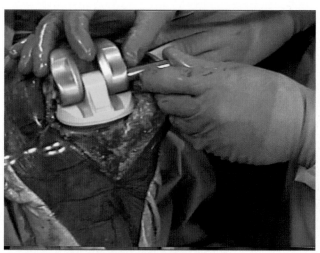

A

B

FIGURE 23-19
Seat bolt connect.

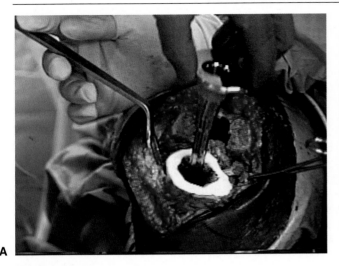

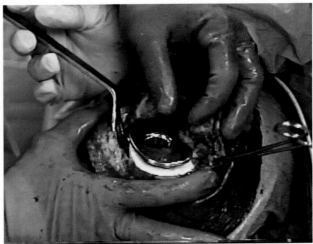

A   B

FIGURE 23-20
Seat tibia, final.

Final assembly of components is accomplished on the back table by matching the positions of the modular trials. Stem-to-implant and metaphyseal sleeve-to-stem fixation is by a secure Morse taper and bolt construct. Particulate auto- or allograft bone can be used to fill metaphyseal defects. The dual articulation of the rotating hinge converts the forces about the knee to compression, encouraging positive bone remodeling. Cement can be used on the undersurfaces of the tibial and femoral components to contain bone graft. Effective fixation comes from the slotted, splined stems matched to the porous coated, stepped sleeves and their fixation with bone (Figs. 23-20 to 23-22) (4,8). Cemented stems and metaphyseal sleeves may be more desirable with some hinged systems, particularly with large metaphyseal defects.

Finally, the extensor mechanism and patella are evaluated. Most contemporary rotating hinges are compatible with patellar components, so preservation is desirable if the polyethylene damage is minimal. Still, release of peripatellar adhesions will help with patellar tracking. Overhanging bone lateral to the polyethylene edge should be excised to assist patellar mobilization. When grossly deformed knees are revised and corrected, the resultant capsular sleeve may fail to close because of contracture. This circumstance may require patella component removal and patelloplasty to decompress the capsular sleeve and to enable secure capsular closure.

After final intraoperative assembly and assessment are completed, capsular closure is performed. The medial proximal tibia area has minimal soft tissue coverage and is prone to subcutaneous hematoma formation. A folded abdominal pad can be placed in the area as a bolster and wrapped with a compressive elastic dressing to prevent fluid collection and enhance healing.

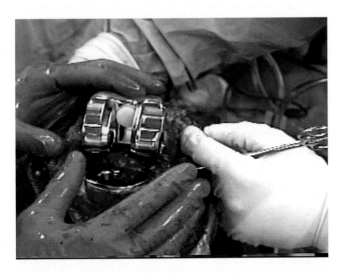

FIGURE 23-21
Seat femur, final.

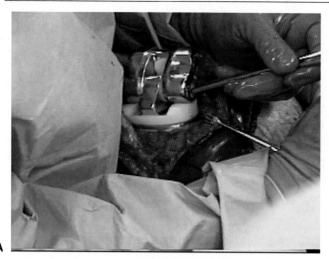
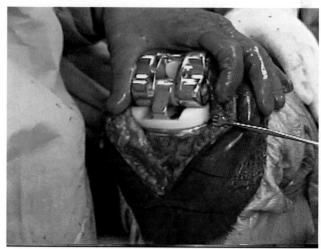

A
B

FIGURE 23-22

Final assembly, axle-yolk mechanism.

POSTOPERATIVE MANAGEMENT

Obtaining and maintaining a stable postoperative wound is paramount. Patients requiring rotating hinges have frequently had multiple interventions, and soft tissue coverage can be tenuous. In such cases, keeping the extremity extended and limiting flexion for 1 to 2 weeks can enhance wound stability and healing. Difficult cutaneous coverage problems should be addressed preoperatively and/or intraoperatively with plastic surgery techniques if flaps are needed.

Some patients with deficient soft tissue support have subluxation or dislocation of the tibial poly post at 90 degrees of flexion. Such patients should have a knee brace with a flexion stop at 75 degrees until soft tissue support is restored (around 3 months). Postoperative weight-bearing status is determined by the security of the intraoperative implant-bone construct. Usually, because of the stem-sleeve-implant stability, the author's patients are full weight bearing in the early recovery phase.

RESULTS

Several recent reports on contemporary rotating hinge TKA systems have shown high complication rates and mixed results in complex revision arthroplasty. Springer et al (9) reported on 69 knees managed with the Kinematic Rotating Hinge (Stryker, Mahwah, NJ). Indications for use of a rotating hinge prosthesis included periprosthetic or acute supracondylar fractures in 27 patients, severe bone loss and/or ligamentous instability in 35, and prior infection in six. Postoperative complications included infection (14.5%), patella dysfunction (13%), and component breakage (10%). Pour et al (10) reported the results in 43 patients who underwent revision TKA with the Kinematic Rotating Hinge (Stryker, Mahwah, NJ) or the Finn rotating hinge (Biomet, Warsaw, IN). Seven knees underwent revision at a mean of 1.7 years for aseptic loosening (four knees), infection (two knees) and periprosthetic fracture (one knee). There were 15 reoperations, including 13 incision and drainage procedures. The prevalence of complications in those two series may reflect the complexity of the patients selected for revision with a hinged TKA or the compromised features of the limb.

Two series reviewed the results with the S-ROM rotating hinge (DePuy, Warsaw, IN) (4,11). One study reported on 65 knees at an average follow-up of 63 months. Statistically significant improvements in Knee Society Clinical scores and range of motion (preoperative, 81 degrees and postoperative, 100 degrees) were reported. There were only three reoperations, two for patella problems and one for recurrent infection. There were no reported mechanical failures (4).

SUMMARY

Modern designs of rotating hinge TKA are necessary when substantial bone or soft tissue defects are encountered during revision TKA. The availability of these implants and reasonable clinical results should encourage surgeons to have increasing confidence in the use of contemporary rotating hinge designs for unique and complex revision situations.

REFERENCES

1. Walldius B. Arthroplasty of the knee using an endoprosthesis: Eight years experience. *ACTA Orthop Scand* 1960;30:137–148.
2. Bargar WL, Cracchiolo A, Amstutz HC. Results with the constrained total knee prosthesis in treating severely disabled patients and patients with failed total knee replacements. *J Bone Joint Surg* 1980;62:504–509.
3. Walker PS, Emerson R, Potter T, et al. The kinematic rotating hinge: biomechanics and clinical application. *Orthop Clin N Am* 1982;13:187–192.
4. Jones RE, Barrack RL, Skedros J. Modular mobile-bearing hinge total knee arthroplasty. *Clin Orthop* 2001;392:306–314.
5. Pradhan NR, Bale L, Kay P. Salvage revision total knee replacement using the endo-model rotating hinge prosthesis. *Knee* 2004;11:469–473.
6. Westrich GH, Mollano AV, Sculco TP, et al. Rotating hinge total knee arthroplasty in severely affected knees. *Clin Orthop* 2000;379:195–208.
7. Hofmann AA, Kurtin SM, Lyons S, et al. Clinical and radiographic analysis of accurate restoration of the joint line in revision total knee arthroplasty. *J Arthroplasty* 2006;21:1154–1162.
8. Jones RE. Mobile bearings in revision total knee arthroplasty. *Inst Course Lect* 2005;54:225–231.
9. Springer BD, Hanssen AD, Sim FH, et al. The kinematic rotating hinge prosthesis for complex knee arthroplasty. *Clin Orthop* 2001;392:283–291.
10. Pour AE, Parvizi J, Slinker N, et al. Rotating hinged total knee replacement: use with caution. *J Bone Joint Surg* 2007;89:1735–1741.
11. Barrack RL. Evolution of the rotating hinge for complex total knee arthroplasty. *Clin Orthop Rel Res* 2001;392:292–299.

ALTERNATIVES TO TOTAL KNEE ARTHROPLASTY

24 Unicompartmental Total Knee Arthroplasty With Conventional Instrumentation

Richard D. Scott

INDICATIONS/CONTRAINDICATIONS

Unicompartmental knee arthroplasty (UKA) is an attractive alternative to proximal tibial osteotomy or tricompartmental arthroplasty in selected osteoarthritic patients with unicompartmental involvement. It should yield a higher initial success rate than osteotomy, with fewer early complications. Additionally, it is a conservative alternative to total knee arthroplasty (TKA) by preserving both cruciate ligaments, the opposite compartment, and the patellofemoral articulation.

Before proceeding with the unicompartmental arthroplasty, a decision has to be made at arthrotomy as to whether the patient is an appropriate candidate. Both cruciate ligaments should be intact, although a deficient anterior cruciate ligament (ACL) is occasionally acceptable if certain criteria are fulfilled. (They include a tibial wear pattern that remains in the anterior two thirds of the tibial plateau. A posterior wear pattern represents an unacceptable ACL deficiency. There should be no evidence of significant medial-lateral tibiofemoral subluxation. Finally, little or no posterior slope should be applied to the tibial resection to discourage a posterior wear pattern from evolving.)

Changes no greater than grade I should be present in the opposite compartment. The patellofemoral compartment can have up to grade III changes, but the presence of eburnated bone is probably a contraindication to the procedure. A significant inflammatory synovitis is a contraindication as is the presence of crystalline disease in the form of gout or pseudogout.

Poor flexion is not an absolute contraindication to unicompartmental arthroplasty (although we prefer a minimum of 90 degrees of flexion), but poor passive extension is, if not correctable to less than 10 to 15 degrees by the procedure. A lax medial collateral ligament (MCL) is a contraindication in the valgus knee with lateral compartment involvement. If this ligament has developed more than 2 mm of laxity, it can stretch even after adequate passive correction of the deformity, causing late failure of the arthroplasty. Varus deformity greater than 10 degrees or valgus deformity greater than 15 degrees are contraindications for UKA unless passively correctable after excision of osteophytes. Finally, morbid obesity is a contraindication as well.

The technique that follows is as generic as possible regarding the implantation of a UKA. Each individual prosthetic design will have its own unique features regarding alignment, cutting jigs, and modes of prosthetic fixation such as lugs or fins.

PREOPERATIVE PLANNING

Preoperative determination of a patient's eligibility for unicompartmental arthroplasty requires confirmation that the pain and arthritis are localized to one of the tibiofemoral compartments, based on the history, physical examination, and radiographs. Pain in another compartment of the knee would discourage unicompartmental arthroplasty and favor an alternative intervention, such as TKA. Radiographs include standing anteroposterior, midflexion posteroanterior, lateral, and sunrise radiographs.

To accomplish a conservative tibia-first preparation, the preoperative anteroposterior (AP) x-rays should be used to plan the level of the resection. A conservative resection line is drawn on the x-ray 90 degrees to the long axis of the tibia (Fig. 24-1). The level of this resection is determined on the lateral side 8 to 10 mm below the joint line. The level of the initial tibial resection should be no lower than this line whether it is for a medial or lateral compartment arthroplasty. For medial compartment

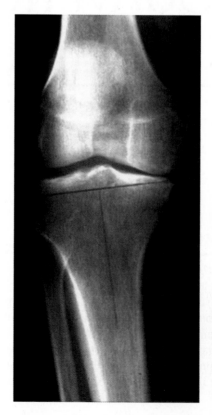
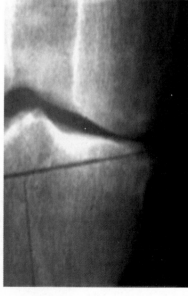

FIGURE 24-1

(A) Preoperative planning involves drawing a conservative resection for a total knee arthroplasty. **(B)** This represents an initial conservative medial resection.

A,B

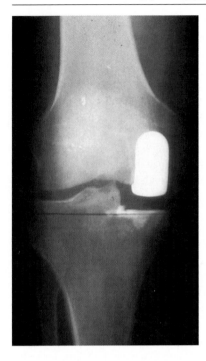

FIGURE 24-2

Postoperative correction can be estimated in degrees by the number of millimeters of plastic added to the tibial resection.

replacement, the resection begins where this line intersects with the most peripheral aspect of the plateau. For most knees, this will be somewhere between 0 and 2 mm of resection. This amount of resection makes sense when one considers that for every millimeter of elevation of the joint line from the periphery of the plateau, 1 degree of correction is obtained. Therefore, if the peripheral resection is 0 and a 7-mm tibial component is used, approximately 7 degrees of correction will be achieved. This would take a typical unicompartmental arthroplasty candidate in 3 degrees of anatomic varus back to 4 degrees of anatomic valgus (Fig. 24-2).

SURGICAL TECHNIQUE

If the prosthetic design and surgical technique remain conservative, bone is preserved in the compartment being resurfaced. My goal is to prepare a unicompartmental replacement in such a way that no augmentation methods will be necessary at the time of any future revision. The only possible deficiency would occur in a medial compartment replacement on the tibial side caused by subsidence of the tibial component. Fortunately, osteolysis compromising bone stock is extremely rare in unicompartmental arthroplasty. The following are my basic principles for unicompartmental arthroplasty.

1. A conservative tibia-first resection
2. Assessment of the resultant extension and flexion gaps
3. Equalization of the gaps
4. Distal femoral resection in the proper alignment and amount
5. Sizing the femur and aligning it relative to the tibia in 90 degrees of flexion
6. Completion of the femoral preparation
7. Sizing, orienting, and completing tibial preparation
8. Confirmation of limb alignment and component orientation with trial implantation of components
9. Implantation of real components

OPERATIVE EXPOSURE

Traditionally, unicompartmental arthroplasty of the medial side was carried out by a standard total knee exposure using a median parapatellar arthrotomy with complete eversion of the patella. Care would be taken not to derange the anterior horn of the lateral meniscus. This exposure gave the surgeon the opportunity to completely explore the knee and make an intra-operative decision as to whether the patient qualified for UKA.

Minimally invasive unicompartmental surgery and exposure is now popular (1). These shorter incisions can allow for a shorter hospital stay and faster recovery. They have several disadvantages, however (2). The limited exposure does not allow a complete assessment of the opposite compartment. It also does not allow a thorough assessment of component orientation, which could lead to malpositioning of components and an increased incidence of both early and late failure of the procedure. There is also concern that the amount of stretching of the skin needed for adequate visualization can lead to an increased incidence of wound healing problems and subsequent infection. I believe that a more rapid recovery associated with minimally invasive unicompartmental arthroplasty is not as much caused by a short incision but rather from the treatment of the quadriceps mechanism. If the patella is subluxed laterally, rather than everted, rapid recovery is possible.

I use a shorter-than-normal skin incision approximately 12 cm in length and begin the arthrotomy approximately 1 cm above the superior pole of the patella. It ends distally at the midportion of the tibial tubercle. Adequate inspection of the joint can usually be accomplished by flexing the knee 30 to 40 degrees and manually subluxing the patella. Digital palpation of the patella allows for the detection of eburnated bone on its surface. A retractor such as a bent Homan is anchored in the intercondylar notch and allows maintenance of the lateral subluxation of the patella during the procedure (Fig. 24-3).

For lateral compartment replacement, many surgeons use a short lateral arthrotomy. My concern with this approach is the fact that a formal lateral parapatellar exposure to the knee would be necessary if the UKA is abandoned for a TKA. My personal preference is to perform a standard median parapatellar approach for a valgus knee requiring lateral compartment replacement. As the arthrotomy approaches the anterior horn of the medial meniscus, the dissection is taken laterally anterior to the coronal ligament to avoid derangement of the medial meniscus (Fig. 24-4). The patella is everted and the knee flexed. Enough fat pad is removed from the anterior aspect of the tibia to expose it for the tibial resection. An incision is made at the midcoronal plane of the lateral plateau just outside the lateral meniscus for placement of a bent Homan retractor. Moist wound towels protect the subcutaneous tissue and the medial compartment throughout the remainder of the procedure.

HELPFUL ELEMENTS OF THE EXPOSURE

Before executing the bony resections, the anatomy should be defined and measures taken to protect the MCL from injury. First, the anterior third of the medial meniscus is removed. This defines an entry point between the deep MCL and the proximal tibial plateau. At this level, the surgeon inserts a curved 1-cm osteotome tangential to the plateau with half of its surface above and the other half below the level of the plateau. It is then tapped with a mallet along the border of the plateau until it reaches the level of the semimembranosus bursa. This creates a pathway for insertion of a retractor that will protect the MCL during tibial preparation.

As noted previously, a bent Homan-type of retractor is placed with its tongue in the intercondylar notch and its blade against the medial border of the patella, subluxing it laterally for adequate

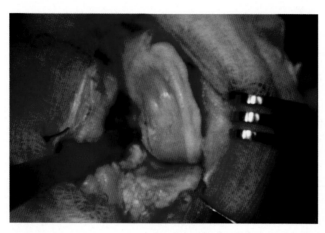

FIGURE 24-3
Excellent exposure is obtained with a short arthrotomy and lateral subluxation of the patella.

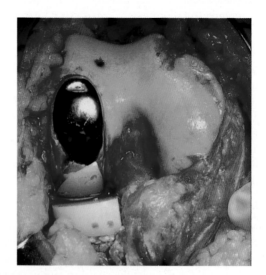

FIGURE 24-4
A medial arthrotomy with preservation of the anterior horn of the medial meniscus provides excellent exposure for a lateral arthroplasty.

exposure of the entire medial femoral condyle. If this exposure is compromised, the arthrotomy can be extended proximally for about a centimeter. Medial and lateral osteophytes are removed to define the true medial-lateral dimension of the condyle. Removal of intercondylar osteophytes relieves any potential impingement between them and the tibial spine and provides a pathway for the resection that will take place along the spine. Removal of medial osteophytes releases the MCL and allows passive correction of the deformity (3).

The chondro-osseous wear pattern on both the femur and tibia is defined with a marking pen or electrocautery. This gives an initial guide to the proper rotatory alignment of the femoral and tibial components (Fig. 24-5). Final rotational alignment of each is confirmed as the bone preparation proceeds.

PREPARATION OF THE TIBIA

Here, I describe the technique for an onlay type of tibial component. The same general principles of preparation apply for an inlay technique.

An external tibial alignment jig is applied with the level of resection based on the preoperative templating for conservative cut (Fig. 24-1). The varus-valgus alignment should be more or less perpendicular to the long axis of the tibia and the amount of initial posterior slope applied between 3 and 5 degrees. The exception to this amount of slope is the rare ACL-deficient knee in which posterior slope is limited to between 0 and 3 degrees.

If the alignment jig is to be stabilized by a fixation pin, I recommend that only one inboard pin should be used. Outboard pins that come close to or infract the medial cortex are associated with postoperative stress fractures as are techniques that call for the application of multiple stabilizing pins (Fig. 24-6) (4). It is important to use a narrow oscillating saw blade for this cut to avoid undercutting the tibial spine or injuring medial soft tissues.

Further protection of the medial tissues is afforded by the placement of a 1.5-cm-wide retractor into the tissue plane created by the curved 1-cm osteotome in the initial exposure (Fig. 24-7). After completion of the horizontal bone cut, a vertical cut is made along the tibial spine with a reciprocating saw that is parallel to the tibial chondro-osseous wear pattern. Removal of the medial femoral osteophyte created a pathway for the saw (Fig. 24-8). The lateral placement of this cut is, in general, halfway up the slope of the medial tibial spine. The resected tibial bone is easier to remove with the knee in extension than in flexion because there is usually cartilage remaining posteriorly on both the femur and the tibia. The resected bone can be grasped with a Kocher clamp while the knee is in flexion and then pulled free when the knee is extended. The resected piece will usually show a wear pattern that is anterior and medial (Fig. 24-9).

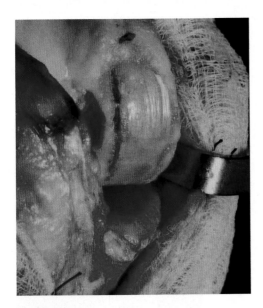

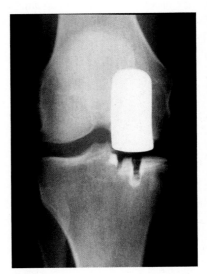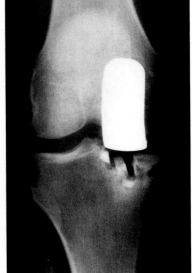

A,B

FIGURE 24-5

The chondro-osseous wear pattern provides a good start for determining the rotational alignment of the components.

FIGURE 24-6

(A) A peripheral pinhole for an alignment jig creates a stress riser.
(B) The result can be a stress fracture through the pinhole.

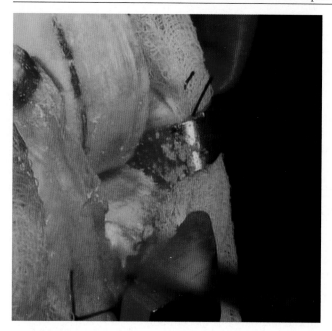

FIGURE 24-7

A well-placed retractor protects the medial collateral ligament from the saw resecting the proximal tibia.

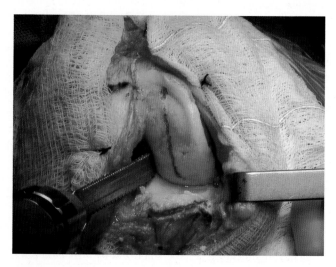

FIGURE 24-8

A reciprocating saw makes the vertical cut on the tibial plateau.

ASSESSMENT OF THE EXTENSION GAP

With the knee now in extension, the thinnest tibial trial is slid into the space created by the tibial resection (Fig. 24-10). If this tibial thickness is correct, the knee should come to full extension, and the anatomic alignment should lie between 2 and 5 degrees of valgus. The knee should be stable to valgus stress. It is permissible for the medial side to spring open 1 or 2 mm with the valgus stress but not remain open this amount when the stress is released. If the alignment is undercorrected or if the medial side is lax, a thicker trial insert is necessary. Alternatively, the distal femoral resection can be less than anatomic to allow tightening of the extension gap. Deciding between these two alternatives depends on the corresponding flexion gap.

For example, if both the extension gap and flexion gap are loose, a thicker tibial insert is appropriate. If the extension gap is loose but the flexion gap is appropriate, diminished distal femoral resection is recommended.

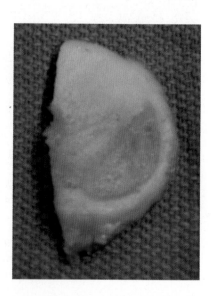

FIGURE 24-9

The typical wear pattern in a varus knee with unicompartmental disease is anterior and medial.

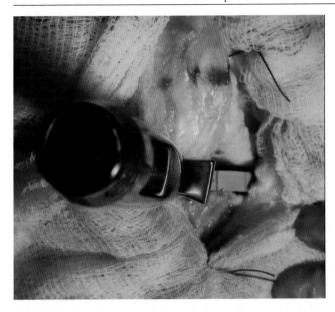

FIGURE 24-10

A trial tibial component is assessed in extension for alignment and stability.

ASSESSMENT OF THE FLEXION GAP

Once the extension gap has been established, the same thickness of tibial component is trialed in flexion. The medial retractor should be relaxed during this test, or it might create a false sense of tightness. Under ideal circumstances, the appropriate trial for extension stability slides in easily under the posterior condyle with the knee flexed 90 degrees (Fig. 24-11). Erring toward the slightly lax side in flexion is better than erring toward the slightly tight side. To relieve flexion tightness for any given tibial thickness, the trial insert is pushed into the flexion space until it engages the posterior condyle (Fig. 24-12). A line is then drawn parallel to the top side of the insert to show the angle and amount of resection that is necessary to increase the flexion space. This resection can be performed with the narrow oscillating saw. It usually amounts to 1 or 2 mm and mainly involves the removal of residual posterior condylar cartilage.

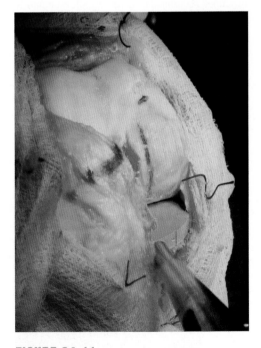

FIGURE 24-11

The same trial is assessed in flexion.

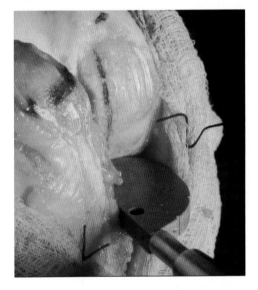

FIGURE 24-12

If the flexion gap is too tight, the trial is pushed up against the posterior condyle to determine the amount of residual cartilage to be removed to equalize the gaps.

If both the flexion and extension spaces are too tight, a little more tibia may be resected, but one must remember to remain as conservative as possible on the tibial side.

If the spacing is fine in flexion but tight in extension, the surgeon can resect a little more than the anatomic amount of distal femur that corresponds with the thickness of the femoral component. If the gap is fine in flexion but loose in extension, the surgeon resects a little bit less than the thickness of femoral component.

DISTAL FEMORAL RESECTION

Distal femoral resection can be guided by intramedullary or extramedullary alignment. The advantage of intramedullary alignment is its accuracy, but the disadvantage is its invasiveness. I prefer an extramedullary technique, which is described here. Regardless of the technique, the goal is to remove an amount of bone equivalent to the thickness of the metal femoral component to attempt to restore the femoral joint line. The ideal angle of resection is probably about 5 degrees of valgus. The forgiveness of varying from this angle depends on the congruency of the femoral-tibial articulation in the coronal plane. For example, a round-on-round articulation forgives any variation. A flat-on-flat articulation demands complete accuracy in the coronal alignment to avoid any edge loading of the articulation. Most articulations are a variation of round on flat with the amount of forgiveness and the amount of contact area dependent on the difference of the radius of curvature between one articulation and the other.

INTRAMEDULLARY FEMORAL ALIGNMENT

With this technique, the medullary canal is entered in a similar way to the technique for TKA. The entry hole is approximately 1 cm above the origin of the posterior cruciate ligament in the intercondylar notch. It is often prejudiced several millimeters to the medial side. In minimally invasive techniques, the intramedullary rod can serve to retract the patella.

EXTRAMEDULLARY DISTAL FEMORAL RESECTION TECHNIQUE

In this technique, the varus-valgus alignment of the femoral component is keyed off its relationship with the previously performed tibial resection. The guide has a rectangular spacer block attached to it that is equivalent to the thickness of the tibial component selected to stabilize the knee in extension. The guide is inserted with the knee somewhere between 5 and 15 degrees of flexion, depending on the amount of posterior slope applied to the tibial resection. Do not hyperextend the knee while pinning the guide because this will impart an extension angle to the resection with resultant extension of the femoral component (Fig. 24-13). Slight flexion can be seen as an advantage because it will enhance metal-to-plastic contact in maximal knee flexion. The guide is pinned to the femur with two fixation pins to create stability. Some surgeons prefer to perform the resection with the

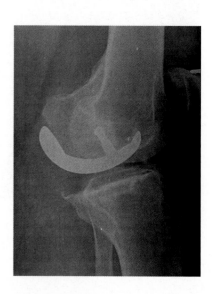

FIGURE 24-13

If the femoral resection is linked to the tibial resection, excessive posterior tibial slope will lead to a hyperextended femoral resection.

knee in extension. A cutting slot in the guide will resect the proper amount of distal condyle to restore the femoral joint line with the femoral component.

An adaptor block can be slid onto the femoral pins to adjust the amount of resection 2 mm proximally or distally depending on the need to either increase or decrease the extension gap.

I prefer to cut the distal femur in flexion to better visualize the progression of the cut. If this technique is chosen in the system I use, the cutting guide that was initially placed in extension must be slid off the pins before the knee is flexed and then slid back into place. Failure to do this may allow the spacer block component of the guide to pry open the knee and possibly avulse the attachment of the ACL.

SIZING OF THE FEMUR

In most unicompartmental arthroplasty systems, any size femur can be articulated with any size tibia. For this reason, they are sized independently. The size is determined by the AP femoral dimension. For medial replacements, I prefer to use the largest possible size that does not protrude anteriorly and permit patellar impingement during flexion. My rationale is that the larger size will better cap the femoral bone providing more surface area for fixation while minimizing the chance for femoral component subsidence or loosening. The anatomic landmark for the leading edge of the femoral component is sometimes obvious as the junction between intact trochlear cartilage and eburnated bone on the distal femoral condyle (Fig. 24-14).

If unclear, this landmark can be determined and confirmed by placing a mark at the estimated spot and then bringing the knee to full extension to confirm that there will be adequate metal-to-plastic contact between the femoral and tibial component with the leg in this position. Virtually all sizing jigs will key off the posterior condyle with the anterior aspect of the guide mimicking the leading edge of actual femoral component.

ROTATIONAL ALIGNMENT OF THE FEMORAL COMPONENT

The patient's chondro-osseous wear pattern will usually suggest the appropriate rotational alignment of the femoral component. Another guide to rotation is to choose an alignment that is perpendicular to the varus-valgus alignment of the tibial component when the knee is flexed to 90 degrees. Choosing this alignment will give maximum congruency between the articulating surfaces in flexion. As in extension, the forgiveness depends on the congruency of the articulating surfaces. As in distal alignment, a flat-on-flat articulation is very unforgiving, whereas a round-on-round articulation is completely forgiving. Most systems are a variation of round on flat with the forgiveness again depending on the difference in radius of curvature between one articulation and the other.

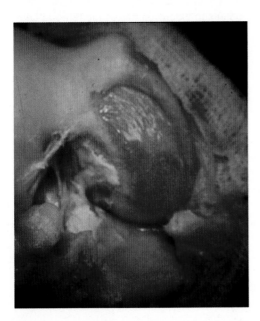

FIGURE 24-14

The leading edge of the femoral component usually extends to the junction between eburnated bone and trochlear cartilage.

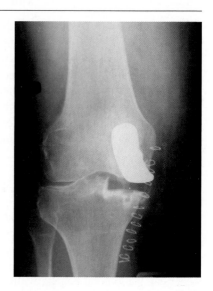

FIGURE 24-15

Internal rotation of the femoral component causes its leading edge to track peripherally.

Another critical aspect of femoral component rotation is its effect on the tracking of the components in full extension. The tibial wear pattern of most varus knees undergoing unicompartmental replacement is anterior and peripheral (9). If the femoral component is placed in internal rotation, its leading edge will ride on the peripheral aspect of the tibial component in extension, possibly promoting premature wear and loosening (Fig. 24-15). For this reason, the surgeon should usually err toward slight external rotation of the femoral component and bring the leading edge of the femur more laterally in extension.

MEDIAL-LATERAL POSITIONING OF THE FEMORAL COMPONENT

As mentioned, the usual wear pattern in early osteoarthritis in the varus knee is anterior and peripheral. To avoid adverse effects on the polyethylene from a return to this wear pattern, the femoral component should be shifted laterally on the condyle (Fig. 24-16). The appropriate amount of shift is determined by checking medial-lateral congruency between the femoral and tibial components in full extension before making any fixation holes or slots.

In lateral compartment arthroplasty, the femoral component should also be shifted laterally for a slightly different reason. The periphery of the lateral plateau extends several millimeters beyond the border of the periphery of the lateral femoral condyle. Most surgeons tend to align the tibial component flush with the peripheral cortex. If this is done in a lateral compartment arthroplasty, there will be medial-lateral incongruency between the components in extension unless the femoral component is shifted laterally (Fig. 24-17). Alternatively, a larger tibial component in the medial-lateral dimension can be used, but in most knees, the shorter AP dimension of the plateau will not accommodate a larger size.

FINAL PREPARATION OF THE FEMUR

Now that the proper size, rotation, and medial-lateral positioning of the femoral component has been determined, the femoral resection can be completed. In most systems, this involves a posterior condylar resection, a posterior chamfer resection, and a partial anterior chamfer resection. In other techniques, a burr is used to prepare a bed for the component, and angle-guided resections are not appropriate. In all cases, a recess must be created for the leading edge of the femoral component to prevent patellar impingement (Fig. 24-18).

This is more critical in a lateral arthroplasty than a medial arthroplasty because of the patella's tendency to track more on the lateral facet during deep flexion. To maximize this recession on the lateral side, the initial distal femoral resection must be adequate enough (Fig. 24-19). Underresection is most likely to occur when there is residual distal femoral cartilage caused by a markedly posterior lateral wear pattern or in an arthroplasty necessitated by a lateral tibial plateau fracture. It is also important

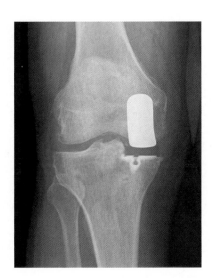

FIGURE 24-16

Erring toward lateral placement of the femoral component improves medial-lateral component congruency.

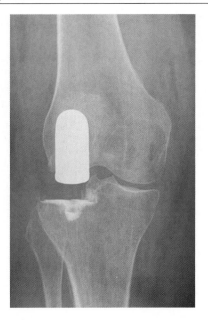

FIGURE 24-17

In a lateral arthroplasty, the femoral component should also be placed laterally for better component congruency.

to err toward undersizing the AP dimension of the femoral component in a lateral arthroplasty to avoid patellar impingement (Fig. 24-20). When undersizing, always check the articulation in full extension to be sure there is adequate metal-to-plastic contact (Fig. 24-21).

The final preparation of the femur involves creating either lug holes or slots for fixation lugs and fins. These are made through instrument templates provided or possibly through holes or slots on a trial component.

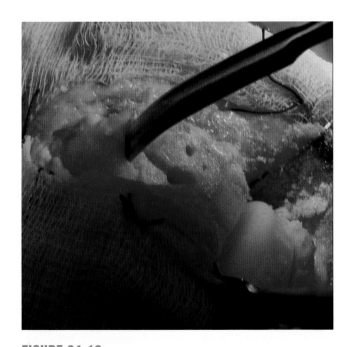

FIGURE 24-18

A recess should be made to countersink the leading edge of the femoral component.

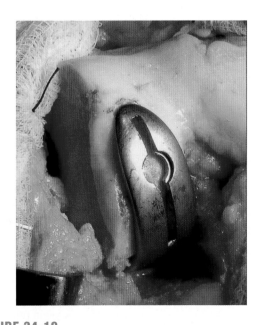

FIGURE 24-19

Failure to remove residual cartilage in a lateral arthroplasty will prevent counter-sinking the leading edge.

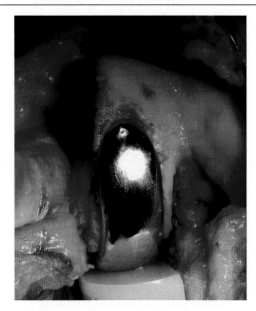

FIGURE 24-20

Undersizing the femoral component in a lateral arthroplasty helps prevent patellar impingement.

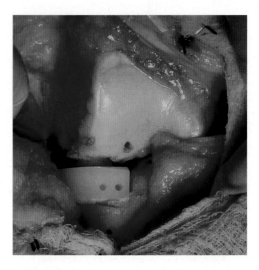

FIGURE 24-21

When undersizing the femur, be sure that there is still adequate metal-to-plastic contact in full extension.

TRIALING OF THE FEMORAL COMPONENT

The trial femur is now slid into place on top of the prepared femoral bed. Some systems provide a shim to pressurize the posterior condyle up against the posterior condylar resection. It is important that a good fit be obtained in this section of the prosthesis to resist forces that may promote femoral component loosening. In some systems, the lug fixation is parallel to the posterior condylar resection so that the component is slid into place without the potential to pressurize the cement. In other systems, femoral lugs are angled so that the posterior condyle is compressed as the component is fully seated. In systems in which the fixation lug is parallel to the posterior condyle, it may be helpful to angle the drill for the lug hole in a slightly anterior direction (Fig. 24-22), which will promote slight flexion of the femoral component and compress the posterior condyle. The drill should never be angled posteriorly because this would drive the femoral component into extension and lift the metallic femoral condyle away from the bone.

Once the femur is fully prepared and the trial is fully seated, it is helpful to take a curved 0.25-inch osteotome and outline the back edge of the metallic condyle to define and eventually remove any retained osteophytes or uncapped posterior condylar bone that may cause impingement on the tibial polyethylene during maximum flexion.

FINAL PREPARATION OF THE TIBIAL COMPONENT

Final sizing of the tibial component can now take place. In most systems, the tibia can be sized independently of the femur. I prefer to use the largest size that does not overhang posteriorly or medially to maximally cap the cut surface of the tibia and decrease focal forces that could promote loosening.

Earlier designs were symmetric so that they could be used on either the medial or lateral compartment in both right and left knees.

Asymmetric components are now the rule to allow maximal capping of the cut surface of the tibia. An asymmetric component also provides more polyethylene anteriorly and peripherally to accommodate the common wear pattern in varus osteoarthritis knees. Final medial-lateral and rotational positioning of the tibial component is determined by a trial reduction. Congruency should be assessed with the knee in full extension (Fig. 24-23). As noted, medial-lateral congruency is altered by medial-lateral placement of the femoral component. Rotational alignment is altered on the tibial side by changing the orientation of the resection along the tibial spine.

If the flexion space is too tight, the tibial component will lift off anteriorly, and/or the femoral component will lift off from the distal femoral condylar resection. This can usually be solved by

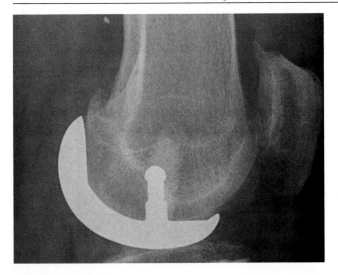

FIGURE 24-22

Angling the drill hole for the fixation lug anteriorly will help pressurize the posterior condyle.

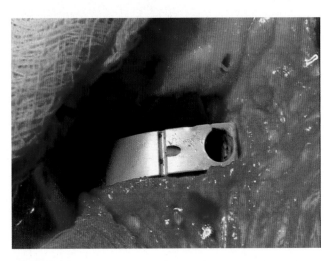

FIGURE 24-23

Make sure there is good component congruency with the trials before making the fixation holes or slots.

applying a little more posterior tibial slope to the tibial resection as long as the surgeon does not exceed a total posterior slope of approximately 10 degrees. Alternatively, tightness in flexion can be resolved by downsizing the femoral component, which will require a little more posterior condylar resection thereby loosening the flexion gap. When doing so, ensure that the smaller component still provides adequate metal-to-plastic contact in full extension. If not, the same size femoral component is shifted anteriorly on the distal femur by resecting more posterior condyle and reorienting the fixation lug(s) to a more anterior location.

TECHNICAL NUANCES IN LATERAL COMPARTMENT ARTHROPLASTY

In my practice, lateral compartment arthroplasties make up only 10% of the UKAs I perform each year. They are technically more difficult and sensitive. It is worth repeating here some technical features of lateral procedures. I believe they are best exposed through a medial arthrotomy that spares the medial meniscus. Other surgeons may prefer a mini-lateral arthrotomy. The distal femur often has residual cartilage that should be removed before the distal femoral resection to avoid underresection that hinders recession of the femoral component's leading edge. This increased distal femoral resection calls for a very conservative initial tibial resection to avoid the need for very thick tibial components. The AP dimension of the femoral component should be undersized to also help avoid patellar impingement. Err toward placing the femoral component laterally and the tibial component medially to maximize congruency between the articulating surfaces.

CEMENTING COMPONENTS

Before actually cementing the real components, they should be tested in the knee as if they are trials because the lugs or fins of the real component may make insertion a little more difficult than that experienced with the lug-free trials. It is better to appreciate and resolve this difficulty before actually committing to the cementing process.

The tibial component is cemented first. Any lug holes or slots are packed under pressure with cement, and little or no cement is placed on the plateau itself (Fig. 24-24). The remaining cement is placed on the undersurface of the real tibial component (Fig. 24-25), which is inserted so that it contacts posteriorly first. This prevents pushing any cement to the back of the knee and allows any extruded cement to come forward as the knee is extended and the anterior aspect of the tibial component seats itself (Fig. 24-26). The femoral component is then cemented using a similar technique. Cement is placed on the distal femoral condyle and pressurized into any lug holes or slots. A thin film of cement is smeared onto the posterior condylar bone for cement intrusion, and the remainder

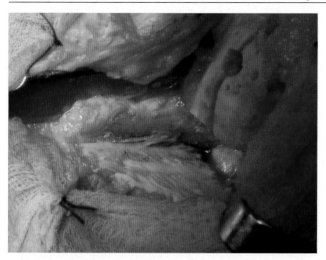

FIGURE 24-24

Put only a thin film of cement on the tibial plateau to prevent posterior cement extrusion.

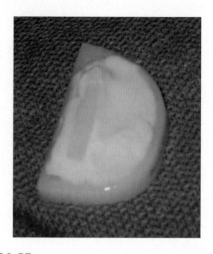

FIGURE 24-25

The remainder of the cement should go on the back of the prosthesis.

of cement is placed on the inside of the femoral component (Fig. 24-27). The knee is slowly extended to pressurize the bone-cement interface (Fig. 24-28). Any extruded cement is brought forward and removed. After terminal extension is achieved, the knee is rested in this position until full polymerization takes place. Flexing and extending the knee during the polymerization process may cause disruption of the prosthesis-cement or bone-cement interface and should be avoided. I leave a little extruded cement anteriorly either on the femur or tibia so it can be tested until it is fully polymerized (the cement will usually harden at a faster rate outside the knee).

After full polymerization, the knee is flexed, and the tourniquet is deflated. Any further extruded cement is removed. I pass an instrument such as a straight pituitary rongeur along the tibial spine to be sure there is no potential impingement between any retained bone or osteophyte. The knee should also be inspected peripherally for any extruded cement that could possibly break off at a later time.

CLOSURE

Two small-caliber drains are inserted and brought out laterally through separate exit points. The wound is closed in layers with monofilament no. 1 PDS sutures (Ethicon, Somerville, NJ) for the capsule, resorbable no. 3–0 sutures for the subcutaneous layer, and interrupted no. 3–0 nylon for the skin.

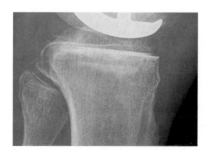

FIGURE 24-26

This x-ray shows good cement penetration into the bone without posterior extrusion.

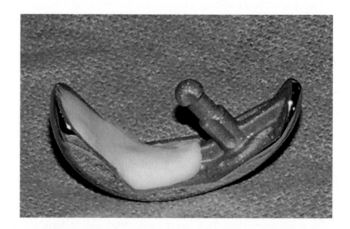

FIGURE 24-27

As recommended on the tibial side, cement is placed on the back of the femoral component to prevent posterior extrusion.

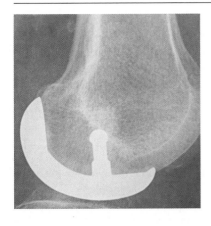

FIGURE 24-28
This femoral component is well seated distally and posteriorly.

Knee flexion against gravity is measured and recorded. The immediate postoperative treatment is the same as TKA except that recovery is often accelerated.

POSTOPERATIVE MANAGEMENT

If tolerated, the continuous passive motion machine is allowed to run continuously throughout the night following surgery, after which it is used at intervals lasting several hours in the morning and once again in the afternoon. Between these intervals, the patient begins quadriceps exercises. Intravenous antibiotics are given at appropriate intervals for a total of 24 hours. Anticoagulation therapy is given for 6 weeks. My preference is warfarin, with a goal of elevating the international normalized ratio to 2.0, in conjunction with bilateral pneumatic compression boots while the patient is hospitalized. At the surgeon's discretion, the patient may be switched to enteric-coated aspirin for 6 weeks upon discharge. Closed-suction knee drainage is monitored, and the drains are removed on the first day after surgery. The dressing is changed on the second day after surgery, and the epidural analgesia is discontinued. Supplementary pain relief can be provided with pills or by injection.

Ambulation begins with a walker, and the patient later graduates to using two crutches. The patient is taught how to perform activities of daily living and to negotiate stairs. Baseline radiographs, including a recumbent AP, lateral, and skyline view are obtained. Discharge plans are made for continued physical therapy at home, a skilled nursing facility, or at a rehabilitation hospital, depending on the patient's individual needs. Recovery following the minimally invasive technique is significantly accelerated, and some surgeons report same-day discharge or just one overnight stay.

The initial postoperative visit occurs 4 to 6 weeks after surgery. At this time, the patient graduates from crutches to a cane outdoors and no support when walking around the house. Permission is now given to drive a car if the right leg was involved (earlier for the left leg). The patient can also begin to ascend stairs with the help of a handrail, using the treated leg and may return to work at a job that can be performed while using a cane. Also at this time, instructions about the use of prophylactic antibiotics during dental and certain medical procedures are reviewed with the patient in the form of a letter.

At 12 weeks, return to full activity is permitted if the patient is ready. Athletic activities such as golf or doubles tennis can be started. The patient is reminded that lifting objects weighing more than 20 pounds (especially from a bent-knee position) should be avoided. Impact forces to the knee, such as those in jumping or jogging, should also be avoided. Single-racquet sports are to be avoided. Downhill skiing is discouraged, but it is not as dangerous as with a bicompartmental replacement because both cruciate ligaments are intact.

COMPLICATIONS

Early Complications

Complications that occur within the first year after surgery are rare. These include inadequate pain relief in approximately 1% or 2% of patients. Deep vein thrombosis may be discovered by venous ultrasound examination in 1% to 5% of patients, and clinically apparent pulmonary embolism occurs in less than 0.5% of cases. The early infection rate in a large series of patients should range from 0.1% to 0.3%. Pes anserinus bursitis is probably the most frequent clinically apparent complication and is noted in 10% of patients in one early series of unicompartmental arthroplasties. In recent series, it has not been reported with as high a frequency. Patients with pes anserinus bursitis present with medial pain just below the joint line, as well as significant local tenderness and possible swelling. The pain is often of a burning nature and occurs at rest as well as with weight bearing. It usually resolves with time, anti-inflammatory medication, or a local steroid injection. The differential diagnosis includes pin-related fracture, insufficiency fracture, osteonecrosis, and loosening, although the latter is an unusual early complication.

Late Complications

Late complications that lead to secondary surgery after unicompartmental arthroplasty occur at the rate of approximately 1% per year of follow-up for the first 10 years after arthroplasty. In the second decade, with earlier prosthetic designs and implantation techniques, late complications have been more frequent. The problems most commonly requiring repeat surgery include loosening or subsidence of one or both components, secondary degeneration of the opposite compartment, wear of the polyethylene articulating surface, or metastatic infection to the joint. The relative incidence of these complications (other than infection) will vary with patient selection, surgical technique, and the prosthetic components that are used. For example, loosening and subsidence are more frequent in heavy, active patients whose deformities have been undercorrected and who have an undersized prosthesis. Secondary degeneration of the opposite compartment is more apt to occur in a heavy, active patient with overcorrection or a previously undiagnosed inflammatory condition such as chondrocalcinosis or a rheumatoid variant. Polyethylene wear is most often seen in metal-backed components with a polyethylene thickness of less than 6 mm and relatively constrained articulating surfaces.

RESULTS

There are several determinants of success after unicompartmental arthroplasty, including patient selection, surgical technique, implant design, and quality of polyethylene. Flaws or imprecision in any of these may compromise the results. In several long-term series assessing both fixed-bearing metal-backed and mobile-bearing implants, 10- to 15-year implant survival was 93% to 96%, with good and excellent results in more than 90% of patients at most recent follow-up (5,6). Mechanisms of failure vary in incidence between studies; however, in general, they include loosening, polyethylene wear, disease progression in the unresurfaced compartment of the knee, and in the case of mobile bearings, bearing dissociation. Contralateral compartment wear is more common with mobile-bearing UKAs, which by nature are put in tighter than fixed- bearing designs to prevent bearing spinout at the peril of overloading the lateral compartment. On the other hand, mechanical wear or loosening may be more common with fixed-bearing UKAs, which tend to be put in looser, thereby avoiding shifting weight to the unresurfaced compartment. Component alignment, body habitus, age, and activity level are also issues that can affect outcomes and should be considered when contemplating, planning, and performing UKA surgery.

REFERENCES

1. Repicci JA, Hartman JF. Minimally invasive unicondylar knee arthroplasty for the treatment of unicompartmental osteoarthritis: an outpatient arthritic bypass procedure. *Orthop Clin North Am* 2004;35:201–216.
2. Scott RD. The mini incision uni: more for less? *Orthopedics* 2004;27:483.
3. Scott RD, Santore RF. Unicondylar unicompartmental knee replacement in osteoarthritis. *J Bone Joint Surg* 1981;63A:536–544.
4. Brumby SA, Carrington R, Zayontz S, et al. Tibial plateau stress fracture: a complication of unicompartmental knee arthroplasty using 4 guide pins. *J Arthrop* 2003;18:809–812.
5. Berger RA, Meneghini RM, Jacobs JJ, et al. Results of unicompartmental arthroplasty at a minimum of 10 years follow-up. *J Bone Joint Surg Am* 2005;87:999–1006.
6. Price AJ, Waite JC, Svard U. Long-term clinical results of the medial Oxford unicompartmental knee arthroplasty. *Clin Orthop* 2005;435:171–180.

25 Robotic Arm-Assisted Unicompartmental Arthroplasty

Jess H. Lonner

INDICATIONS/CONTRAINDICATIONS

Unicompartmental knee arthroplasty (UKA) preserves the articular cartilage, bone, and menisci in the unaffected compartments, as well as the cruciate ligaments, thus preserving proprioception and more normal kinematics in the knee than total knee arthroplasty (TKA). For some, it is a bridging procedure before TKA becomes necessary; therefore, it is important to preserve bone during implantation of the UKA. For other patients, it is the definitive procedure that will last their lifetimes.

The classic indications and contraindications for UKA (1) are equally appropriate when considering use of robotic-arm technology, although expanding indications for UKA, in general, continue to be evaluated (2–5). The classic recommendations are attributed to Kozinn and Scott who advocated restricting UKA to low-demand patients older than age 60 with unicompartmental osteoarthritis or focal osteonecrosis. Additionally, they recommended that patients weigh less than 82 kg (181 lbs), have a minimum 90-degree flexion arc and flexion contracture of less than 5 degrees, an angular deformity not exceeding 10 degrees of varus or 15 degrees of valgus (both of which should be correctable to neutral passively after removal of osteophytes), an intact anterior cruciate ligament (ACL), and no pain or exposed bone in the patellofemoral or opposite tibiofemoral compartment (1).

More recently, the indications for UKA have expanded to include younger and more active patients, without substantial compromise in outcomes or implant survivorship (2–5), making it a legitimate alternative to periarticular osteotomy or TKA in younger patients. Obese patients have been shown to have compromised outcomes, although UKA is a reasonable option for patients who are only mildly obese (6). I would not advocate the procedure in morbidly obese patients. Incompetence of the ACL may cause abnormal knee kinematics, and anterior tibial subluxation will typically result in posterior tibial wear. However, although ACL insufficiency had historically been considered an absolute contraindication to UKA, it is now considered a reasonable option if there is limited functional instability, if the area of femoral contact on the tibia in extension and the tibiofemoral arthritis is anterior (3). Minimizing the tibial slope in the ACL-deficient knee is critical, however, to ensure durability (7).

If subchondral bone loss is significant—caused, for instance, by a large cyst or extensive focal osteonecrosis with structural compromise—then I advise against UKA because this may predispose to component subsidence. Additionally, this procedure should be restricted to patients without inflammatory arthritis and crystalline arthropathy (e.g., gout and chondrocalcinosis), as these ailments can increase the risk of pain and accelerated degeneration of the remaining compartments of the knee. If there are areas with grade IV chondromalacia in the other compartments of the knee, I would not recommend UKA. Lesser stages of chondromalacia are not contraindications to UKA, however, unless the patient complains of pain in those compartments.

There are no specific contraindications to the use of robotic assistance for UKA, although the added duration of surgery early in the learning curve may make robotic assistance undesirable for some patients in whom a briefer anesthetic time is desirable. Anesthetic times are typically approximately 2 hours during the initial few cases with robotic assistance but quickly decrease soon thereafter to approximately 1 hour, as the surgical team becomes more proficient with the setup, preparation, and nuances of the surgical procedure.

RATIONALE FOR ROBOTICS IN UKA

The results of UKA are affected by a variety of factors including the underlying diagnosis, patient selection, prosthesis design, polyethylene quality, and implant alignment and fixation. If we assume that patients are appropriately selected and an implant of sound design with good polyethylene is used, then the accuracy of implantation is likely the most important variable having an impact on whether an implant will perform well and survive as long as expected.

An excessive posterior tibial slope; or tibial component or mechanical axis varus malalignment predisposes the prosthesis to early failure (7–9). Studies have shown that using conventional approaches and instrumentation, it is difficult to consistently accurately align the tibial component in UKA (8,10,11). Outliers beyond 2 degrees of the preoperatively planned alignment may occur in as many as 40% to 60% of cases using conventional methods (11,12). Additionally, the range of component alignment varies considerably, even in the hands of skilled knee surgeons (8). The problem is compounded when using minimally invasive surgical approaches, which is how most contemporary UKAs are likely performed (10,13). One study analyzing the results of 221 consecutive UKAs performed through a minimally invasive surgical approach found a large range of tibial component alignment, with a mean of 6 degrees (SD ± 4) and a range from 18 degrees varus to 6 degrees valgus (10).

Computer navigation was introduced in an effort to reduce the number of outliers and improve the accuracy of UKA. Even with computer navigation, however, the number of outliers (beyond 2 degrees of the preoperatively planned implant position) may approach 15% (11). Robotic guidance was therefore introduced to capitalize on the improvements seen with computer navigation but also to further refine and enhance the accuracy of bone preparation, even with minimally invasive techniques (12).

Finally, the complexity of revision of the failed UKA to TKA, and the results of the revision, partially depend on the extent of bone compromise. When greater bone resection has been performed during the UKA, revision is more challenging, and the need for augments to fill bone defects is greater. With robotic assistance, the intention is not only to make component position more consistent but also to limit bone resection and reduce the thickness of the tibial polyethylene inserts needed to balance the knee.

SYSTEM DESCRIPTION

The Tactile Guidance System (TGS) Robotic Arm (MAKO Surgical Inc., Ft. Lauderdale, FL) is a surgeon-interactive robotic arm that uses preoperative images of the patient's lower extremity to allow accurate preoperative planning, intraoperative navigation, and robotic assistance to prepare bone for implantation of UKA components (Fig. 25-1). The system provides a stereotactic interface that constrains the surgeon in the preparation of the femur and the tibia. Stereotactic boundaries are virtual walls created by the software and implemented through the robotic arm hardware to restrict the cutting tip to within a predefined resection volume.

The TGS technology is an alternative to standard UKA instrumentation with their intra- and extramedullary guides, pinned cutting blocks and jigs, and saws. In their place are burrs of varying sizes, which have reduced inventory and further optimized the application of minimally invasive approaches to UKA without having to squeeze miniaturized, but still bulky, instruments into a small wound (Fig. 25-2). The TGS robotic arm is enabling technology that has improved the accuracy and the performance of UKA through a minimally invasive approach.

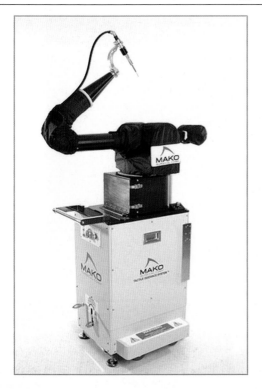

FIGURE 25-1

Tactile Guidance System Robotic Arm (MAKO Surgical Inc., Ft. Lauderdale, FL).

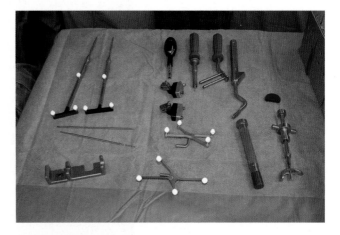

FIGURE 25-2

Display of the array of instruments needed for robotic arm-assisted unicompartmental arthroplasty. Cutting blocks and saws are unnecessary with this system.

PREOPERATIVE PLANNING

The preoperative history and physical examination should demonstrate pain and dysfunction limited to either the medial or lateral tibiofemoral compartments. Additionally, standard radiographs including standing anteroposterior, standing midflexion posteroanterior, lateral, and sunrise views should show localized tibiofemoral arthritis or focal osteonecrosis (Fig. 25-3). Once the patient is considered a candidate for UKA, the preoperative planning becomes focused on the robotic arm and TGS software and technology. A preoperative computed tomography scan is performed of the patient's hip, knee, and ankle to gather the patient-specific data on limb alignment (mechanical axis) and anatomic features so that the operative plan for resection can be developed (Fig. 25-4). The TGS software converts the computed tomography scan data into segmented slices, which creates the patient-specific bone model from which the surgeon can determine the operative plan before surgery. The TGS software allows manipulation and coordination of the collected data to model the limb and accurately plan the implant size, alignment, and corresponding volume and orientation of bone resection (Figs. 25-5 and 25-6).

PROCEDURE

After confirmation of the preoperative plan, anesthesia is administered. I typically prefer to use spinal anesthesia, which provides reasonable pain control for the duration of the surgical procedure but allows early recovery of motor function so that physical therapy may commence on the day of surgery in most patients. The patient is positioned supine on the operating table, and the surgical limb is positioned in a table-mounted leg holder. The limb is sterilely prepped and draped. The robotic arm is then sterilely draped and brought into the surgical field (Fig. 25-7). A 6-mm burr is attached to the "hand" of the robotic arm, also called the *end effector*. An end-effector optical array is used to register the robotic arm tactile-guided system (Fig. 25-8A,B).

Bicortical partially threaded pins are drilled into the proximal tibia and distal femur after making small stab incisions in the skin. The parallel tibial pins are inserted approximately 4 cm inferior to the tibial tubercle, just off the tibial crest (Fig. 25-9). The femoral bicortical pins are inserted

(text continues on p. 332)

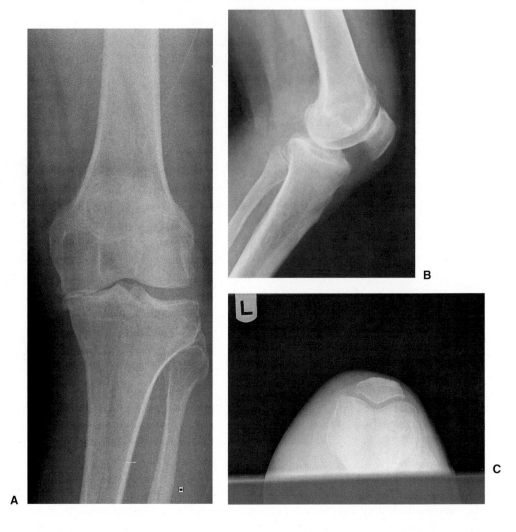

FIGURE 25-3

Standing anteroposterior, lateral, and sunrise radiographs showing advanced medial compartment arthritis.

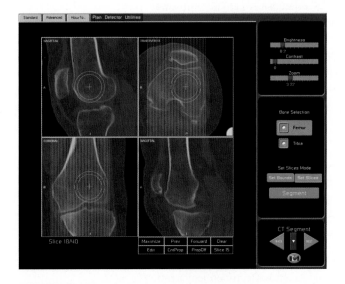

FIGURE 25-4

Preoperative computed tomography scan is input into the computer where TGS software allows segmentation of the images to create a patient-specific bone model.

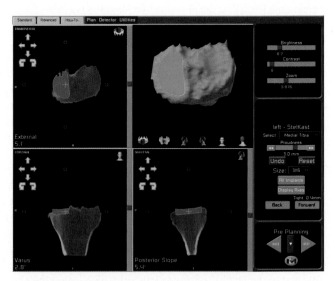

FIGURE 25-5

The tibial component is virtually templated preoperatively, including selection of size, alignment, and position within the proximal tibia.

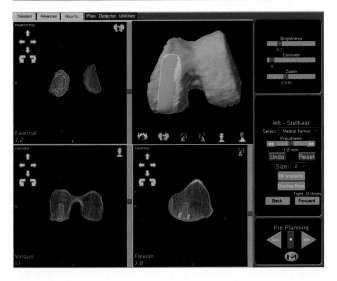

FIGURE 25-6

The femoral component is similarly templated.

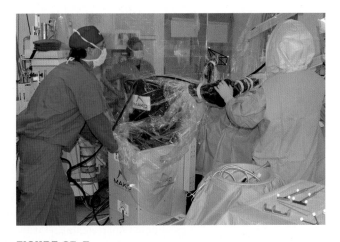

FIGURE 25-7

The robotic arm is sterilely draped and moved next to the operating table and patient.

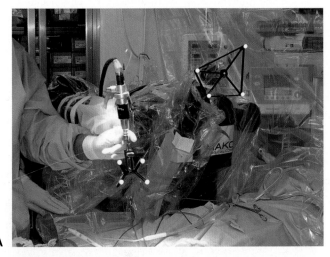

A

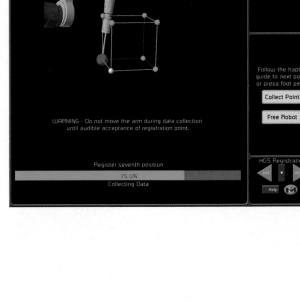

B

FIGURE 25-8

(A,B) The end-effector array registers the robotic arm.

FIGURE 25-9

Parallel bicortical tibial pins are inserted 4 cm inferior to the tibial tubercle.

approximately 4 cm above the patella with the knee hyperflexed to approximately 135 degrees to avoid placing the pins into the suprapatellar pouch, which could cause synovial irritation or synovial sinus tract formation. Optical tracking arrays are clamped to the respective pins, approximately 1 cm above the skin surface (Fig. 25-10). It is then confirmed that the camera can visualize the robotic arrays and the femoral and tibial arrays in all degrees of flexion and extension. The hip center is determined by circumducting the limb until adequate registration is achieved (Fig. 25-11).

For medial compartment arthritis, the knee joint is exposed using a minimally invasive quadriceps-sparing incision that extends along the medial border of the patella to approximately 1 cm below the tibial plateau, with slight modifications depending on the size of the limb and complexity of the case (Fig. 25-12). For tight or well-muscled knees, a secondary capsular incision can be made approximately 1 cm below the vastus medialis through the capsule to enhance exposure, making a "T" in the capsule, or a mini-midvastus or mini-subvastus approach could be used. A partial resection of the infrapatellar fat pad can be performed to enhance exposure of the knee. The medial capsule and deep fibers of the medial collateral ligament (MCL) are elevated from the proximal tibia using a periosteal elevator. A more extensive release is typically neither advocated nor necessary. The medial meniscus is excised. The joint is inspected to ensure that there is isolated unicompartmental arthritis. The integrity of the anterior and posterior cruciate ligaments is also assessed. More extensive arthritis may be more appropriately treated either with a bicompartmental arthroplasty or TKA.

Next, surface landmarks, including the medial and lateral malleoli, medial and lateral epicondyles, and numerous points along the articular cartilage of the knee and periarticular surfaces of the distal femur and proximal tibia, are identified and registered using optical probes (Fig. 25-13A,B). A femoral checkpoint is inserted along the medial femoral condyle just off the condylar surface, and a tibial checkpoint is inserted on the anteromedial tibia approximately 1.5 cm beneath the articular surface. These checkpoints ensure that the registration of the robotic arm relative to the knee remains accurate during the procedure. Their positions are confirmed using blunt optical probes to have an error of less than 1 mm (Figs. 25-14 and 25-15). The TGS integrates the registration points and preoperative computed tomography data.

Once the registration has been completed and the osteophytes tethering the MCL are removed and the deep MCL (meniscotibial ligament) is released, a dynamic soft–tissue-balancing algorithm is

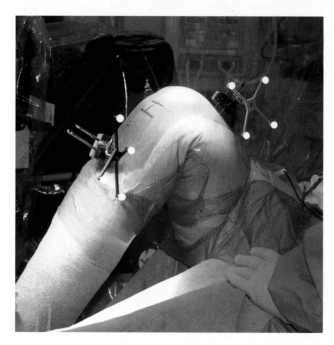

FIGURE 25-10

Optical tracking arrays are mounted on the femoral and tibial pins. The femoral pins are inserted approximately 4 cm proximal to the patella with the knee hyperflexed to avoid insertion through the knee joint.

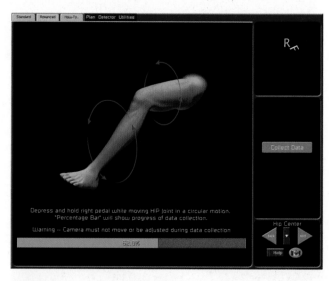

FIGURE 25-11

The hip center is determined by circumducting the limb until adequate registration is achieved.

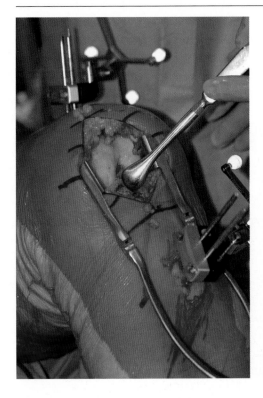

FIGURE 25-12

A quadriceps-sparing approach is often adequate to expose the medial compartment of the knee and allow inspection of the remainder of the joint. A periosteal elevator can be used to elevate the fibers of the meniscotibial ligament.

initiated. The virtual modeling of the patient's knee and intraoperative tracking allows real-time adjustments to obtain correct knee kinematics and soft tissue balancing. With an applied valgus stress to tension the MCL, the three dimensional position of the femur and the tibia are captured throughout a passive range of knee motion. By providing a virtual representation of flexion and extension gap spacing, an assessment can be made of whether the planned position of the femoral and tibial components is appropriate through a full range of motion.

With each planned position of the implants, a visual representation of the tightness or looseness of the knee is displayed at every captured flexion angle. The distance between planned components

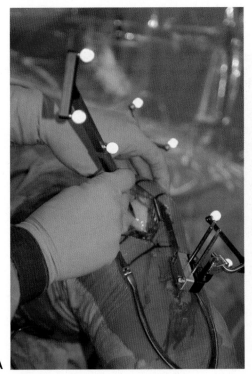

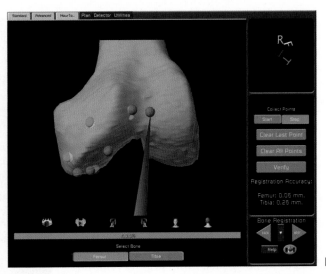

FIGURE 25-13

(A,B) An optical probe is used to identify and register landmarks around the knee.

A

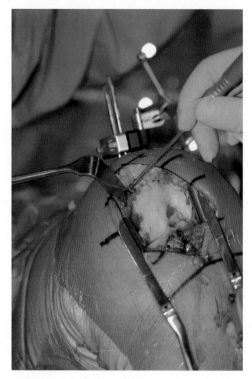

FIGURE 25-14

Femoral and tibial checkpoints in place. An optical probe is in the femoral checkpoint, confirming an accuracy of 0.1 mm.

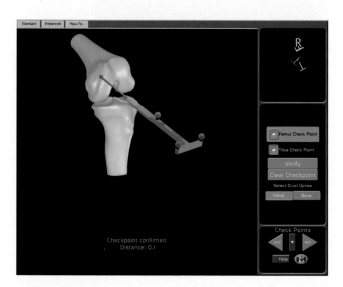

FIGURE 25-15

Femoral and tibial checkpoints in place. An optical probe is in the femoral checkpoint, confirming an accuracy of 0.1 mm.

is displayed on a bar graph at the corresponding flexion angles captured (Fig. 25-16). Each bar represents relative knee tightness or laxity between the femoral and tibial components at a particular degree of knee flexion. By adjusting the implant position, the flexion and extension gaps can be planned a priori to achieve the desired postsurgical values.

When the operative plan is finalized, the end of the robotic arm is equipped with a burr that is used to resect the bone. The robotic arm facilitates controlled bone resection by applying stereotactic

FIGURE 25-16

The bar graph shows relative tightness or laxity of the knee in different degrees of flexion based on where the femoral and tibial components are preoperatively templated. Adjustments can be made to tighten or loosen the knee in different areas by adjusting the virtual position of the components.

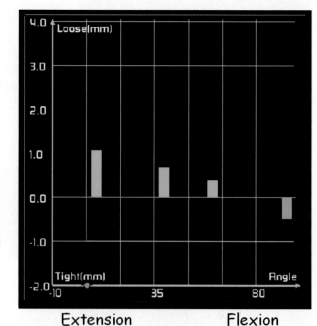

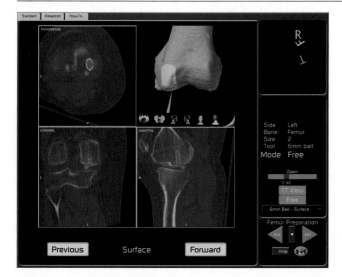

FIGURE 25-17

The 6-mm burr (represented by the round bull's-eye) is being moved on the femoral condyle to confirm that the bone to be removed corresponds to the templated region. On the virtual images, the outer edge of the burr is perfectly flush with the nonarticulating surface of the implant.

boundaries to a cutting burr. If a surgeon attempts to move the cutting burr past the predefined volume in burring mode, the arm applies a force simulating contact with a rigid wall, thereby confining the tip to the correct region in space. While inside the volume of bone to be resected, the robotic arm operates without offering any resistance. Thus, the robotic arm effectively acts as a three-dimensional virtual instrument that precisely executes the preoperative plan.

Before beginning to remove bone, the 6-mm burr can be moved along the femoral condyle or tibial plateau to confirm that the depth, alignment, and volume of resection correspond to the preoperative plan (Fig. 25-17). The femur is addressed first and is resected at varying degrees of flexion and extension to gain access to different parts of the condyle (Fig. 25-18A,B). For preparation of the anterior aspect of the femur, the knee is brought into a relatively greater amount of midextension. Deep flexion helps gain exposure for preparation of the posterior femoral condyle. The bone is removed methodically with the 6-mm burr followed by a 2-mm burr, which is used to prepare the trough for the femoral keel (Fig. 25-19A,B). An optical probe can then be used to confirm that the depth and orientation of resection correspond to the virtual plan (Fig. 25-20) and adjustments can be made as needed.

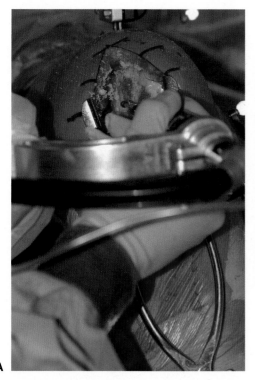

A

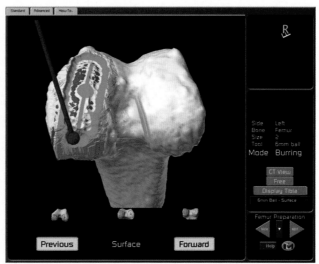

B

FIGURE 25-18

(A,B) Femoral preparation as seen in real life and real-time virtual imaging.

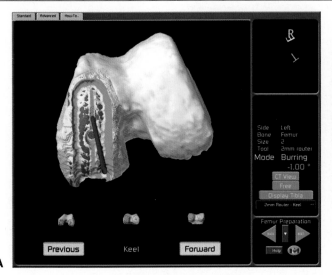
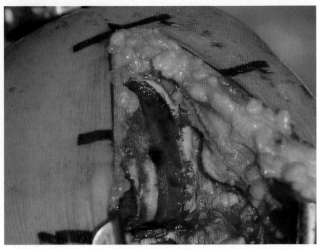

A

B

FIGURE 25-19

(A,B) Virtual real-time image during preparation for the femoral keel. The surface of the distal femur has been adequately prepared with burrs. Notch osteophytes will be removed before implantation of the final components.

Preparation of the proximal tibia is performed in a similar fashion using a 6-mm burr (Fig. 25-21A,B). My preference with this current system is an inlay tibial component, which is oriented with a varus and posterior slope that match the native slope and alignment of the patient's proximal tibia. This ensures that the component is inserted perpendicular to the trabecular bone of the proximal medial tibia and minimizes the amount of bone resection. This type of design requires sufficient subchondral sclerotic bone of the medial tibial plateau to support the inlay component without the direct support of the cortical rim (14). The alternative, an onlay-style component, would be implanted perpendicular to the long axis of the tibia. Once again, after removal of the tibial bone, bone preparation is grossly assessed, and confirmation can be achieved by placing the optical probe at various positions along the floor of the prepared bone bed (Fig. 25-22). An assessment of range of

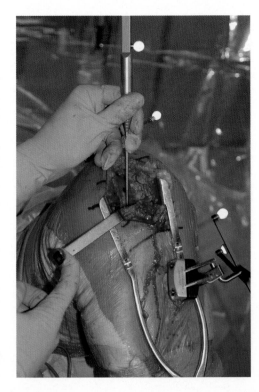

FIGURE 25-20

An optical probe is used to confirm that the depth and orientation of bone preparation match the preoperative plan.

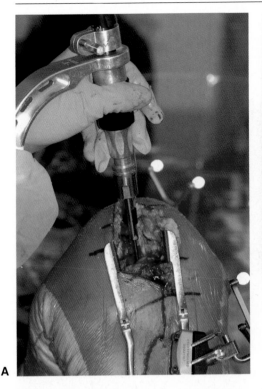

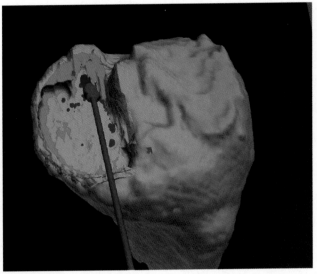

A

B

FIGURE 25-21

(A,B) Tibial preparation.

motion and stability is made after the trial femoral and tibial components are provisionally implanted. Optical probes are used once again to trace the surfaces of the prostheses to ensure that the position matches the preoperative plan (Fig. 25-23A–C). Knee motion, kinematics, and alignment are also assessed.

Once satisfactory alignment and stability are achieved and if no additional adjustments are needed, the bony surfaces are irrigated with pulsatile lavage and dried. Cement is mixed with 500 mg of vancomycin. The components are cemented into place, and extruded cement is removed (Fig. 25-24A–C). Before closure, the soft tissues are injected with a mixture of Duramorph and Marcaine and sprayed with a hemostatic agent to minimize postoperative bleeding (Figs. 25-25 and 25-26).

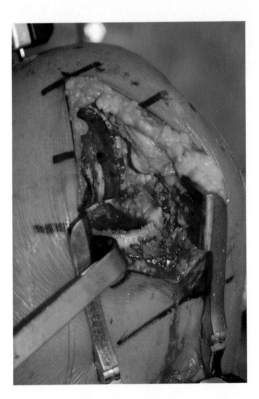

FIGURE 25-22

The distal femoral and proximal tibial bones have been adequately prepared.

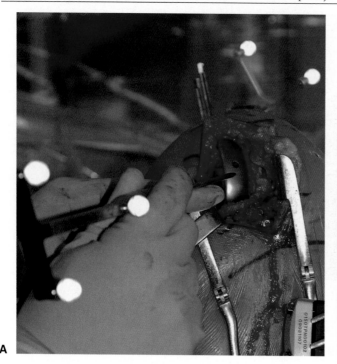

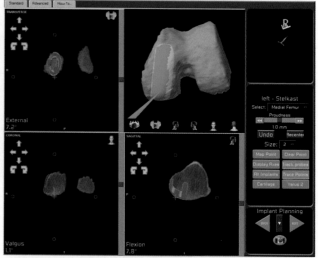

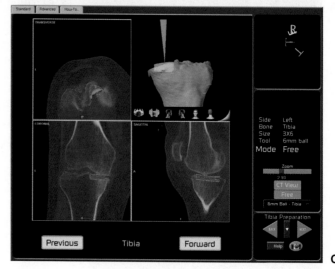

FIGURE 25-23

(A–C) Trialing of the components is performed, and an optical probe is used to trace the articulating surfaces of the femoral and tibial components to ensure that their positions match the preoperative plan. In these images **(B,C)**, the tip of the probe, represented by the cross hairs, is perfectly aligned with the preoperative plan.

POSTOPERATIVE MANAGEMENT

Physical therapy is typically commenced on the day of surgery, once the spinal anesthetic has worn off. Patients are encouraged to ambulate immediately with a cane, crutches, or a walker. Range-of-motion exercises begin immediately, and patients are most often discharged 1 day after surgery. Use of a cane can be terminated once the patient recovers adequate balance and strength. Most patients have been able to ambulate without a cane as soon as 1 to 2 weeks after surgery.

RESULTS

To date, more than 400 TGS robotic arm-assisted UKAs have been performed at several sites throughout the United States, with a registry prospectively tracking the clinical results. The early clinical outcomes of unicompartmental arthroplasties performed with the robotic arm were compared to a matched group performed with conventional instrumentation, both with minimally invasive surgical technique. There were no significant differences in average Knee Society scores or change in Knee Society scores between the two groups at 3-, 6-, or 12-week follow-up. Furthermore, there were no significant differences in the measures that comprise these scores, such as range of

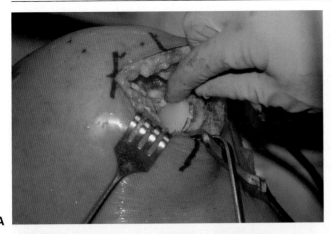

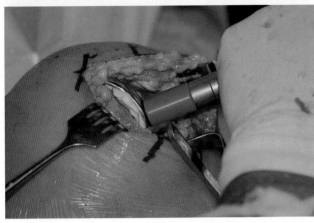

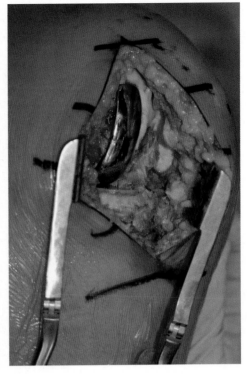

FIGURE 25-24

(A–C) The components are cemented in place, and extruded cement is removed.

motion, pain, and use of assistive devices. These clinical results show no detrimental effects early in the learning curve with this new technology.

The goal of three-dimensional preoperative planning and robotic arm-assisted bone resection is to improve the accuracy of component positioning. A comparison of matched groups undergoing unicompartmental arthroplasties using minimally invasive approaches with either standard manual instrumentation or the robotic arm-guided implantation system, found that the root mean square error of the tibial slope was 2.5 times greater, and the variance was 2.8 times greater with the manual technique than the robotic arm-guided technique. In the coronal plane, the average error was 3.3 degrees

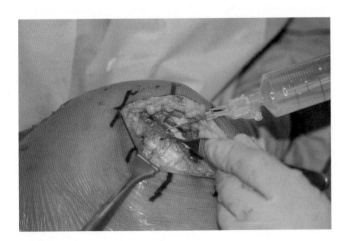

FIGURE 25-25

The soft tissues are injected with a combination of Duramorph and Marcaine.

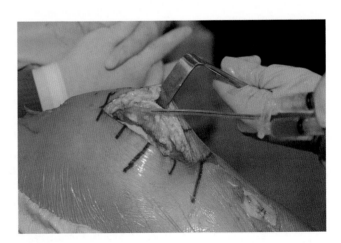

FIGURE 25-26

A hemostatic agent is applied to the soft tissues and exposed bone surfaces.

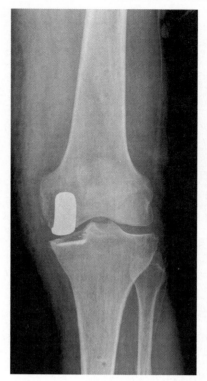 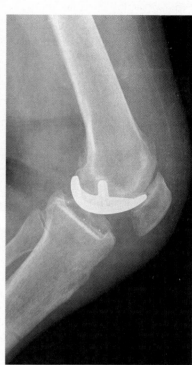

FIGURE 25-27

(A,B) Postoperative anteroposterior and lateral radiographs show a well-aligned implant that corresponds to the preoperative plan.

A,B

using manual instruments compared to 0.1 degree when using robotic arm assistance. Additionally, consistently less bone is removed from the proximal tibia, and thinner polyethylene inserts are used when surgery is performed with TGS compared to conventional instrumentation. These data show that tibial component alignment is significantly more accurate and less variable using robotic guidance compared to manual, jig-based instrumentation through minimally invasive surgical approaches (Fig. 25-27A,B).

COMPLICATIONS

Surgical complications resulting from robotic arm-assisted UKA are identical to those encountered with surgical navigation, in general. The pin sites create a stress riser in the cortical bone, which poses a risk for fracture. The use of bone pins for the optical arrays has not led to bleeding complications in the initial 400 cases; however, inadvertent pin placement could theoretically cause arterial or venous laceration.

Typical complications after UKA, in general, can also occur with robotic arm assistance, including loosening of the prostheses, polyethylene wear, progressive osteoarthritis of the unresurfaced compartments of the knee, infection, stiffness, instability, and thromboembolic complications.

REFERENCES

1. Kozinn SC, Scott RD. Unicondylar knee arthroplasty. *J Bone Joint Surg Am* 1989;71A:145–150.
2. Berend KR, Lombardi AV Jr, Adams JB. Obesity, young age, patellofemoral disease, and anterior knee pain: identifying the unicondylar arthroplasty patient in the United States. *Orthopedics* 2007;30(5 Suppl):19–23.
3. Borus T, Thornhill T. Unicompartmental knee arthroplasty. *J Am Acad Orthop Surg* 2007;15:9–18.
4. Pennington DW, Swienckowski JJ, Lutes WB, et al. Unicompartmental knee arthroplasty in patients sixty years of age or younger. *J Bone Joint Surg Am* 2003;85A:1968–1973.
5. Schai PA, Suh JT, Thornhill TS, Scott RD. Unicompartmental knee arthroplasty in middle aged patients: a two to six year follow-up evaluation. *J Arthrop* 1998;13:365–372.
6. Berend KR, Lombardi AV Jr, Mallory TH, et al. Early failure of minimally invasive unicompartmental knee arthroplasty is associated with obesity. *Clin Orthop* 2005;435:171–180.
7. Hernigou P, Deschamps G. Posterior slope of the tibial implant and the outcome of unicompartmental knee arthroplasty. *J Bone Joint Surg Am* 2004;86A:506–511.
8. Collier MB, Eickmann TH, Sukezaki F, et al. Patient, implant, and alignment factors associated with revision of medial compartment unicondylar arthroplasty. *J Arthrop* 2006;21(Suppl):108–115.

9. Hernigou P, Deschamps G. Alignment influences wear in the knee after medial unicompartmental arthroplasty. *Clin Orthop* 2004;423:161–165.
10. Hamilton WG, Collier MB, Tarabee E, et al. Incidence and reasons for reoperation after minimally invasive unicompartmental knee arthroplasty. *J Arthrop* 2006;21(Suppl):98–107.
11. Keene G, Simpson D, Kalairajah Y. Limb alignment in computer-assisted minimally-invasive unicompartmental knee replacement. *J Bone Joint Surg Br* 2006;88B:44–48.
12. Cobb J, Henckel J, Gomes P, et al. Hands-on robotic unicompartmental knee replacement. *J Bone Joint Surg Br* 2006;88B:188–197.
13. Fisher DA, Watts M, Davis KE. Implant position in knee surgery: a comparison of minimally invasive, open unicompartmental, and total knee arthroplasty. *J Arthrop* 2003;18(Suppl):2–8.
14. Romanowski MR, Repicci JA. Minimally invasive unicondylar arthroplasty: eight-year follow-up. *J Knee Surg* 2002;15:17–22.

26 Patellofemoral Arthroplasty

Jess H. Lonner

Epidemiological studies show that isolated patellofemoral arthritis may occur in as many as 9% of patients over the age of 40 and in 15% of patients 60 and older (1). Women who present with symptomatic knee arthritis are more likely than men to have the degeneration localized to the patellofemoral compartment. In patients over the age of 55, arthritis may be restricted to the patellofemoral compartment in 24% of women compared to 11% of men (2). These patients frequently seek orthopedic treatment.

Many cases of patellofemoral arthritis are typically treated adequately with measures such as activity modification, physical therapy, oral medications, and injections. However, patellofemoral arthroplasty (PFA) may be beneficial when nonoperative interventions are ineffective. Other surgical alternatives to PFA have had inconsistent success managing patellofemoral arthritis. Arthroscopic lavage and debridement, with or without marrow stimulation, has had satisfactory short-term results in only approximately 40% to 60% of patients (3). "Biologic" approaches for isolated patellofemoral arthritis, including autologous chondrocyte implantation and fresh osteochondral allografting, as well as tibial tubercle unloading procedures (direct anteriorization and anteromedialization) have had 25% to 30% unsatisfactory results at short-term follow-up (4–7). Patellectomy reduces knee extension power, and tibiofemoral joint reaction forces have been shown to increase as much as 250% after patellectomy, which increases the risk for the development of tibiofemoral arthritis (8). Variable pain relief, substantial residual quadriceps weakness, secondary instability, an early failure rate as high as 45% after patellectomy, and a tendency for relatively poor outcomes after total knee arthroplasty (TKA) in patients who had previously undergone patellectomy (9,10), have led to the abandonment of the procedure except perhaps in very unusual circumstances. TKA is an effective treatment option for elderly patients with isolated patellofemoral arthritis; however, it may not be desirable for all patients (11). In many patients with isolated patellofemoral arthritis and no tibiofemoral disease, I prefer to perform PFA because of its conservative nature, kinematic preservation, quick recovery, and clinical success.

INDICATIONS/CONTRAINDICATIONS

The success of PFA is, in part, contingent on appropriate patient selection. After a reasonable attempt at nonoperative measures, the procedure can be considered for patients with isolated patellofemoral osteoarthritis, posttraumatic arthritis, or advanced chondromalacia (Outerbridge grade IV) on either or both the trochlear and patellar surfaces. PFA is very effective in the presence of patellar or trochlear dysplasia (12,13), although some implant designs are more appropriate in the setting of dysplasia than others (14,15). Slight patellar tilt or subluxation observed on preoperative tangential radiographs or intraoperatively (with a normal Q angle) can usually be addressed effectively with a lateral retinacular release, medialization of the patellar component, and resection of the lateral patellar facet.

In the past, my personal preference was to restrict PFA to patients younger than 55 or 60 (12,14). Subsequently, however, I have treated a number of patients between the ages of 60 and 85, and the results of PFA have been excellent in that cohort. Additionally, there are no published data showing that the results differ in younger and older patients.

PFA is contraindicated in patients with considerable medial and lateral joint line pain. Any evidence of tibiofemoral arthritis or advanced chondromalacia is a contraindication to the use of isolated PFA, although combining PFA with chondral resurfacing for focal defects of the weight-bearing condylar surfaces or with unicompartmental arthroplasty for more advanced tibiofemoral arthrosis are emerging strategies (12,16). It is not appropriate for patients with inflammatory arthritis or those with chondrocalcinosis of the menisci or weight-bearing surfaces of the tibiofemoral compartments. I would also avoid this in patients who have severe coronal deformity unless corrected, because it may negatively affect patellar tracking and predispose to early development of tibiofemoral arthritis. The patellofemoral prosthesis cannot be expected to stabilize a highly malaligned patellofemoral articulation; therefore, the presence of a very high Q angle is a relative contraindication to PFA unless a tibial tubercle anteromedialization is performed before or simultaneous with PFA. Patients with inappropriate expectations regarding the extent of pain relief, duration of recovery, and allowable activities after they have recovered from PFA may not be suitable candidates for the procedure (12).

It is unknown at this time whether obesity or cruciate ligament insufficiency have deleterious effects on the outcomes of PFA. Intuitively, the former condition may predispose to implant wear or loosening, and both conditions may predispose to early tibiofemoral arthritis. I have successfully performed PFA in mildly obese patients but not morbidly obese patients, particularly because in my experience, morbidly obese patients often tend to have tibiofemoral pain in addition to patellofemoral pain, even when radiographically, the preponderance of arthritis affects the patellofemoral compartment.

PREOPERATIVE PLANNING

It is necessary to ensure that the pain and arthritis are, in fact, localized to the patellofemoral compartment, which can be done primarily by taking a thorough history and performing a meticulous physical examination. Patients will typically report anterior knee pain and crepitus (often retropatellar and medial and lateral peripatellar), which is exacerbated when sitting with the knee flexed, standing from a seated position, walking up and down hills and stairs, and squatting. There is typically much less or even no pain when walking on level ground. A key detail of the patient's history should include whether there was previous trauma to the knee, a history of patellar dislocation, or prior patellofemoral problems. A history of recurrent atraumatic patellar dislocations may suggest considerable malalignment, which may need to be corrected before PFA.

On physical examination, there is pain on patella inhibition testing, patellofemoral crepitus, and retropatellar knee pain with squatting. Any medial or lateral tibiofemoral joint line tenderness raises my suspicion of more diffuse chondral disease (even in the presence of relatively normal radiographs), and I consider this a contraindication to PFA except in circumstances when the pain appears to be referred from the arthritic patellofemoral surfaces. Other potential sources of anterior knee pain, such as pes anserinus bursitis, patellar tendonitis, and prepatellar bursitis, or pain referred from the ipsilateral hip or back, should be excluded.

Generally, weight-bearing radiographs are ample imaging studies to aid in the diagnostic evaluation and subsequent surgical planning (Fig. 26-1A–D). Standing anteroposterior (AP) and midflexion posteroanterior radiographs will not allow visualization of the patellofemoral compartment of the knee, but they help establish the presence or absence of tibiofemoral arthritis. The standing midflexion posteroanterior view is particularly useful in showing whether there is posterior condylar wear, especially in patients who may have occasional tibiofemoral pain. Axial and lateral radiographs will demonstrate the presence of patellofemoral arthritis, whether there is patella alta or baja, and whether there is patella tilt or subluxation. Occasionally, the axial radiograph will underestimate the extent of patellofemoral arthritis if the full-thickness cartilage defects are shouldered by relatively intact cartilage on both the trochlear and patellar surfaces in the angle at which the radiograph is taken. Occasionally, subchondral sclerosis and facet "flattening" may be the only radiographic clues that there is patellofemoral arthritis. Computed tomography scan and magnetic resonance imaging are not typically necessary. Occasionally, patients have had prior arthroscopic intervention, and photographs and surgical reports from these procedures provide important information regarding the extent of patellofemoral arthritis and the status of the tibiofemoral compartments.

Assessment of patellar tracking and the Q angle is also important. It is my opinion that an excessive Q angle (more than 20 degrees in women and 15 degrees in men) needs to be corrected either

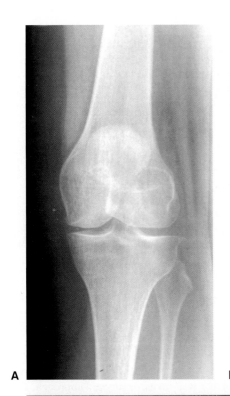

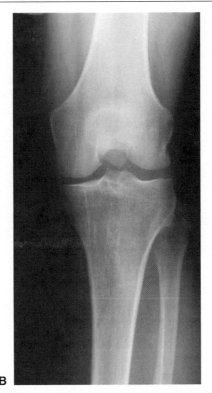

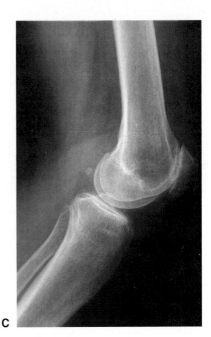

A   B   C

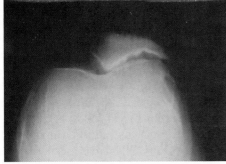

D

FIGURE 26-1

(A–D) Standing anteroposterior, midflexion posteroanterior, lateral, and sunrise radiographs of the left knee show isolated patellofemoral arthritis.

before or simultaneous with PFA. If the choice is made to correct the Q angle with a tibial tubercle anteromedialization at the time of PFA, provisions need to be made beforehand to have an appropriate set of drills and screws available for tubercle fixation, as well as fluoroscopic imaging.

If a small area of full-thickness chondromalacia is found on the weight-bearing surfaces of the femoral condyles during PFA, autologous osteochondral grafting can be performed, harvesting an osteochondral plug from either a relatively unaffected area of the trochlea that is being removed for the trochlear implant or from the edge of the intercondylar notch (16). Therefore, a cylindrical osteochondral plug harvesting system should be available during the procedure, and the surgical consent form should reflect the possibility of this additional procedure. Additionally, occasionally patients are advised that an intraoperative decision may be made to combine the PFA with a unicompartmental arthroplasty or to perform a TKA instead. These alternatives are appropriate if there is more extensive medial and/or lateral arthritis than anticipated (although typically this would be predictable beforehand, based on the physical examination and radiographs). In cases when these additional or alternative procedures may be necessary, the surgical consent should reflect these possibilities, and additional implant systems and sets should be ordered in advance.

SURGICAL TECHNIQUE

The knee is approached through a midline or anteromedial skin incision and a medial arthrotomy (Fig. 26-2A,B). My preference is a minimally invasive approach, although I recommend that early in a surgeon's experience, the skin incision should be a traditional extensile length incision with a

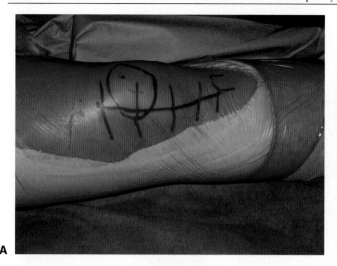
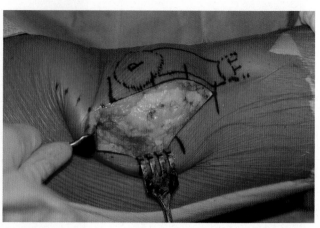

FIGURE 26-2

(A) An anteromedial incision is made from 1 to 2 cm proximal to the proximal medial edge of the patella to 1 to 2 cm proximal to the tibial tubercle. **(B)** The fascia over the vastus medialis is exposed for a midvastus incision.

standard arthrotomy to achieve ample exposure and become familiar with the nuances of the surgical technique and instrumentation without being distracted by a less-invasive surgical approach. The skin incision I use typically extends from 1 to 2 cm above the tibial tubercle to 1 to 2 cm proximal to the patella, but it can be extended liberally depending on the challenge of the procedure and appearance of the proximal and distal skin edges. I typically use either a mini-midvastus or mini-subvastus arthrotomy (Fig. 26-3A,B). The infrapatellar fat pad can be partially excised to facilitate exposure, while taking care to avoid cutting normal articular cartilage, menisci, or the intermeniscal ligament at the time of arthrotomy (Fig. 26-4). Before proceeding with PFA, carefully inspect the entire joint to make sure that the arthritis is restricted to the patellofemoral compartment and the tibiofemoral compartments are free of disease (Figs. 26-5 and 26-6; see Figs. 26-13 and 26-28). If a minimally invasive approach is used, a "mobile window" concept is utilized, adjusting retraction on the soft tissues to visualize separately either the medial or lateral compartments. With broader exposure, visualization of all compartments of the knee is achievable at once. Release of the lateral patellofemoral synovial ligaments facilitates patellar eversion, if the surgeon prefers to do so, and it removes a

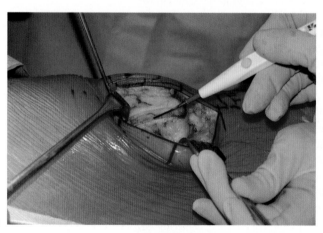
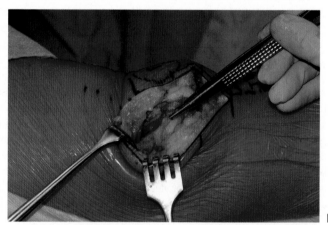

FIGURE 26-3

(A) The capsular aspect of the arthrotomy is made, taking care not to inadvertently cut the articular cartilage, menisci, or transverse intermeniscal ligament during arthrotomy. **(B)** The vastus medialis muscle is split 2 to 3 cm in length, in line with its fibers from the proximal medial edge of the patella.

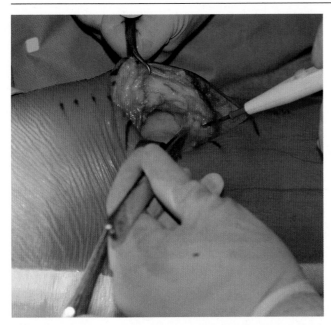

FIGURE 26-4

The infrapatellar fat pad can be partially excised to facilitate exposure, but the incision should not incise the menisci or transverse intermeniscal ligament. The extent of arthritis is assessed.

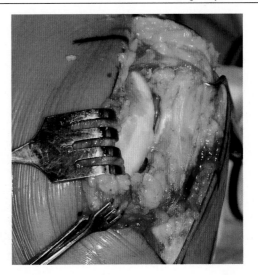

FIGURE 26-5

The mobile window strategy can be used to assess the tibiofemoral articular surfaces if a minimally invasive approach is used. Here, the medial femoral condyle is noted to be intact. Alternatively, if a slightly more extensile arthrotomy is used, broad visualization of both condyles simultaneously is possible (see Fig. 26-8).

potential lateral tether on the patella. This is not a lateral retinacular release, although it may also help to optimize patellar tracking (Fig. 26-7).

If a femoral condylar defect is noted in addition to the patellofemoral arthritis, an osteochondral plug can be harvested from a relatively healthy area of the trochlear surface or from around the intercondylar notch. The size of the condylar lesion is determined, and it is removed with a cylindrical coring system. A second cylindrical harvester with a diameter measuring approximately 1 mm larger than the defect is used to harvest the donor osteochondral plug, which is then implanted into the recipient site, leaving it flush with the surrounding articular cartilage (Figs. 26-8 to 26-11).

The proximal extent of the trochlea is demarcated using electrocautery, anterior synovial tissue excised from the area on which the trochlear component will be implanted, and osteophytes removed from the intercondylar notch (Fig. 26-12). One of the more critical components of the procedure is ensuring that the trochlear component is externally rotated perpendicular to the AP axis (Whiteside's line) of the distal femur. The AP axis is a line drawn from the low point of the anterior surface of the trochlear groove to the highest point of the intercondylar notch (Fig. 26-13). If the trochlear surface

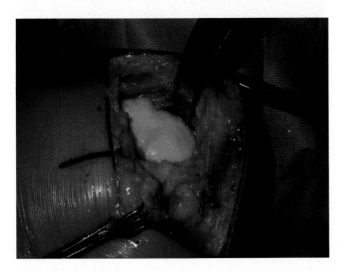

FIGURE 26-6

The mobile window has been moved laterally showing healthy articular cartilage on the lateral femoral condyle.

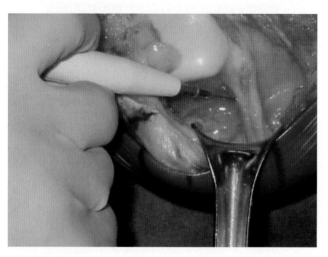

FIGURE 26-7

With the knee in extension, release of the lateral patellofemoral synovial ligament may help mobilize the patella during exposure and releases a potential lateral tether that may affect patellar tracking. This is not a lateral retinacular release, which may be necessary in some cases.

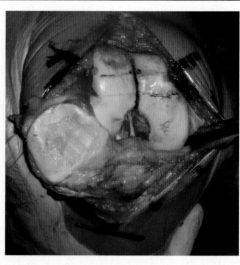

FIGURE 26-8

A knee with advanced patellofemoral arthritis and a 10-mm × 7-mm focal full-thickness chondral defect on the medial femoral condyle. Despite the small size of the condylar defect, it was considered amenable to autologous osteochondral grafting.

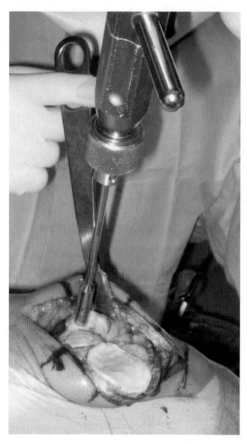

FIGURE 26-9

An osteochondral donor plug is harvested from a healthy surface of the trochlea that has no apparent arthritis.

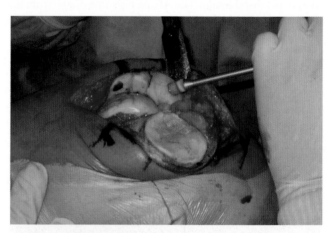

FIGURE 26-10

The autologous osteochondral plug is implanted into the prepared recipient site on the medial femoral condyle.

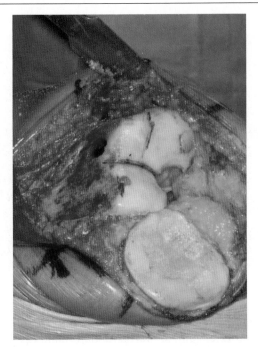

FIGURE 26-11

The osteochondral plug is in place, flush with the surrounding articular cartilage. The anterior trochlear surface has been resected. The donor harvest site will be covered by the implant and filled with bone graft or cement.

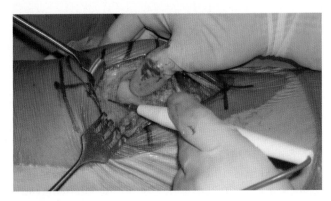

FIGURE 26-12

The proximal extent of the femoral trochlea is demarcated using electrocautery.

is extremely dysplastic, and if the sulcus of the trochlear groove is indeterminable, the trochlear component is implanted parallel to the transepicondylar axis. This is a line drawn from the sulcus of the medial epicondyle to the prominence of the lateral epicondyle. A slightly more extensile incision may be necessary to identify these landmarks.

I prefer to use an onlay-style trochlear component, which is implanted flush with the anterior femoral cortex. The alternative is an inlay-style component, which is inset into the anterior trochlear surface, but unlike the onlay variety, these cannot accommodate all trochlear sizes or shapes and has a higher tendency for patellar maltracking (14,15). An intramedullary system is used to prepare the anterior trochlear surface. With the knee in flexion, a drill hole is made in the center of the inter-condylar region of the trochlear groove, approximately 1 to 2 cm anterior to the roof of the in-tercondylar notch (Fig. 26-14). The marrow elements are suctioned to minimize the risk of fat embolization when the fluted rod of the anterior cutting guide is inserted into the medullary canal of

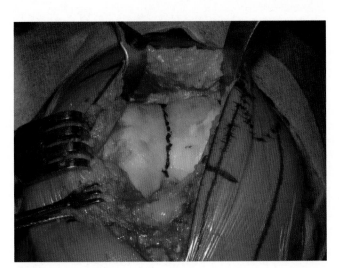

FIGURE 26-13

Advanced trochlear arthritis is noted, particularly laterally. The medial and lateral condylar surfaces show no gross evidence of degeneration. The anteroposterior axis of the femur has been drawn from the lowest point of the trochlear sulcus to the roof of the intercondylar notch.

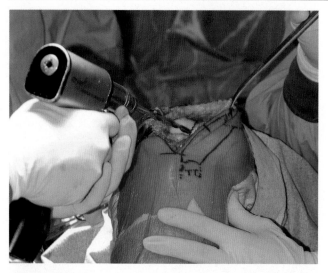

FIGURE 26-14

An entry hole for the intramedullary anterior trochlear cutting guide is drilled in the center of the trochlear groove, 1 to 2 cm above the roof of the intercondylar notch.

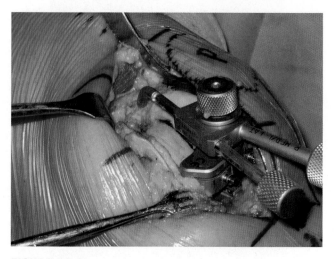

FIGURE 26-15

The outrigger boom is attached to the anterior trochlear cutting guide and rests on the lateral slope of the anterior femoral cortex to determine the depth of anterior resection.

the femur. The cutting guide is inserted until it rests against the distal condylar surfaces. An outrigger boom is then applied to the cutting guide to determine the depth of the anterior resection (Fig. 26-15). The guide is adjusted up or down to achieve an anterior resection that is flush with the anterior femoral cortex. Anteriorization of the cut will result in overstuffing of the patellofemoral compartment; overly aggressive resection will cause notching of the anterior femur. The anterior cutting guide is rotated so that its cutting slot is perpendicular to the AP axis of the femur (or parallel to the transepicondylar axis) (Fig. 26-16). Once the rotational alignment and depth of resection are confirmed, the guide is pinned into place, and an oscillating saw used to resect the anterior trochlear surface (Fig. 26-17). The surgeon then confirms that the depth and rotational alignment of resection are appropriate (Fig. 26-18); subtle adjustments can be made if necessary.

The next step involves sizing of the trochlear component and preparation of the intercondylar surface. I prefer to use a milling system that can accurately prepare this area. In the system I use,

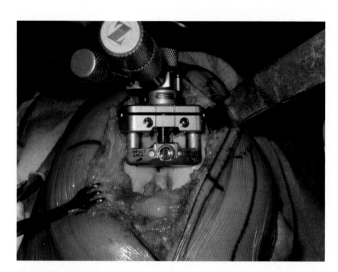

FIGURE 26-16

The anterior cutting guide is in place, externally rotated so that the cutting slot is perpendicular to the anteroposterior axis of the femur. The vertical reference lines on the guide are parallel to the marked anteroposterior axis.

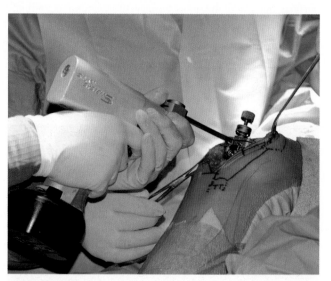

FIGURE 26-17

An oscillating saw is used to resect the anterior trochlear surface.

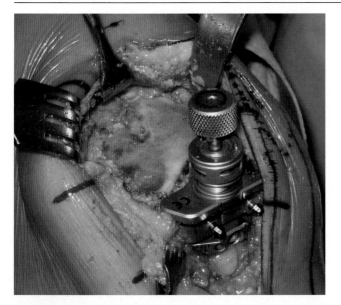

FIGURE 26-18

The depth of the anterior trochlear resection is checked. The goal is a resection flush with the anterior cortex. If the medial aspect of the anterior cortex is deficient, then the resection should be flush with the anterolateral aspect of the cortex to avoid notching the femur.

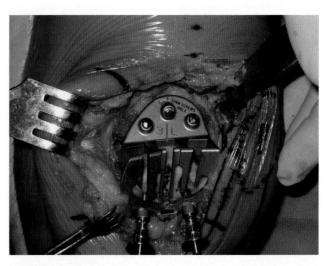

FIGURE 26-19

The milling guide serves as a sizing template. The outer edges of the guide correspond to the outer geometry of the implant. The appropriate size is selected. I prefer to leave 1 to 3 mm of bone exposed anteriorly to avoid mediolateral overhang and reduce the risk of synovial irritation on the edges of the trochlear prosthesis.

the outer border of the milling guide corresponds to the outer geometry of the trochlear prosthesis; therefore, it is also used to select the appropriately sized component. An implant size is selected that maximizes coverage of the resected anterior trochlear surface, but which leaves approximately 1 to 3 mm of bone exposed on either side of the anterior surface of the trochlear component. This optimizes the surface for patellar tracking while also reducing the risk of mediolateral trochlear component overhang or synovial irritation (Fig. 26-19). It is also important to check that the templated trochlear component does not encroach on the weight-bearing surfaces of the tibiofemoral articulations or overhang into the intercondylar notch (Fig. 26-20). The varus-valgus alignment of the trochlear component (and milling guide) is determined by the orientation of the femoral condylar surfaces, because in the region of transition into the intercondylar area, the component edges must be flush with or 1 mm recessed relative to the adjacent condylar articular cartilage. The

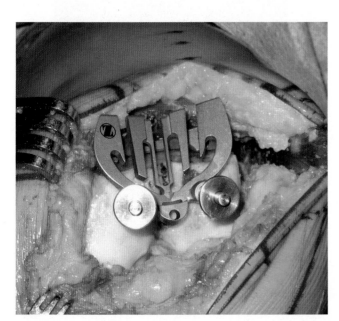

FIGURE 26-20

When the trochlear template/milling guide is applied to the distal femur in the appropriate position, it should not extend onto the articular surfaces of the femoral condyles or overhang into the intercondylar notch.

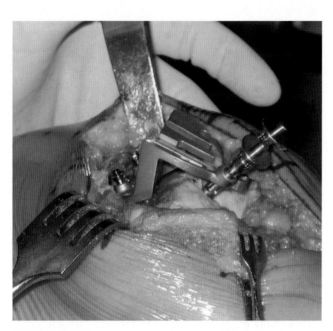

FIGURE 26-21

The milling guide is resting flush on the resected anterior surface, and the "feet" are touching the articular cartilage of the intercondylar region of the knee.

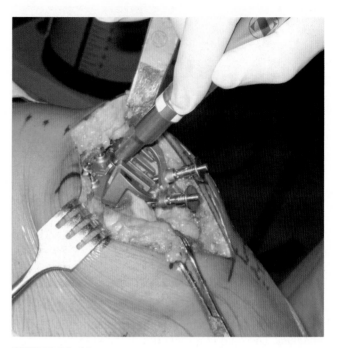

FIGURE 26-22

A milling burr is used to prepare the intercondylar surface.

milling guide is applied so that it is flush anteriorly against the resected trochlear surface, it is centered or slightly lateralized anteriorly, and its "feet" are resting on the articular cartilage of the intercondylar surfaces (Fig. 26-21). The intercondylar surface is then prepared with a milling burr, and the guide is removed (Fig. 26-22). The quality of bone preparation is assessed (Fig. 26-23). The appropriately sized trochlear template is then inserted into the prepared bed of bone, fixed with screw pins, and the lug holes are drilled (Figs. 26-24 and 26-25). The trial

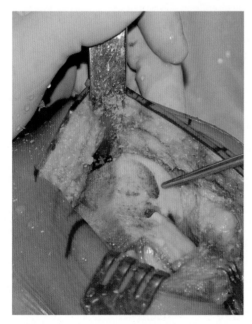

FIGURE 26-23

Trochlear bone preparation has been completed.

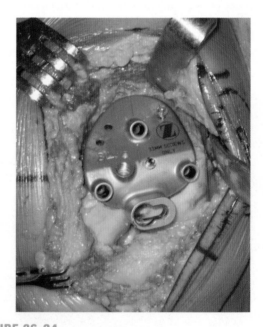

FIGURE 26-24

The correctly sized trochlear drill guide is secured to the prepared bone surface.

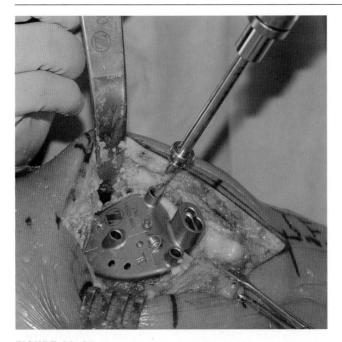

FIGURE 26-25
The trochlear lug holes are drilled.

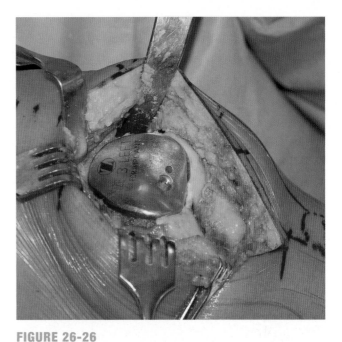

FIGURE 26-26
The trial component is in place. The intercondylar edges are flush with the adjacent condylar cartilage or recessed 1 mm relative to it. There is appropriate anterior coverage, with approximately 2 mm of bone exposed on either side of the anterior portion of the implant.

trochlear component is then impacted into place (Fig. 26-26). Once again, check that it is appropriately oriented, resting flat on the resected bone anteriorly and flush with or 1 mm recessed from the condylar surfaces.

Next, attention is turned to the preparation of the patella. The patella is resurfaced by the same principles followed in TKA. The periphery of the patella is cleared of synovial tissue to define its margins and eliminate from the undersurface of the quadriceps tendon a potential source of soft tissue impingement and crepitus (Fig. 26-27). The maximal pre-resection patellar thickness is measured using calipers, as the objective of resurfacing is to restore the native patellar thickness (Fig. 26-28). I prefer to perform a freehand transverse patellar osteotomy, removing the articular surface from the medial to lateral patellar facets (Fig. 26-29). The resection should parallel the

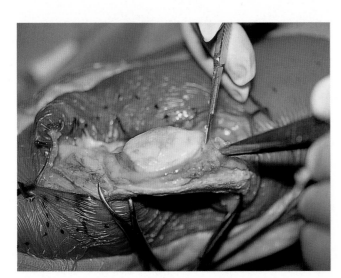

FIGURE 26-27
Peripatellar synovium around the periphery of the patella and undersurface of the quadriceps tendon is excised to define the margins of the patella and eliminate a potential source of synovial impingement on the trochlear implant.

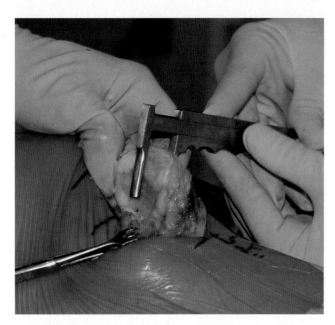

FIGURE 26-28

The thickness of the patella is measured with calipers before resection.

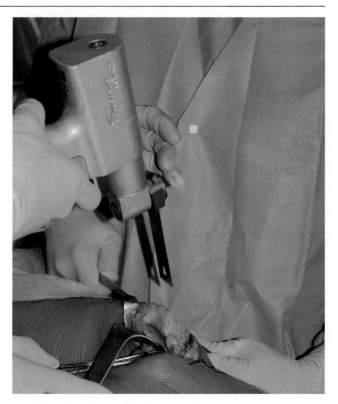

FIGURE 26-29

Transverse resection of the articular surface of the patella is performed from the medial to the lateral facets using an oscillating saw. This can be performed without everting the patella (shown here) or with it.

anterior patellar cortex, and the thickness of the remaining patella typically is approximately 9 to 10 mm thinner than prior to resection, depending on the thickness of the patellar component selected and how much resection the native patella can accommodate (Fig. 26-30). The patellar component size is selected using a guide applied medially. The guide should rest on the medial edge of the patella and not overhang beyond the margins of the bone. Three lug holes are drilled,

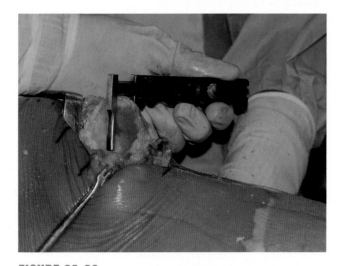

FIGURE 26-30

The thickness of the patella and symmetry of the resection are assessed. Typically, the remaining patellar bone should be 12 to 15 mm thick depending on its original dimension.

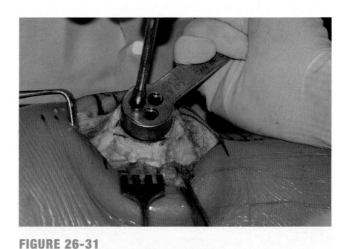

FIGURE 26-31

The patella sizing guide is applied to the medial edge of the patella, and three lug holes are drilled. The lateral edge of the guide, which corresponds to the lateral edge of the patellar prosthesis, is traced with a methylene blue marker.

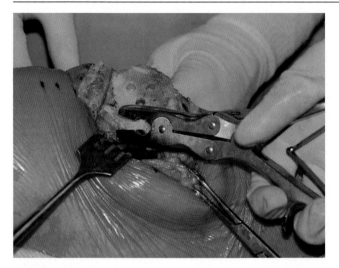

FIGURE 26-32

The bone from the lateral patellar facet that will not be covered by the patellar prosthesis is removed to avoid a source of bone impingement.

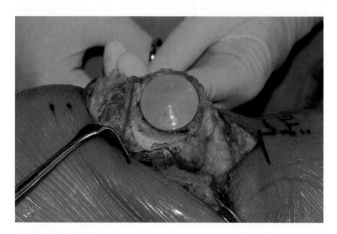

FIGURE 26-33

The trial patellar prosthesis is applied to the prepared surface. The composite thickness of the remaining patella and the patellar prosthesis is measured. The composite should be equivalent to or 1 mm less than the original thickness of the patella.

and the lateral edge of the guide or patellar prosthesis is traced with a methylene blue marker (Fig. 26-31). The portion of the lateral patellar facet that is not covered by the patellar component should be removed to avoid a potential source of painful bone impingement that could occur if it were to articulate against either the trochlear implant or articular cartilage (Fig. 26-32). The patellar trial is applied. The composite patellar thickness (prosthetic component and residual patellar bone) should be measured and adjustments made if necessary (Fig. 26-33). Typically, the goal is to have the composite thickness of the remaining patella and the patellar prosthesis equal the original patella thickness. Assessment of patellar tracking is performed with the trial components in place (Fig. 26-34). Attention is paid to identify patellar tilt, subluxation, or catching of the components. Patellar tilt and mild subluxation can usually be addressed successfully by a lateral retinacular release. As stated earlier, more severe extensor mechanism malalignment would require a tibial tubercle realignment if there is an excessive Q angle or a proximal realignment if the Q angle is normal. Catching of the patella on the trochlear component may often be resolved by subtle alterations in bone bed preparation, lateral release or patellar realignment, or adjustment in trochlear component position. Often, it is related to implant design, occurring more frequently with inlay-style implants and resolved with onlay designs (12,15,27).

After satisfactory trialing, the prepared recipient sites are irrigated with pulsatile lavage and dried. Methylmethacrylate is mixed and applied directly to the prepared bone surfaces in a doughy state. The cement is pressurized into the trabeculae, and the components are implanted. Manual pressure

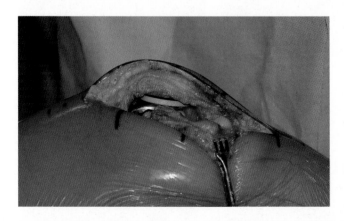

FIGURE 26-34

With the trial components in place and the patellar prosthesis reduced over the trochlear implant, there is no evidence of patellar tilt or subluxation with the "no-thumbs" technique. If subluxation or tilt is present, check for component malposition or soft tissue imbalance. If necessary, a lateral retinacular release is performed at this stage.

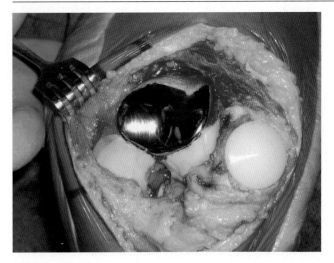

FIGURE 26-35

Intraoperative photograph of the patellofemoral prosthesis after cementation of the components shows appropriate positioning of the components.

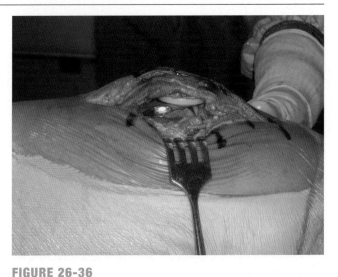

FIGURE 26-36

Patellar tracking is once again checked after the prosthesis has been implanted and the cement is hardened.

is applied to the trochlear component, and a patellar clamp is used for the patellar component until the cement cures. Extruded cement is removed (Fig. 26-35). Once again, patellar tracking is reassessed, and the need for a lateral release or recession is determined (Fig. 26-36). The wound is irrigated and sutured in layers. Postoperative radiographs confirm implant position and alignment (Fig. 26-37A–C).

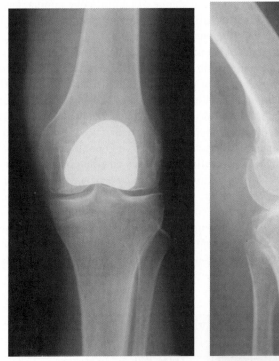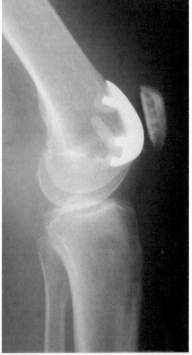

A,B

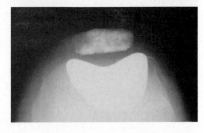

FIGURE 26-37

(A–C) Postoperative standing anteroposterior, lateral, and sunrise radiographs showing a successful patellofemoral arthroplasty.

C

POSTOPERATIVE MANAGEMENT

Isometrics and range-of-motion exercises are started immediately. A continuous passive motion machine during hospitalization (average, 1 or 2 days) may be used at the surgeon's discretion. Full weight bearing is permitted immediately, with support of crutches and a cane until there is adequate recovery of quadriceps strength. In some circumstances, full recovery of quadriceps strength can take 6 months or longer if there was severe preoperative quadriceps atrophy. I might protect the weight bearing during the initial 6 weeks after surgery if an osteochondral autologous grafting is performed, depending on the recipient site. Thromboembolism prophylaxis is used for 4 to 6 weeks; I prefer enteric-coated aspirin (325 mg twice daily) for most patients unless they pose an unusually high risk for thromboembolism, in which case I use warfarin. Twenty-four hours of perioperative antibiotics is advisable, and appropriate precautions regarding antibiotic prophylaxis for dental procedures or other interventions should follow the standard recommendations of the American Academy of Orthopaedic Surgeons (17). Once fully recovered, patients are allowed unrestricted activities, although I discourage excessive loading in deep flexion and lower extremity weight lifting.

PEARLS AND PITFALLS

- Patient selection is a key determinant of success in PFA. Restrict the procedure to patients with arthritis and symptoms localized to the patellofemoral compartment.
- Standing radiographs that include a midflexion posteroanterior view are useful in evaluating patients for PFA, particularly if they have mild joint line tenderness.
- Tibial tubercle anteromedialization should be performed before or simultaneous with PFA if the patient has a high Q angle (more than 20 degrees in women and 15 degrees in men).
- Although an inlay design (which is inset into the trochlea) is highly conservative in its bone preparation, onlay trochlear designs (implanted flush with the anterior femoral cortex) are more applicable for all trochlear shapes, regardless of the extent of trochlear dysplasia and have a predictable track record and a lower incidence of patellar snapping, catching, and subluxation than the inlay designs.
- Combining PFA with autologous osteochondral transplantation for a focal femoral condylar defect may preserve the tibiofemoral compartment.

CLINICAL RESULTS

Most series have reported good and excellent results in roughly 80% to 90% of cases at short- and midterm follow-up. However, clinical results of PFA are affected by trochlear component design features, as well as patient selection and surgical technique (12,14,15,23). Outcomes and patellofemoral performance have improved, and the need for secondary soft tissue surgery to enhance patellar tracking after PFA has decreased, because of trochlear design improvements that have occurred as we have moved from first- to second- and now to third-generation implants (14,15). The radius of curvature, width, tracking angle, and extent of constraint of the trochlear component have been shown to have an impact on patellar tracking and outcomes. Contemporary designs have substantially reduced the incidence of patellofemoral complications, leaving tibiofemoral arthritis as the major source of failure of PFAs (14,15).

Blazina et al reported 81% good results after a follow-up period of less than 2 years in 55 knees using a first-generation PFA with a trochlear implant constrained with a sharp trochlear groove (18). Thirty subsequent procedures were necessary in their series to either realign the extensor mechanism or to revise malpositioned components. Although the investigators credited technical errors as the reason for most secondary surgeries, component design (i.e., trochlear constraint, an obtuse radius of curvature, and narrow implant width) most certainly contributed to the failures as well.

Cartier et al had 85% good or excellent results in 72 first-generation PFAs followed for an average of 4 years (19). There were numerous concomitant surgical procedures performed to enhance patellar tracking, including soft tissue realignment or tibial tubercle transfer. Longer-term follow-up of those patients, at a mean of 10 years (range, 6 to 16 years) after surgery, found that results deteriorated over time, primarily because tibiofemoral arthritis had developed. That is not surprising, given the average patient age of 60 at the time of the initial PFA in that series. At most recent follow-up, 80% of patients who retained their patellofemoral prostheses were pain-free and 20% had moderate or severe pain, primarily from tibiofemoral arthritis. Stair ambulation was considered normal in 91%

of patients. No cases of patellar or trochlear loosening were identified. The authors noted that early failures peaked at 3 years and were related to inappropriate indications for the surgery and presumably to patellar maltracking problems that could likely be traced to implant design quirks. They identified a later peak in failures in the 9th and 10th years that corresponded to the development of symptomatic tibiofemoral osteoarthritis. The authors reported a survivorship of 75% at 11 years (20). Kooijman et al reported an 86% long-term success rate with the same first-generation PFA, although early secondary soft tissue surgery was necessary in 18% of patients, and revision of the PFA was necessary for catching, imbalance, or malposition in 16% (26).

In a consecutive series of 30 first-generation implants and 25 second-generation implants, this author found that results varied depending on which trochlear design was used (14). The incidence of patellofemoral dysfunction, subluxation, catching, and substantial pain was reduced from 17% with the earlier design to less than 4% with the more contemporary product. In another series, the same first-generation patellofemoral implants were revised to a second-generation implant that had a more favorable topography for patellar tracking. The etiologies of primary procedure failure were component malposition, subluxation, polyethylene wear, or overstuffing. After revision, there was statistically significant improvement in knee scores and patellar tracking at a mean 5-year follow-up. Mild femorotibial arthritis (Ahlbach stage I) predicted a poorer clinical outcome. At most recent follow-up, there was no evidence of wear, loosening, or subluxation. This study showed that significant improvement can be obtained when revising the failed PFA with a more accommodating implant design, provided there is no tibiofemoral arthritis (27).

Ackroyd reported on 306 second-generation PFAs and found that patellar tracking was substantially improved compared a to first-generation implant. In that series, patellar subluxation occurred in 3% of patients, and residual anterior knee pain was noted in 4%. Four percent required revision to TKA, mostly for tibiofemoral arthritis and none for mechanical loosening or wear (21).

Argenson reported on 66 second-generation PFAs in patients with a mean age of 57 and with a mean follow-up of 16 years (22). Although most patients had substantial and sustained pain relief, 25% were revised to TKA for tibiofemoral arthritis (at a mean of 7.3 years after PFA) and 14% for aseptic trochlear component loosening, many of which were uncemented (at a mean of 4.5 years after PFA). The authors reported the best results when the procedure was performed for posttraumatic patellofemoral arthritis or patellar subluxation, and the least favorable in those with primary degenerative arthritis. The development of tibiofemoral arthritis was the most frequent cause of failure; however, at the time of initial PFA, 14% had concomitant tibiofemoral osteotomies for early arthritis, which confounds the results. In those who retained their PFAs at most recent follow-up, there were significant improvements in Knee Society scores. The authors continue to advocate for the procedure as an intermediate stage before TKA in the absence of tibiofemoral arthritis or coronal plane malalignment (22).

My experience with more than 120 PFAs includes the use most recently of the third-generation implant presented in this chapter. In a series of 28 PFAs performed during a 6-month period using this particular implant, all patients have had substantial improvement in anterior knee pain and their ability to climb up and down stairs and stand from a chair, and there has been statistically significant improvement in Knee Society scores. There has been only one case of slight patellar subluxation noted on routine postoperative radiographs, caused by chronic weakness of the vastus medialis; this improved by 6 months postoperatively with an appropriate strengthening program. There have been no failures from patellar catching, instability, or clinically apparent subluxation. There have been no mechanical failures at short-term follow-up.

COMPLICATIONS

Early designs had a high incidence of patellar snapping and instability, requiring secondary surgery to realign the soft tissues or revise the trochlear prosthesis. These problems were often related to trochlear implant design features, as well as soft tissue imbalance or extensor mechanism malalignment. Contemporary designs have substantially reduced the tendency for patellar maltracking or dysfunction because prosthetic trochlear geometries are more accommodating of patellar tracking.

Residual anterior knee pain and dysfunction from patellar instability, resulting from soft tissue imbalance or component malalignment, were the major reported etiologies of failure with early PFA designs, but these are much less common now. A small percentage of patients will have mild anterior knee pain from soft tissue impingement, but this problem occurs with a similar frequency that we see in TKA. Late failures from component subsidence, polyethylene wear, or loosening may eventually develop in the long term, but these issues occur in less than 1% of published cases combined. Trochlear component loosening may be more common in cementless designs (22).

The development of tibiofemoral arthritis is the most common failure mechanism, occurring in approximately 20% of knees at 15 years (20,26). This is more common when the underlying diagnosis is primary osteoarthritis and less common in patellofemoral dysplasia or posttraumatic arthritis (22). In the event that revision to TKA is necessary to treat progressive arthritis, typically the all-polyethylene patellar component can be retained if not worn or loose, and standard total knee components can be used without the need for stems, augments, or bone graft, without compromising the results (28).

As with any arthroplasty procedure, infection and thromboembolism complications are potential complications, and standard prophylactic strategies should be followed.

REFERENCES

1. Davies AP, Vince AS, Shepstone L, et al. The radiologic prevalence of patellofemoral osteoarthritis. *Clin Orthop* 2002;402:206–212.
2. McAlindon RE, Snow S, Cooper C, Dieppe PA. Radiographic patterns of osteoarthritis of the knee joint in the community: the importance of the patellofemoral joint. *Ann Rheum Dis* 1992;51:844–849.
3. Federico DJ, Reider B. Results of isolated patellar debridement for patellofemoral pain in patients with normal patellar alignment. *Am J Sports Med* 1997;25:663–669.
4. Bugbee WD. Fresh osteochondral allografts. *Semin Arthrop* 2000;11:221–226.
5. Minas T, Chiu R. Autologous chondrocyte implantation. *Am J Knee Surg* 2000;13:41–50.
6. Maquet P. Advancement of the tibial tuberosity. *Clin Orthop* 1976;115:225.
7. Fulkerson JP, Becker GJ, Meaney JA, et al. Anteromedial tibial tubercle transfer without bone graft. *Am J Sports Med* 1990;18:490–497.
8. Dinham JM, French PR. Results of patellectomy for osteoarthritis. *Postgrad Med* 1972;48:590.
9. Ivey FM, Blazina ME, Fox JM, Del Pizzo W. Reoperation following patellectomy for chondromalacia. *Orthopedics* 1979;2:134.
10. Laskin RS, Palletta G. Total knee replacement in the patient who had undergone patellectomy. *J Bone Joint Surg* 1995;77A:1708–1712.
11. Laskin RS, Van Steijn M. Total knee replacement for patients with patellofemoral arthritis. *Clin Orthop* 1989;367:89–95.
12. Lonner JH. Patellofemoral arthroplasty. *J Am Acad Orthop Surg* 2007;15:495–506.
13. Argenson JN, Guillaume JM, Aubaniac JM. Is there a place for patellofemoral arthroplasty? *Clin Orthop* 1995;321:162–167.
14. Lonner JH. Patellofemoral arthroplasty. Pros, cons, and design considerations. *Clin Orthop* 2004; 428:158–165.
15. Lonner JH. Patellofemoral arthroplasty: the impact of design on outcomes. *Orthop Clin N Am* 2008;39:347–354.
16. Lonner JH, Mehta S, Booth RE. Ipsilateral patellofemoral arthroplasty and autogenous osteochondral femoral condylar transplantation. *J Arthrop* 2007;22:1103–1136.
17. Hanssen AD, Osmon DR, Nelson CL. Prevention of deep periprosthetic joint infection. *J Bone Joint Surg* 1996;78A:458–471.
18. Blazina ME, Fox JM, Del Pizzo W, et al. Patellofemoral replacement. *Clin Orthop* 1979;144:98–102.
19. Cartier P, Sanouiller JL, Grelsamer R. Patellofemoral arthroplasty. *J Arthrop* 1990;5:49–55.
20. Cartier P, Sanouiller JL, Khefacha A. Long-term results with the first patellofemoral prosthesis. *Clin Orthop* 2005;436:47–54.
21. Ackroyd CE, Newman JH, Evans R, et al. The Avon patellofemoral arthroplasty. Five-year survivorship and functional results. *J Bone Joint Surg* 2007;89B:310–315.
22. Argenson JNA, Flecher X, Parratte S, Aubaniac JM. Patellofemoral arthroplasty: an update. *Clin Orthop* 2005;440:50–53.
23. Australian Orthopaedic Association National Joint Replacement Registry. Available at: http://www.aoa.org.au/docs/njrrrep06.pdf.
24. Sisto DJ, Sarin VK. Custom patellofemoral arthroplasty of the knee. *J Bone Joint Surg* 2006;88A: 1475–1480.
25. Merchant AC. Early results with a total patellofemoral joint replacement arthroplasty prosthesis. *J Arthrop* 2004;19:829–836.
26. Kooijman HJ, Driessen APPM, van Horn JR. Long-term results of patellofemoral arthroplasty. *J Bone Joint Surg* 2003;85-B:836–840.
27. Hendrix MRG, Ackroyd CE, Lonner JH. Revision patellofemoral arthroplasty: 3–7 year follow-up. *J Arthrop* 2008.
28. Lonner JH, Jasko JG, Booth RE. Revision of a failed patellofemoral arthroplasty to a total knee arthroplasty. *J Bone Joint Surg* 2006;88A:2337–2342.

27 Opening-Wedge Proximal Tibial Osteotomy

Michael J. Stuart

INTRODUCTION

Limb malalignment results in an imbalance of force transmission to the knee joint. A varus deformity is most common, because osteoarthritis typically involves the medial compartment. Articular cartilage, bone, and medial meniscus loss combined with lateral collateral ligament stretching cause an increased tibial condylar-plateau angle. The resultant load concentration at the medial portion of the joint contributes to arthritis pain.

A valgus-producing tibial osteotomy can redistribute the weight-bearing forces, lessen the medial compartment load, and reduce the varus knee moment. The goals of this procedure are to relieve pain, buy time before an arthroplasty is necessary, and decrease forces on ligament, meniscus, and osteochondral grafts. Unicompartment or total knee arthroplasty have supplanted realignment osteotomy as a primary treatment for many middle-aged patients with gonarthrosis. However, the indications for an osteotomy have actually broadened to include younger patients or athletes with ligament deficiencies, chondral defects, absent menisci, or post-traumatic degenerative arthritis. An osteotomy should also be performed in combination with ligament reconstruction, articular cartilage regeneration, or meniscal transplantation in a knee with associated limb malalignment.

The lateral closing-wedge osteotomy of the proximal tibia was popularized by Coventry in the 1960s (1,2). Appropriate patient selection and sufficient postoperative correction have been correlated with a 90% success rate at more than 10 years after surgery (3–5). Worsening of results is caused by recurrent pain, arthritis progression, and occasionally, recurrence of varus deformity (6). In recent years, a medial opening-wedge osteotomy of the proximal tibia has gained popularity as new instrumentation and implants have become available (7–9).

The advantages of the opening-wedge technique include:

- no violation of the proximal tibiofibular joint
- no change in the fibular collateral ligament length
- a more precise intraoperative correction
- easier biplanar correction
- same incision for concomitant procedures (anterior cruciate ligament reconstruction, osteochondral allografts, etc.) or subsequent knee arthroplasty
- avoidance of metaphyseal-diaphyseal offset deformity common in closing-wedge proximal tibial osteotomy

Disadvantages of the opening-wedge technique include:

- lengthening of the patellar tendon and elevation of the tibiofemoral joint line (10)
- increased tension in the medial collateral ligament (MCL)

- distal translation of the patella and lateral translation of the tibial tubercle
- bone graft requirement
- slower healing and longer protection from weight bearing

INDICATIONS

A valgus-producing osteotomy of the proximal tibia is primarily indicated for pain relief in patients with medial compartment arthritis and/or mechanical axis correction as an adjunct to other reconstructive knee procedures. Patients should have pain and tenderness localized to the medial joint line, less than 10 degrees of terminal knee extension loss, and greater than 90 degrees of knee flexion. Osteotomy can be performed in patients with:

- varus mechanical axis and medial unicompartmental tibiofemoral arthrosis
- chronic posterolateral instability and varus thrust
- varus mechanical axis and anterior or posterior cruciate ligament reconstruction
- varus mechanical axis and meniscus transplantation
- varus mechanical axis and subchondral bone microfracture, autologous chondrocyte implantation, or osteochondral transplantation

CONTRAINDICATIONS

Osteotomy should be avoided in patients with (11):

- diffuse knee pain and tenderness
- knee stiffness (greater than 10 degrees of terminal knee extension loss and/or less than 90 degrees of knee flexion)
- bicompartmental or tricompartmental arthritis
- severe deformity
- medial tibial bone loss
- pronounced joint line obliquity
- lateral tibial subluxation
- varus angulation of the proximal tibia combined with excessive valgus angulation of the distal femur
- uncorrected ligamentous laxity and functional knee instability
- obesity
- previous meniscectomy in contralateral compartment
- inflammatory arthropathy
- unrealistic patient expectations

PREOPERATIVE PLANNING

Gait observation and physical examination of the knee will identify a lateral thrust and pathologic collateral ligament laxity that may not be apparent on standing radiographs. The desired angle of correction is determined by static analysis of full-length standing roentgenograms (51 × 14 inches). The mechanical axis of the limb is the angle formed between a line drawn from the hip center to the knee center (femoral mechanical axis) and a line drawn from the knee center to the ankle center (tibial mechanical axis). The normal mechanical axis is approximately 1.2 degrees of varus (12). A valgus-producing proximal tibial osteotomy performed for medial compartment arthritis typically overcorrects the mechanical axis to 3 to 5 degrees of valgus. The Weight-Bearing Line Method is a simple and reproducible technique for determining the desired coronal plane correction angle (Fig. 27-1) (13).

1. Divide the lateral tibial plateau from 0% to 100% from the medial to the lateral margin.
2. Draw lines from the center of the femoral head and the center of the tibiotalar joint to the desired coordinate depending on the indication for the procedure (typically 62% [range, 50% to 75%]).
3. The angle formed by these two lines equals the angle of correction.
4. The use of standing radiographs can overestimate the magnitude of correction because of osseous defects and/or attenuated ligaments. Each millimeter of lateral tibiofemoral joint separation

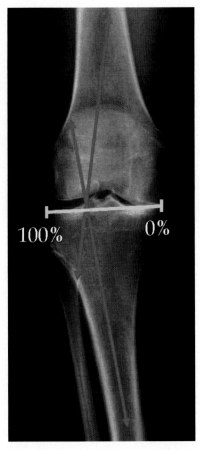

FIGURE 27-1

Detail of the knee from a full-length standing radiograph of the right lower extremity. The Weight-Bearing Line Method divides the lateral tibial plateau from 0% to 100% from the medial to the lateral margin. Lines drawn from the center of the femoral head and the center of the tibiotalar joint intersect at the 62% coordinate to form the desired angle of correction.

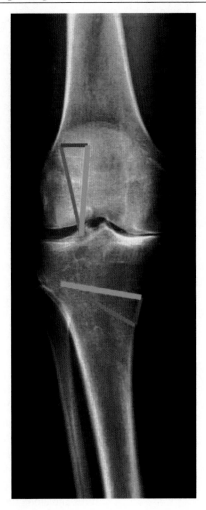

FIGURE 27-2

The medial tibial cortex opening in millimeters is determined by measuring "like triangles" on the film according to the desired angle of correction.

causes approximately 1 degree of varus angular deformity. Compare the amount of lateral joint space opening (in millimeters) with the contralateral knee and subtract the difference from the calculated angle (1 degree per mm) to avoid overcorrection.

5. Once the desired angle of correction has been calculated, determine the medial tibial opening in millimeters by measuring "like triangles" on the film (Fig. 27-2) or by performing a cutout using tracing paper.

6. Study the lateral radiograph to appreciate the sagittal plane geometry of the tibial plateau. The osteotomy should maintain a neutral tibial slope, unless a sagittal plane correction is desired. Increase in the posterior tibial slope will cause excessive anterior cruciate ligament graft strain but may be advantageous for a posterior cruciate ligament-deficient knee. Increase in the anterior tibial slope will cause excessive posterior cruciate ligament graft strain but may be desired in an anterior cruciate ligament-deficient knee.

SURGICAL TECHNIQUE

1. Setup:
   Place the patient supine on a radiolucent operating room table. Check the fluoroscope to ensure clear visualization of the femoral head, knee, and talus.

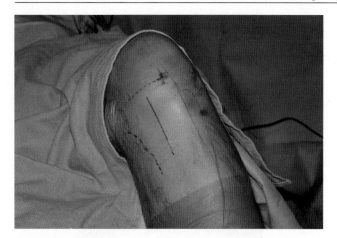

FIGURE 27-3

The skin incision is centered between the medial border of the tibial tubercle and the posteromedial margin of the tibia, extending from below the joint line for a distance of approximately 7 cm.

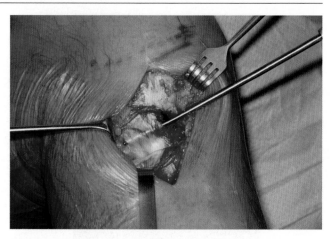

FIGURE 27-4

The sartorius fascia is split, gracilis and semitendinosus tendons are retracted distally, and the superficial medial collateral ligament identified with a probe.

2. Exposure:

Exsanguinate the leg and inflate the tourniquet. Make a vertical incision, centered midway between the tibial tubercle and the posteromedial border of the tibia, beginning 1 cm distal to the joint line extending distally for approximately 7 cm (Fig. 27-3). Split the sartorius fascia diagonally between its fibers and identify the superficial MCL (Fig. 27-4). Retract the gracilis and semitendinosus tendons distally or transect the tendons for later repair. Incise the superficial MCL distally, subperiosteally elevate, but preserve the proximal 2 cm of its tibial attachment. Flex the knee to 90 degrees and extend the subperiosteal dissection along the anterior and posterior tibial cortices. Place a malleable or Z retractor along the posterior tibial cortex to protect the neurovascular structures and along the anterior tibial cortex to protect the patellar tendon (Fig. 27-5).

3. Guide pin placement:

Insert a guide pin in place under fluoroscopic guidance, beginning 4 cm distal to the joint line, angled proximally toward the tip of the fibular head, approximately 2 cm distal to the lateral joint line (Fig. 27-6). Verify that the guide pin traverses just proximal to the patellar tendon at-

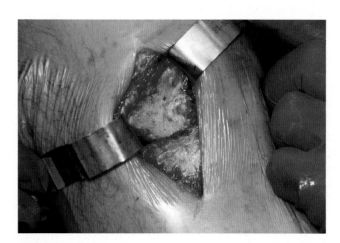

FIGURE 27-5

With the knee flexed to 90 degrees, malleable retractors are placed along the anterior and posterior tibial cortices to protect the neurovascular structures and patellar tendon.

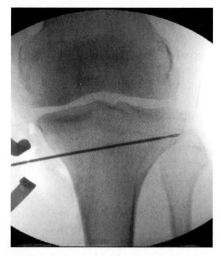

FIGURE 27-6

A guide pin is placed under fluoroscopic guidance beginning 3 cm distal to the joint line angled proximally toward the tip of the fibular head up to the lateral tibial cortex.

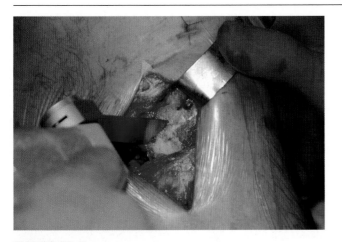

FIGURE 27-7

An oscillating saw cuts distally along the guide pin while replicating the posterior slope of the tibia.

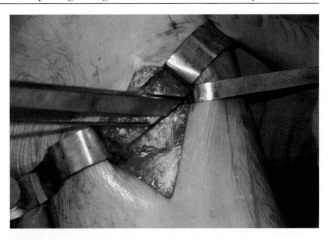

FIGURE 27-8

The anterior and posterior tibial cortices are transected, and the osteotomy is continued to within 1 cm of the lateral tibial cortex using an osteotome.

tachment at the tibial tubercle. An alternative technique is to place a second parallel guide pin to replicate the posterior slope of the tibial plateau.

4. Saw/osteotome:

Use an oscillating saw to cut along the guide pin distally while replicating the posterior slope of the tibia (Fig. 27-7). Cut across two thirds of the tibia with the saw and then continue with an osteotome to within 1 cm of the lateral tibial cortex. Complete the osteotomy of the anterior and posterior tibial cortices with an osteotome (Fig. 27-8).

5. Distractor device:

Insert the distractor device or lamina spreaders while carefully preserving the medial tibial cortical bone (Fig. 27-9). Gradually open the osteotomy to the desired distance under fluoroscopic guidance.

6. Verify correction:

With the distractor or an opening-wedge osteotomy plate in place, verify the desired coronal plane correction with an anterior-posterior view and the tibial slope with a lateral view. Use fluoroscopy to place a metal rod or the cautery cord from the center of the femoral head to the center of the talus (Fig. 27-10). Hold the knee in full extension and apply a slight valgus stress to the knee and an axial load to the foot. Visualize the position of the rod at the knee joint us-

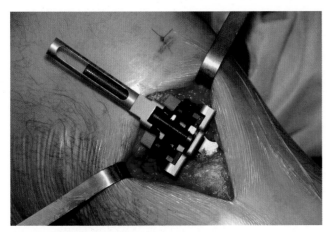

FIGURE 27-9

A distractor device or lamina spreader is used to gradually open the osteotomy to the desired distance.

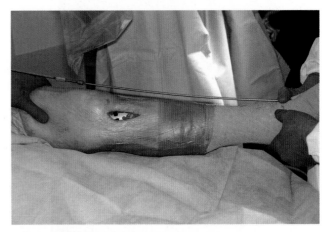

FIGURE 27-10

A metal rod or the cautery cord is positioned between the centers of the femoral head and the talus to verify the desired coronal plane correction with an anterior-posterior fluoroscopic view.

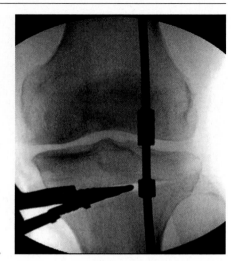

FIGURE 27-11

The knee is held in full extension while applying a slight valgus stress and an axial load to the foot to visualize the position of the rod at the knee joint.

ing fluoroscopy (Fig. 27-11). Adjust the amount of correction to match the preoperative plan (the desired weight-bearing line).

7. Osteotomy plate/screws:

Insert the appropriate size opening-wedge osteotomy plate, and then remove the distractor. Ensure that the plate is seated flush against the cortex of the tibia (Fig. 27-12). Secure the plate with two cancellous screws proximally and two bicortical screws distally. Verify the plate position and screw length with fluoroscopy (Fig. 27-13).

8. Auto- or allogeneic graft:

Deflate the tourniquet and achieve hemostasis. Pack the tibial defect with bone graft: cancellous allograft mixed with the patient's platelet-rich plasma gel (Fig. 27-14), allograft wedges, or iliac crest autograft.

9. Wound closure:

Insert a drain if bleeding is present. Loosely repair the superficial MCL and reapproximate the fascia to cover the plate (Fig. 27-15). Close the wound with monofilament absorbable interrupted subcutaneous sutures, a running monofilament absorbable subcuticular suture, and Steri-Strips.

10. Brace:

Apply an elastic dressing and a rehabilitation brace locked in full extension (Fig. 27-16).

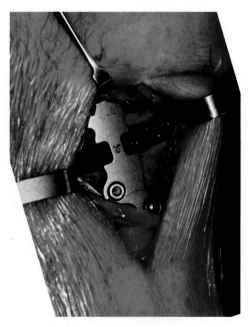

FIGURE 27-12

The appropriate-size opening-wedge osteotomy plate is inserted, and the distractor is removed.

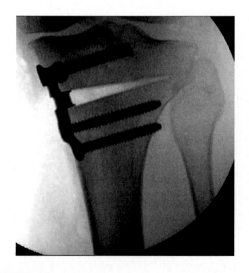

FIGURE 27-13

Satisfactory plate position and screw length are verified with fluoroscopy.

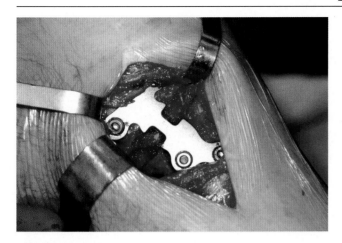

FIGURE 27-14

The tibial defect is packed with cancellous allograft mixed with the patient's platelet-rich plasma gel.

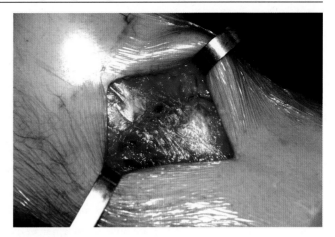

FIGURE 27-15

The superficial medial collateral ligament and sartorius fascia are loosely reapproximated to cover the plate.

PEARLS AND PITFALLS

Protect the patellar tendon and neurovascular structures:

- Flex the knee when using the saw and osteotome.
- Place malleable retractors along the anterior and posterior tibial cortices to protect the patellar tendon and neurovascular structures.

Prevent intra-articular fracture:

- Use fluoroscopic guidance to determine the depth of osteotome penetration.
- Maintain 1 cm of intact lateral tibial bone.
- Gradually open the osteotomy.
- If the osteotomy does not open, use an osteotome to ensure that the anterior and posterior tibial cortices have been cut.

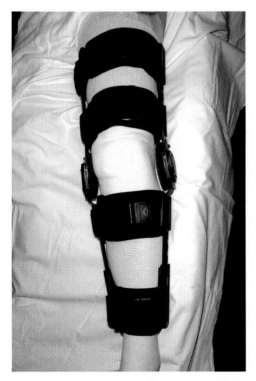

FIGURE 27-16

An elastic dressing and a rehabilitation brace locked in full extension are applied.

Avoid increased posterior slope (unless desired for a posterior cruciate-deficient knee):

- Place the plate as posterior as possible.
- The anterior tibial gap should be approximately two thirds of the posterior tibial gap (14).

Ensure a stable construct:

- Allow osteoclasis of the lateral tibial cortex to maintain an intact periosteal hinge.
- Preserve the medial tibial cortex at the site of the plate tines.
- Consider bicortical autograft or allograft wedges for added stability if large correction is required.

Avoid hematoma or compartment syndrome:

- Release the tourniquet before bone grafting to obtain hemostasis.
- Insert a drain if necessary.

Prevent loss of correction or nonunion:

- Irrigate bone when using an oscillating saw.
- Ensure stable internal fixation.
- Toe-touch weight bearing only for 6 to 8 weeks.
- Discontinue protected weight bearing at 12 weeks if radiographic documentation of osteotomy union (Fig. 27-17).

POSTOPERATIVE MANAGEMENT

The rehabilitation brace is worn full time, except for bathing. Touch weight bearing (20 to 30 pounds) using crutches is allowed with the brace locked in full extension. The brace is unlocked for full, active range-of-motion exercises three times daily. The patient is also instructed on ankle pumps, quadriceps sets, and straight-leg lifts. The knee is re-examined 2 weeks after surgery to inspect for wound healing, swelling, and range of motion. At 8 weeks following surgery, anteroposterior and lateral knee radiographs are performed. Patients are allowed to remove the brace when not walking, bear progressive weight with the brace unlocked, and wean from crutches. At 12 weeks following surgery, knee examination and repeat radiographs (anteroposterior, lateral, and full-length standing views) are performed to document bone healing and limb alignment. Progressive resistance strengthening exercises and nonimpact aerobic conditioning are started.

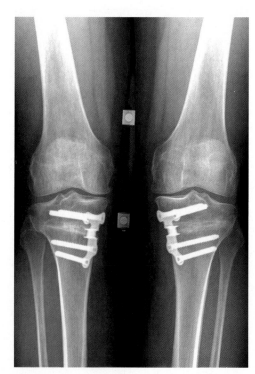

FIGURE 27-17

Anteroposterior radiograph verifies no change in position of the plate and screws along with consolidation of bone graft at the osteotomy site.

COMPLICATIONS

Complications can be averted by careful patient selection, precise preoperative planning, and meticulous surgical technique (15–17). Complications include:

- Malalignment (undercorrection or overcorrection)
- Loss of correction/malunion (Fig. 27-18)
- Neurologic injury
- Vascular injury
- Tourniquet palsy
- Compartment syndrome
- Intra-articular tibial plateau fracture (Fig. 27-19)
- Delayed union or nonunion
- Deep venous thrombosis
- Infection
- Instability
- Persistent pain

RESULTS

Hernigou reported on 93 osteotomies performed on patients with medial compartment arthritis and varus deformity. Excellent or good results were identified in 90% of patients at 5 years and 45% at 10 years. Failures occurred at an average of 7 years after surgery because of recurrent knee pain. The importance of adequate correction was evidenced by the observation that the best results were obtained in a subgroup of 20 knees with a resultant mechanical axis of +3 to +6 degrees of valgus (7). A retrospective radiographic analysis of 32 osteotomies by Marti and colleagues stressed the challenge of achieving the desired limb alignment. In the coronal plane, only 50% were adequately corrected, 31% were undercorrected, and 19% overcorrected. In the sagittal plane, mean posterior tibial slope increased 2.7 degrees (range, −8 degrees to 10 degrees) (8). Naudie reported on 17 opening-wedge osteotomies performed for a hyperextension-varus thrust. At a mean of 4.5 years after surgery,

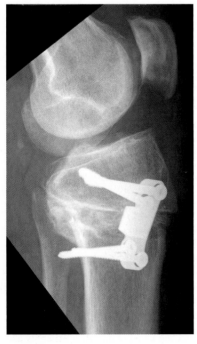

FIGURE 27-18

Postoperative lateral radiograph depicting excessive posterior tibial slope as a result of construct failure and loss of correction.

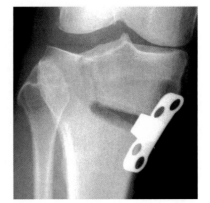

FIGURE 27-19

Intraoperative anteroposterior radiograph of an intra-articular lateral tibial plateau fracture resulting from an incomplete osteotomy.

15 of the 16 patients were satisfied. The femorotibial axis was corrected to a mean of 6 degrees of valgus; the posterior tibial slope increased 8 degrees on average, and the patellar height ratio decreased to a mean of 0.17. Despite the persistent pathologic ligament laxity, further ligament surgery was avoided in 11 of the 16 patients (~70%) (9). A prospective cohort study by Arthur and colleagues examined the outcome of a valgus-producing proximal tibial opening-wedge osteotomy to treat combined grade 3 posterolateral instability and varus malalignment. Eight of the 21 patients (38%) had sufficient improvement, and a subsequent posterolateral reconstruction was not necessary (18). Noyes et al published a case series of 55 consecutive patients treated with an opening-wedge osteotomy using autologous iliac crest bone graft (19). Full weight bearing was achieved at a mean of 8 weeks after surgery. The posterior tibial slope remained unchanged. Although union occurred in all patients, three had a delayed union, and one patient had a loss of correction. A human cadaver study, using a material-testing machine and pressure-sensitive film, quantified tibiofemoral contact pressures in varus, neutral, and valgus alignments. After performing a valgus-producing opening-wedge proximal tibial osteotomy, high medial compartment pressures were maintained despite the fact that the loading axis was shifted into the lateral compartment. Both realignment and complete release of the distal fibers of the MCL were required to produce a decompression of the medial compartment (20). Miller combined 61 proximal tibial opening-wedge osteotomies with microfracture in patients with varus malalignment and chondral defect. Nineteen patients also had grade 3 or 4 chondromalacia of the patella. At a minimum 2-year follow-up, the mean Lysholm score improved from 49.9 to 75.4, and the mean satisfaction score was 7.6 (range, 0 to 10) (21).

CONCLUSIONS

The valgus-producing proximal tibial osteotomy remains a viable option for medial unicompartmental arthritis and varus malalignment. Clinical studies document a 10-year survival without the need for arthroplasty of approximately 70%. The indications for osteotomy are expanding because correction of varus malalignment is an essential adjunct for ligament reconstruction, medial meniscus transplantation, and medial femoral condyle cartilage restoration procedures. Success depends on careful patient selection, precise preoperative planning, and meticulous surgical technique. The valgus-producing proximal tibial opening-wedge method offers some distinct advantages. Future trends may incorporate computer-assisted navigation, improved plate designs, and biological bone graft enhancement.

REFERENCES

1. Coventry M. Osteotomy of the upper portion of the tibia for degenerative arthritis of the knee: a preliminary report. *J Bone Joint Surg* 1965;47A:984–990.
2. Coventry M. Stepped staple for upper tibial osteotomy. *J Bone Joint Surg* 1969;51A:1011.
3. Coventry MB. Osteotomy about the knee for degenerative and rheumatoid arthritis. *J Bone Joint Surg* 1973;55A:23–48.
4. Coventry MB. Proximal tibial varus osteotomy for osteoarthritis of the lateral compartment of the knee. *J Bone Joint Surg* 1987;69A:32–38.
5. Coventry M, Ilstrup D, Wallrichs S. Proximal tibial osteotomy. A critical long-term study of eighty-seven cases. *J Bone Joint Surg* 1993;75A:196–201.
6. Stuart MJ, Grace JN, Ilstrup DM, et al. Late recurrence of varus deformity after proximal tibial osteotomy. *Clin Orthop* 1990;260:61–65.
7. Hernigou P, Medevielle D, Debeyre J, et al. Proximal tibial osteotomy for osteoarthritis with varus deformity. A ten to thirteen-year follow-up study. *J Bone Joint Surg* 1987;69:332–354.
8. Marti CB, Gautier E, Wachtl SW, et al. Accuracy of frontal and sagittal plane correction in open-wedge high tibial osteotomy. *Arthroscopy* 2004;20:366–372.
9. Naudie DD, Amendola A, Fowler PJ. Opening wedge high tibial osteotomy for symptomatic hyperextension-varus thrust. *Am J Sports Med* 2004;32:60–70.
10. Chae DJ, Shetty GM, Lee DB, et al. Tibial slope and patellar height after opening wedge high tibial osteotomy using autologous tricortical iliac bone graft. *Knee* 2005;15:128–133.
11. Morrey BF. Upper tibial osteotomy for secondary osteoarthritis of the knee. *J Bone Joint Surg* 1989;71B:554–559.
12. Hsu RWW, Himeno S, Coventry MB, et al. Normal axial alignment of the lower extremity and load-bearing distribution at the knee. *Clin Orthop* 1990;255:215–227.
13. Dugdale TW, Noyes FR, Styer D. Preoperative planning for high tibial osteotomy. The effect of lateral tibiofemoral separation and tibiofemoral length. *Clin Orthop* 1992;274:248–264.
14. Song EK, Seon JK, Park SJ. How to avoid unintended increase of posterior slope in navigation-assisted open-wedge high tibial osteotomy. *Orthopedics* 2007;30(10 Suppl):S127–131.

15. Kettelkamp DB, Leach RE, Nasca R. Pitfalls of proximal tibial osteotomy. *Clin Orthop* 1975;106:232–241.
16. Engel GM, Lippert FG. Valgus tibial osteotomy: avoiding the pitfalls. *Clin Orthop* 1981;160:137–143.
17. Rubens F, Wellington JL, Bouchard AG. Popliteal artery injury after tibial osteotomy: report of two cases. *Can J Surg* 1990;33:294–297.
18. Arthur A, LaPrade RF, Agel J. Proximal tibial opening wedge osteotomy as the initial treatment for chronic posterolateral corner deficiency in the varus knee: a prospective clinical study. *Am J Sp Med* 2007;35:1844–1850.
19. Noyes FR, Mayfield W, Barber-Westin SD, et al. Opening wedge high tibial osteotomy: an operative technique and rehabilitation program to decrease complications and promote early union and function. *Am J Sports Med* 2006;34:1262–1273.
20. Agneskirchner JD, Hurschler C, Wrann CD, et al. The effects of valgus medial opening wedge high tibial osteotomy on articular cartilage pressure of the knee: a biomechanical study. *Arthroscopy* 2007;23: 852–861.
21. Miller BS, Joseph TA, Barry EM, et al. Patient satisfaction after medial opening high tibial osteotomy and microfracture. *J Knee Surg* 2007;20:129–133.

28 Distal Femoral Osteotomy

Eugenio Savarese, Bryce Bederka, and Annunziato Amendola

INDICATIONS/CONTRAINDICATIONS

Limb alignment plays a critical role in the development of arthritis and overload syndromes. An osteotomy involves opening or removing a wedge of bone to alter the mechanical axis of that bone in an effort to reduce overloaded areas of a joint surface. Osteotomy about the knee surgically reshapes bone, realigning the mechanical axis of the limb away from the affected compartment. This strategy has the distinct advantage of joint preservation that may be particularly attractive for younger and more active patients with unicompartmental arthritis. Varus malalignment is most commonly corrected with a high tibial osteotomy. In contrast, valgus malalignment is most commonly corrected with a supracondylar femoral osteotomy, using either an opening- or closing-wedge osteotomy (1). Small valgus correction may be carried out with a tibial osteotomy as well, but larger corrections will lead to significant obliquity in the joint line if performed through the proximal tibia.

Distal femoral osteotomy is indicated in:

- moderate corrections up to 17.5 degrees for opening wedge (2)
- larger corrections from 12 degrees to 27 degrees for closing wedge (3)
- mild–to-moderate osteoarthritis (OA) (2)
- lateral condyle cartilage lesions (with or without cartilage grafting) (2)
- lateral meniscal transplants (2)
- individuals younger than 65 years

Distal femoral osteotomy is contraindicated in:

- extreme valgus deformity associated with a fixed subluxation of the tibia (4)
- severe medial compartment OA (3)
- severe tricompartmental OA (3)
- severe patellofemoral osteoarthritis (4) (relative contraindication)
- inflammatory disease (1)
- severe osteoporosis (5)
- high body mass index (4) (relative)
- individuals older than 65 years (relative)

PREOPERATIVE PLANNING

The standard evaluation begins with assessing the extent of knee arthrosis and lower extremity alignment. Standard radiographic assessment includes bilateral weight-bearing anteroposterior views in full extension, bilateral weight-bearing posteroanterior tunnel views at 30 degrees of flexion, lateral, and skyline views, and a bilateral full-length standing alignment film (Fig. 28-1). The most common deformity seen in the valgus knee is located in the femur. The normal lateral distal femoral angle is 84 degrees, with angles less than that being considered abnormal (Fig. 28-2). Magnetic resonance

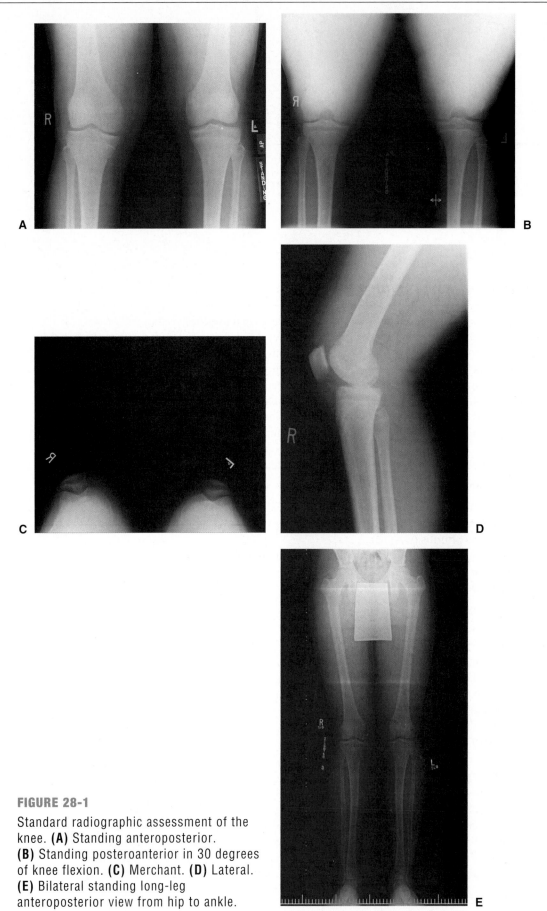

FIGURE 28-1

Standard radiographic assessment of the
knee. **(A)** Standing anteroposterior.
(B) Standing posteroanterior in 30 degrees
of knee flexion. **(C)** Merchant. **(D)** Lateral.
(E) Bilateral standing long-leg
anteroposterior view from hip to ankle.

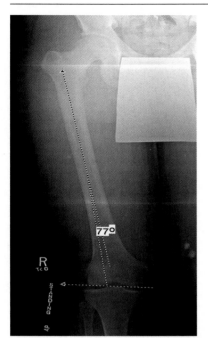

FIGURE 28-2

The lateral distal femoral angle is the acute angle between a line drawn down the femoral shaft and a line drawn across the femoral condyles. The normal angle is 84 degrees, with smaller angles associated with a valgus deformity. In this case, the angle measures 77 degrees.

imaging is useful in the preoperative assessment when significant intra-articular chondral or meniscal pathology is suspected based on history or exam with mechanical findings (4).

The required correction is calculated according to the method described by Dugdale at al (6). The osteotomy is planned so that it will place the weight-bearing line (center of the femoral head to the center of the tibiotalar joint) to fall at a selected position approximately through the tip of the medial tibial spine (Fig. 28-3). In case of significant medial joint line opening on weight-bearing radiographs, the total amount of correction should be measured from a supine or a varus stress radiograph

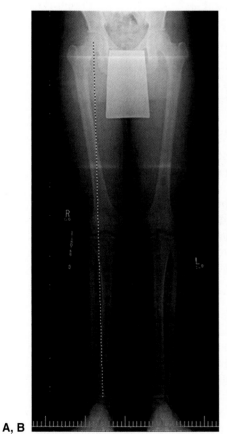

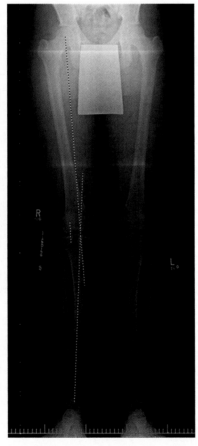

FIGURE 28-3

Radiographic planning of a distal femoral osteotomy according to the method described by Dugdale et al (6). **(A)** A native weight-bearing line is drawn on the bilateral standing full-length anteroposterior radiograph. **(B)** Planned axes of tibia and femur are drawn through the point of correction. *(continued)*

A, B

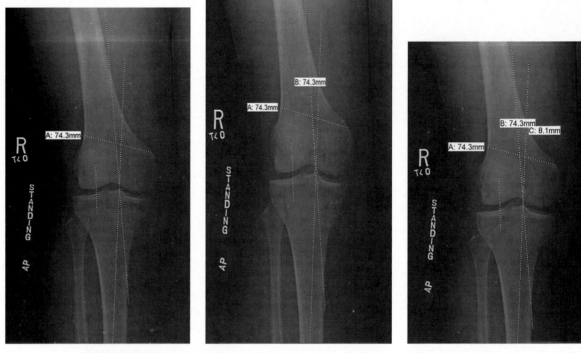

C–E

FIGURE 28-3 *(Continued)*

(C) The planned osteotomy is marked, and the length is taken. **(D)** The length is transferred to the new femoral weight-bearing line. **(E)** The horizontal distance between the lines equals the size of the corrective osteotomy.

to take out the deformity from ligamentous laxity, which would be corrected by soft tissue reconstruction. Overcorrection to varus is absolutely contraindicated if an optimal long-term result is to be gained (2,4).

SURGICAL TECHNIQUE

A distal femoral valgus osteotomy can be performed using two surgical techniques: (1) distal femoral medial closing-wedge osteotomy and (2) distal femoral lateral opening-wedge osteotomy.

Distal Femoral Medial Closing-Wedge Osteotomy

The patient is placed in the supine position on a radiolucent operating table. A tourniquet is used on the proximal thigh. A fluoroscopic C-arm is available to obtain films of the hip, knee, and ankle joints during the procedure.

After diagnostic or operative arthroscopy, a longitudinal medial incision is made along the femur, beginning from just distal to the joint line across the adductor tubercle approximately 10 cm proximal along the line of the posterior aspect of the vastus medialis (Fig. 28-4). The fascia over the vastus medialis is incised, and the muscle is dissected from the medial septum and reflected anteriorly and laterally to expose the medial part of the femoral cortex and the medial femoral condyle (Figs. 28-5 and 28-6). The neurovascular bundle is posterior to the septum proximal to this incision.

Using fluoroscopic guidance, the surgeon places a guidewire parallel to the joint line from the adductor tubercle across the distal femur (Fig. 28-7). A second guidewire is placed 2 cm distal, and a slot for a blade plate is prepared parallel to the guidewire (Fig. 28-8). The osteotomy is then fashioned at the level of the adductor tubercle (Fig. 28-9). We use a 100-degree offset dynamic compression blade plate, which is driven across the distal femur with the blade in the blade slot (Fig. 28-10) as described by McDermott et al (7). A varus manual reduction is performed, allowing the medial spike of the proximal part to dig into the distal cancellous bone (Fig. 28-11). Fixation is performed with large-fragment cortical screws using standard AO technique. The first screw is placed closest to the osteotomy and in

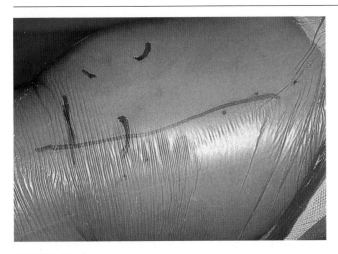

FIGURE 28-4

The skin incision is medial at the margin of the vascular medialis proximally and progresses distally over the adductor tubercle, ending approximately 2 cm distal to the joint line.

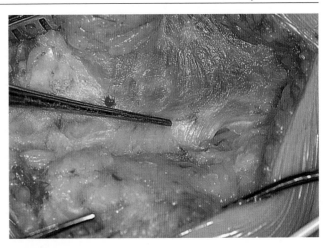

FIGURE 28-5

The posterior aspect of the vastus medialis is identified and elevated.

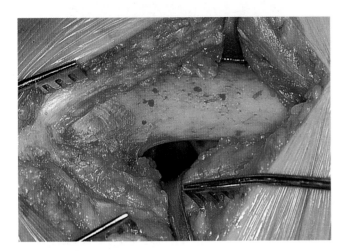

FIGURE 28-6

By elevating the vastus medialis, the distal medial aspect of the femoral shaft is identified.

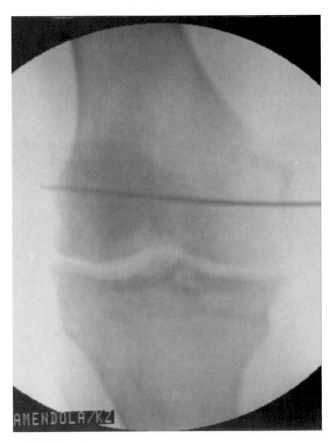

FIGURE 28-7

Using fluoroscopic guidance, a guidewire is drilled parallel to the joint line from the adductor tubercle across the distal femur.

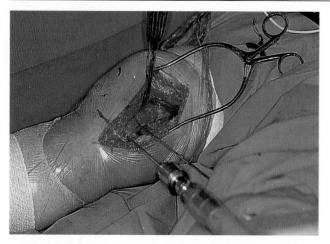

FIGURE 28-8

A fluoroscope is used to accurately place the pin just distal to the adductor tubercle and in the 10-degree varus alignment referable to the joint surface of the femoral condyles. This accommodates the 100-degree plate, which I prefer.

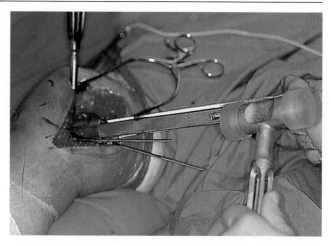

FIGURE 28-9

The osteotome follows a guide pin placed distal to the adductor tuberosity. The position is verified with a fluoroscopic spot film.

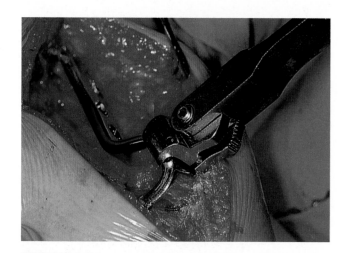

FIGURE 28-10

The 100-degree AO plate is driven across the distal femur.

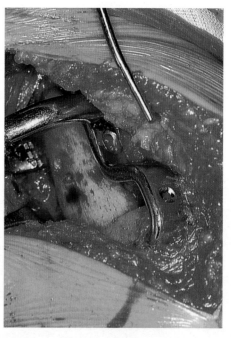

FIGURE 28-11

The medial spike of the proximal part of the femur is buried into the metaphyseal segment until the plate is resting flush against the femoral cortex.

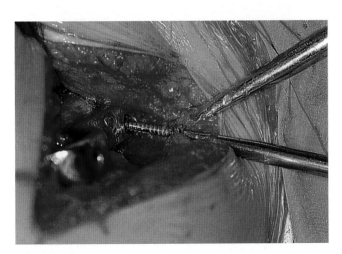

FIGURE 28-12

With the osteotomy reduced, screws are inserted routinely. The first is used in a compression mode.

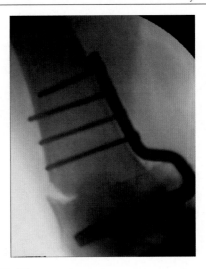

FIGURE 28-13

Fluoroscopic imaging is used to confirm accurate alignment and reduction of the osteotomy.

compression mode (Fig. 28-12). The fixation is achieved with the anatomic knee axis of 0 degrees. Fixation and alignment are again confirmed radiographically (Fig. 28-13). The tourniquet is released, and hemostasis is obtained. For wound closure, the vastus medialis obliquus is sewn to the intermuscular septum (Fig. 28-14). The wound is closed in layers, usually without a drain (2,5).

Distal Femoral Lateral Opening-Wedge Osteotomy

The distal femoral lateral opening-wedge osteotomy is the author's preferred technique. The patient is placed in the supine position on a radiolucent operating table. A tourniquet is used on the proximal thigh. A fluoroscopic C-arm is positioned to obtain films of hip, knee, and ankle joints during the procedure.

After diagnostic or operative arthroscopy, a distal midlateral thigh incision is used (Fig. 28-15). The incision is carried down to the iliotibial band. The iliotibial band is split in line with the incision down to the level of the joint line. The vastus lateralis is retracted anteriorly, and blunt dissection is

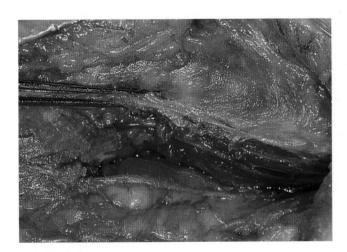

FIGURE 28-14

The vastus medialis obliquus is brought down over the plate, and closure is routine.

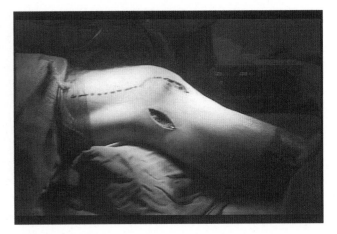

FIGURE 28-15

For a valgus opening-wedge osteotomy, a distal midlateral thigh incision is used, incising the iliotibial band down to the level of the joint line. In this case, a smaller additional lateral joint incision is present for a lateral meniscal transplantation.

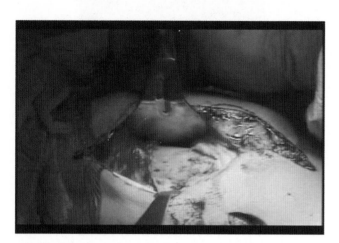

FIGURE 28-16

The vastus lateralis is dissected off the intermuscular septum and retracted anteriorly with a Bennett retractor.

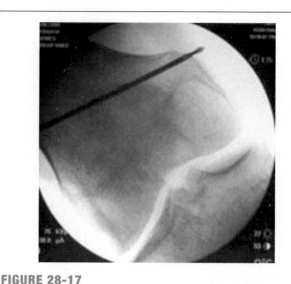

FIGURE 28-17

With the knee in extension, a guidewire is inserted from lateral and proximal to medial and distal. The medial exit point should be at or just proximal to the medial epicondyle.

carried anterior to the intermuscular septum to the femur (Fig. 28-16). A Bennett retractor is used to retract the quadriceps anteriorly, and blunt dissection is carried anterior to the intermuscular septum to the femur. The joint capsule is left intact. Cautery is used to cut the periosteum down to bone at the metaphyseal level. Subperiosteal dissection is used and retracted anteriorly and posteriorly just at the level of the osteotomy. Fluoroscopy is used to determine the level of the osteotomy. With the knee in extension, a guidewire is inserted from lateral and proximal to medial and distal (Fig. 28-17). The medial exit point should be at or just proximal to the medial epicondyle. The guidewire is kept in place during the osteotomy to protect the osteotomy from going too distal. A thin microsagittal saw is used to cut only the lateral cortex, and then a sharp and thin osteotome is used to osteotomize the femur along the proximal aspect of the guidewire under fluoroscopic guidance. (Fig. 28-18A,B). The osteotomy is continued medially to just within 1 cm of the medial cortex, a depth usually of 60 mm. At this point, the osteotomy site should open slightly with manual varus stress, indicating that the wedge opener may be inserted. The wedge opener is inserted with a mallet, slowly and carefully,

A,B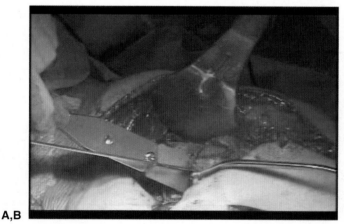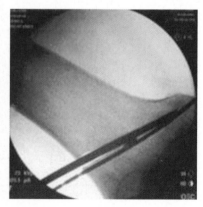

FIGURE 28-18

(A,B) The guidewire is kept in place during the osteotomy to protect the osteotomy from going too distal. A thin microsagittal saw is used to cut only the lateral cortex, and then a sharp and thin osteotome is used to osteotomize the femur along the proximal aspect of the guidewire under fluoroscopic guidance. The osteotomy is continued medially to just within 1 cm of the medial cortex.

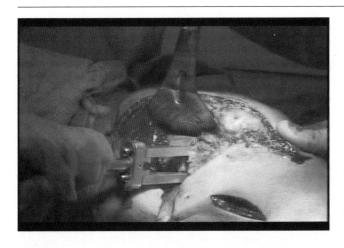

FIGURE 28-19

The osteotomy site is opened slightly with manual varus stress and the wedge opener is inserted with a mallet, slowly and carefully, to the desired amount of correction.

to the desired amount of correction (Fig. 28-19). Fluoroscopy is used to assess the opening and the limb correction. The distal femoral osteotomy T-shaped plate (Arthrex, Naples, FL) is inserted and fixed with three 6.5-mm cancellous screws distally and with four 4.5-mm cortical screws proximally (Fig. 28-20). Fixation and alignment are again confirmed radiographically (Fig. 28-21). We then insert fashioned wedges of femoral head allograft and morselized cancellous graft into the osteotomy site. Alternatively, autogenous tricortical iliac crest graft may be used. The tourniquet is released, and hemostasis is performed. The wound is closed in layers without a drain (2).

POSTOPERATIVE MANAGEMENT

Postoperatively, the knee is protected in a hinged brace in full extension or in slight flexion for 6 weeks, with range of motion from 0 to 90 degrees for therapy. Continuous passive motion is allowed on the first postoperative day. The patient is kept partial weight bearing within the maximum limit of 25 pounds with crutches for 6 weeks postoperatively. When postoperative knee pain and effusion are minimal, range of motion, flexibility, and isometric strengthening exercises are commenced. If there is radiographic evidence of union at 6 weeks, the patient is advanced to weight bearing as tolerated, and the brace and crutches are discontinued. A bicycle is used for conditioning, and resistance training is initiated as tolerated. At 12 weeks, with appropriate evidence of radiographic healing, a jogging program is initiated. Sport-specific training is begun from 5 to 6 months if range of motion is full and if symptoms have resolved.

The exercise program should also integrate core strengthening, which requires that patients maintain continual balance between protection and function (2,4).

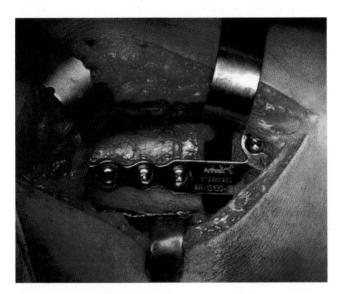

FIGURE 28-20

The plate is secured to the femur cortex with two (rarely three) distal cancellous screws and all four cortical screws. (Reprinted with permission from Jackson DW. *Master Techniques in Orthopaedic Surgery: Reconstructive Knee Surgery.* Philadelphia: Lippincott Williams & Wilkins; 2007.)

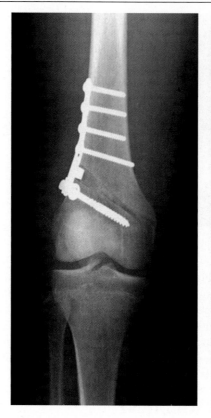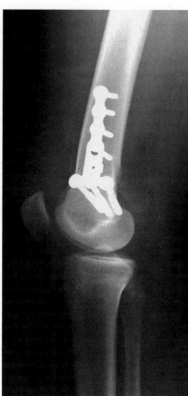

FIGURE 28-21

Post-operative AP and lateral radiographs demonstrating the osteotomy and fixation with a Puddu plate. The osteotomy gap is filled with structural graft from femoral head allograft at the cortex, with morselized graft placed in the medullary defect. Alignment is restored.

COMPLICATIONS

The risk of intra-articular fracture is always present if the guidewire is positioned too close to the joint. Otherwise, intra-articular fracture may result from failure to completely osteotomize the posterior or anterior cortex.

Subluxation or instability of the osteotomy can occur when the surgeon does not leave a sufficient hinge of intact bone. This problem can be avoided by stopping the cut 1 cm short of the opposite cortex to ensure creating a hinge allowing angular correction.

The plate should be completely in contact with the femoral shaft to avoid impaired fixation and screw or plate failure, collapse of the osteotomy, and malunion or nonunion (4).

The risk of distal femoral osteotomy nonunion is approximately 5% of cases; consolidation may be slow and can take up to 6 months (5).

Thrombophlebitis and infection are complications common to all surgical procedures performed on the lower limb and should be treated with prophylaxes or in accordance with usual standards.

Neurovascular injury is uncommon in these procedures, but extreme care must be taken during the procedure to protect the posterior neurovascular structures with a retractor and avoid inadvertent penetration posteriorly with the saw or osteotome.

Screw breakage or failure arises when weight bearing is allowed too early in the postoperative period prior to union of the osteotomy.

RESULTS

Backstein et al reviewed a series of 40 distal femoral osteotomies for a mean of 10 years (range, 3 to 12 years). Patient age at the time of distal femoral varus osteotomy (DFVO) was 44 years (range, 20 to 67 years). At most recent follow-up, there were 60% good and excellent results and 15% fair and poor results. Two thirds of the patients in the fair/poor group were awaiting total knee arthroplasty and 20% had already been converted to total knee arthroplasty. The 10-year survival rate was 82%, and the 15-year survival rate was 45%, showing clear deterioration over time. Despite deteriorating results, the investigators felt that the procedure was indicated for relatively young patients with isolated lateral compartment arthritis and valgus deformity.

The results of total knee arthroplasty after a varus distal femoral osteotomy are compromised compared with those of primary arthroplasty performed in a patient without a prior femoral osteotomy (8). Surgical exposure, retained hardware, extra-articular deformity, and metaphyseal-diaphyseal offset make the approach difficult, ligament balancing challenging, and compromise the ability to use stems.

REFERENCES

1. Segal NA, Buckwalter JA, Amendola A. Other surgical techniques for osteoarthritis. *Best Pract Res Clin Rheumatol* 2006;20:155–176.
2. Phisitkul P, Wolf BR, Amendola A. Role of high tibial and distal femoral osteotomies in the treatment of lateral-posterolateral and medial instabilities of the knee. *Sports Med Arthrosc Rev* 2006;14:96–104.
3. Wang JW, Hsu CC. Distal femoral varus osteotomy for osteoarthritis of the knee. *J Bone Joint Surg Am* 2006;88-A(Suppl 1):100–108.
4. Puddu G, Cipolla M, Cerullo G, et al. Osteotomies: the surgical treatment of the valgus knee. *Sports Med Arthrosc Rev* 2007;15:15–22.
5. Edgerton BC, Mariani EM, Morrey BF. Distal femoral varus osteotomy for painful genu valgum. A five- to 11- year follow-up study. *Clin Orthop Relat Res* 1993;288:263–269.
6. Dugdale TW, Noyes FR, Styer D. Preoperative planning for high tibial osteotomy. *Clin Orthop* 1992;274:248–264.
7. McDermott AG, Finklstein JA, Farine I. Distal femoral varus osteotomy for valgus deformity of the knee. *J Bone Joint Surg Am* 1988;70-A:110–116.
8. Nelson CL, Saleh KJ, Kassim RA, et al. Total knee arthroplasty after varus osteotomy of the distal part of the femur. *J Bone Joint Surg Am* 2003;85-A:1062–1065.

29 Periprosthetic Femur and Tibia Fractures After Total Knee Arthroplasty

Richard Iorio, Robert Trousdale, and William L. Healy

EPIDEMIOLOGY

The population of the United States is projected to increase 33% to 400 million people by 2043. The number of people over the age of 45 is expected to increase 37% to 150 million by 2030, and Americans over the age of 65 will increase 74% to 61 million people by 2025. (1) As the population ages and increases, more patients will develop painful arthritic knees, and the demand for surgical treatment of the knee will continue to increase. In 2005, the number of primary total knee arthroplasty (TKA) procedures reached 523,000, and the number of revision TKA procedures reached 37,000 (2). By 2030, the number of primary TKA procedures is expected to reach 3.48 million annually, an increase of 565%, and the number of revision TKA procedures is expected to reach 268,000 annually, an increase of 601% (3).

Periprosthetic fractures above and below TKA are becoming more prevalent because of the aging population, the increasing number of TKA operations, and the increasing time in situ of the implant. Periprosthetic supracondylar fractures above a TKA occur in 0.3% to 2.5% of patients (4). Periprosthetic tibial fractures associated with TKA occur in 0.39% to 0.5% of patients. Periprosthetic fractures around TKA can occur both intraoperatively and postoperatively. Complication rates associated with the treatment of these injuries have been reported to be as high as 25% to 75% (6). Recognition and appropriate intervention are critical to the successful treatment of these injuries.

Risk factors commonly associated with intraoperative fractures complicating TKA include osteopenia, revision operation, the use of canal fitting, press fit, stemmed components, and inadequate removal of retained cement (7). Risk factors associated with periprosthetic fracture after TKA operation include osteopenic bone, osteolysis, inflammatory arthritis, female gender, increasing age, corticosteroid use, neurologic disorder, previous revision knee surgery, and constrained implants (6–8).

Minimal trauma can lead to postoperative fractures following TKA. Additionally, major trauma, seizure activity, and the manipulation of a TKA for inadequate motion can also lead to periprosthetic fractures. Anterior notching of the distal femur can be a predisposing factor to periprosthetic TKA fracture in osteopenic bone (4–8). It has been suggested that violation of the anterior cortex of the distal femur and osteopenic bone can predispose to perioperative fracture, and these deficiencies should be bypassed by a stemmed femoral component to avoid postoperative periprosthetic fractures (4).

PREOPERATIVE CLASSIFICATION AND PLANNING

Several classifications have been developed to aid in the treatment of periprosthetic fractures around TKA. The goal of fracture classification is to develop an algorithm for treatment that is reproducible and easily implemented. The classification system of Lewis and Rorabeck accomplishes these goals (Table 29-1) (9). The system can be applied equally to the femur and tibia. Preoperative planning requires methodical assessment of the fracture pattern, determination of whether the implant is stable or loose, and appraisal of the quality of bone. Ordering of appropriate fixation devices or implants is necessary beforehand to avoid being ill prepared for the challenges of fracture surgery, which are often unpredictable.

Type I fractures are nondisplaced, and the implant is stable. Successful treatment can be operative or nonoperative depending on the patient's general health, prefracture ambulatory status, bone quality, fracture pattern, fracture stability, and type of implant. Although early motion and prevention of displacement or malunion are advantages of operative intervention with internal fixation, there are patients who may be better served with nonoperative treatment. Patients who may not be able to tolerate anesthesia, surgical blood loss, wound healing, infection, and loss of fixation may be candidates for nonoperative treatment. Nonoperative treatment options include skeletal traction (rarely used), casting, or bracing (4). When surgical intervention is not indicated, the fracture is usually immobilized in extension for 4 to 6 weeks, and weight bearing is protected.

Type II fractures are displaced, and the prosthesis is intact with no evidence of loosening. The goals of treatment are restoration of prefracture alignment, achievement of fracture stability with stable, internal fixation, and the restoration of early motion and function. There are many techniques available to achieve these goals. Advantages of surgical treatment include anatomic (or near anatomic) fracture reduction, early range of motion of the knee, and prevention of late fracture displacement.

TABLE 29-1. Total Knee Arthroplasty Periprosthetic Fracture Classification

Type I	Undisplaced fractures; prosthesis intact
Type II	Displaced fracture; prosthesis intact
Type III	Displaced or undisplaced fracture; prosthesis loose or failing

Reprinted with permission from Lewis PL, Rorabeck CH. Periprosthetic Fractures. In: Eng GA, Rorabeck CH, eds. *Revision Total Knee Arthroplasty.* Baltimore, MD: Williams & Wilkins; 1997:275–295.

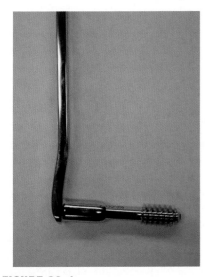

FIGURE 29-1
Distal condylar screw and side plate.

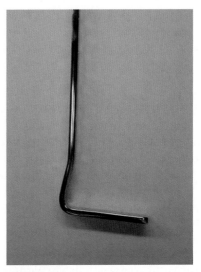

FIGURE 29-2
Ninety-five-degree angled blade plate.

Type III fractures may or may not be displaced, but the implant is not stable and requires revision to achieve a functional knee. Bone quality and fracture pattern will determine how the bone stock is restored. If there is missing bone and structural integrity cannot be achieved with internal fixation combined with a revision TKA operation, then additional allograft bone may be necessary or a bone-replacing prosthesis may be used.

SURGICAL TECHNIQUES FOR PERIPROSTHETIC FEMORAL FRACTURES AROUND TKA

Operative treatment of displaced periprosthetic femur fractures around TKA has been shown to offer the best patient outcome as defined by a well-aligned, well-functioning, stable implant after fracture healing (4,10–12). There are five surgical treatment options for treating type II fractures including a distal condylar screw and side plate, a 95-degree blade plate, a condylar buttress plate, a locking periarticular plate (i.e., less-invasive stabilization system plating), and a retrograde supracondylar intramedullary nail (Figs. 29-1 to 29-4). Obstacles to obtaining stable fixation of these fractures include osteopenic bone, fracture comminution, the amount and quality of bone left in the distal condylar fragment attached to the implant, and the design of the femoral component.

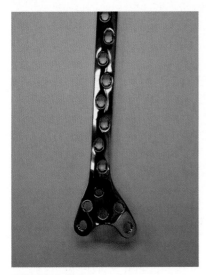

FIGURE 29-3
Condylar buttress plate.

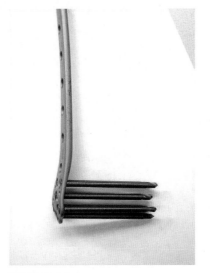

FIGURE 29-4
Periarticular locking plate.

FIXED-ANGLE PLATING

Open reduction with plate fixation using a 95-degree blade plate or distal condylar screw and side plate has provided predictable fixation when treating these fractures. It is imperative that radiographs identify the degree of comminution and any intercondylar extension of the fracture. Multiple oblique views of the distal femur along with true anterior-posterior and lateral projections are a must. Three-dimensional reconstructions of these injuries on computed tomography scan may be helpful in delineating fracture lines obscured by the implant. Depending on the geometry of the distal fragment and the quality of bone, stable fracture fixation can be obtained, which allows early motion and restoration of knee function. In severely osteopenic bone, polymethylmethacrylate or allograft bone can be used to augment fixation in the distal condylar fragment.

At times, the distal condylar fragment is too small to accommodate a distal condylar screw and side plate. A blade plate will preserve distal bone for fixation (Figs. 29-5 to 29-7). If intercondylar extension is present, adjunct fixation with large screws can be added adjacent to the blade and may be placed prior to the seating chisel to prevent further fracture displacement. Orthogonal, anterior-posterior screws can provide a second plane of fixation to increase stability. Should fixation with the blade plate fail to provide a stable construct, then the distal condylar screw and side plate can be used if there is sufficient distal bone, or adjunctive polymethylmethacrylate can be added.

Advantages of traditional plate fixation include stable internal fixation and the restoration of alignment. Disadvantages of traditional distal plate fixation include the need for extensive soft tissue dissection and fracture exposure, potential loss of distal fixation, and varus collapse and difficulty with some posterior stabilized knee implant designs. The presence of the box that accommodates the post in a posterior stabilized knee design may limit the amount of bone available for distal fixation with plates. Measurement of construct stiffness has shown that the distal condylar screw, side plate, and the blade plate were more rigid than the condylar buttress plate for supracondylar fracture above TKA (13).

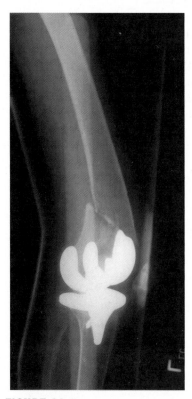

FIGURE 29-5

Supracondylar periprosthetic femur fracture above a posterior cruciate-retaining implant.

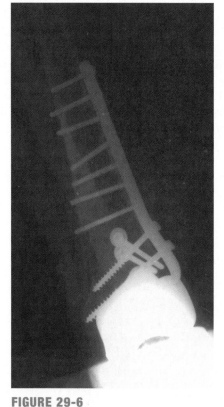

FIGURE 29-6

Anterior/posterior radiographs of a 95-degree angled blade plate fixing a supracondylar femur fracture.

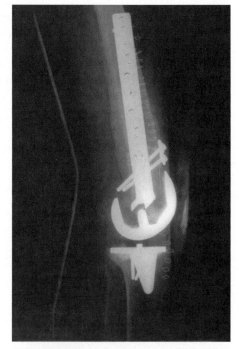

FIGURE 29-7

Lateral radiograph of a 95-degree angled blade plate fixing a supracondylar femur fracture.

RETROGRADE SUPRACONDYLAR INTRAMEDULLARY NAIL

Intramedullary retrograde supracondylar femoral nails have been used to treat periprosthetic distal femur fractures. Retrograde nailing is an attractive concept because of limited soft tissue dissection and exposure and a theoretically rigid construct. If there is a sufficient distal fragment to allow two rigid distal interlocking screws (generally 2 to 3 cm of distal bone above the prosthesis), then a retrograde supracondylar intramedullary nail can be used. These retrograde nails can be placed through a relatively small medial parapatellar arthrotomy, if there is a posterior cruciate-retaining implant in place (Figs. 29-8 and 29-9). Most cruciate-retaining knee designs can accommodate rod diameters from 11 to 20 mm (4,6–8,11). Some cruciate-substituting designs have boxes with holes that allow access to the femoral canal. These holes can be opened and will allow small 8- to 10-mm nail diameters to pass. If the box is solid or the opening is too small to accommodate the nail, a diamond-tip burr can be used to open the box. This approach generates a lot of metal debris, however, and may compromise the intra-articular integrity of the arthroplasty if care is not taken to remove all of the debris (4,6–8,11,14).

Disadvantages of retrograde intramedullary supracondylar femoral fixation include the limits of distal fixation if the distal fragment is not large enough to accommodate two rigid locking screws and the difficulties encountered with posterior-substituting designs. Additionally, controlling alignment with intramedullary fixation is difficult because of the limitation and sizes of the supracondylar nails as well as the large variability in the positions of the distal fragment in reference to the nail. Nonunion, locking-screw loosening, nail migration, valgus drift, and decreased range of motion are all reported complications. Although the union rate is high, maintenance of acceptable alignment can be difficult. Retrograde intramedullary supracondylar rod fixation should be reserved for fractures with 2 to 3 cm of bone above the prosthesis, relatively good distal bone stock that allows rigid fixation of at least two distal locking screws, and minimal proximal comminution to allow maintenance of alignment with a good diaphyseal fit (11,15). Intramedullary fixation is not as stable as blade plate or distal condylar screw and side plate fixation (13).

PERIARTICULAR LOCKING PLATES

Periarticular locking plates, also known as less-invasive stabilization system plating, are characterized by threaded screw holes in the plate that "lock" the screws to the plate (16,18). These locking screws transform the plate-screw construct into a fixed-angle device (Figs. 29-4 and 29-10). It is possible to insert these plates and screws through small incisions without exposing the fracture directly. Screw placement can be performed percutaneously and/or through the use of a jig. The periarticular locking plates allow multiple points of fixation with angular stability, and the construct can function like an internalized external fixator. The internalized external fixation function allows periarticular

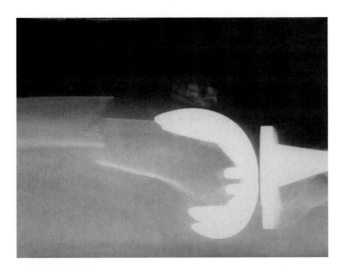

FIGURE 29-8

Lateral radiograph of a supracondylar periprosthetic femur fracture in a posterior cruciate-retaining implant.

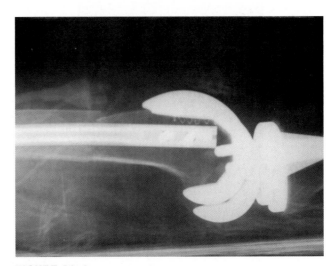

FIGURE 29-9

Lateral radiograph of an intramedullary supracondylar femoral nail fixing a periprosthetic femur fracture.

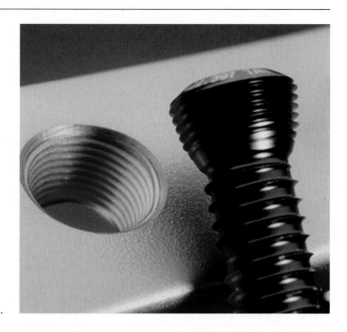

FIGURE 29-10

Periarticular locking plate with locking screw.

locked plates to act as a bridge over metaphyseal comminution with minimal fragment stripping and the maintenance of alignment (Figs. 29-11 to 29-14).

Advantages of periarticular locking plates for the treatment of periprosthetic, distal femur fractures include the achievement of coronal plane stability and maintenance of alignment, the ability to vary the points of fixation distally, the potential for screws to miss lugs, boxes, and stems of the femoral implant, making distal fixation easier to achieve with very distal fractures (Figs. 29-15 to 29-20).

Disadvantages of periarticular locking plates include a reduction in torsional stability compared with retrograde intramedullary nails when anterior and posterior loads are applied to comminuted fractures. Additionally, early models of the periarticular locking plate did not vary the trajectory of the distal locking screws, thus making distal fixation more difficult to attain with osteoporotic bone (Fig. 29-21). More recent variations of the periarticular locking plates allow variable distal screw trajectory with the ability to add a larger-diameter locking screw that resembles a distal condylar screw (Fig. 29-22), and which can be helpful for treating comminuted osteoporotic fractures after TKA (Fig. 29-3).

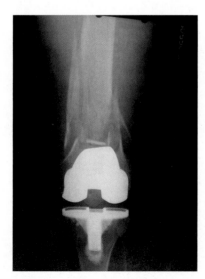

FIGURE 29-11

Anteroposterior radiograph of a periprosthetic femur fracture in a posterior cruciate-substituting implant.

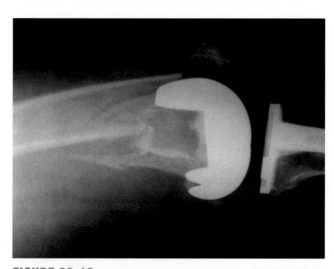

FIGURE 29-12

Lateral radiograph of a periprosthetic femur fracture in a posterior cruciate-substituting implant.

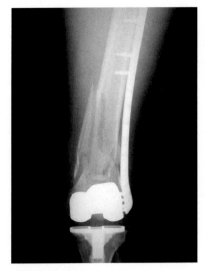

FIGURE 29-13

Anteroposterior radiograph of a periarticular locking plate bridging metaphyseal comminution.

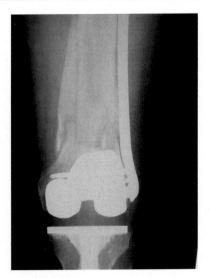

FIGURE 29-14

Healed anteroposterior radiograph of a periarticular locking plate bridging metaphyseal comminution.

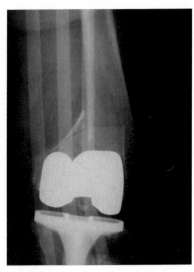

FIGURE 29-15

Anteroposterior radiograph of a supracondylar periprosthetic femur fracture with distal extension.

PEARLS AND PITFALLS

Intraoperative Techniques for Periarticular Locking Plates

Regardless of which method of fixation is used, patient setup can be standardized. A radiolucent table is used, and the patient is positioned supine with a small rolled towel or sheet under the buttock to internally rotate the limb slightly. The limb is prepared and draped, so access high up on the thigh is achieved. The upper thigh, anterior hemipelvis, and buttock should be accessible to ensure that the necessary areas of the upper thigh are not draped out of the field. A sterile tourniquet is helpful so that proximal exposure is achievable. Fluoroscopic imaging is used.

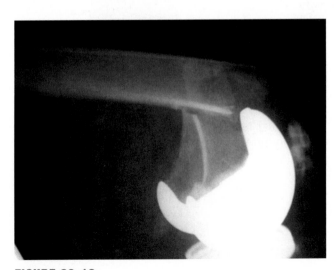

FIGURE 29-16

Lateral radiograph of a supracondylar periprosthetic femur fracture with distal extension.

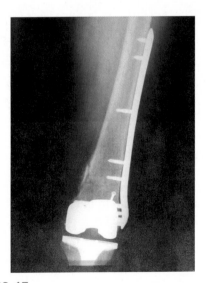

FIGURE 29-17

Periarticular locking plate illustrating a healed periprosthetic supracondylar femur fracture with distal extension.

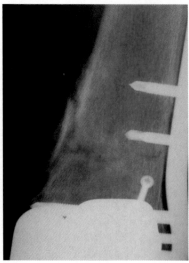

FIGURE 29-18

Anteroposterior radiographic close-up of a healed supracondylar periprosthetic femur fracture with distal extension.

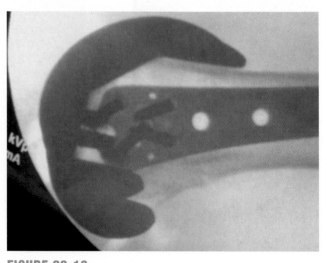

FIGURE 29-19

Intraoperative lateral fluoroscopic image illustrating the ability of a periarticular locking plate to bypass distal lugs and obtain distal fixation in a fracture with distal extension.

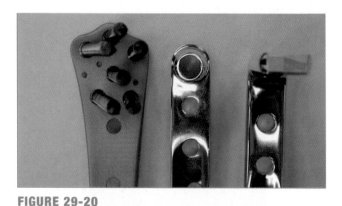

FIGURE 29-20

A comparison of distal fixation of a periarticular locking plate, a distal condylar screw, side plate, and a 95-degree blade plate. Note the ability of the periarticular locking plate to obtain fixation in multiple different locations.

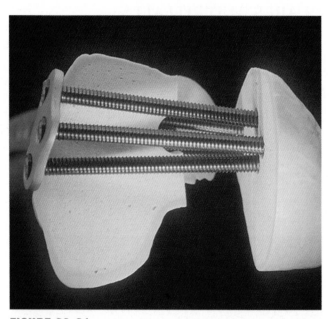

FIGURE 29-21

Periarticular locking plate without variable screw trajectory for distal fixation.

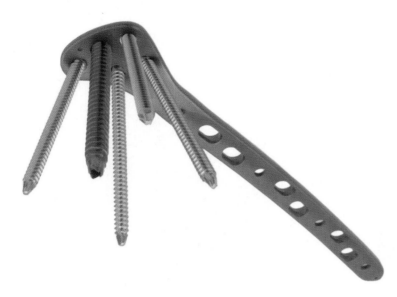

FIGURE 29-22

Screw pattern of a variable trajectory periarticular locking plate.

The well leg is positioned out of the penetration field of a horizontally placed fluoroscopy beam. The fractured extremity is placed on a bump underneath the injured knee and in slight flexion (Figs. 29-24 to 29-26). The bump is then placed under the fracture, and reduction is confirmed fluoroscopically. Gentle longitudinal manual traction may be necessary to assist reduction (Fig. 29-26). Flexion of the knee will relax the pull of the gastrocnemius muscles on the distal femoral fragment, counteracting the tendency of the distal fragment to flex.

Through a limited lateral approach, the plate is placed distally and slid up along the femoral shaft proximally with the alignment jig attached. Limited distal fixation is obtained (Figs. 29-27 to 29-30). The plate is locked proximally. Reduction is confirmed and adjusted as needed. Additional fixation is added to maintain alignment and ensure stability (Figs. 29-31 and 29-32). Medial metaphyseal comminution may predispose to collapse into varus. Femoral or fibular strut allografts may be applied to the regions of comminution and secured with cerclage wire or cables to buttress the compromised cortex and reduce the risk of collapse (Fig. 29-33). Fluoroscopic visualization is critical to allow minimal fracture exposure and maximal use of percutaneous fixation (Figs. 29-34 to 29-39). Although minimally invasive approaches are attractive in their ability to preserve vascularity of the fracture fragments, the basic principles of hardware selection, fracture reduction, and stabilization are typically applied through a more extensile approach and should be used by surgeons with less experience with the limited-incision approaches.

(text continues on p. 398)

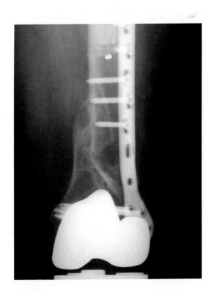

FIGURE 29-23

Anteroposterior radiograph showing a healed periprosthetic supracondylar femur fracture above a total knee replacement and below a total hip replacement with metaphyseal bridging and healing with good alignment of a comminuted fracture.

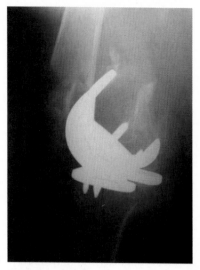
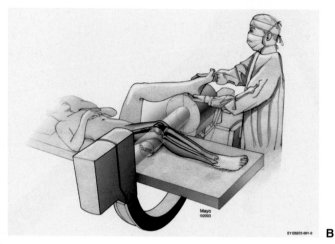

FIGURE 29-24

(A) Lateral radiograph of displaced supracondylar periprosthetic femur fracture with distal extension. **(B)** Optimal intraoperative positioning of the patient in slight flexion over a bump at the fracture site with positioning of the fluoroscopy equipment for visualization in both the anteroposterior and lateral projections. Note the positioning of the well leg to obtain optimal lateral visualization.

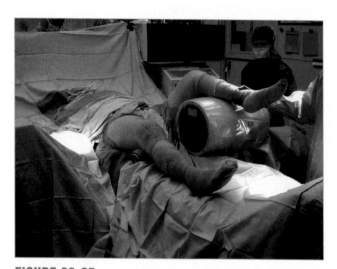

FIGURE 29-25

Actual intraoperative positioning for reduction and internal fixation of a supracondylar periprosthetic fracture.

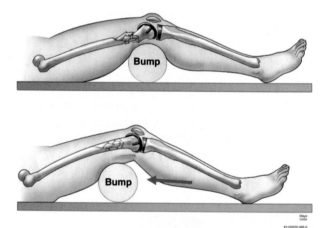

FIGURE 29-26

Using a bump under the fracture site to reduce the fracture with gentle traction and slight flexion.

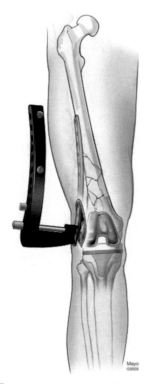

FIGURE 29-27

Insertion of a periarticular less-invasive locking plate with the screw jig attached. Note the minimal distal fracture exposure and a minimally invasive approach to placing proximal screws.

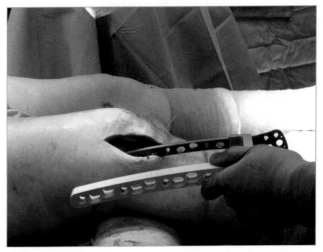

FIGURE 29-28

Intraoperative photograph of insertion of a periarticular locking plate using minimally invasive techniques.

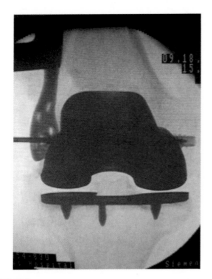

FIGURE 29-29

Intraoperative fluoroscopic imaging of an anteroposterior view obtained while distal fixation is confirmed.

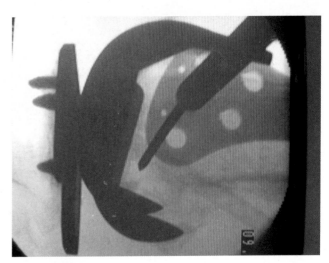

FIGURE 29-30

Lateral fluoroscopic imaging of distal fixation with a periarticular locking plate.

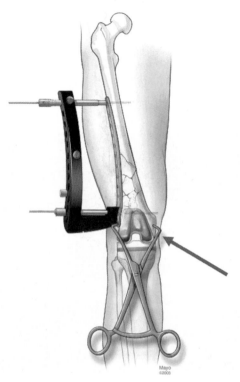

FIGURE 29-31

The interlocking jig obtains proximal locking of the less-invasive periarticular locking plate.

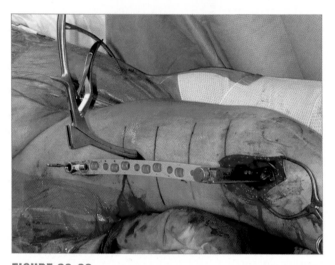

FIGURE 29-32

Intraoperative photograph of periarticular plate-locking jig being used to obtain proximal locking-plate fixation.

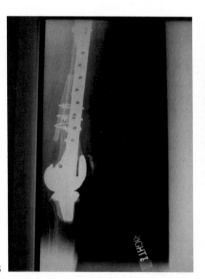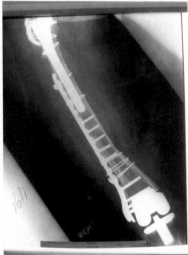

A,B

FIGURE 29-33

(A,B) Anteroposterior and lateral radiographs after ORIF of a comminuted periprosthetic femur fracture in a patient with severe osteoporosis and rheumatoid arthritis. Medial and posterior fibular strut allografts were used to buttress areas of comminution, in addition to the condylar buttress plate.

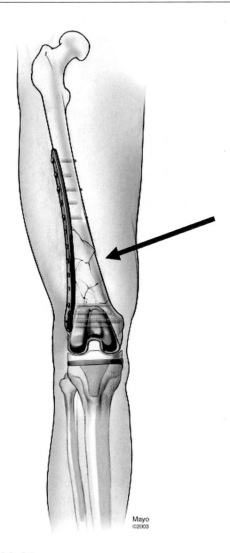

FIGURE 29-34

A distally and proximally locked periarticular plate that bridges metaphyseal comminution.

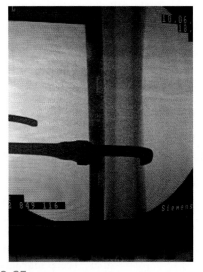

FIGURE 29-35

Intraoperative fluoroscopic image of a periarticular locking plate being seated adequately above the fracture site.

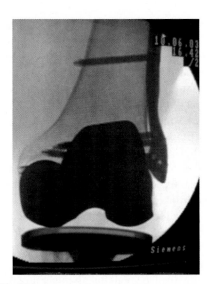

FIGURE 29-36

Distal anteroposterior fluoroscopic imaging of a periarticular locking plate.

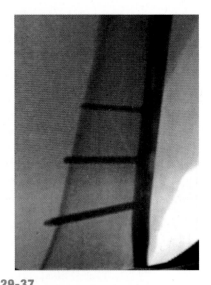

FIGURE 29-37

Fluoroscopic imaging of proximal interlocking screws in a well-seated periarticular locking plate.

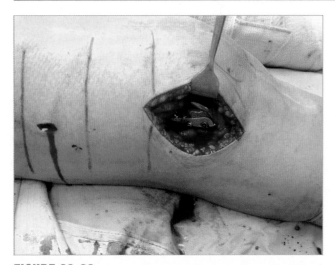

FIGURE 29-38

Intraoperative photograph of a minimal distal incision used to expose a supracondylar periprosthetic femur fracture.

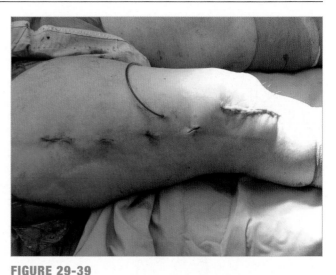

FIGURE 29-39

Intraoperative photograph of the extent of the less-invasive approach associated with a periarticular locking plate used to fix a supracondylar periprosthetic femur fracture.

TYPE III PERIPROSTHETIC DISTAL FEMUR FRACTURES

Type III periprosthetic distal femur fractures have a loose femoral component. These complex fractures require a fracture stabilization operation and revision TKA operation. If the distal fragment is large, and if the epicondyles and medial and lateral ligamentous attachments are intact, revision TKA operation with a stemmed component and conventional revision prosthesis is possible.

In type III fractures, in which the quality of the distal bone will not support a conventional prosthesis, two options are available: (a) distal femoral replacement or (b) an allograft-prosthesis composite. Distal femoral replacement is reserved for elderly or sedentary individuals with poor bone stock. These implants are by definition highly constrained and are not optimal in high-demand, younger patients. An allograft-prosthetic composite allows a one-stage operation with early mobilization. The allograft-prosthetic composite option is technically more demanding and has a higher degree of morbidity in the perioperative period than the distal femoral replacement, which is considered the more expedient operation (Figs. 29-40 to 29-43) (19,21).

SURGICAL TECHNIQUES FOR PERIPROSTHETIC TIBIAL FRACTURES AROUND TKA

Fractures of the tibia can occur during the performance of a TKA operation or postoperatively. Intraoperative fractures can occur during component removal, preparation of the tibia for a stemmed component, impaction/insertion of a keeled or stemmed component, or trial reduction. Postoperative fractures can be secondary to high- or low-velocity trauma and may be associated with loosening, osteolysis, malalignment, or stress risers around the implant (6,8,23–25). Stress fractures after unicompartmental knee arthroplasty and navigated TKA have been reported because of pin use for alignment jigs or navigation transmitters. Care must be taken to avoid diaphyseal placement of navigation pins and the propagation of fractures from the tibial keel to the cortical interruption from pins in the tibial plateau after unicompartmental knee arthroplasty (26–28).

Type I tibial periprosthetic fractures occurring after TKA not associated with malalignment or instability can be treated with traditional fracture management techniques (6). Tibial metaphyseal fractures are not as frequent as those seen in the femur (29). Non-displaced fractures with an intact, well-fixed implant can be managed with bracing or casting.

Type II tibial periprosthetic fractures with fracture displacement but an intact prosthesis can be managed by buttress plating or periarticular locked plating. Technical pitfalls include avoiding the

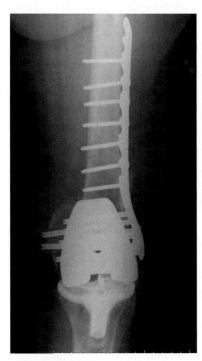

FIGURE 29-40

Anteroposterior radiograph of a comminuted periprosthetic supracondylar femur fracture with a loose implant.

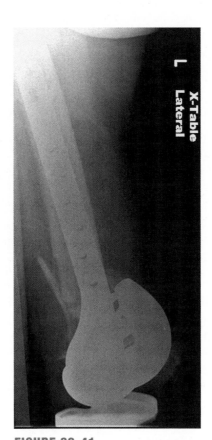

FIGURE 29-41

Lateral radiograph of a periprosthetic supracondylar femur fracture with a loose implant.

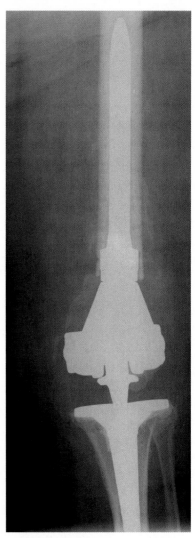

FIGURE 29-42

An anteroposterior radiograph of a distal femoral replacement.

tibial keel proximally with anterior and posterior screws and preserving the integrity of the proximal cement mantle in an intact prosthesis. Stable fixation and maintenance/restoration of alignment is the goal of managing periprosthetic fractures of the tibia. Tibial tubercle osteotomy can be a risk factor leading to tibial periprosthetic fracture after revision TKA (Figs. 29-44 to 29-46) (8,25).

Diaphyseal extension can be managed by extending a plate distally or by revising the tibial implant to a stemmed component and using the stem component as an intramedullary rod to bypass the fracture. Adjunctive fixation can be added as needed to stabilize the diaphyseal shaft around the implant stem. Periarticular locking plates can be helpful in managing diaphyseal extension in a less-invasive manner than traditional diaphyseal plating with buttress plates.

Type III tibial periprosthetic fractures involve a loose implant. The implant and cement are removed; the fracture is reduced, and the fracture is bypassed with a stemmed tibial component. Distally, cementless stems are used to prevent cement intrusion into the fracture and disruption of fracture healing. Additional internal fixation is added as needed to supplement reduction, alignment, and support of the implant (Figs. 29-47 to 29-50) (8,25,29).

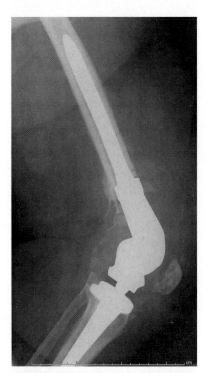

FIGURE 29-43
Lateral radiograph of a distal femoral replacement.

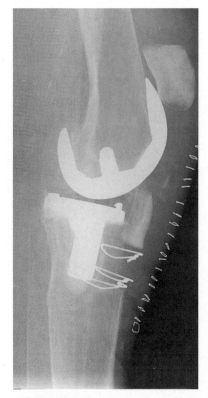

FIGURE 29-44
Lateral radiograph of a metaphyseal periprosthetic tibia fracture secondary to a fracture through a tibial tubercle osteotomy.

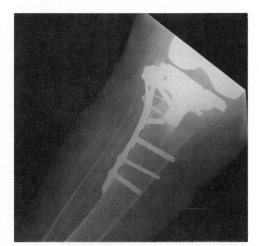

FIGURE 29-45
Anteroposterior radiograph of a healed periarticular locking plate used to internally fix a metaphyseal periprosthetic tibia fracture.

COMPLICATIONS

Soft tissue management of tibia fractures can be difficult when arthroplasty is involved. Avoiding extensive soft tissue disruption on the anterior surface of the tibia and the extensor surface of the knee decreases the risk of postoperative wound problems. An intramedullary stem and periarticular less-invasive locking plates minimize the extent of soft tissue disruption and subsequent postoperative infection. Preservation of the extensor mechanism is critical to the eventual function of the TKA. Prophylactic fixation of the tibial tubercle in the presence of metaphyseal fracture with anterior extension may be advised to prevent postoperative disruption of the extensor function. Nonunion and malunion may occur if inadequate fixation of a tibial fracture causes displacement and loss of alignment.

RESULTS

The management of periprosthetic fractures after TKA can be challenging. Union rates with nonoperative treatment of nondisplaced supracondylar femoral fractures and intact implants have been reported in the range of 65% to 100% of patients (30). Success with operative intervention for these injuries has varied widely (30% to 100% union rate) and depends on stability of fixation, maintenance of alignment, and degree of fracture shortening. The combination of fracture fixation and TKA revision has not been well discussed in the literature, and success rates are not available. Tibia fractures, in association with TKA, are rare and also have not been well discussed in the literature. The addition of less-invasive management techniques such as periarticular locking plates and intramedullary supracondylar nails have made soft tissue management of these injuries less difficult. It remains to be seen if nonunion or malunion rates will be affected.

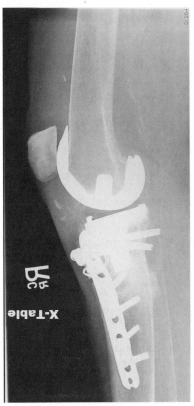

FIGURE 29-46

Lateral radiograph of a periarticular locking plate used to internally fix a metaphyseal periprosthetic tibia fracture.

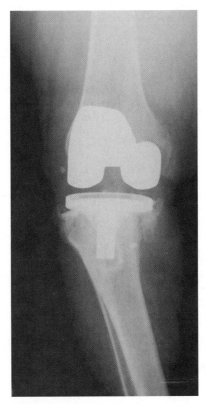

FIGURE 29-47

Anteroposterior radiograph of a medial tibial plateau fracture and a loose tibial implant.

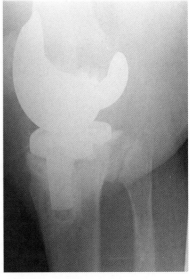

FIGURE 29-48

Lateral radiograph of a loose tibial implant and a medial tibial plateau fracture.

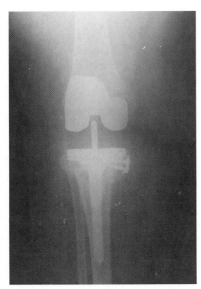

FIGURE 29-49

Anteroposterior radiograph of a revision tibial component with intramedullary stem and internal fixation of a tibial plateau fracture.

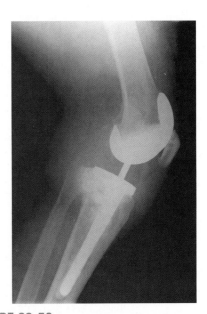

FIGURE 29-50

Lateral radiograph of a revision stemmed tibial implant with ORIF of a tibial plateau fracture.

REFERENCES

1. Frankowski JJ, Watkins-Castillo S. Primary Total Knee and Hip Arthroplasty Projections for the United States Population to the Year 2030. AAOS Dept of Research and Scientific Affairs. Rosemont, IL 2002:1–8.

2. Mendenhall S. 2006 hip and knee implant review. *Orthopaedic Network News* 2006;17:1–3.

3. Kurtz SM, Lau E, Zhao K, et al. Projections of primary and revision hip and knee arthroplasty in the United States from 2005–2030. *J Bone Joint Surg* 2007;89:780–785.

4. Su ET, Dewal H, Decesare PE: Periprosthetic femoral fractures above total knee replacement. *J Am Acad Orthop Surg* 2004;12:12–20.

5. Burnett RS, Bourne RB. Periprosthetic fractures of the tibia and patella in total knee arthroplasty. *AAOS Instr Course Lect* 2004;53:217–235.

6. Dennis DA. Revision total knee arthroplasty: periprosthetic fractures following total knee arthroplasty: the good, bad, and ugly. *Orthopaedics* 1998;21:1048–1050.

7. Rorabeck CH. Problems following total knee arthroplasty, periprosthetic fractures: a problem on the rise. *Orthopaedics* 2000;23:989–990.

8. Callaghan JJ, Hanssen AD. Periprosthetic fractures following total knee arthroplasty. In: *Masters Techniques in Orthopaedic Surgery: Knee Arthroplasty*, 2nd ed. Philadelphia, PA: Williams & Wilkins; 2002:421–434.

9. Lewis PL, Rorabeck CH. Periprosthetic Fractures. In: Eng GA, Rorabeck CH, eds. *Revision Total Knee Arthroplasty*. Baltimore, MD: Williams & Wilkins; 1997:275–295.

10. Healy WL, Siliski JM, Incavo SJ. Operative treatment of distal femoral fractures in proximal and total knee replacements. *J Bone and Joint Surg Am* 1993;75:27–34.

11. Gliatis J, Megal P, Panagiotopoulos E, Lambiris E. Midterm results of treatment with a retrograde nail for supracondylar periprosthetic fractures of the femur following total knee arthroplasty. *J Orthop Trauma* 2005;19:164–170.

12. Ricci WM, Loftus J, Cox C, Barelli J. Locked plates combined with minimally invasive insertion technique for the treatment of periprosthetic supracondylar femur fractures above a total knee arthroplasty. *J Orthop Trauma* 2006;20:190–196.

13. Cusick RP, Lucas GL, McQueen DA, Graber CD: Construct stiffness of different fixation methods for supracondylar femoral fractures above total knee prosthesis. *Amer J Orthop* 2000;29:695–699.

14. Manior RN, Umlas ME, Rodriguez JA, Ranawat CS. Supracondylar femoral fracture above a PFC posterior cruciate substituting total knee arthroplasty treated with supracondylar nailing: a unique technical problem. *J Arthroplasty* 1996;11:637–639.

15. Bezwada HP, Neubauer P, Baker J, Israelite CL, Johanson, N: Periprosthetic supracondylar femur fractures following total knee arthroplasty. *J Arthroplasty* 2004;19:453–458.

16. Althausen PL, Lee MA, Finkemaier CG, et al. Operative stabilization of supracondylar femur fractures above total knee arthroplasty: a comparison of four treatment methods. *J Arthroplasty* 2003;18:834–839.

17. Koval KJ, Kummer FJ, Sue T, et al. Comparison of LISS and a retrograde-inserted supracondylar intramedullary nail for fixation of a periprosthetic distal femur fracture proximal to a total knee arthroplasty. *J Arthroplasty* 2002;17:876–881.

18. Thuroni R, Nakasone C, Vince KG. Periprosthetic fractures after total knee arthroplasty. *J Arthroplasty* 2005;20:27–32.

19. Gross AE. Periprosthetic fractures of the knee: puzzle pieces. *J Arthroplasty* 2004;19:47–50.

20. Kalsab M, Zalzal P, Azores GMS, et al. Management of periprosthetic femoral fractures after total knee arthroplasty using a distal femoral allograft. *J Arthroplasty* 2004;19:361–368.

21. Kim KI, Egol KA, Hozack WJ, Parvizi J. Periprosthetic fractures after total knee arthroplasties. *Clin Orthop Relat Res* 2006;446:167–175.

22. Stuart MT, Hanssen AD: Total knee arthroplasty periprosthetic tibial fractures. *Orthopaed Clin N Am* 1999;30:279–286.

23. Healy WL. Tibial fractures below total knee arthroplasty. In: Insall JN, Scott WN, Scuderi GR, eds. *Current Concepts and Primary and Revision Total Knee Arthroplasty*. Philadelphia: Lippincott-Raven Publishers; 1996:163–167.

24. Burnett RS, Bourne RB. Periprosthetic fractures of the tibia and patella in total knee arthroplasty. *AAOS Instructional Course Lectures* 2004;53:217–235.

25. Felix NA, Stuart MT, Hanssen AD. Periprosthetic fractures of the tibia associated with total knee arthroplasty. *Clin Orthop Relat Res* 1997;345:113–124.

26. Rudol G, Jackson MP, James SE. Medial tibial plateau fractures complicating unicompartmental knee arthroplasty: case report. *J Arthroplasty* 2007;22:148–156.

27. Van Loon P, DeMunnynck D, Belleman J. Periprosthetic fracture of the tibial plateau after unicompartmental knee arthroplasty: case report. *Acta Orthop Belg* 2006;72:369–374.

28. Ossendorf C, Fuchs B, Koch P. Femoral stress fracture after computer navigated total knee arthroplasty: short communication. *The Knee* 2006;13:397–399.

29. Backstein D, Safri O, Gross AE. Periprosthetic fractures of the knee. *J Arthroplasty* 2007;22:45–49.

30. Kim KI, Egol KA, Hozack WJ, Parvizi J: Periprosthetic fractures after total knee arthroplasties. *Clin Orthop Relat Res* 2006;446:167–175.

30 Management of Patella Fractures After Total Knee Arthroplasty

Charles Nelson

INTRODUCTION

Patella fractures following total knee arthroplasty (TKA) are very different from traumatic patella fractures. Whereas traumatic patella fractures in nonarthroplasty patients tend to be associated with reasonably good outcomes with internal fixation, TKA patients tend to be older, have by definition had at least one prior surgical procedure to the knee that likely disrupted at least a portion of the patellar blood supply, and if they underwent patellar resurfacing, have less patellar bone stock, with less area for internal fixation and less surface area for healing. Additionally, osteonecrosis may be present because of disruption of the geniculate blood flow as well as from thermal necrosis caused by the exothermic reaction of polymerizing PMMA cement. Furthermore, TKA alters normal knee kinematics and proprioception under optimal conditions. In the setting of malrotation or malalignment, TKA may further alter kinematics and joint forces, predisposing to patellar fracture and patellar dislocation or subluxation. When malalignment and malrotation following TKA are not corrected during surgical management of a post-arthroplasty patella fracture, these abnormal forces may lead to failure of an otherwise excellent repair or reconstruction.

Indications

Patella fractures are often noted incidentally following TKA. Fractures noted incidentally on postoperative radiographs without associated symptoms may be successfully treated without surgery. Acute patellar fractures with a minimally displaced transverse component (typically displacement <5 mm) but with an intact extensor mechanism and no patellar component loosening are best managed in a locked brace or cast. In the setting of an acute fracture, immobilization in extension for approximately 6 weeks is recommended. For asymptomatic fractures noted incidentally with an intact extensor mechanism and well-fixed patellar component, observation alone is indicated (Fig. 30-1).

Although it is preferable to treat many patella fractures nonoperatively, there are some patients for whom surgery provides the only opportunity to achieve satisfactory outcomes. Indications for surgical treatment of periprosthetic patella fracture after TKA include displaced fractures with a disruption of the extensor mechanism (often manifest by displacement >5 to 10 mm and an extensor lag >20 degrees or a complete inability to extend the leg) and symptomatic fractures associated with patellar component loosening. Unfortunately, for patients who require surgical management for patella fractures after TKA, the outcomes of surgical management have often been poor (1–5).

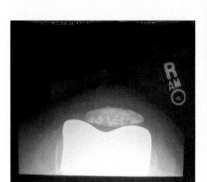
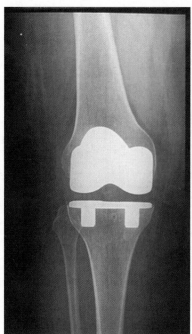
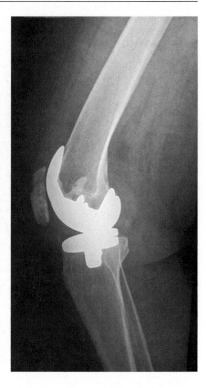

FIGURE 30-1

Incidental patella fracture noted during routine follow-up of a 47-year-old female. The patient is asymptomatic, the anterior knee is not tender, and she has full active extension, no lag, and excellent strength. There is no evidence of patellar loosening, and there is good patellar tracking. Observation alone is recommended.

CONTRAINDICATIONS

Surgical intervention is not indicated for the following fractures:

- Asymptomatic and symptomatic periprosthetic patellar stress fractures
- Asymptomatic fractures noted incidentally on radiographs
- Nondisplaced fractures
- Displaced transverse, longitudinal, and comminuted fractures with an intact extensor mechanism, well-fixed patellar implant, good function, and no or minimal pain
- Most vertical fractures
- Even in the setting of patellar component loosening, surgical intervention is generally not recommended if the extensor mechanism is intact when the patient has no or minimal symptoms, although retrieval of the patella component is recommended in this rare situation once fracture healing has occurred.

PREOPERATIVE PREPARATION

Preoperative evaluation of any patient in whom surgical management is indicated with a patella fracture after TKA includes an assessment of the femoral, tibial implants and patellar implants. A clinical and radiographic evaluation is performed to rule out infection, component loosening, instability, stiffness, neuropathic pain, and referred pain. It is important to pay particular attention to femoral and tibial component alignment and rotation. Many patients who develop patella fractures following TKA have component malalignment, malposition, and/or malrotation, as well as overstuffing of the patellofemoral compartment, which must be corrected to ensure success of surgical treatment of periprosthetic patella fractures (6,8).

Anteroposterior and lateral radiographs on a long cassette or 3-foot film are most useful for evaluating component alignment. Tangential patella views allow assessment of patellar tracking and may provide clues related to femoral and tibial rotation. Both lateral radiographs and

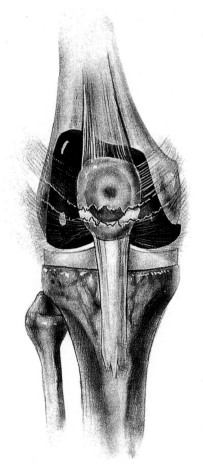

A

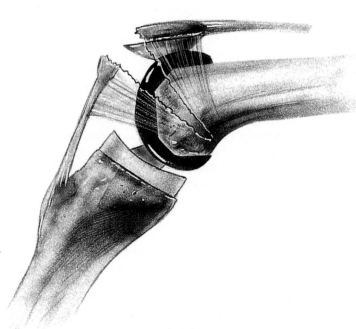

B

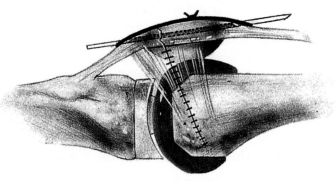

D

C

FIGURE 30-2

(A) Anterior view of a displaced transverse patellar fracture after a total knee arthroplasty. **(B)** Lateral view of a displaced patellar fracture (bone-cement interface intact). **(C)** Anterior view of the left knee after repair of the patellar fracture and retinacular repair with Kirschner wires and suture tension band before cutting and bending wires. **(D)** Lateral view of the left knee after repair of the patellar fracture and the retinacular structures.

tangential patellar views may allow analysis of whether the patellofemoral joint has been over-stuffed, particularly when compared with preoperative radiographs or the contralateral knee. Computerized tomography is particularly valuable in evaluating appropriate femoral and tibial component rotation.

Ortiguera and Berry proposed a classification scheme that is helpful in the management of patellar fractures after TKA (Table 30-1) (1). An algorithm has been recommended based on this classification scheme (1,8). For type 1 fractures, nonoperative management with either observation or immobilization in extension is recommended. For type II fractures, extensor mechanism repair with partial or complete patellectomy or open reduction with internal fixation is recommended. For type III fractures, operative treatment has been recommended if the patient is sufficiently symptomatic. For type IIIa fractures, patelloplasty with either patellar component revision or resection arthroplasty has been recommended. For type IIIb, patellar component removal with patelloplasty or complete patellectomy has been advised. Extensor mechanism allografting can be performed early for type III fractures or later if other treatment methods have failed (8).

The surgical options for treating periprosthetic patella fractures include open reduction and internal fixation, partial or complete patellectomy with extensor mechanism repair or reconstruction, and patellar component removal with or without resurfacing. Preoperative planning requires that the surgeon make certain the instruments, implants, and allograft tissues (when appropriate) needed for primary and contingency treatment plans are available. Contingency plans should include revision femoral and tibial implants and instrument sets in case femoral and/or tibial component revision is necessary.

TECHNIQUE

Because of the varied pathology encountered in the setting of periprosthetic patella fracture post-TKA, there is no single surgical technique that applies to all of the clinical presentations. The following are the author's preferred techniques for five different surgical methods of management. It is important that femoral and/or tibial component revision is performed in concert with these procedures when necessary for malalignment, malposition, malrotation, or loosening. The details of revision arthroplasty are beyond the scope of this chapter.

Regardless of the fracture treatment, the surgical approach is similar. The limb is prepared and draped, and the knee is approached through the original scar used for the TKA. Skin flaps are minimized, although large flaps may be necessary if there is disruption of the medial and lateral retinacula, in which case the flaps are made subfascial to minimize devascularization of the skin. The joint is exposed through the fracture site and the retinacular tears; a vertical arthrotomy should not be made in most cases. Hematoma is evacuated and the joint lavaged. The patella prosthesis and cement are removed if it is loose. It is retained if it is not loose.

Open Reduction and Internal Fixation

Although open reduction and internal fixation of patella fractures after TKA is often not recommended, it may be reasonable in the setting of a displaced transverse fracture with a notable extensor lag, when there is sufficient bone stock. Tension band wiring technique is used, typically using two 0.625-mm Kirschner wires (K-wires), although if residual bone is thick enough, two 4.0-mm longitudinal cannulated screws may be considered (11). Retrograde drilling of a K-wire from the fracture to the periphery proximally, and from the fracture site to the periphery distally, allows more

TABLE 30-1. Classification of Management of Patellar Fractures After Total Knee Arthroplasty
Type 1: Stable patellar component and intact extensor mechanism
Type 2: Disrupted extensor mechanism
Type 3a – Loose patellar component with good patellar bone stock
Type 3b – Loose patellar component with poor patellar bone stock
Reprinted with permission from Ortiguera C, Berry DJ. Patellar fractures after total knee arthroplasty. *J Bone Joint Surg Am* 2002;84-A:535–540.

accurate positioning of the K-wires in the thinner-than-normal patellar bone so frequently encountered in the management of post-TKA patellar fractures. The fracture is reduced in place, and two 0.625-mm K-wires wires are passed longitudinally at a right angle to the fracture. The wires are anterior to the patellar prosthesis and cement mantle but obviously posterior to the anterior patellar cortex. If the patella is too thin or avascular, an alternative repair technique is considered, such as partial patellectomy. Stainless steel wire or heavy nonabsorbable suture (no. 5 Tycron) are passed around the ends of the K-wires and wrapped around the anterior aspect of the patella in a figure-of-eight fashion, tensioning the construct (Fig. 30-2). The proximal and distal ends of the K-wires are bent posteriorly to avoid skin prominence and irritation. Standard closure is performed. Drains can be used at the discretion of the surgeon, although they are typically unnecessary. When there is comminution or small fragments for which stable internal fixation is not possible, a partial patellectomy with extensor mechanism repair or reconstruction should be performed, given the high failure rates with open reduction and internal fixation.

Partial and/or Complete Patellectomy With Extensor Mechanism Repair

In patients in whom the patella fracture is comminuted and not reconstructable, or when there is a small distal or proximal fragment, complete or partial patellectomy, respectively, and extensor mechanism repair is an option (Fig. 30-3A–D). Care is taken to attempt to preserve the largest and most central patellar fragments with attached extensor mechanism. The joint is exposed through the fracture site and retinacular tears. The retinacula can be incised longitudinally to increase exposure. The larger fragment is preserved. This is often the proximal fragment and typically retains the patellar component. The patellar component is retained if it is stable, and the smaller fragments are removed with sharp dissection. Longitudinal drill holes are passed retrograde through the patella, between the patella prosthesis/cement surface and the anterior patellar cortex. A heavy nonabsorbable (no. 5 Tycron) suture is passed through the patella drill holes and tied to the patella tendon using a running Krackow weave to anchor the repair to the patellar tendon (or quadriceps tendon if the larger fragment is distal). When there is insufficient tissue for a solid repair, the repair may be supplemented with autograft or allograft tissue. Options for use of autograft include use of semitendinosus, gracilis, or iliotibial band. Allograft Achilles tendon is an option as well, but I have not used the technique (12).

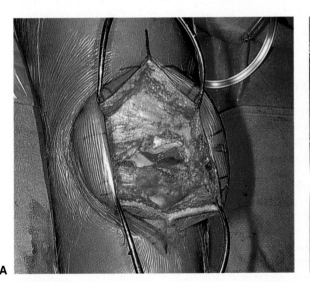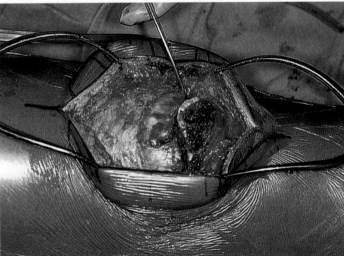

A   B

FIGURE 30-3

(A) The joint is exposed through the fracture site and retinacular tears. The retinacula can be incised longitudinally to increase exposure. **(B)** The larger fragment is preserved. This is often the proximal fragment and typically retains the patellar component. The patellar component is retained if it is stable. The smaller fragments are removed with sharp dissection. *(continued)*

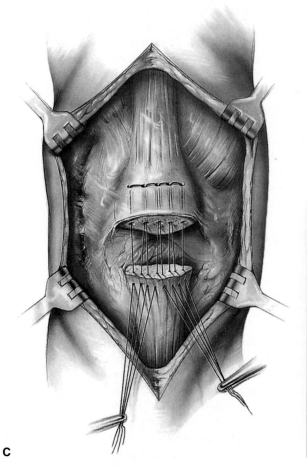

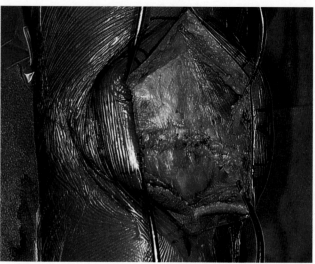

C

D

FIGURE 30-3 *(Continued)*

(C,D) Longitudinal drill holes are passed retrograde through the patella, between the patella prosthesis/cement surface, and the anterior patellar cortex. Heavy nonabsorbable (no. 5 Tycron) suture is passed through the patella drill holes and tied to the patella tendon. Often, a Krackow weave is used to anchor the repair to the patellar tendon. (Reprinted with permission from Jackson DW. *Master Techniques in Orthopaedic Surgery: Reconstructive Knee Surgery*, 3rd ed. Philadelphia: Lippincott Williams and Wilkins; 2008.)

Complete Patellectomy and Extensor Mechanism Reconstruction

Extensor mechanism reconstruction after complete patellectomy is occasionally necessary for acute fracture management, when the fracture is not amenable to fixation or primary repair, or for late treatment of failed management of periprosthetic patella fractures. Refer to the chapter on extensor mechanism reconstruction for a more detailed description of the procedure (see Chapter 31).

Patella Component Removal With Revision of Patellar Resurfacing

Traditionally, patellar revision has been indicated for type IIIa fractures with good remaining patellar bone stock, whereas patellar component removal with patellar resection arthroplasty or patellectomy has been preferred for type IIIb fractures with poor residual bone. In my experience, patellar resurfacing/revision may be feasible after patellar component removal in both type IIIa and type IIIb fractures (10). When there is a large patellar fragment of at least 10- to 12-mm thickness, a small cemented all-polyethylene button allows stable resurfacing in nearly every case. In the setting of even comminuted fractures, we have noted good outcomes for patients with type IIIb fractures undergoing patellar resurfacing (Fig. 30-4A–C) using a porous tantalum patellar shell.

The surgical technique involves reaming the remaining patellar shell, a step I prefer to do with the tourniquet deflated to assess patellar vascularity. The appropriately sized porous tantalum patellar shell is held in its desired location with a clamp while it is sutured to the fractured patellar bony shell and soft tissues. A 1.6- or 2.0-mm drill and Keith needle facilitates passage of heavy braided

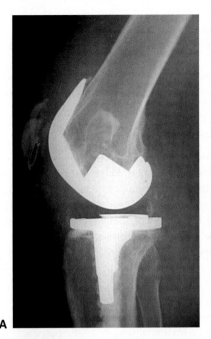

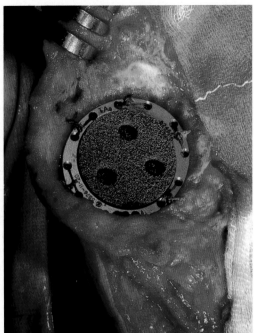

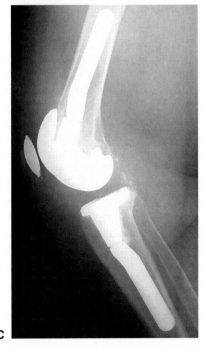

A

B

C

FIGURE 30-4

(A) Lateral preoperative radiographs of a post-total knee arthroplasty with a comminuted patella fracture with a loose patellar button and an intact extensor mechanism. **(B)** Intraoperative photograph of trabecular metal shell sewn into prepared bed of prepared patella, over fragmented patella. **(C)** Postoperative lateral radiograph after revision of the femoral and tibial components, and patellar component revision using a porous tantalum patellar shell.

nonabsorbable sutures (no. 2 or no. 5) through the patellar shell. Once the porous tantalum patellar shell is well fixed to the fractured patella (Fig. 30-4B), an all-polyethylene patella can be cemented to the porous tantalum shell (Fig. 30-4B,C).

Patellar Component Removal With Patella Resection Arthroplasty

Patellar component removal with patella resection arthroplasty is indicated for type IIIb fractures when patellar resurfacing/revision is not feasible because of poor bone stock or osteonecrosis. Partial patellectomy may be performed, with the goal of maintaining as much viable patellar bone as possible. The technique of partial patellectomy is discussed in detail previously and shown in Figure 30-3.

PEARLS AND PITFALLS

- Nonoperative management is strongly recommended for post-TKA patella fractures with well-fixed implants and intact extensor mechanisms.

- When surgical intervention is necessary for a satisfactory outcome, internal fixation must be highly stable, or it will fail.
- If excellent stability of the fracture cannot be achieved with internal fixation, partial patellectomy with extensor mechanism repair or reconstruction is preferable to less-than-optimal internal fixation.
- Although surgery is generally best avoided for management of post-TKA patella fractures, when surgical intervention is necessary, the best outcomes are associated with optimizing knee component alignment and rotation.

POSTOPERATIVE MANAGEMENT

Postoperative management depends on the surgical procedure performed. When surgical intervention is necessary secondary to disruption of the extensor mechanism, immobilization in extension following surgery is recommended for all patients during weight bearing for at least 6 weeks. The decision to immobilize in extension after repair is at the discretion of the surgeon based on the strength of the repair. Given the high failure rates in these patients, recommendations are to err to longer periods of immobilization. The goal is extensor mechanism union and healing, even if it comes at the expense of flexibility.

COMPLICATIONS

- Nonunion: The rate of nonunion in one systematic literature review of periprosthetic patellar fractures was as high as 92% following open reduction and internal fixation prompting the authors to not recommend open reduction and internal fixation for any patients with periprosthetic patella fractures (8).
- Patella dislocation: Patellar dislocation may lead to failure of even a very stable patellar internal fixation or extensor mechanism reconstruction. The occurrence of patellar dislocation should alert the evaluating physician that there is likely malrotation of the femoral and/or tibial components.
- Infection: Any surgery carries an additional risk of infection, particularly if revision arthroplasty is necessary, the vascularity of the extensor mechanism is compromised, or if allograft is used. Infection after treatment of periprosthetic patella fracture must be treated aggressively with debridement. Ultimately, these patients are at elevated risk for arthrodesis if the extensor mechanism is lost as a result of infection.
- Osteonecrosis: Osteonecrosis after periprosthetic patella fractures has been confirmed histologically (9). Factors contributing to osteonecrosis include performance of a lateral retinacular release following a medial parapatellar arthrotomy, resection of the patellar fat pad, which carries an anastomotic geniculate branch between the inferior medial and inferior lateral geniculate vessels, (9) and necrosis secondary to heat during the exothermic polymerization of PMMA cement.

RESULTS

The outcomes of open reduction and internal fixation for displaced periprosthetic patellar fractures with disruption of the extensor mechanism are often unsatisfactory. Better outcomes appear to be associated with partial patellectomy and extensor mechanism repair (1,8).

Because of the relative infrequency of patellar fractures following TKA, particularly the subgroup requiring surgical intervention, it is very difficult to analyze the results. In one of the larger reviews of post-TKA patellar fractures, Ortiguera and Berry reviewed the results of 78 periprosthetic patella fractures following TKA from a cohort of 12,464 total knee procedures for a prevalence of 0.68% (1). Of 38 type I fractures, 37 were simply observed, braced, or casted. In this group, 74% (27) remained asymptomatic, one patient required excision of a symptomatic nonunion, one developed arthrofibrosis, and in one, the patellar implant eventually loosened. One type I fracture was initially treated operatively. In patients with type II fractures, 11 of 12 were treated with extensor mechanism repair and partial patellectomy, or open-reduction and internal fixation. One patient was treated in a brace and remained asymptomatic at 5-year follow-up, despite a 5-degree extension lag. Five of six patients managed with open reduction and internal fixation of the fracture and extensor mechanism repair failed treatment. The other five fractures were treated with partial patellectomy and extensor mechanism repair. There were no results specified for this group of patients. There was a 50% complication rate in the management of type II fractures, which required revision operation in five of 11 patients. Six of 12 patients with type II fractures were treated operatively and had instability, pain, or weakness at last follow-up. Type III fractures (with patellar implant loosening) occurred in 24 patients and were treated operatively if the patient was symptomatic. The type of operation selected was based on the quality of the remaining bone stock. Twelve type IIIa fractures (implant loose, good remaining bone stock) received both component resection and patelloplasty or component revision, while 12 type IIIb fractures (implant loose, poor remaining bone stock) underwent partial or complete patellectomy. Thirteen complications following treatment of type III fractures occurred, including failure of fixation, an extensor lag in excess of 15 degrees, nonunion, infection, instability, and arthrofibrosis. Three patients required a revision operation.

Although the numbers were small, one series evaluating outcomes of patellar resurfacing/revision using a porous tantalum patellar shell in three patients with comminuted type IIIb patellar fractures had good results. Further follow-up of the technique and technology are required before broad endorsement of the approach to type IIIb periprosthetic patella fractures.

REFERENCES

1. Ortiguera C, Berry DJ. Patellar fractures after total knee arthroplasty. *J Bone Joint Surg Am* 2002;84-A:535–540.
2. Keating EM, Haas G, Meding JB. Patella fracture after post total knee arthroplasty. *Clin Orthop Relat Res* 2003:93–97.
3. Parvizi J, Kim K, Oliashirazi A, et al. Periprosthetic patellar fractures. *Clin Orthop Rel Res* 2006;446:161–166.
4. Hozack WJ, Goll SR, Lotke PA, et al. The treatment of patellar fractures after total knee arthroplasty. *Clin Orthop Rel Res* 1988;236:123–127.
5. Windsor RE, Scuderi GR, Insall JN. Patellar fractures in total knee arthroplasty. *J Arthrop* 1989;4(Suppl):S63–67.
6. Figgie HE III, Goldberg VM, Figgie MP, et al. The effect of alignment of the implant on fractures of the patella after condylar total knee arthroplasty. *J Bone Joint Surg Am* 1989;71-A:1031–1039.
7. Goldberg VM, Figgie HE III, Inglis AE, et al. Patella fracture type and prognosis in condylar total knee arthroplasty. *Clin Orthop Rel Res* 1988;236:115–122.
8. Sheth NP, Pedowitz DI, Lonner JH. Current concepts review: periprosthetic patellar fractures. *J Bone Joint Surg Am* 2007;89:2285–2296.
9. Scapinelli R. Blood supply of the human patella. Its relation to ischaemic necrosis after fracture. *J Bone Joint Surg Br* 1967;49-B:563–570.
10. Nelson C, Lonner J, Lahiji A, et al. Use of a porous metal shell for management of marked bone loss during revision total knee arthroplasty. *J Arthrop* 2003;18(Suppl):37–41.
11. Szyszkowitz R, Allgöwer M, Burch HP, et al. Patella and tibia. In: Müller M, Allgöwer M, Schneider R, Willenegger H, eds. *Manual of Internal Fixation*. New York: Springer-Verlag; 1991.
12. Crossett LS, Sinha RK, Sechriest VF, Rubash HE. Reconstruction of a ruptured patellar tendon with Achilles tendon allograft following total knee arthroplasty. *J Bone Joint Surg Am* 2002;84:1354–1361.

31 Extensor Mechanism Allograft

Alexander P. Sah, Craig J. Della Valle, and Aaron G. Rosenberg

INDICATIONS

Extensor mechanism failure in the setting of a total knee arthroplasty can be a devastating complication that is difficult to manage. The extensor mechanism can be disrupted by tibial tubercle avulsion, patellar tendon rupture, patella fracture, or quadriceps tendon rupture (Fig. 31-1). Whether occurring intraoperatively or postoperatively, primary repair of the extensor mechanism is associated with a substantial rate of failure and associated complications (1–3).

Failure of a primary repair is often the result of compromised blood supply or significant soft tissue loss or damage. In this setting, an extensor mechanism allograft reconstruction may be indicated. A fresh-frozen allograft is composed of an intact allograft extensor mechanism including tibial tuberosity, patellar tendon, patella, and quadriceps tendon (Fig. 31-2). Although various reconstructive procedures such as medial gastrocnemius flaps or Achilles allografts have been described (4,5), we have found that the use of a complete extensor mechanism allograft has most reliably been associated with a successful outcome (6,7). We believe the success of this procedure is related to the surgeon's ability to obtain robust fixation both proximally and distally as well as the ability to completely cover the allograft with native soft tissue in most cases. An extensor mechanism allograft may also be indicated in the treatment of severe heterotopic ossification of the extensor mechanism, severe patella baja, or conversion of a previous knee arthrodesis to a total knee with a fibrosed or deficient extensor mechanism.

CONTRAINDICATIONS

- Active infection or repeated unsuccessful staged reimplantation surgeries with infection are contraindications to the procedure.
- Patient inability to comply with postoperative immobilization and participation in a suitable rehabilitation program is a contraindication to the procedure.
- In the setting of a problematic total knee arthroplasty (aseptic loosening, malalignment, instability), extensor mechanism reconstruction is likely to fail unless the knee is revised.
- For patients not meeting the criteria for extensor mechanism allograft, bracing or knee arthrodesis are alternative options.

PREOPERATIVE PREPARATION

Preoperative planning includes an appropriate history, physical examination, and radiographic evaluation. Information regarding previous procedures or surgeries is useful to estimate the amount and type of host soft tissue available. The affected knee must be tested for both active and passive range of motion. Flexion contractures are common in total knee replacements with extensor mechanism

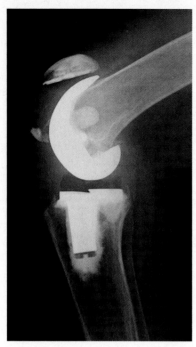

FIGURE 31-1

Preoperative lateral radiograph showing avulsion fracture of the inferior pole of the patella, resulting in extensor mechanism incompetence.

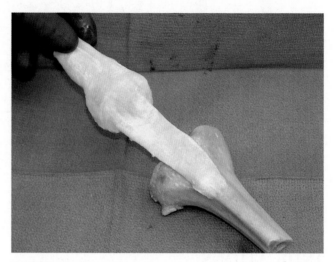

FIGURE 31-2

The fresh-frozen, nonirradiated extensor mechanism allograft includes quadriceps tendon, patella, patellar tendon, and proximal tibia.

disruption. It must be determined whether a contracture can be addressed with soft tissue procedures or if component revision is required. Left untreated, a flexion contracture will predispose to failure of the extensor mechanism reconstruction. In addition, the tibial and femoral components should be evaluated for any signs of malalignment or loosening, which would also warrant component revision. A computed tomography scan may be useful to thoroughly evaluate component rotation (8). Hardware in the area of the tibial tubercle should be recognized, and the proper equipment should be available for possible removal. Preoperative workup for infection, including erythrocyte sedimentation rate, C-reactive protein, and complete blood count with differential are useful, followed by a knee aspiration if any of these values are elevated. Medical comorbidities or immunosuppressive therapy that may affect soft tissue healing must be taken into consideration.

Early planning is required to ensure that a fresh-frozen, nonirradiated extensor mechanism allograft (Allosource, Centennial, CO) is available that matches the affected side. For instance, it is not advisable to use a right-sided allograft in a left lower extremity. Furthermore, although resurfacing of the allograft patella may address tracking issues, cementing a patella button onto allograft bone may lead to increased complications (9). Five cm of quadriceps tendon is necessary for sufficient soft tissue fixation and overlap with the host tissue. If the allograft tibia is not delivered in its entirety, a minimum 5 cm of tuberosity bone length must be available for sufficient distal graft fixation. The allograft should be inspected and deemed appropriate before the patient enters the operating room.

TECHNIQUE

The patient is placed supine with a bump under the ipsilateral hip. The lower extremity is prepped with draping placed as proximal as possible to allow proximal thigh exposure if necessary. In a short obese thigh, the use of a sterile tourniquet may be useful to maximize proximal exposure. Previous skin incisions are marked, and hash marks are made transversely along the planned incision to assist during closure (Fig. 31-3).

A midline incision is made through the previous skin incision. If multiple incisions exist, an attempt is made to use the most lateral incision to avoid added disruption of the vascular supply to the skin. Full-thickness subfascial skin flaps are raised on either side of the incision to preserve skin vascularity. The host extensor mechanism is evaluated, and the patella is outlined (Fig. 31-4). The host

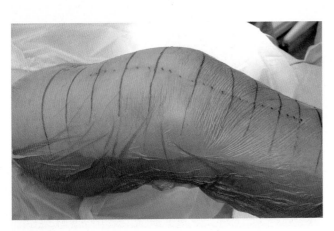

FIGURE 31-3

Previous skin incisions are identified, and hash marks are placed to assist in soft tissue closure.

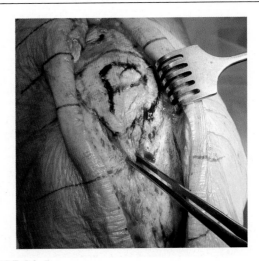

FIGURE 31-4

The patella is identified, and the host extensor mechanism is exposed.

extensor mechanism, from the quadriceps tendon through the patellar tendon, is incised in the midline (Fig. 31-5). The patella is shelled out from the host tissue and can be divided in half longitudinally in line with the extensor mechanism arthrotomy with an oscillating saw to facilitate this process (Fig. 31-6). The surrounding soft tissue is preserved in continuity with the medial and lateral flaps. This approach provides equal soft tissue on the medial and lateral sides for eventual closure over the extensor allograft. The medial and lateral gutters as well as the suprapatellar pouch are re-established (Fig. 31-7). If there is tendinous tissue at the actual site of the host tuberosity, it is removed by sharp dissection, as it is critical in allowing proper visualization for preparing the host tibial trough.

Excellent exposure of both the femoral and tibial components is possible with this approach (Fig. 31-8). Component revision is now performed if necessary. If a stemmed tibial component is chosen, the host tibial bone trough is prepared, and drill holes and fixation wires are placed before inserting the revision tibial component.

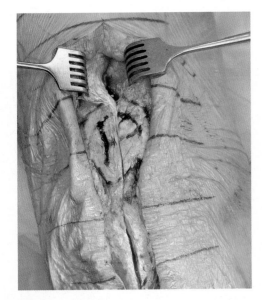

FIGURE 31-5

The extensor mechanism is incised in the midline.

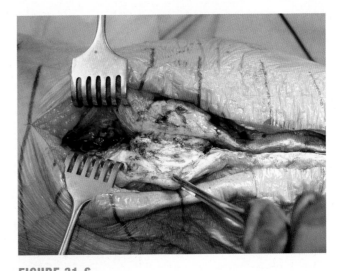

FIGURE 31-6

The patella is divided with an oscillating saw in line with the arthrotomy. The patella halves are shelled out of the surrounding soft tissues.

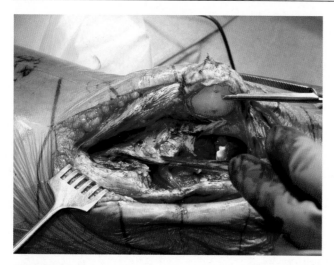

FIGURE 31-7

A thorough synovectomy is performed during re-establishment of the medial and lateral gutters and suprapatellar pouch.

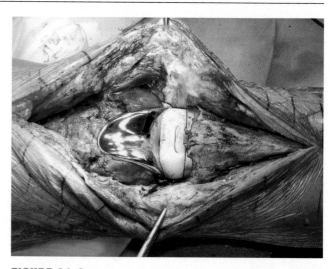

FIGURE 31-8

Excellent exposure of existing knee arthroplasty components is possible with this approach.

Allograft Preparation

A separate team can prepare the allograft during arthroplasty component revision. The allograft bone block is harvested from the allograft tibia with the extensor mechanism carefully secured on the back table. The tibial tubercle of the allograft is carefully measured to dimensions of approximately 5 × 2 × 2 cm (Fig. 31-9). The allograft is made slightly larger than the host insertion site because it can be easily trimmed down to obtain a press-fit at the time of insertion. The patellar tendon must be carefully protected during allograft tibial tubercle preparation so it is not damaged by the oscillating saw. The proximal portion of the tubercle is dovetailed in a distal/anterior to proximal posterior fashion, just proximal to the patellar tendon insertion. The dovetail is outlined with a pen in a 30- to 40-degree angle with a 20- to 25-mm length (Fig. 31-10). The allograft is securely stored until ready for implantation.

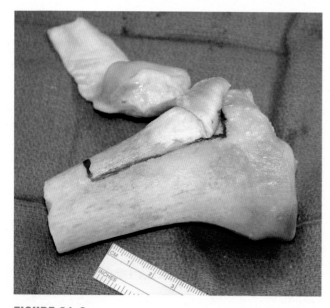

FIGURE 31-9

The tibial tubercle allograft is measured and outlined to be at least 5 × 2 × 2 cm.

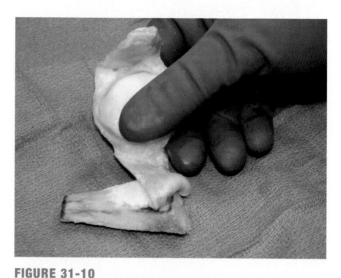

FIGURE 31-10

The dovetail at the proximal end of the tibial allograft allows secure distal fit.

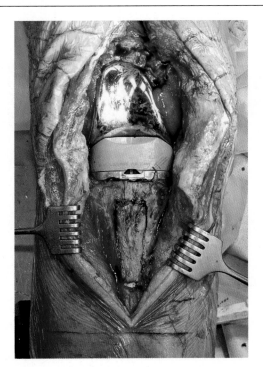

FIGURE 31-11
The host tibial tubercle trough is planned and outlined.

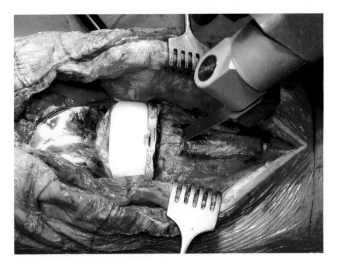

FIGURE 31-12
A thin, small oscillating saw is used to create the host tibial trough.

Host Tibial Preparation

The host site is outlined in pen to dimensions just less than the $5 \times 2 \times 2$ cm of the graft to facilitate eventual press-fit fixation (Fig. 31-11). The bone trough is made either at or slightly medial to the site of the native tibial tubercle. Its vertical position is determined by laying the allograft on the front of the fully extended knee so that the patella is positioned such that the inferior pole is just proximal to the distal edge of the femoral component. An oscillating saw is used to make the longitudinal cuts, and a narrow, thin oscillating saw is used to make the proximal and distal ends (Fig. 31-12). The surgeon uses an osteotome to gently and carefully remove the bone block (Fig. 31-13). A bevel is made at the proximal portion of the host trough to accept the allograft dovetail. A small curette may be useful to undermine the bevel in the proximal trough (Fig. 31-14). At least 15 mm of host bone below the tibial component is recommended to resist proximal graft escape. Maintenance of this bevel helps augment the strength of the allograft fixation to the host tibia and to minimize proximal migration of the graft, but it may not be possible in cases when proximal tibial bone loss has occurred. It is critical

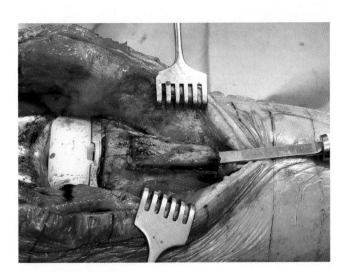

FIGURE 31-13
The bone block is removed carefully with protection of the proximal tibia bone bridge.

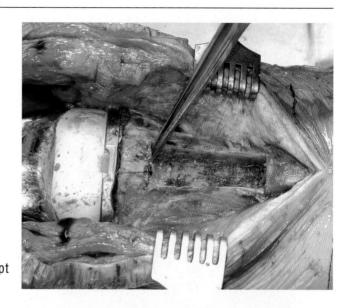

FIGURE 31-14

A small curette is useful to undermine the bevel to accept the graft dovetail.

to protect the bone bridge extending from the tibial plateau to the bevel to prevent fracture. Fracture is most likely to occur during creation of the bevel or during impaction of the tibial allograft.

Fixation of the graft is achieved with three 16- or 18-gauge stainless steel wires placed through drill holes in the tibia created from a medial-to-lateral direction. These wires may pass deep to the bone trough, and if a stemmed tibial component is used, the wires are placed with the trial components in place to ensure that they will pass anterior to the revision stem. Alternately, the wires may be passed directly into the host trough to be passed through the allograft tubercle segment.

Extensor Allograft Fixation

The tibial bone block is gently inserted in an up-and-in fashion to achieve a press-fit and engage the dovetail into the bevel (Fig. 31-15). The wires are then twisted, tightened, cut, and bent over bone on the lateral tibia to maximize soft tissue coverage and prevent soft tissue irritation (Fig. 31-16).

The extensor mechanism allograft must be tensioned tightly with the knee in full extension. This technique is essential to provide adequate postoperative extension. Despite concerns for knee stiffness, total knees managed with extensor mechanism allografts in this fashion do not have difficulty regaining adequate flexion (6). The allograft quadriceps tendon is sutured to the host tissue with a no. 5 nonabsorbable suture (FiberWire, Arthrex, Naples, FL) placed in a modified Krackow fashion along both the medial and lateral aspects of the tendon (Fig. 31-17). The sutures are used to pull the

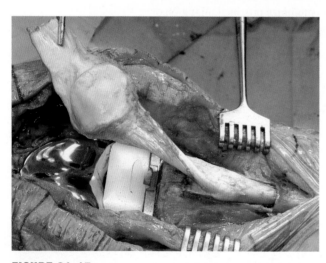

FIGURE 31-15

The graft is press-fit into place, and the dovetail and bevel are engaged.

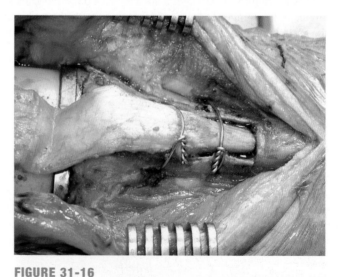

FIGURE 31-16

Wires are passed through drill holes to provide additional fixation to the distal graft.

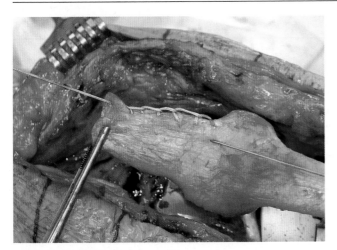

FIGURE 31-17

Modified Krackow sutures are placed in the allograft quadriceps tendon.

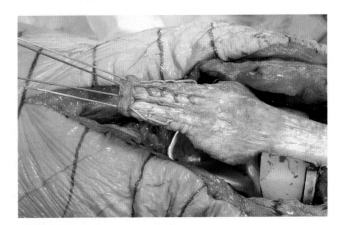

FIGURE 31-18

The sutures are used to both place tension and secure the allograft tendon to host tissue.

graft proximally with the knee in extension during repair (Fig. 31-18). The host quadriceps tissue is pulled tightly distally with modified Krackow sutures or with a Kocher clamp during repair to maximize tension in the reconstructed extensor mechanism (Fig. 31-19). The remaining allograft is then sutured in place below the host quadriceps tendon in a vest-over-pants fashion over a drain. The repair is continued distally so that the host retinacular tissues cover the entire allograft with multiple sutures placed through both the allograft and the remaining native tissue (Fig. 31-20).

The extensor mechanism reconstruction is not tested intraoperatively, and the knee is not put through a range of motion to maintain the integrity of the tensioned repair. With the knee in extension, the subcutaneous tissues and skin are closed in routine fashion. After application of a sterile dressing, a plaster splint is applied to the knee to maintain full extension after surgery. The patient should not be awakened from anesthesia until the plaster is completely hard to prevent knee flexion upon awakening.

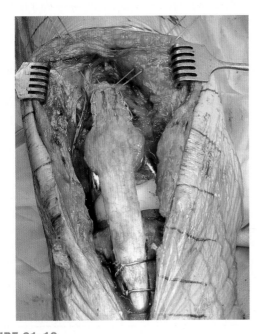

FIGURE 31-19

The fixation of the allograft to the host extensor mechanism is performed with the knee in extension with tension on the graft.

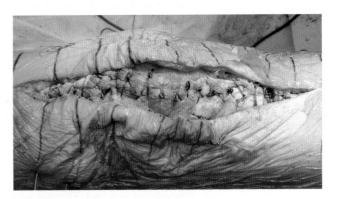

FIGURE 31-20

The entire allograft mechanism is covered by host tissue.

PEARLS AND PITFALLS

Pearls

- A direct midline arthrotomy and shelling out of the patella provides excellent soft tissue coverage over the allograft.
- Full knee extension is necessary with the previous arthroplasty components or with revision trials in place to ensure the ability to adequately tension the extensor mechanism allograft.
- The dovetail and bevel trough provide a press-fit as well as resistance to proximal graft escape.
- The quadriceps tendon should be sutured with the knee in full extension and tightly tensioned to optimize postoperative extension.
- The stainless steel wires should be bent toward the lateral side of the tibia to maximize coverage and minimize soft tissue irritation.
- Complete coverage of the allograft with host tissues minimizes contact of the allograft with the subcutaneous tissues and may reduce the risk of infection.
- Strict knee extension beginning from skin closure should be maintained during patient awakening from anesthesia, to transfer to recovery, to postoperative day 3 for cast change, until 6 weeks follow-up.

Pitfalls

- An improper allograft that does not have a sufficient tibial bone block or quadriceps tendon will jeopardize distal or proximal fixation, respectively.
- Making the tibial allograft bone block too small will not allow a press-fit into the host bone trough and may compromise the dovetail-bevel mechanism.
- Gentle graft impaction allows an excellent press-fit, but overzealous impaction or an imperfect fit will risk host tibial trough or bone bridge fracture.
- Testing the repair or moving the knee can attenuate the tissues and loosen the reconstruction.
- Improper maintenance of knee extension beginning at skin closure until 6-week follow-up can jeopardize results.

POSTOPERATIVE MANAGEMENT

The plaster splint and dressing are changed on postoperative day 3, when a long leg cast is applied for 3 weeks at which point the wound is checked, sutures are removed, and a new cast is applied for an additional 3 weeks (total immobilization for 6 weeks). Touchdown weight bearing is allowed in the cast. Isometric static quadriceps contractions are encouraged during this period. Knee motion begins after cast removal at 6 weeks with placement of a hinged knee brace locked from 0 to 30 degrees to allow active flexion and extension under supervision of a physical therapist. Passive flexion performed by the therapist is not allowed. The patient's brace is adjusted to allow for an additional 10 degrees of flexion per week, and quadriceps strengthening is initiated. Weight bearing as tolerated with the brace locked in extension is allowed at this time when the patient is ambulating. At 3 months postoperatively, the brace is removed, and active flexion is not restricted.

COMPLICATIONS

Extensor lag is the most common complication of this procedure. Reconstruction with the allograft loosely tensioned results in extensor lag as well as clinical failure (10). Tightening of the extensor mechanism allograft in full extension is useful to prevent or minimize this complication. Other rare complications include nonunion of the tibial tubercle allograft in the tibial trough, failure of proximal soft tissue incorporation, and infection.

RESULTS

Emerson et al reported promising early clinical results with extensor mechanism allograft, but further follow-up revealed extensor lag of 20 to 40 degrees in one third of patients (9). Nazarian and Booth modified the technique by tightly tensioning the graft in full extension and reported successful clinical results (7). At minimum 2-year follow-up, Burnett et al directly compared the two techniques and

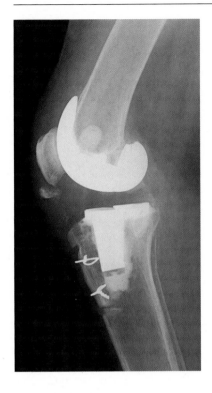

FIGURE 31-21

Postoperative lateral radiograph 3 months after extensor mechanism reconstruction using extensor mechanism allograft.

found improved knee extension and clinical outcomes in knees in which the graft was tensioned tightly in full extension (Fig. 31-21) (6).

In a case report of a histological evaluation of an extensor mechanism allograft used in a total knee arthroplasty, the graft was incorporated into the tibial bone and remained in continuity with the host retinaculum proximally (11).

REFERENCES

1. Dobbs RE, Hanssen AD, Lewallen DG, Pagnano MW. Quadriceps tendon rupture after total knee arthroplasty. Prevalence, complications, and outcomes. *J Bone Joint Surg* 2005;87:37–45.
2. Goldberg VM, Figgie HE, Inglis AE, et al. Patellar fracture type and prognosis in condylar total knee arthroplasty. *Clin Orthop Relat Res*1988;236:115–122.
3. Rand JA, Morrey BF, Bryan RS. Patellar tendon rupture after total knee arthroplasty. *Clin Orthop Relat Res*1989;244:233–238.
4. Busfield BT, Huffman GR, Nahai F, et al. Extended medial gastrocnemius rotational flap for treatment of chronic knee extensor mechanism deficiency in patients with and without total knee arthroplasty. *Clin Orthop Relat Res* 2004;428:190–197.
5. Crossett LS, Sinha RK, Sechriest VF, Rubash HE. Reconstruction of a ruptured patellar tendon with Achilles tendon allograft following total knee arthroplasty. *J Bone Joint Surg* 2002;84:1354–1361.
6. Burnett RS, Berger RA, Paparosky WG, et al. Extensor mechanism allograft reconstruction after total knee arthroplasty—a comparison of two techniques. *J Bone Joint Surg* 2004;86:2694–2699.
7. Nazarian DG, Booth RE. Extensor mechanism allografts in total knee arthroplasty. *Clin Orthop Relat Res* 1999;367:123–129.
8. Berger RA, Crossett LS, Jacobs JJ, Rubash HE. Malrotation causing patellofemoral complications after total knee arthroplasty. *Clin Orthop Relat Res* 1998;356:144–153.
9. Emerson RH, Head WC, Malinin TI. Extensor mechanism reconstruction with an allograft after total knee arthroplasty. *Clin Orthop Relat Res* 1994;303:79–85.
10. Burnett RS, Berger RA, Della Valle CJ, et al. Extensor mechanism allograft reconstruction after total knee arthroplasty—surgical technique. *J Bone Joint Surg* 2005;87:175–194.
11. Burnett RS, Fornasier VL, Haydon CM, et al. Retrieval of a well-functioning extensor mechanism allograft from a total knee arthroplasty—clinical and histological findings. *J Bone Joint Surg Br* 2004;86:986–990.

32 Management of the Stiff Total Knee Arthroplasty

Raymond H. Kim and Douglas A. Dennis

INTRODUCTION

Although total knee arthroplasty (TKA) has been a successful procedure with excellent survivorship and functional outcomes (1–4), it is not without complications. One of these possible complications is postoperative stiffness. One analysis of knee motion demonstrated a requirement of 67 degrees of flexion for the swing phase of gait, 83 degrees to ascend stairs, 84 degrees to descend stairs, and at least 93 degrees to rise from a chair (5). It is reasonable to describe a stiff TKA as a knee that limits activities of daily living secondary to lack of motion. In a study on stiffness following TKA, Kim and Lotke et al reviewed 1,000 consecutive knees (6). At 32 months postoperatively, there was a 1.3% prevalence of stiffness, defined as a flexion contracture of greater than or equal to 15 degrees or maximal flexion less than 75 degrees.

This chapter to reviews the etiologies, evaluation strategies, and management options for patients who develop stiffness after undergoing a TKA.

ETIOLOGY

The etiology of stiffness after TKA is multifactorial and can be attributed to three general causes: patient factors, technical errors, and surgical complications. Although technical errors and surgical complications may be treatable causes of stiffness by manipulation, scar excision, or revision total knee arthroplasty, patient-related factors are less effectively treated with revision surgery and should most often be avoided.

Patient Factors

Numerous patient factors can contribute to postoperative restriction of knee motion. Multiple studies have shown that the primary determinant of postoperative ROM is preoperative ROM (7–11). This is likely because of patients' individual anatomy, particularly their soft tissues, as well as the severity and chronicity of their arthritic disease. Ritter and Stringer reviewed 145 consecutive TKA patients and found that the degree of postoperative flexion was determined by the preoperative flexion, particularly if the degree of flexion was less than 75 degrees (7,8). Obesity often limits postoperative knee motion because of increased lower extremity girth, resulting in earlier calf-thigh impingement (12). Cutaneous factors include scarring from multiple incisions, burns, and previous radiation therapy, which can all lead to superficial restriction of flexion (Fig. 32-1).

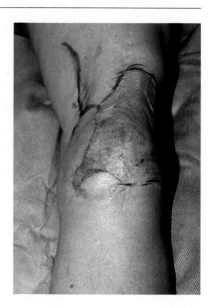

FIGURE 32-1

Photograph demonstrating excessive cutaneous scarring of the anterior aspect of the knee.

Another significant patient factor involves inadequate postoperative rehabilitation. The patient's understanding of the postoperative recovery should be cultivated preoperatively by providing detailed education preoperatively ("prehabilitation"). Emphasis on early mobilization, diligence in attending physical therapy sessions, and goal setting is critical.

Adequate pain control perioperatively also influences patient compliance with therapy participation. Pre-emptive analgesics, regional nerve blocks, and postoperative pain control should be optimized to maximize the patient's efforts when performing knee ROM exercises (13,14). Diligence with anticoagulation monitoring is critical to prevent hemarthroses that can result in painful swelling and significantly delay gains in knee motion during the postoperative rehabilitation period.

Psychiatric comorbidities affecting postoperative pain and functional outcome (eg, history of depression) have been recently identified (15–17). Psychiatric consultation may prove valuable to address perioperative antidepressants.

Technical Errors Limiting Extension

Good surgical technique is the most critical factor in the surgeon's ability to minimize the incidence of postoperative stiffness. Intraoperative technical errors can result in either decreased extension (flexion contracture) and/or decreased flexion. Decreased extension can result from poor balancing of the flexion-extension gaps, failure to remove posterior osteophytes, or failure to release a tight posterior capsule.

An excessively tight extension gap will often result in lack of full extension. Assuming the level of resection for the tibial cut was appropriate, one cause of a tight extension gap is an inadequate distal femoral resection. For patients with a preoperative flexion contracture, the surgeon can anticipate the need to resect an additional couple of millimeters of distal femur when setting the distal femoral cutting block to ensure an adequate extension gap. After the distal femur and proximal tibial cuts are made, the extension gap should be assessed for the gap height as well as the symmetry of the gap medially and laterally. This can be performed using spacer blocks, laminar spreaders, or other tensioning device. If the extension gap is asymmetric medially compared to laterally, appropriate releases should be performed at this time to obtain a balanced extension gap.

Large, posterior osteophytes on the femoral condyles can tent the posterior capsule and mechanically inhibit full extension. Osteophytes are most simply removed after making the anterior and posterior condylar resections on the distal femur. To remove the osteophytes, the knee can be placed at 90 degrees of flexion with a laminar spreader in the lateral compartment. A three-quarter-inch curved or angled osteotome can then be used to sharply chisel off the medial posterior osteophyte at the osteochondral junction (Fig. 32-2). This can then be repeated in the lateral compartment after switching the laminar spreader to the opposite side. The flexion and extension gaps can then be reassessed to determine if further balancing is required. In cases with massive posterior compartment osteophytes, it is often wise to attempt to remove them before extensive soft tissue releases are

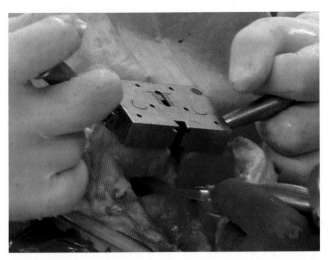

FIGURE 32-2

Intraoperative photograph demonstrating removal of posterior femoral osteophytes using a curved osteotome.

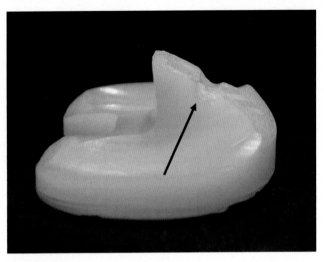

FIGURE 32-3

Photograph demonstrating anterior postimpingement secondary to excessive femoral component flexion in conjunction with increased posterior tibial slope.

performed, because removal of large osteophytes can have a dramatic effect on both the coronal and sagittal plane balance.

Premature extension impingement of the femoral and tibial components can occur if components of a posterior stabilized knee are malpositioned in the sagittal plane. Excessive flexion of the femoral component or a tibia prepared with too much posterior slope will result in prosthetic mechanical impingement of the intercondylar portion of the femoral component against the anterior aspect of the tibial stabilizing post that will inhibit extension and could potentially result in accelerated post wear (Fig. 32-3). Care should be taken to avoid flexing the distal femoral cut by ensuring that the entry hole for the intramedullary distal femoral cutting guide is not placed too posteriorly. Slope of the extramedullary tibial cutting guide should be carefully checked before making the proximal tibial cut to make sure excessive posterior slope is avoided.

In patients with long-standing significant preoperative flexion contractures, the posterior capsule of the knee is often significantly contracted. If adequate distal femoral resection has been performed, yet a tight extension gap persists, a posterior capsular release should be performed. The authors prefer to perform this bluntly with a Cobb elevator, gently elevating the posterior capsule directly off of the posterior femur. Care should be taken not to stray off of the bone with instruments to minimize the risk of harming neurovascular structures. Assistants should also avoid holding the leg behind the knee to prevent ballottement of the neurovascular bundle anteriorly as the posterior capsular release is performed.

Technical Errors Limiting Flexion

Technical errors known to limit flexion after TKA include flexion-extension gap imbalance, retention of posterior femoral condylar osteophytes, failure to restore posterior femoral condylar offset, and substantial elevation of the joint line. Excessive flexion gap tension typically leads to limited motion and can result from multiple errors such as insufficient bone resection, use of oversized components (18), inadequate ligamentous release, or component malposition. Conversely, leaving a flexion gap too loose in a posterior cruciate ligament (PCL)-retaining TKA often results in paradoxical femoral translation, which anteriorizes the axis of knee flexion, results in earlier posterior impingement of the femur on the tibial component, and decreased weight-bearing flexion (19–21).

If a knee is unbalanced with an excessively tight flexion gap relative to the extension gap, and a tibial insert is selected to accommodate the extension gap, then the knee will resist flexion because of an overstuffed flexion space. Excessive flexion gap tightness can also result from placement of the tibial component with an anterior slope or from errors associated with femoral component position or size. Placing the femoral component too posteriorly tightens the flexion gap and may limit flexion. If the femoral component is placed in excessive flexion, the anterior flange tightens the extensor mechanism and can cause chronic tendinous irritation. Finally, if the femoral component is placed in internal rotation, arthrofibrosis has been shown to occur, possibly by asymmetrically tightening the medial aspect of the flexion gap. Boldt et al identified and analyzed 38 TKA subjects with postoperative arthrofibrosis from a cohort of 3,058 consecutive mobile-bearing patients (22). They compared these stiff TKA patients with a matched control group of 38 asymptomatic, mobile-bearing TKA subjects without arthrofibrosis. Computerized axial tomography scans were obtained in both groups. The surgical epicondylar axis was compared with the posterior condylar axis of the femoral prosthesis. Femoral components in the arthrofibrosis group were significantly internally rotated relative to the transepicondylar axis by a mean of 4.7 degrees (SD, 2.2 degrees; range, 10 degrees internal to 1 degree external rotation). In the control group, the femoral components were positioned at a mean of 0.3 degrees internal rotation relative to the transepicondylar axis (SD, 2.3 degrees; range, 4 degrees internal to 6 degrees external rotation).

Excessive femoral component flexion can be avoided by ensuring that the entry hole for the intramedullary distal femoral cutting guide is not placed too posteriorly. To avoid oversizing the femoral component, preoperative templating is helpful to estimate the femoral component size on appropriately scaled lateral radiographs. Most TKA systems determine femoral component sizing based on a guide referencing the anterior cortex of the femur and the posterior condyles. When using the sizing guide, care should be taken to clearly identify the anterior cortex. Failure to identify the anterior cortex because of overlying hypertrophic synovium can lead to oversizing the femoral component.

In addition to varus-valgus ligamentous balance, balance of the PCL has been shown to be an important determinant of knee flexion following PCL-retaining TKA. Leaving a PCL too tight will inhibit flexion by creation of an overly tight flexion gap. Conversely, overreleasing of the PCL, particularly in minimally constrained PCL-retaining TKA designs, may result in paradoxical anterior femoral translation during deep, weight-bearing flexion resulting in a reduction in knee flexion as previously discussed (19,23). Because of the paradoxical anterior sliding, posterior femoral rollback is inhibited, which is necessary to avoid posterior impingement and to allow higher magnitudes of knee flexion.

Technical errors resulting in failure to obtain symmetry (rectangular gap) of either the flexion or extension gap can similarly result in diminished flexion. Matsuda et al evaluated coronal plane (varus-valgus) stability following TKA by applying a 150 Newton load using a Telos arthrometer (Fa Telos; Medizinisch-Technische GmbH, Griesheim, Germany) (24). Knees were judged to be balanced if the difference in varus and valgus laxity was less than 2 degrees. In the balanced TKA group (n = 69 TKA), mean flexion improved 10 degrees postoperatively ($p < .0001$), whereas in the unbalanced TKA group (n = 11 TKA), mean postoperative flexion was reduced by 8.3 degrees ($p = .0061$), emphasizing the importance of having a balanced extension gap.

A well-balanced flexion gap is one that is not only equivalent in height to the extension gap, but one that is also symmetric medially and laterally, thus creating a rectangular flexion gap. Because of the association of femoral component malrotation with arthrofibrosis previously discussed, the authors prefer to use a gap-balancing technique as opposed to the measured-resection technique to ensure proper balancing of the flexion and extension gaps. The critical step in this technique involves placement of the anterior-posterior cutting block, which determines the rotation of the femoral component. The anterior-posterior distal femoral cutting block is positioned anteriorly or posteriorly to ensure the flexion gap height is equal to the extension gap height with the collateral ligaments equally tensioned with laminar spreaders or another tensioning device. The rotation of the anterior-posterior cutting block is then appropriately adjusted rotationally to also ensure that the flexion gap space itself is symmetric medially and laterally and parallel to the tibial cut with each collateral ligament equally tensioned (Fig. 32-4). Secondary checks are then performed to ensure reasonable rotational orientation relative to the transepicondylar and anteroposterior axes. Using this technique facilitates obtaining balanced flexion and extension gap heights as well as a rectangular flexion gap that is symmetric medially and laterally.

Although retention of large posterior femoral osteophytes can result in postoperative flexion contracture as previously discussed, numerous reports have documented that retention of these osteophytes reduces knee flexion as well (25–27). Failure to remove these osteophytes leads to earlier posterior impingement of the femur on the posterior aspect of the tibial component. Goldstein et al studied the effects of retained posterior femoral osteophytes on TKA flexion in a computer simulation in which a geometric model was created of a midsize TKA (PFC Sigma Cruciate Retaining TKA; DePuy, Inc., Warsaw, IN) (25). The geometric model showed that a retained posterior femoral

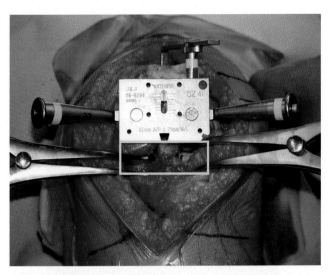

FIGURE 32-4

Intraoperative photograph demonstrating placement of the anterior-posterior femoral cutting block in appropriate external rotation to create a rectangular flexion gap.

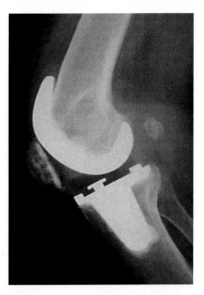

FIGURE 32-5

Lateral radiograph demonstrating substantial postoperative joint line elevation with secondary patellar baja.

osteophyte with a radius smaller than 2.87 mm permitted 120 degrees of knee flexion, whereas a retained osteophyte larger than 6.48 mm resulted in only 105 degrees of TKA flexion before posterior impingement.

Finally, elevation of the joint line and secondary patellar baja following TKA has been shown to adversely affect postoperative knee flexion and clinical scores (28,29). This may be related to patellar-tibial component impingement, midflexion instability typically associated with excessive joint line elevation, or caused by creation of excessive tension in the PCL when the joint line is significantly elevated (Fig. 32-5).

Technical Errors Involving the Extensor Mechanism

Technical errors regarding the extensor mechanism can occur as a result of functional shortening of the extensor mechanism, which can occur by overstuffing the patella, anteriorizing the femoral component, excessive femoral component flexion resulting in chronic quadriceps tendon irritation, or excessive tightening of the extensor mechanism secondary to a nonanatomic arthrotomy closure.

Several principals should be kept in mind during patellar preparation to avoid postoperative problems with flexion. Bengs and Scott performed 31 consecutive TKAs in which custom trial patellar components that were thicker than the standard trial by 2-mm increments (2 to –8 mm) were inserted intraoperatively, and the effect on flexion was assessed. Passive TKA flexion intraoperatively decreased 3 degrees for every 2-mm increment increase in patellar component thickness (30). Mihalko et al evaluated the effect of increasing trochlear groove thickness beyond anatomic trochlear groove height in a cadaveric model (31). They observed that a 2-mm increase in trochlear height resulted in a 1.3 ± 1.2-degree decrease in passive flexion ($p = .007$), whereas a 4-mm increase in trochlear height decreased passive flexion by 4.8 ± 3.2 degrees ($p = .001$). Therefore, overstuffing of the patellofemoral joint during TKA may have adverse effects on postoperative knee flexion.

A reasonable approach to avoid overstuffing the patella is to measure the prepatellar resection height. After the patellar resection and placing the trial patellar component, the composite height can be measured and compared. By reproducing the previous patellar height, the surgeon can be ensured that the patella is not overstuffed. Caution should be taken to not overresect the patella, which increases the risk of patella fracture (32).

The patellofemoral compartment can also be overstuffed secondary to anteriorization of the femoral component (Fig. 32-6). Although avoiding notching is a good practice to prevent increased risk of supracondylar fracture (33,34), excessive anteriorization will result in diminished flexion. If

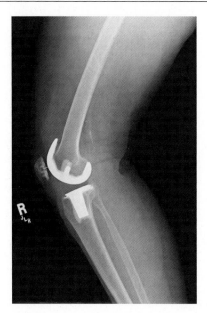

FIGURE 32-6

Lateral radiograph demonstrating excessive anterior femoral component placement.

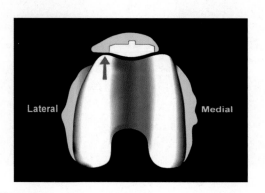

FIGURE 32-7

Diagram demonstrating a medialized inset patellar component with lateral facet impingement on the lateral flange of the femoral component.

the femoral component appears to be anteriorized because of the necessity of creating a larger flexion gap for balancing, the surgeon should consider downsizing the femoral component.

Arthrotomy closure can also affect postoperative flexion. Closure with the knee in flexion may allow a more anatomic closure, which will avoid functional shortening of the extensor mechanism. Closure of the arthrotomy with excessive tension of the extensor mechanism may result in limited postoperative motion.

Problems with postoperative pain secondary to extensor mechanism complications such as instability, fracture, clunk, or crepitus can result in guarding and inhibited flexion as can lateral facet pain generated from direct contact of an "uncovered" lateral facet with the femoral component. The authors have observed this most frequently with the use of a small inset patellar component placed in a medialized position (Fig. 32-7).

Implant Design and Kinematics

The implant design and the subsequent kinematic patterns also contribute to the ROM and may have an impact on reducing postoperative stiffness. A kinematic analysis of various TKA designs performed in the authors' research laboratory evaluated knees with high weight-bearing flexion (greater than 125 degrees) and knees with low weight-bearing flexion (less than 90 degrees) using video fluoroscopy (35). Patients who underwent TKA and who had limited flexion showed substantially less posterior femoral translation (Fig. 32-8). A similar correlation between the amount of posterior femoral translation and subsequent postoperative knee flexion was observed by Banks et al in a fluoroscopic kinematic analysis of 93 subjects (121 TKA) implanted with 16 different articular TKA

FIGURE 32-8

Histogram demonstrating the magnitudes of posterior femoral translation occurring in high-flexion versus low-flexion knees.

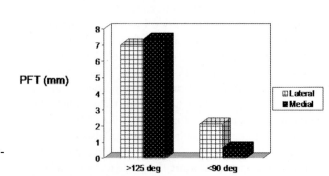

surface designs (36). They observed a mean increase of 1.4 degrees of knee flexion per millimeter of posterior femoral translation (R = 0.64, $p < .001$). The importance of posterior femoral translation is supported by studies that have shown higher flexion levels with the use of cruciate-substituting versus cruciate-retaining TKA designs (21). The etiology of reduced knee flexion with lesser amounts of posterior femoral translation is likely multifactorial. Posterior impingement of the femoral component on the tibial component occurs in a lesser degree of flexion as the femorotibial contact point is shifted anteriorly. Additionally, as the femoral component translates anteriorly with progressive flexion, tightening of the extensor mechanism occurs, which may limit maximum knee flexion.

Insertion of femoral components, which fail to restore the posterior femoral offset of the native femur will result in limited flexion. Bellemans et al performed a fluoroscopic review of 29 TKA patients during a deep squatting maneuver and found that 72% demonstrated direct posterior impingement of the tibial insert against the distal femur resulting in a mechanical block to further flexion (37). In a subsequent clinical review of 150 consecutive TKA subjects, the magnitude of posterior femoral condylar offset correlated with the final amount of knee flexion. Massin and Gournay performed a study using radiographic templating as well as in vivo TKA procedures using a computer navigation system (38). They analyzed the relationship between posterior condylar offset and the value of knee flexion in which posterior impingement of the distal femur and tibial component occurred. A 7- to 10-degree reduction in knee flexion was found when the posterior condylar offset was reduced by 3 mm.

PERIOPERATIVE COMPLICATIONS

Numerous perioperative complications can result in stiffness after a TKA. Infection, hemarthroses secondary to excessive anticoagulation, component loosening, periprosthetic fracture, reflex sympathetic dystrophy, and heterotopic ossification can all lead to postoperative stiffness and compromise the functional outcome.

Evaluation of the Stiff TKA

As with any medical evaluation, meticulous gathering of the patient history, physical examination, as well as radiographic and laboratory analysis is important. Pertinent history includes symptoms of infection, history of trauma, and the timing of the onset of stiffness. Early stiffness can often be attributed to either lack of appropriate physical rehabilitation or an intraoperative technical error. Late stiffness, after an extended period of good TKA motion should lead to suspicion of infection, component loosening, or failure.

Physical examination should include assessment of the skin, presence of effusion, ROM, stability, and evaluation of the extensor mechanism. Skin examination must include assessment for erythema, suggesting the presence of infection, signs of reflex sympathetic dystrophy (cutaneous hyperhydrosis, hypothermia, etc.), and for the presence of extensive scarring. Cutaneous adhesions warrant a plastic surgery consultation and consideration for implantation of soft tissue expanders (Fig. 32-9) (39). Stability examination is helpful in determining the overall balance of the knee with regard to the flexion and extension gaps. Examination of the extensor mechanism is important to rule out peripatellar sources of pain such as facet impingement, patellar subluxation, or patellar clunk or crepitus, which may result in guarded flexion.

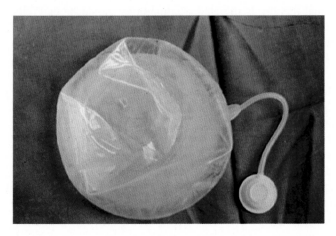

FIGURE 32-9

Photograph of a soft tissue expander used preoperatively in total knee arthroplasty cases with complex skin problems.

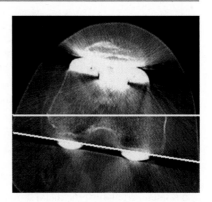

FIGURE 32-10

Computed tomography scan utilized to assess femoral component rotation versus the transepicondylar axis demonstrating undesirable internal rotation of the femoral component.

Radiographic evaluation begins with standard anterior-posterior, lateral, and merchant views (40). The lateral view is particularly helpful for evaluating femoral component size, sagittal alignment, and component positioning, tibial slope, the presence of posterior femoral osteophytes, heterotopic ossification, component loosening, level of the joint line, and patellar baja. The merchant view allows assessment of facet impingement and patellar tracking. If plain radiographs are noncontributory, bone scans may be helpful for identifying component loosening or infection. Computed tomography scans can be used to evaluate component malrotation (22,41). Thin axial cuts through the knee will allow assessment of femoral component rotation relative to the transepicondylar axis (Fig. 32-10). Tibial component rotation can also be assessed with reference to the tibial tubercle.

Laboratory analysis is focused on measures to identify the presence of infection. Hematologic evaluation should include obtaining a complete blood count with differential, erythrocyte sedimentation rate, and C-reactive protein. If a knee effusion is present, it is wise to perform an aspiration for cell count with differential (42), gram stain, and cultures.

MANAGEMENT OF THE STIFF TKA

Treatment of the stiff TKA depends, in part, on when the stiffness is diagnosed.

Early Postoperative Diagnosis

Early in the postoperative period, aggressive physical therapy is critical for achieving good motion. Communication between the physical therapist and the surgeon is important so that the physical therapist understands the expectations and protocols of the surgeon, and the surgeon can be made aware if the patient is having difficulty regaining knee motion. Adequate analgesics are important to ensure that the patient is reasonably comfortable while participating in the postoperative physical therapy program. Patients who have difficulties with extension should be splinted at night in extension. Close patient follow-up is imperative to assess the progress of motion.

Manipulation under anesthesia: Patients struggling with TKA motion at 4 to 8 weeks postoperatively should be considered candidates for a closed manipulation under anesthesia. Placing an epidural catheter or a regional nerve block is a good option for providing adequate pain control during and after the procedure. It is not unreasonable to anticipate overnight admission to continue with pain control as aggressive physical therapy is initiated. Radiographs should be carefully examined before the procedure to evaluate for osteopenia and anterior femoral notching, to heighten the awareness for periprosthetic fracture potential during manipulation. The procedure should be documented photographically to allow the patient to understand the pre- and postprocedure motion capabilities. The camera used for arthroscopy provides a nice vehicle for taking pictures and printing hard copies for both the patient and his or her physical therapist (Fig. 32-11).

Manipulation for flexion should be performed with gentle pressure applied with one hand on the proximal tibia and one hand on the anterior aspect of the patient's thigh. The surgeon should avoid manipulating the knee by holding the leg down by the ankle, which places excessive amounts of force on the end of a long lever arm. This leads to generating extreme forces that can potentially result in periprosthetic fracture or tendinous avulsion.

The surgeon can perform manipulation for extension by placing a bolster posterior to the lower leg. Gentle anterior pressure can then be applied with one hand on the proximal tibia and one hand on the distal femur. Dynamic splinting can also be used to aid maintaining extension after

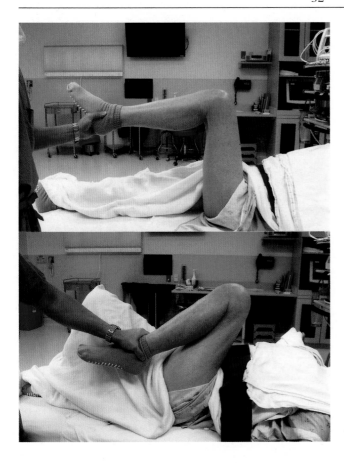

FIGURE 32-11

Premanipulation (top) and postmanipulation (bottom) photographs provided to the patient following closed manipulation under anesthesia to demonstrate the flexion gained from the manipulation.

manipulation. At the completion of a manipulation, radiographs should be performed to rule out fracture or component failure.

Late Postoperative Diagnosis

Patients with chronic motion problems (greater than 3 months postoperatively) usually require surgical intervention as capsular healing is complete. Flexion of less than 90 degrees or flexion contractures of greater than 15 degrees result in significant functional limitations. Many of these patients by this point have already undergone a closed manipulation under anesthesia. The type of surgical treatment depends on the source of stiffness. If the preoperative workup demonstrates appropriate component sizing, alignment, and TKA stability, arthrolysis without component revision is a reasonable option. This can be performed arthroscopically or with an open procedure if more radical debridement is required. An aggressive evaluation to rule out infection is critical before any surgical intervention is considered.

Although an arthroscopic arthrolysis can be performed to address intra-articular adhesions and arthrofibrosis (43,44), it is not generally recommended because of the risks of scratching the femoral component surfaces within the very tight scarred joint space. If attempted, the medial and lateral gutters should be débrided as well as the suprapatellar pouch. In a cruciate-retaining knee, the PCL can be released (44). This procedure should also be coupled with a concomitant manipulation. Bocell et al reported that only three of seven (43%) subjects with arthrofibrosis treated arthroscopically obtained improvement in motion (43), whereas Williams and Windsor et al noted an average improvement from preoperative flexion of 73.9 degrees to 104.5 degrees postoperatively in 10 cases treated with arthroscopic arthrolysis, PCL recession, and manipulation (44).

An open debridement is recommended and can be performed with extensive arthrolysis as required or if component exchange is anticipated. Exposure is often difficult and may require extensile exposure techniques such as a quadriceps snip (45–47), V-Y turndown (48–51), or a tibial tubercle osteotomy (45,52–55) to gain mobilization of the extensor mechanism. Radical scar excision should be performed to reestablish the medial and lateral gutters and the suprapatellar pouch, which are typically obliterated in the stiff TKA. A longer arthrotomy is wise, and a lateral release may be helpful to un-tether the extensor mechanism. A quadricepsplasty can also be performed to

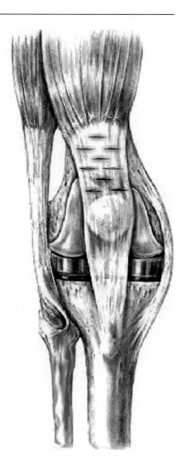

FIGURE 32-12
Pie-crusting of the quadriceps tendon enhances total knee arthroplasty flexion.

functionally lengthen the extensor mechanism through a V-Y lengthening or pie-crusting of the quadriceps tendon (Fig. 32-12).

COMPONENT REVISION

If the preoperative workup demonstrates component malpositioning, loosening component failure, improper sizing, an incorrect joint line level, marked instability, or inadequate bone resection, revision TKA is indicated after failure of nonoperative intervention. The same principles apply regarding radical scar excision as mentioned previously. Particular attention should be focused on the status of the femoral component. Errors in femoral component positioning, rotation, or sizing should not be accepted, and revision should be considered even in the setting of a well-fixed component. An isolated polyethylene insert exchange to a thinner insert without addressing the other components is rarely successful (56,57). During a revision procedure, after addressing component position, a decision must be made regarding tibial insert thickness during trialing of components. Particularly for patients with anticipated aggressive scar formation, it is reasonable to select a slightly thinner polyethylene insert thickness that is more conducive to obtaining greater flexion or extension as long as stability is not compromised. Patellar composite thickness should be carefully assessed and measured. If determined to be too thick because of inadequate resection, component revision should be performed to reduce patellar composite thickness to prearthroplasty levels. Posterior cruciate-retaining knees can be revised to a posterior-stabilized design, which mechanically guarantees posterior femoral rollback to enhance flexion and is less sensitive to alterations of the joint line level (58). Postoperative care is critical with emphasis on aggressive ROM accompanied by optimized pain control. Clinical results show modest gains in motion with component revision. Kim and Lotke et al reported 56 knee arthroplasties revised for stiffness. An increase in mean arc of motion from 54.6 to 82.2 degrees was obtained (6).

CONCLUSION

There are multiple causes of stiffness after a TKA including patient factors, technical errors, and perioperative complications. As with most issues in medicine, prevention is the best form of treatment. Patient factors should be addressed with preoperative education to promote diligent participation in physical therapy regimens. Technical errors should be avoided by focusing on proper flexion and extension gap balancing, accurate component positioning and sizing, and appropriate handling of the extensor mechanism. Stiffness should be thoroughly evaluated to discern the etiology. Acute postoperative stiffness can be treated with aggressive physical therapy with appropriate analgesics. Subacute stiffness can be managed with a manipulation under anesthesia. Chronic stiffness, which significantly inhibits activities of daily living, usually requires operative intervention. In the presence of component malposition, malrotation, or improper sizing, revision TKA should be performed. Although stiffness after a TKA is a known possible complication, attention to prevention and appropriate management will minimize the incidence and magnitude of stiffness.

REFERENCES

1. Colizza WA, Insall JN, Scuderi GR. The posterior stabilized total knee prosthesis: assessment of polyethylene damage and osteolysis after a ten-year-minimum follow-up. *J Bone Joint Surg Am* 1995;77:1713.
2. Dennis DA, Clayton ML, O'Donnell S, et al. Posterior cruciate condylar total knee arthroplasty. Average 11-year follow-up evaluation. *Clin Orthop Relat Res* 1992;281:168–176.
3. Ranawat CS, Luessenhop CP, Rodriguez JS. The press-fit condylar modular total knee system: four to six year results with a posterior-cruciate-substituting design. *J Bone Joint Surg Am* 1997;79:342.
4. Laubenthal KN, Smidt GL, Kettlekamp DB. A quantitative analysis of knee motion during activities of daily living. *Phys Therapy* 1972;52:34–43.
5. Kettlekamp DB, Johnson RJ, Smidt GL, et al. An electrogoniometric study of knee motion in normal gait. *J Bone Joint Surg Am* 1970;52:775–790.
6. Kim J, Nelson CL, Lotke PA. Stiffness after total knee arthroplasty. *J Bone Joint Surg Am* 2004; 86:1479–1494.
7. Ritter MA, Stringer EA. Predictive range of motion after total knee replacement. *Clin Orthop Relat Res* 1979;143:115–119.
8. Ritter MA, Campbell ED. Effect of range of motion on the success of a total knee arthroplasty. *J Arthrop* 1987;2:95–97.
9. Parsley BS, Engh GA, Dwyer KA. Preoperative flexion. Does it influence postoperative flexion after posterior-cruciate-retaining total knee arthroplasty? *Clin Orthop Relat Res* 1992;275:204–210.
10. Lizaur A, Marco L, Cebrian R. Preoperative factors influencing the range of movement after total knee arthroplasty for severe osteoarthritis. *J Bone Joint Surg Br* 1997;4:626–629.
11. Harvey IA, Barry K, Kirby SPJ, et al. Factors affecting the range of movement of total knee arthroplasty. *J Bone Joint Surg Br* 1993;75:950–955.
12. Shoji H, Solomonow M, Yoshino S, et al. Factors affecting postoperative flexion in total knee arthroplasty. *Orthopedics* 1990;13:643–649.
13. Horlocker TT, Kopp SL, Pagnano MW. Analgesia for total hip and knee arthroplasty: a multimodal pathway featuring peripheral nerve block. *J Am Acad Orthop Surg* 2006;14:126–135.
14. Hebl JR, Kopp SL, Ali MH, et al. A comprehensive anesthesia protocol that emphasizes peripheral nerve blockade for total knee and total hip arthroplasty. *J Bone Joint Surg Am* 2005;87(Suppl 2):63–70.
15. Brander V, Gondek S, Martin E, Stulberg SD. Pain and depression influence outcome 5 years after knee replacement surgery. *Clin Orthop Relat Res* 2007;464:21–26.
16. Ayers DC, Franklin PD, Ploutz-Snyder R, et al. Total knee replacement outcome and coexisting physical and emotional illness. *Clin Orthop Relat Res* 2005;440:157–161.
17. Ayers DC, Franklin PD, Trief PM, et al. Psychological attributes of preoperative total joint replacement patients: implications for optimal physical outcome. *J Arthroplasty* 2004;19(7 Suppl 2):125–130.
18. Lo CS, Wang SJ, Wu SS. Knee stiffness on extension caused by an oversized femoral component after total knee arthroplasty: a report of two cases and a review of the literature. *J Arthroplasty* 2003;18:804–808.
19. Dennis DA, Komistek RD, Colwell CW, et al. In vivo anteroposterior femorotibial translation of total knee arthroplasty: a multicenter analysis. *Clin Orthop Relat Res* 1998;356:47–57.
20. Dennis DA, Komistek RD, Mahfouz MR, et al. Multicenter determination of in vivo kinematics after total knee arthroplasty. *Clin Orthop Relat Res* 2003;416:37–57.
21. Dennis DA, Komistek RD, Stiehl J, et al. Range of motion following total knee arthroplasty: The effect of implant design and weight-bearing conditions. *J Arthrop* 1998;13:748–752.
22. Boldt JG, Stiehl JB, Hodler J, et al. Femoral component rotation and arthrofibrosis following mobile-bearing total knee arthroplasty. *Int Orthop* 2006;30:420–425.
23. Dennis DA, Komistek RD, Hoff WA, et al. In vivo knee kinematics derived using an inverse perspective technique. *Clin Orthop Relat Res* 1996;331:107–117.
24. Matsuda Y, Ishii Y, Noguchi H, et al. Varus-valgus balance and range of movement after total knee arthroplasty. *J Bone Joint Surg Br* 2005;87:804–808.
25. Goldstein WM, Raab DJ, Gleason TF, et al. Why posterior cruciate-retaining and substituting total knee replacements have similar ranges of motion. The importance of posterior condylar offset and clean out of posterior condylar space. *J Bone Joint Surg Am* 2006;88:182–188.
26. Kurosaka M, Yoshiya S, Mizuno K, Yamamoto T. Maximizing flexion after total knee arthroplasty: the need and the pitfalls. *J Arthrop* 2002;17(4 Suppl):59–62.

27. Ritter MA, Harty LD, Davis KE, et al. Predicting range of motion after total knee arthroplasty. Clustering, log-linear regression, and regression tree analysis. *J Bone Joint Surg Am* 2003;85-A:1278–1285.

28. Figgie HE 3rd, Goldberg VM, Heiple KG, et al. The influence of tibial-patellofemoral location on function of the knee in patients with the posterior stabilized condylar knee prosthesis. *J Bone Joint Surg Am* 1986;68:1035–1040.

29. Partington PF, Sawhney J, Rorabeck CH, et al. Joint line restoration after revision total knee arthroplasty. *Clin Orthop Relat Res* 1999;367:165–171.

30. Bengs BC, Scott RD. The effect of patellar thickness on intraoperative knee flexion and patellar tracking in total knee arthroplasty. *J Arthrop* 2006;21:650–655.

31. Mihalko W, Fishkin Z, Krakow K. Patellofemoral overstuff and its relationship to flexion after total knee arthroplasty. *Clin Orthop Relat Res* 2006;449:283–287.

32. Ortiguera CJ, Berry DJ. Patellar fractures after total knee arthroplasty. *J Bone Joint Surg Am* 2002;84:532–540.

33. Lesh ML, Schneider DJ, Deol G, et al. The consequences of anterior femoral notching in total knee arthroplasty. A biomechanical study. *J Bone Joint Surg Am* 2000;82:1096.

34. Ritter MA, Faris PM, Keating EM. Anterior femoral notching and ipsilateral supracondylar femur fracture in total knee arthroplasty. *J Arthrop* 1988;3:185–187.

35. Dennis DA, Komistek RD, Scuderi GR, et al. Factors affecting flexion after total knee arthroplasty. *Clin Orthop Relat Res* 2007;464:53–60.

36. Banks S, Bellemans J, Nozaki H, et al. Knee motions during maximum flexion in fixed and mobile-bearing arthroplasties. *Clin Orthop Relat Res* 2003;410:131–138.

37. Bellemans J, Banks S, Victor J, et al. Fluoroscopic analysis of the kinematics of deep flexion in total knee arthroplasty. Influence of posterior condylar offset. *J Bone Joint Surg Br* 2002;84:50–53.

38. Massin P, Gournay A. Optimization of the posterior condylar offset, tibial slope, and condylar roll-back in total knee arthroplasty. *J Arthrop* 2006;21:889–996.

39. Manifold SG, Cushner FD, Craig-Scott S, et al. Long-term results of total knee arthroplasty after the use of soft tissue expanders. *Clin Orthop Relat Res* 2000;380:133–139.

40. Merchant AC, Mercer RL, Jacobsen RH, et al. Roentgenographic analysis of patellofemoral congruence. *J Bone Joint Surg Am* 1974;56:1391–1396.

41. Berger RA, Crossett LS, Jacobs JJ, et al. Malrotation causing patellofemoral complications after total knee arthroplasty. *Clin Orthop Relat Res* 1998;356:144–153.

42. Mason JB, Fehring TK, Odum SM, et al. The value of white blood cell counts before revision total knee arthroplasty. *J Arthrop* 2003;18:1038–1043.

43. Bocell JR, Thorpe CD, Tullos HS. Arthroscopic treatment of symptomatic total knee arthroplasty. *Clin Orthop Relat Res* 1991;271:125–134.

44. Williams RJ, Westrich GH, Siegel J, et al. Arthroscopic release of the posterior cruciate ligament for stiff total knee arthroplasty. *Clin Orthop Relat Res* 1996;331:185–191.

45. Della Valle CJ, Berger RA, Rosenberg AG. Surgical exposures in revision total knee arthroplasty. *Clin Orthop Relat Res* 2006;446:59–68.

46. Garvin KL, Scuderi GR, Insall JN. Evolution of the quadriceps snip. *Clin Orthop Relat Res* 1995;321:131–137.

47. Younger AS, Duncan CP, Masri BA. Surgical exposures in revision total knee arthroplasty. *J Am Acad Orthop Surg* 1998;6:55–64.

48. Aglietti P, Buzzi R, D'Andria S, Scrobe F. Quadricepsplasty with the V-Y incision in total knee arthroplasty. *Ital J Orthop Traumatol* 1991;17:23–29.

49. Coonse K, Adams JD. A new operative approach to the knee joint. *Surg Gynecol Obstet* 1943;77:344–347.

50. Scott RD, Siliski JM. The use of a modified V-Y quadricepsplasty during total knee replacement to gain exposure and improve flexion in the ankylosed knee. *Orthopedics* 1985;8:45–48.

51. Trousdale RT, Hanssen AD, Rand JA, et al. V-Y quadricepsplasty in total knee arthroplasty. *Clin Orthop Relat Res* 1993;286:48–55.

52. Dolin MG. Osteotomy of the tibial tubercle in total knee replacement. A technical note. *J Bone Joint Surg Am* 1993;65:704–706.

53. Ries MD, Richman JA. Extended tibial tubercle osteotomy in total knee arthroplasty. *J Arthroplasty* 1996;11:964–967.

54. Whiteside LA, Ohl MD. Tibial tubercle osteotomy for exposure of the difficult total knee arthroplasty. *Clin Orthop Relat Res* 1990;260:6–9.

55. Wolff AM, Hungerford DS, Krackow KA, et al. Osteotomy of the tibial tubercle during total knee replacement. A report of twenty-six cases. *J Bone Joint Surg Am* 1989;71: 848–852.

56. Babis GC, Trousdale RT, Morrey BF. The effectiveness of isolated tibial insert exchange in revision total knee arthroplasty. *J Bone Joint Surg Am* 2002;84:64–68.

57. Engh GA, Koralewicz LM, Pereles TR. Clinical results of modular polyethylene insert exchange with retention of total knee arthroplasty components. *J Bone Joint Surg Am* 2000;82:516–523.

58. Dennis DA, Komistek RD, Mahfouz MR. In vivo fluoroscopic analysis of fixed-bearing total knee replacements. *Clin Orthop Relat Res* 2003;410:114–130.

33 Prolonged Drainage, Skin Necrosis, and Wound Problems

Michael D. Ries

INTRODUCTION

Serous wound drainage after total knee arthroplasty (TKA) is not uncommon, but prolonged drainage is associated with an increased risk of developing infection. If infection is suspected, early irrigation and debridement is indicated to prevent chronic infection involving the prosthetic components.

Skin necrosis can rapidly lead to exposure of the implant and deep infection of the TKA. The risk of skin necrosis can be reduced by utilizing previous scars and more lateral incisions in the multiply scarred knee when possible, and maintaining full-thickness skin and subcutaneous flaps during surgical exposure, as well as limiting early knee range of motion (ROM) after surgery. If full-thickness necrosis occurs, with resultant exposure of the TKA, prompt debridement and soft tissue coverage is necessary. Most soft tissue defects can be covered successfully with a medial gastrocnemius muscle flap transposition.

POSTOPERATIVE WOUND DRAINAGE

Blood drainage from the wound after TKA is common during the first few days after surgery. Once the wound is sealed and the skin begins to epithelialize, drainage should diminish considerably. However, serous fluid drainage can continue for up to a week in some patients. The fluid may originate from edema, blood debris, and ischemia in the subcutaneous tissues. When drainage is present, the wound is at a higher risk of developing infection (1,2). Infection is more likely to occur in patients with poor vascularity of the soft tissues, diabetes, immunosuppressive disorders, malnutrition, steroid use, and in obese patients with large subcutaneous tissue planes exposed during surgery (3,4).

Surgical technique can affect the vascularity to the skin and subcutaneous layer. Ideally, the skin incision is placed in close proximity to the arthrotomy incision to avoid elevating soft tissue flaps. However, prior scars often restrict the location of the surgical incision so that flaps are required to expose the medial retinaculum and permit use of a medial parapatellar arthrotomy. Blood vessels perforate through the fascia to form an anastomosis deep to the subcutaneous layer, which supplies circulation to the subcutaneous tissue and skin (Fig. 33-1) (5). Dissection of the subcutaneous tissue should be performed along the subfascial plane between the deepest portion of the subcutaneous layer and deep fascia. If full-thickness skin and subcutaneous soft tissue flaps are dissected from the fascial layer, relatively large flaps can be raised without compromising soft tissue vascularity. If dissection is carried out into the subcutaneous plane and subcutaneous tissue is left attached to the fascia, however, the overlying soft tissue can become devascularized and lead to ischemia or necrosis (Fig. 33-2).

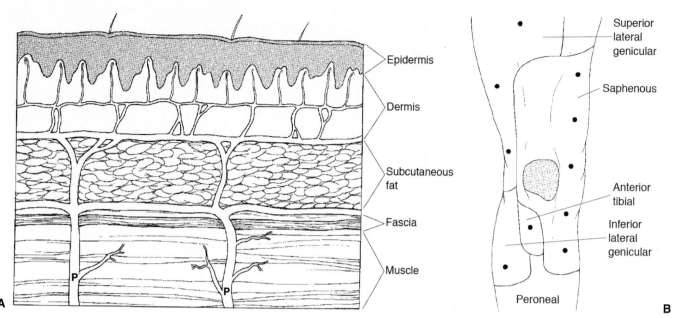

Epidermis

Dermis

Subcutaneous fat

Fascia

Muscle

A

Superior lateral genicular

Saphenous

Anterior tibial

Inferior lateral genicular

Peroneal

B

FIGURE 33-1

(A) The microvascular circulation to the skin and subcutaneous tissue consists of deep perforating vessels (P) that penetrate the fascia and form an anastomosis along the deep portion of the subcutaneous layer. Skin flaps should be raised by dissection along the fascial plane to maintain the anastomotic blood supply to the subcutaneous tissue and skin. **(B)** The areas of the skin over the knee supplied by the deep perforators are shown. Most of the blood supply comes from the medial side, so the lateral skin flap will be more hypoxic than the medial skin flap, and using a more medial incision may increase the risk of skin necrosis. (Reprinted with permission from Younger ASE, Duncan CP, Masri BA. Surgical exposures in revision total knee arthroplasty. *J Am Acad Orthop Surg* 1998;6:55–64.)

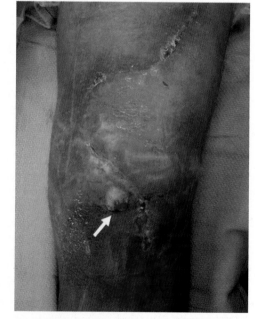

FIGURE 33-2

A 54-year-old man underwent total knee arthroplasty for posttraumatic arthritis. Three weeks after surgery, a small amount of drainage developed lateral to the surgical incision. Surgical exploration demonstrated deep infection.

TABLE 33-1. Summary of Types of Acute Postoperative Wound Drainage

Diagnosis	Source of Drainage	Signs	Infected (yes/no)	Treatment
Type 1 Superficial serous drainage	Edema caused by surgical trauma and ischemia of subcutaneous soft tissues.	After initial onset, serous drainage volume decreases daily. No cellulitis, or wound induration.	No	Daily sterile dressing changes. Oral or IV antibiotics if drainage excessive to prevent wound colonization.
Type 2 Superficial infection	Abscess fluid in subcutaneous layer.	Serous drainage, volume increases daily. Cellulitis around wound. Fever, erythema, and induration may be present.	Yes	Joint aspiration to confirm absence of deep infection. If drainage is minimal, treat with IV antibiotics and dressing changes. If drainage persists, then I and D of subcutaneous layer.
Type 3 Deep serous drainage	Intra-articular blood and joint fluid expressed into subcutaneous layer through a fascial defect.	Serous drainage, increases with activity. No fever, erythema, or induration.	No	I and D of joint, place drains, repair fascial defect if possible, use postoperative antibiotics.
Type 4 Deep postoperative infection	Infected hematoma or abscess fluid expressed into subcutaneous layer through a fascial defect.	Thick serous or purulent drainage. Fever, erythema, and induration may be present.	Yes	I and D with tibial insert exchange. Closure of fascial defect over drains. Six weeks post-operative IV antibiotic therapy.

I and D, irrigation and debridement; IV, intravenous.

Wound drainage management depends on the location of fluid accumulation (superficial or deep) and presence or absence of infection (Table 33-1). Serous drainage originating from edema in the subcutaneous layer does not necessarily represent infection, but the expression of fluid through the surgical incision indicates that the wound is not sealed. Incomplete wound healing indicates that the wound does not provide a complete barrier to contamination from the skin. Sterile dressings should be maintained on the wound and changed daily as often as necessary to collect wound drainage.

When drainage is present, the wound is at risk of developing infection from skin contamination (1,2). If the drainage volume decreases daily and clinical signs of infection (fever, erythema, and induration) are absent, however, then the drainage can be treated with dressing changes alone and without antibiotics or surgical debridement. Antibiotics can be used to manage a noninfected draining surgical wound as a prophylactic measure to prevent infection because the wound is incompletely sealed and exposed to skin contamination. However, antibiotic therapy alone for treatment of a deep post-operative infection is not an appropriate method to eradicate infection. If there is a clinical suspicion that deep infection is present and the source of wound drainage is not clear, then use of antibiotics may suppress an infection and make the diagnosis more difficult to establish. Therefore, the distinction between a wound that is not infected and draining from the subcutaneous tissues and one that is infected or draining from the knee joint into the subcutaneous layer is important.

IRRIGATION AND DEBRIDEMENT FOR PROLONGED DRAINAGE

Indications

Irrigation and debridement (I and D) is indicated for deep wound drainage originating within the knee draining out of the skin incision (type 3 or 4, Table 33-1). Drainage from a sinus outside of the surgical incision indicates that drainage is occurring from within the knee joint and surgical debridement is necessary (Fig. 33-3). I and D is also appropriate for superficial infection (type 2, Table 33-1). I and D is not necessary to treat serous fluid drainage resulting from edema or ischemia of the subcutaneous tissue that is not infected (type 1, Table 33-1). However, type 1 drainage may

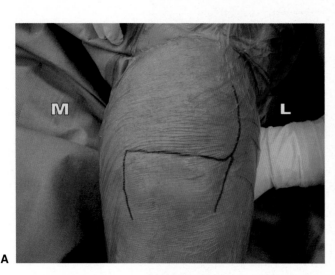

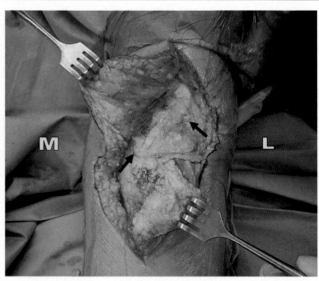

FIGURE 33-3

(A) A previous S-shaped scar was present in a patient who required total knee arthroplasty. The medial (M) and lateral (L) sides of the knee are indicated. **(B)** The previous incision was used, which required elevation of skin and subcutaneous soft tissue flaps from the fascia. Subcutaneous tissue has been left attached to the fascia and detached from the skin flap (*arrows*) indicating that dissection extended into rather than deep to the subcutaneous layer. As a result, a portion of the overlying skin and subcutaneous soft tissue may become ischemic.

convert to type 2 drainage. A period of observation is appropriate for type 1 drainage. If the drainage is decreasing each day and if clinical signs of infection are not present, then the drainage should resolve as wound healing occurs in the subcutaneous layer.

Contraindications

There are virtually no contraindications to I and D for wound drainage suspected to originate from within the knee (type 3 or 4, Table 33-1) or associated with a superficial infection (type 2, Table 33-1). If infection is suspected, I and D is the most appropriate treatment. If I and D is performed during the early postoperative period, however, primary wound closure may be associated with excess skin tension caused by edema and contracture of the soft tissues over the knee. If the wound is closed under tension, limiting early knee ROM after surgery can be beneficial to allow wound healing to occur (6). If primary wound closure is not possible after I and D, additional soft tissue flap coverage is necessary. The integrity of the soft tissues and any potential difficulty with primary wound closure should be carefully assessed prior to I and D.

Technique

If I and D is performed for treatment of superficial infection (type 2, Table 33-1), the fascial layer will be intact, and debridement is limited to the skin and subcutaneous layer. Fluid and soft tissue specimens should be obtained for culture. After debridement, the wound should be closed over a subcutaneous drain.

For debridement of deep wound drainage (type 3 or 4, Table 33-1), the wound should be adequately exposed during I and D to provide access to all areas of the knee including the posterior compartment. The surgeon can perform debridement as an open procedure or arthroscopically. Arthrotomy provides wide exposure of the knee, permits exchange of the tibial insert, and direct exposure of the metallic components to determine whether they are well fixed. Tibial insert exchange allows exposure and debridement of the tibial base plate surface and better exposure of the posterior compartment of the knee. Successful results have also been reported with arthroscopic debridement (7), but it is difficult to access completely all regions of the knee joint and to perform a thorough debridement or exchange the polyethylene. Therefore, it is not typically advocated. Arthroscopic instruments should be inserted into the knee carefully to avoid damage to the prosthetic articular surfaces. With either open or arthroscopic debridement, fluid and soft tissue specimens should be obtained for culture. Thorough irrigation and debridement of any loose, necrotic, or potentially infected soft tissue should be performed and the wound closed over a deep drain.

Postoperative Management

Intravenous antibiotics are generally continued for 3 weeks after I and D of superficial infection and 6 weeks after I and D for deep infection. The selection and duration of antibiotics depends on many factors, however, including the specific bacterial organism(s) identified, duration of known or suspected infection, immune status of the host, appearance of the wound and amount of soft tissue inflammation observed during debridement, vascularity to the bone and surrounding tissues, and integrity of soft tissue coverage over the knee. An infectious disease consultation is appropriate and usually helpful to determine the optimal antibiotic treatment.

Drains should be used for several days after I and D until drainage is minimal. Knee ROM can be started immediately if the soft tissue flaps are well vascularized and closed without tension. Otherwise, ROM exercises should be delayed for several days until vascularity of the wound has improved.

RESULTS

Results of I and D for superficial infection (type 2, Table 33-1) are very successful because the knee joint is not involved. Occasional recurrent superficial infections may develop, however, probably related to underlying fat necrosis in the subcutaneous layer or incompletely treated areas of infection. Additional antibiotic therapy or debridement may be necessary to treat recurrent superficial infection.

In the setting of deep periprosthetic infection, failure rates of greater than 50% have been reported for I and D with retention of the components after TKA (8,9). Results of I and D for deep postoperative infection (type 4, Table 33-1) are more successful if performed early (within the first 4 weeks) after TKA (8,10). Results are also less favorable for infections caused by *Staphylococcus aureus* (9). Failure of I and D leads to chronic deep infection, requiring removal of the prosthetic components to adequately treat the infection. Because of the relatively low morbidity rate associated with debridement and retention of the components, this treatment is appropriate in the acute postoperative period although the success rate may be low.

SKIN NECROSIS

Necrosis of the skin after TKA is a rare complication but can rapidly lead to full-thickness soft tissue loss, with exposure and infection of the prosthetic components. Risk factors for the development of skin necrosis include poor soft tissue vascularity, rheumatoid arthritis, steroid use, immunosuppression, malnutrition, peripheral vascular disease, and multiple prior scars. Lengthy tourniquet times, particularly in patients with other risk factors for developing wound complications may also be a contributing factor. The preoperative nutritional status can influence the risk of wound complications. Greene et al found that patients with a preoperative lymphocyte count less than 1500 cells/mm^3 had a five times greater frequency of developing major wound complications, and patients with an albumin count of less than 3.5 g/dL had a seven times greater frequency (3).

Vascularity of the skin over the knee will affect the rate of healing postoperatively and risk of necrosis. Skin tension can also affect the vascularity. A medial parapatellar incision is more parallel to the skin cleavage lines than a vertical midline incision and is associated with less tension during flexion (11). Because most of the circulation to the skin over the knee originates medially, however, a more medial incision can compromise circulation to the lateral skin edge (Fig. 33-1B).

Knee flexion increases soft tissue tension that can decrease perfusion to the soft tissues (12). Yashar et al reported that high flexion constant passive motion (70 to 100 degrees flexion started in the recovery room) was associated with increased knee flexion during hospitalization, but wound necrosis requiring medial gastrocnemius coverage occurred in one of 104 patients (13). Kim et al observed skin necrosis in 13 of 27 patients who underwent TKA for bony ankylosis (14). Henkel et al reported skin necrosis requiring muscle flap coverage in two of seven patients who were converted from arthrodesis to TKA (15). Patients with soft tissue atrophy or contracture caused by

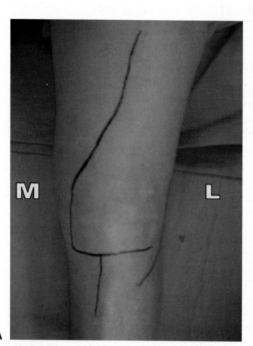
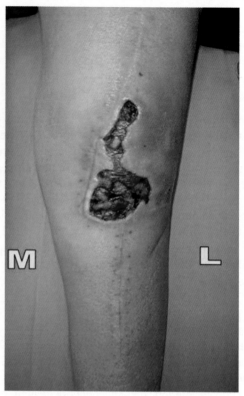

FIGURE 33-4

(A) Multiple scars were present over the knee in a patient with a history of cigarette smoking and prior knee arthrodesis who then underwent conversion to total knee arthroplasty. The prior medial (M) and lateral (L) scars have been outlined. **(B)** An incision was made through the prior anteromedial scar, and full-thickness skin and subcutaneous tissue flaps were elevated. However, skin necrosis developed along the lateral skin flap. (Reprinted with permission from Ries MD, Bozic KJ. Medial gastrocnemius flap coverage for treatment of skin necrosis after total knee arthroplasty. *Clin Orthop* 2006;446:186–192.)

long-standing restricted knee motion may have increased skin tension during ROM after TKA that can lead to necrosis (Fig. 33-4). Particularly for patients with multiple risk factors for developing wound complications, avoidance or delayed use of constant passive motion and early ROM exercises may be beneficial in reducing the development of skin necrosis.

Transcutaneous skin oxygen tension decreases for the first 2 to 3 days after surgery and then increases (12). In addition, the lateral skin edge is more hypoxic than the medial edge (12). When necrosis occurs, it is more likely to develop along the lateral skin flap (Fig. 33-4), suggesting that when multiple prior scars are present, the most vertical lateral incision should be used to minimize skin hypoxia (Fig. 33-5).

DEBRIDEMENT AND SOFT TISSUE COVERAGE

Indications

If skin necrosis occurs after TKA, early recognition of the problem and treatment will minimize the risk of deep infection of the prosthetic components. When skin necrosis is present, the underlying subcutaneous tissue is also likely to be necrotic, but the circulation to the subcutaneous tissue and skin is separate from the deep fascia. The deep fascia and muscle under the necrotic skin may be viable and provide a source of vascularity to support a skin graft or granulation tissue. Because the proximal portion of the knee contains more muscle and fascia than the distal portion, necrosis of the proximal wound including the area over the patella may be treated by local wound care and skin grafting (6). However, the deep tissues at the distal aspect of the knee, particularly the patellar

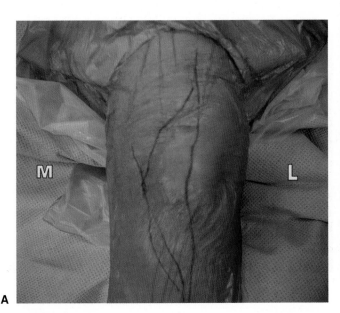
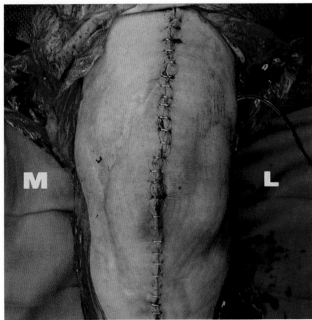

FIGURE 33-5

(A) Prior medial parapatellar and midline scars were present over the knee. The medial (M) and lateral (L) sides are indicated. Although the medial parapatellar incision is associated with less skin tension than a midline incision, the lateral skin edge has less vascularity than the medial skin edge. If the medial scar is used, necrosis could develop along the lateral edge of the incision in between the two scars. **(B)** The more lateral vertical scar was used, and the skin edges remained well vascularized.

ligament and tibial tubercle are not well vascularized. If this area is exposed as a result of necrosis of the overlying skin and subcutaneous tissue, infection of the patellar ligament can occur and lead to avulsion of the extensor mechanism. Necrosis over the tibial tubercle or patellar tendon requires muscle flap coverage to prevent infection involving the patellar tendon and extensor mechanism disruption (Figs. 33-6 and 33-7).

CONTRAINDICATIONS

When full-thickness skin necrosis occurs, the TKA can become contaminated with skin bacteria and rapidly lead to a deep infection of the prosthetic components. Therefore, if skin necrosis develops after TKA, prompt debridement and soft tissue coverage is indicated. If full-thickness skin necrosis occurs, the exposed TKA should be treated as if there is an acute deep infection, with debridement of contaminated and potentially infected periarticular soft tissues, exchange of the tibial insert, and soft tissue transfer procedures to obtain coverage over the TKA. I and D with retention of the prosthetic components is most effective if surgical treatment is performed soon after the onset of infection (8,10). If chronic infection is present, however, and involves the prosthetic components, then salvage of the TKA is not likely, and debridement and soft tissue coverage alone can be expected to have a high risk of failure.

PEARLS AND PITFALLS

Very small areas of necrosis particularly over the patella or proximal wound in which the underlying muscle or fascia is likely to remain vascularized can be treated with local wound care. Restricting knee flexion will diminish skin tension and may prevent further ischemia. For larger areas of necrosis or those over the distal wound, however, debridement of the necrotic soft tissue and soft tissue flap coverage is necessary (Figs. 33-4, 33-6, and 33-7).

Treatment of an infected TKA with loss of soft tissue coverage requires both removal of the prosthetic components and soft tissue coverage (16). The TKA should be removed, an antibiotic-

(text continues on p. 444)

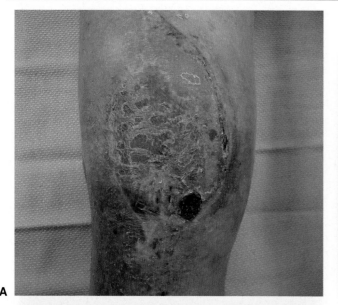

A

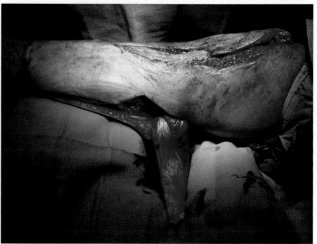

B

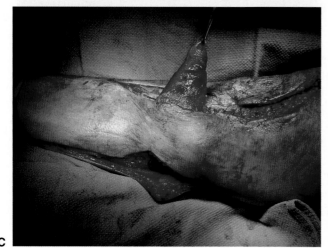

C

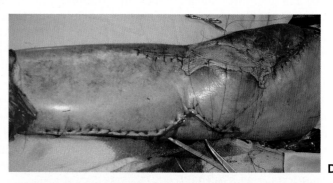

D

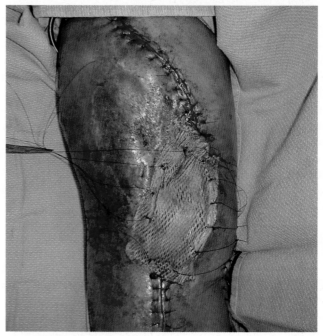

E

FIGURE 33-6

(A) A 62-year-old man presented with an infected total knee arthroplasty. The skin is atrophic with a prior skin graft and necrosis along the medial inferior wound overlying the proximal tibia. **(B)** The medial gastrocnemius was dissected and detached distally. **(C)** The muscle is transposed under a skin bridge to the anterior knee wound. (Reprinted with permission from Ries MD. Skin necrosis after total knee arthroplasty. *J Arthrop* 2002;17:S74–S77.) **(D)** The medial gastrocnemius donor site incision is closed primarily. **(E)** A skin graft was required to cover the muscle over the anterior knee wound. *(continued)*

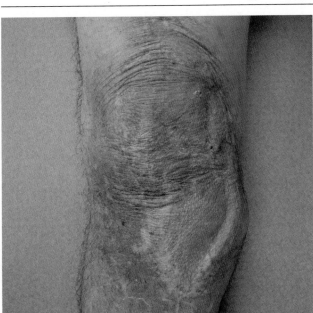

F

FIGURE 33-6 *(Continued)*

(F) One year after reconstructive surgery, the knee wounds are well healed with minimal deformity.

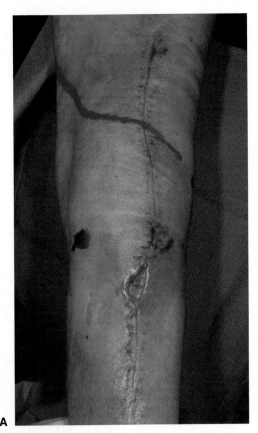

A

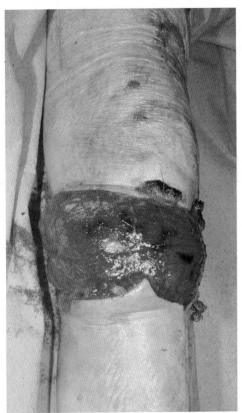

B

FIGURE 33-7

(A) Skin necrosis developed over the tibial tubercle in an 80-year-old woman who underwent total knee arthroplasty for posttraumatic arthritis. **(B)** Medial gastrocnemius flap transposition was performed to cover the defect. *(continued)*

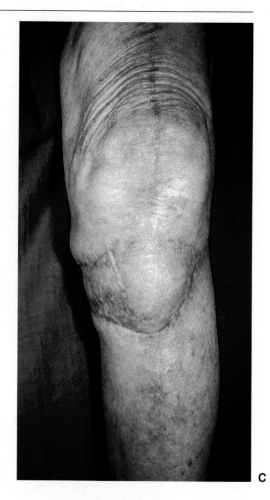

C

FIGURE 33-7 *(Continued)*

(C) One year after muscle flap coverage, the wounds are well healed, range of motion is 0 to 90 degrees, and the patient ambulates without support. (Reprinted with permission from Ries MD, Bozic KJ. Medial gastrocnemius flap coverage for treatment of skin necrosis after total knee arthroplasty. *Clin Orthop* 2006;446:186–192.)

impregnated cement spacer placed, and soft tissue coverage should be obtained as a single procedure (Fig. 33-8) (17). The patient is also treated with IV antibiotic therapy usually for 6 weeks during which time the soft tissue flap can heal. A second-stage revision TKA is then performed.

At the second-stage revision TKA, the skin incision should follow the lateral border of the transposed medial gastrocnemius flap. The flap is then mobilized in a lateral-to-medial direction to preserve its medial-based pedicle with blood supply to the flap. The entire thickness of the muscle

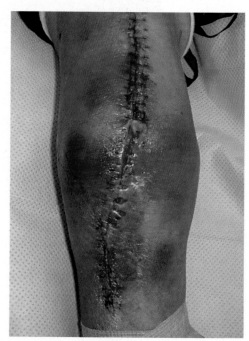

A

FIGURE 33-8

(A) A 32-year-old HIV-positive man with hemophilia developed infection after revision total knee arthroplasty with necrosis along the skin incision. *(continued)*

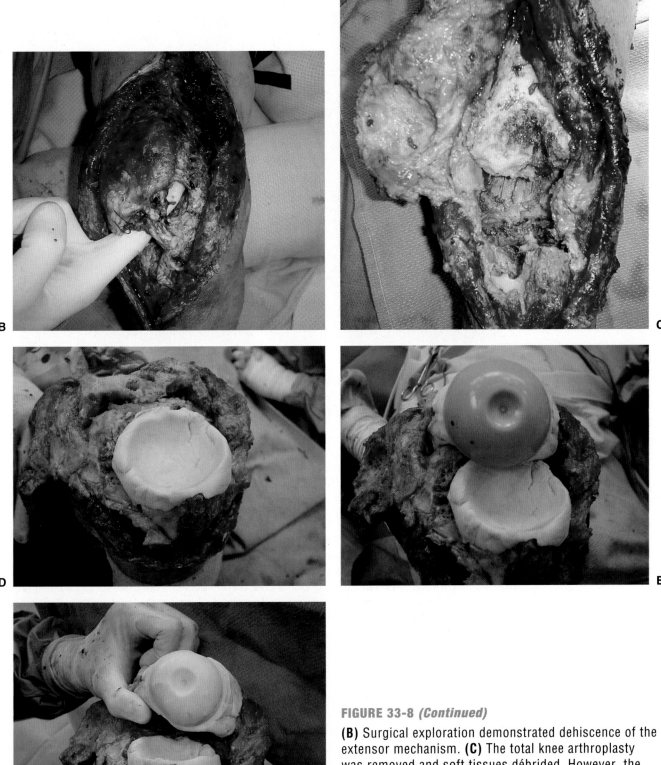

FIGURE 33-8 *(Continued)*

(B) Surgical exploration demonstrated dehiscence of the extensor mechanism. **(C)** The total knee arthroplasty was removed and soft tissues débrided. However, the patellar ligament attachment was avulsed. **(D)** An articulated antibiotic cement spacer was placed. A bipolar hip 55-mm trial component was used as a mold to form a concave tibial surface. **(E)** The bulb portion of an irrigation syringe was used to form a convex femoral surface. **(F)** The "ball-and-socket" articulated spacer permitted knee range of motion and stability between the femoral and tibial surfaces. *(continued)*

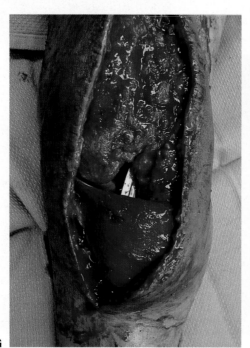

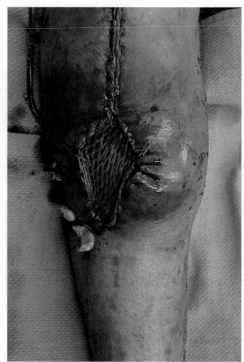

G

H

FIGURE 33-8 *(Continued)*
(G) A medial gastrocnemius transposition was performed to cover the anterior knee wound and re-establish continuity of the tibia to the proximal extensor mechanism.
(H) A skin graft was placed over the transposed muscle.

is elevated from the deep fascial layer or bone to expose the extensor mechanism retinaculum and permit a medial arthrotomy to be performed (Fig. 33-9).

Technique of Soft Tissue Flap Coverage

Soft tissue flaps options include fasciocutaneous, muscle transposition, and free flaps (6, 15,16,18,19). Muscle flaps contain a rich blood supply, and most defects can be covered well with a medial gastrocnemius transposition flap. If the patellar tendon is not viable and the extensor mechanism is disrupted, the medial gastrocnemius flap can also be used to augment the extensor mechanism (20). More lateral defects may be better treated with a lateral gastrocnemius flap, and a soleus flap can be helpful to extend the coverage proximally. Skin grafts are needed during muscle flap transposition. The skin graft can be placed directly onto the transposed muscle overlying the knee. Alternatively, the muscle and overlying skin are transposed together as a vascularized musculocutaneous flap, which leaves a skin defect at the donor site requiring skin graft coverage. Free flaps are indicated for very large defects that cannot be covered adequately with local flaps (Fig. 33-10). However, this requires microvascular anastomoses with a risk of flap necrosis that is much less of a concern with local transposition flaps. Donor site morbidity is also a concern with use of muscle flaps, but the loss of strength after medial gastrocnemius flap transposition appears to significantly impair functional activity in the TKA patient population (16). Fasciocutaneous flaps avoid loss of donor site function but do not carry the rich vascularity of muscle and may result in cosmetic defects. Flaps may be used in combination to optimize soft tissue coverage. The choice of flap coverage depends on many factors including the location and size of the defect, vascularity of the local tissue and donor site options, potential donor site morbidity, and functional demands and medical status of the patient.

POSTOPERATIVE MANAGEMENT

The primary objective of soft tissue coverage procedures is to seal the knee and prevent or limit infection. Motion is often sacrificed to ensure wound healing. The knee is immobilized until soft tissue healing has been achieved. Antibiotic therapy may be necessary; the class and duration are

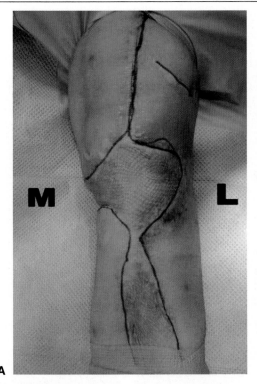
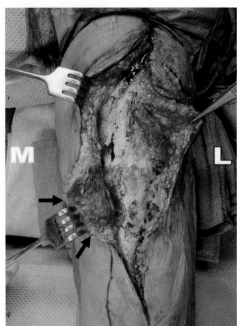

A   B

FIGURE 33-9

(A) Prior medial (M) and lateral (L) scars are present after previous medial gastrocnemius muscle flap coverage of the knee. **(B)** The lateral incision is used, and the medial gastrocnemius flap (arrows) is elevated in a lateral (L) to medial (M) direction to preserve the medial-based blood supply to the flap.

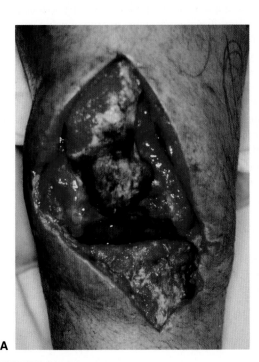
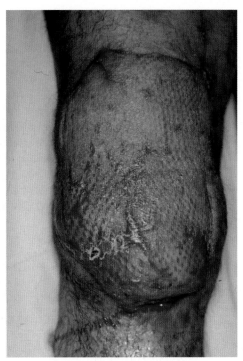

A   B

FIGURE 33-10

(A) A 68-year-old man with diabetes mellitus developed infection after total knee arthroplasty with extensive skin and soft tissue necrosis and loss of the distal extensor mechanism. **(B)** The patient refused amputation and was treated with debridement, insertion of an antibiotic cement spacer, and latissimus free-flap coverage. Drainage occurred along the inferior margin of the wound. *(continued)*

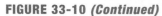

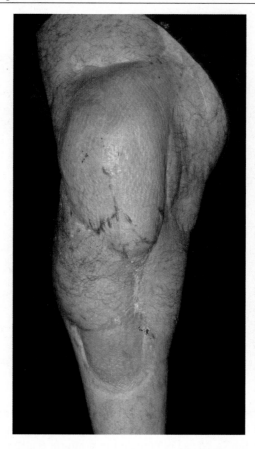

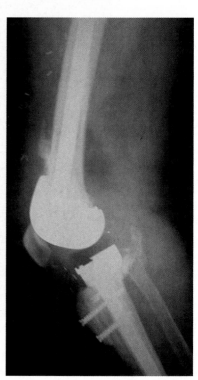

C-D

FIGURE 33-10 *(Continued)*
(C) The antibiotic cement spacer was exchanged, and the inferior wound was covered with a medial gastrocnemius transposition flap, which resulted in wound healing.
(D) Delayed revision total knee arthroplasty was performed with reconstruction of the extensor mechanism using a whole patellar allograft (Parts A, C, and D reprinted with permission from Ries MD, Bozic KJ. Medial gastrocnemius flap coverage for treatment of skin necrosis after total knee arthroplasty. *Clin Orthop* 2006;446:186–192.)

determined on the basis of intraoperative cultures, duration that the wound was open, and postoperative course. Consultation with an infectious diseases specialist may be of value, even in the absence of known infection.

RESULTS

When skin necrosis occurs and the TKA is exposed, the arthroplasty is at high risk of becoming infected. Factors influencing the results of treatment include the location and extent of necrosis, presence and duration of deep infection involving the prosthesis, vascularity of the surrounding soft tissues, and choice and technique of the specific soft tissue coverage procedure used. Failure to obtain soft tissue coverage or to control deep infection can require above-knee amputation. However, prompt debridement and medial gastrocnemius flap coverage for treating skin necrosis with exposure of the TKA is associated with an arthroplasty salvage rate of over 90% (16).

REFERENCES

1. Patel VP, Walsh M, Sehgal B, et al. Factors associated with prolonged wound drainage after primary total hip and knee arthroplasty. *J Bone Joint Surg* 2007;89A:33–38.
2. Saleh K, Olson M, Resig S, et al. Predictors of wound infection in hip and knee replacement: results from a 20-year surveillance program. *J Orthop Res* 2002;20:506–515.
3. Greene KA, Wilde AH, Stulberg BN. Preoperative nutritional status of total joint patients. Relationship to postoperative wound complications. *J Arthrop* 1991;6:321–325.
4. Vince K, Chivas D, Droll KP. Wound complications after total knee arthroplasty. *J Arthrop* 2007;22 (Suppl 1):39–44.
5. Younger ASE, Duncan CP, Masri BA. Surgical exposures in revision total knee arthroplasty. *J Am Acad Orthop Surg* 1998;6:55–64.
6. Ries MD. Skin necrosis after total knee arthroplasty. *J Arthrop* 2002;17:S74–S77.
7. Ilahi OA, Al-Habbal GA, Bocell JR, et al. Arthroscopic debridement of acute periprosthetic septic arthritis of the knee. *Arthroscopy* 2005;21:303–306.
8. Hartman MB, Fehring TK, Jordan L, Norton HJ. Periprosthetic knee sepsis: the role of irrigation and debridement. *Clin Orthop* 1991;273:113–118.

9. Deirmengian C, Greenbaum J, Lotke PA, et al. Limited success with open debridement and retention of components in the treatment of acute *Staphylococcus aureus* infections after total knee arthroplasty. *J Arthrop* 2003;18(Suppl 1):22–26.

10. Mont MA, Waldman B, Banerjee C, et al. Multiple irrigation, debridement, and retention of components in infected total knee arthroplasty. *J Arthrop* 1997;12:426–433.

11. Johnson DP. Midline or parapatellar incision for knee arthroplasty. *J Bone Joint Surg* 1986;70B:656–658.

12. Johnson DP. The effect of continuous passive motion on wound healing and joint mobility after knee arthroplasty. *J Bone Joint Surg* 72(A):421–426.

13. Yashar AA, Venn-Watson E, Welsh T, et al. Continuous passive motion with accelerated flexion after total knee arthroplasty. *Clin Orthop* 1997;345:38–43.

14. Kim YH, Cho SH, Kim JS. Total knee arthroplasty in bony ankylosis in gross flexion. *J Bone Joint Surg* 1999;81B:296–300.

15. Henkel TR, Boldt JG, Drobny TK, Munzinger UK. Total knee arthroplasty after formal knee fusion using unconstrained and semiconstrained components: a report of 7 cases. *J Arthroplasty* 16;768–776.

16. Ries MD, Bozic KJ. Medial gastrocnemius flap coverage for treatment of skin necrosis after total knee arthroplasty. *Clin Orthop* 2006;446:186–192.

17. MacAvoy M, Ries MD. The ball and socket articulating spacer for infected total knee arthroplasty. *J Arthrop* 2005;20:757–762.

18. Ikeda K, Morishita Y, Nakatani A, et al. Total knee arthroplasty covered with pedicle peroneal flap. *J Arthrop* 1996;11:478–481.

19. Lian G, Cracchiolo III A, Lesavoy M. Treatment of major wound necrosis following total knee arthroplasty. *J Arthrop* 1989;4(Suppl 1):S23–S32.

20. Busfield B, Huffman R, Nahai F, et al. Extended medial gastrocnemius rotational flap for treatment of chronic knee extensor mechanism deficiency in patients with and without total knee arthroplasty. *Clin Orthop* 2004;428:190–197.

34 Arthrodesis for the Chronically Infected Total Knee Arthroplasty

Stephen J. Incavo and Michael R. Dayton

INDICATIONS

Knee arthrodesis is a salvage operation used when staged revision has failed to resolve infection after total knee arthroplasty (TKA), when the extensor mechanism is unreconstructable, or when soft tissue coverage is inadequate for further revision arthroplasty. Its goals are the eradication of infection and a successful fusion resulting in a stable and pain-free knee.

Arthrodesis does not guarantee resolution of infection. In fact, given the chronicity of infection in some patients, the risk of post-fusion sepsis or osteomyelitis likely remains elevated (supporting the role of chronic suppressive antibiotic therapy in many of these patients). Even if successful arthrodesis is achieved, recurrent local infection may cause chronic pain and pose a systemic threat.

CONTRAINDICATIONS

Successful fusion requires not only bone healing but also reasonable soft tissue coverage. Therefore, a fusion may not be feasible in patients who have compromised and unreconstructable soft tissue coverage. Plastic surgery consultation should be sought early to determine the feasibility of flap coverage in the setting of chronic knee infection with wound breakdown.

Arthrodesis is also contraindicated in most nonambulatory patients who might be served better with resection arthroplasty or above-knee amputation. Fusion may be contraindicated in the presence of overwhelming or persistent sepsis, particularly when arthroplasties are present in other joints, because they would be at increased risk for metachronous infection.

Patients with unreconstructable severe vascular insufficiency may be better candidates for an above-knee amputation.

In the presence of severe bone deficiency, successful arthrodesis may be untenable, although emerging fusion devices or future biologic options may expand the indications for fusion. Chronically infected knees treated previously with hinged implants with metaphyseal-filling or segmental-replacing metal augments may not be amenable to fusion; in such cases, above-knee amputation may be a more appropriate solution.

There are unusual situations that may render the patient an unsuitable candidate for knee arthrodesis, although it is unclear whether these criteria are as appropriate in patients requiring salvage of a chronically infected TKA as they are in patients considering arthrodesis for primary or secondary arthritis of the knee. These include patients with a contralateral above-knee amputation or knee or hip arthrodesis, or those with ipsilateral hip or ankle arthritis.

FIXATION OPTIONS

A variety of fixation options exist for knee arthrodesis. These include either cephalomedullary or modular intramedullary nails, external fixation, and internal plate fixation. Traditionally, external fixation with circular frames or multiplanar fixation and internal fixation using plates and screws have had lower fusion rates than intramedullary techniques. This statistic may, in fact, be changing with the use of modern locking plates, which provide improved stability. External fixators have the unique risks of pin tract problems and a relatively limited capacity for compression. Fusion rates are relatively low with external fixation compared to alternative methods and is therefore used less frequently than the other methods of fusion.

Plate fixation and external fixators have the advantage of limiting the fusion procedure to the knee, and intramedullary techniques theoretically carry a potential risk of spreading a residual infection up and down the femoral or tibial intramedullary canals. Despite this theoretical concern regarding intramedullary fixation, however, the meticulous attention placed on the eradication of infection prior to knee arthrodesis surgery has limited its occurrence in most contemporary reports on intramedullary techniques of knee fusion (1). Intramedullary techniques are also facilitated with the use of improved intramedullary nail systems. Long intramedullary nails are easily removed should further surgery be necessary. On the other hand, although short intramedullary fusion nails are appealing because they are relatively easily inserted and assembled through the knee, they can be very difficult to remove if infection recurs once the joint is successfully fused, unless an osteotomy or large bony window is made in the knee.

In the absence of ipsilateral hip problems or "obstacles" (such as a total hip arthroplasty), we prefer to use intramedullary nail fixation; therefore, the remainder of this chapter focuses on the insertion technique of long cephalomedullary nails, with a brief discussion on double plating.

PREOPERATIVE PREPARATION

Arthrodesis for salvage of the chronically infected TKA should be preceded by aggressive treatment of the infection, including removal of implants, cement debris and necrotic tissue, an appropriate course of antibiotics (perhaps even chronic antibiotic suppressive therapy), and a period of treatment with antibiotic-impregnated spacers (Fig. 34-1). Ideally, the serum C-reactive protein and erythrocyte sedimentation rate should be normalized, and there should be negative cultures of fluid from a joint aspiration or tissue biopsy. If evidence exists of residual infection or necrotic tissue, further debridement and attempts at eradication of the infection should be performed before attempting arthrodesis.

The history should determine whether the patient has ipsilateral hip, ankle, or foot problems that would influence the decision to proceed with arthrodesis and the choice of technique for fusion. Determine whether the patient has a hip replacement, previous hip fracture, or hardware in place. Examine the ipsilateral hip and ankle to make sure range of motion is adequate to sustain the patient following the arthrodesis. Determine if there are other problems related to the ipsilateral hip or femur, such as deformity, which would have an impact on knee arthrodesis. Document the neurovascular status of the limb. Make sure the patient has an adequate vascular supply to heal skin incisions at the knee. Examine the skin integrity to determine whether muscle flaps are present from previous reconstructions that need special consideration during surgical exposure.

Anteroposterior and lateral radiographs of the affected knee and entire lower extremity from hip to ankle are necessary to identify existing deformity, assess bone stock, and ensure that no unexpected findings are present through the entire length of the femur and tibia (such as extra-articular deformity or retained hardware) that would preclude the use of intramedullary fixation. Apparent obstructions, such as fracture malunion, callus or deformity, ipsilateral hip arthroplasty, or retained hardware require an alternative to intramedullary fixation (such as plating or external fixation). A long, standing radiograph from hips to ankles with radiographic magnification markers is helpful to determine the overall limb alignment, to identify whether there are bony deformities of the femur or tibia, and to plan for fixation device dimensions. If fusion with a long antegrade intramedullary nail is anticipated, calculate the proper nail length and diameter; this calculation needs to take into account the radiographic magnification. The measurement should extend from the tip of the greater trochanter to within 8 cm from the tibial plafond. The calculation should also account for the gap between the distal femur and the proximal tibia that will be closed at arthrodesis and the bone that will be removed as the distal femur and proximal tibia are trimmed to optimize apposition during

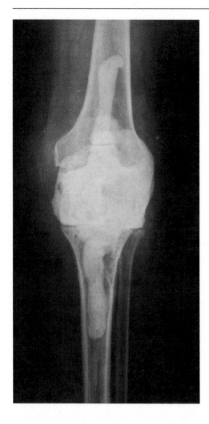

FIGURE 34-1

Preoperative x-ray showing the presence of a spacer block in a patient's knee after multiple attempts at salvage of a chronically infected total knee arthroplasty.

arthrodesis. Lateral radiographs of the femur and tibia with radiographic markers are helpful to determine the proper diameters of the femoral and tibial portions of the rod. Restoring limb length after failed treatment of infection after TKA is less important than maximizing bone apposition and achieving successful fusion. Therefore, use of structural graft to restore lost bone mass and length is not generally advised.

TECHNIQUE

Setup

Placement of an intramedullary device for knee arthrodesis requires a radiolucent operating room table with a single C-arm fluoroscopic unit. The C-arm is best positioned over the patient (not under the operating room table). The patient is placed in a lateral decubitus position with the affected limb up (Fig. 34-2). Alternatively, the patient could be positioned semi-supine with a bump under the ipsilateral hip. The affected limb should be prepared and draped free from the gluteal region, torso, anterior hemipelvis, and buttock down to the ankle. This optimizes positioning, access to the

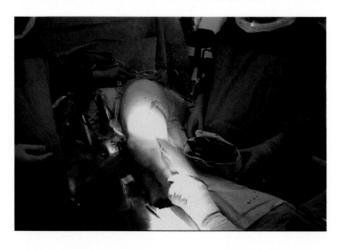

FIGURE 34-2

Patient positioned in the lateral decubitus position.

hip area, and maneuverability while the guide, reamer, and nail are passed antegrade through the hip. Do not use an ipsilateral arm board, as this will get in the way during passage of the guidewire, reamers, and the long nail. A sterile tourniquet may be placed on the thigh during knee exposure. Prior to starting surgery, confirm that the starting point for antegrade intramedullary nailing is accessible. Also confirm that the distal part of the leg is accessible where a distal interlocking screw may be inserted.

Procedure

The knee is approached through the standard anterior arthrotomy. If that is not possible, use the same criteria for choosing incisions as one would for revision knee arthroplasty. Be sure to maintain full-thickness skin flaps and avoid devascularization of the skin. If the patella is still present, perform either a straight midline or a medial parapatellar arthrotomy, and elliptically excise the patella. Obtain adequate exposure to débride the knee. Remove antibiotic-impregnated cement spacer blocks if present and débride soft tissue from the metaphyseal bone ends. Remove only the minimum amount of bone necessary to obtain adequate contact between the surfaces of the femur and tibia. The goal is to cut the femur and tibia perpendicular to the long axis of the medullary canal of each with no posterior slope. The distal femoral and proximal tibial canals are identified (Fig. 34-3A). The tibia is reamed in an antegrade fashion under direct vision with flexible intramedullary reamers, the last of which matches the size of the tibial portion of the nail (Fig. 34-3B). This determines nail diameter. At this point, the guidewire is passed retrograde into the femur, across the isthmus, and into the greater trochanter (Fig. 34-3C). Using fluoroscopic guidance, the guidewire is gently advanced through the tip of the greater trochanter and then retrieved through a small stab incision in the buttock (Fig. 34-4A–C).

The surgeon makes an incision at the level of the greater trochanter, centered over the guidewire and extended proximally and slightly posteriorly on the buttock. The incision should be large enough to identify the greater trochanter and piriformis fossa. To initiate an opening proximally in the tip of the greater trochanter, an awl or small guidewire and cannulated drill may be used. Once optimal

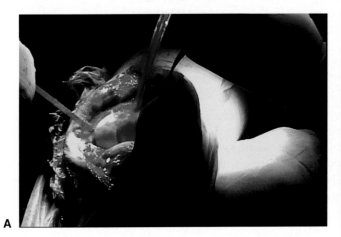

A

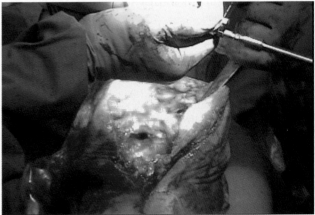

B

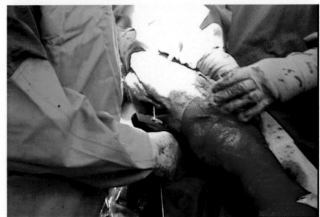

C

FIGURE 34-3

(A) Removal of antibiotic-impregnated spacer. **(B)** Reaming of the tibia (antegrade). **(C)** Guidewire introduced into the femur (retrograde).

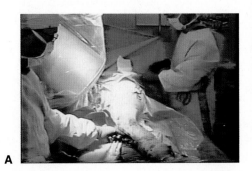

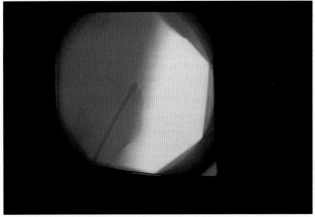

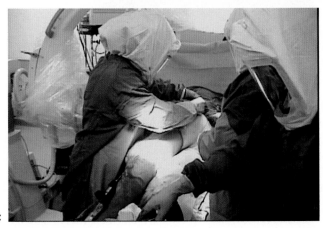

FIGURE 34-4

(A) Advancing guidewire retrograde into the femur.
(B) Fluoroscopic view of the guidewire passed retrograde into the tip of the greater trochanter.
(C) Retrieving the guidewire at the hip region.

position has been established, the opening is made, and a guidewire is passed down the femoral canal and recovered through the anterior knee incision at the level of the distal femoral canal. The guidewire is directed across the joint, introduced into the proximal tibia, and passed to the level of the distal tibial physeal scar.

Femoral reaming commences in an antegrade fashion (Fig. 34-5). In the event the reamer is of insufficient length to ream the tibia antegrade from the hip incision, reaming the tibia can be performed through the knee incision. The femur is reamed 2 mm larger than the size of the nail to accommodate the bow of the implant. It is helpful to use fluoroscopic visualization at the level of the knee when passing the reamer (and eventually the nail) across the knee (Fig. 34-6A). This step will ensure that the tibia is positioned under the femur on both the anteroposterior and lateral views.

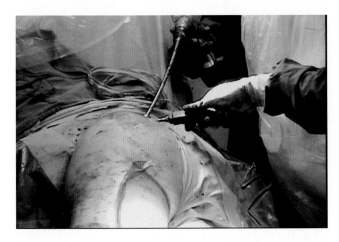

FIGURE 34-5
Femoral reaming (antegrade).

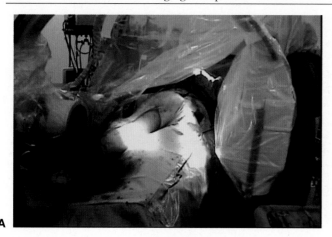

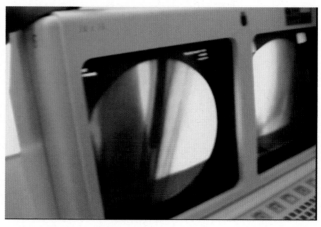

A   B

FIGURE 34-6

(A) Advancing the nail. The fluoroscopy arm is positioned at the level of the knee to observe the nail going across the knee into the tibia. **(B)** Fluoroscopic view confirming passage of the nail into the tibia.

The rod is selected and mounted on the proximal targeting guide/inserter. It is introduced antegrade into the femur through the starting hole in the greater trochanter and carefully advanced by tapping the inserter handle. The advancement of the nail is viewed fluoroscopically (Fig. 34-6B). As the nail exits the distal femur, it is particularly important to ensure that the tibial and femoral canals are aligned for nail passage into the tibial metaphysis. Once the nail enters the tibial metaphysis, it is critically important to select the final rotational position of the foot. It is more difficult to adjust the rotation once the nail is seated beyond the tibial isthmus. Try to align the limb so that the rotation of the foot is similar to the foot progression angle on the contralateral limb, typically between 0 and 5 degrees of external rotation. Carefully, the rod seating is completed with frequent fluoroscopic views.

Femoral and tibial bone at the fusion site need not always be grafted (2). In cases with poor femoral-tibial bone apposition, preparation of the proximal tibia with a convex reamer and the distal femur with a concave reamer has been described to allow the bone ends to key together (3). However, try to avoid further shortening of the lower extremity. Gaps in bone contact can be grafted with a small amount of autograft or fresh-frozen allograft morsels.

The femoral nail should be seated such that the proximal tip is flush with the tip of the greater trochanter, thus making for correct placement of the proximal interlocking screw. Proximal interlocking of the nail is then performed using the previously attached and secured insertion/targeting guide (Fig. 34-7A,B). At this stage, final alignment and fusion site compression are assessed. A

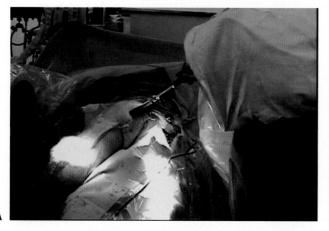

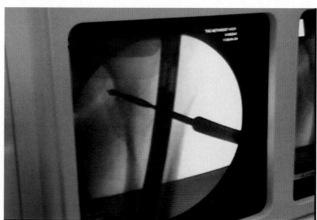

A   B

FIGURE 34-7

(A) Proximal interlocking of the nail is performed using the previously attached and secured insertion/targeting guide. **(B)** Fluoroscope screen showing drill bit passed through the proximal interlocking slot in the nail.

distal interlocking screw is not always necessary in the tibia; however, it may be helpful if a very tight fit in the tibial isthmus is not achieved. If a distal interlocking screw is used, the distal interlock may be placed first, then the nail is backslapped to provide optimal apposition of the bone ends and minimize bone distraction at the knee. If distal interlocking screws are not used, a small amount of distraction of the bone ends is permissible, with subsequent weight bearing providing the necessary compression for union. Incision closure may then be performed over the trochanteric region and anterior knee (Fig. 34-8).

A recognized complication of knee arthrodesis with hardware fixation is recurrent infection. During nail placement, it may be helpful to avoid burying the interlocking screws or the nail tip into the bone. Hole coverage of the proximal nail may be provided as recommended by the manufacturer for subsequent removal, if this is indicated for resolution of infection and irrigation and debridement.

PEARLS AND PITFALLS

Preoperative Planning

- During the preoperative planning process, make sure the proposed intramedullary rod diameter and length are appropriate. Be particularly careful with mathematics involved in calculating radiographic magnification. Be careful not to make the rod too long by failing to allow for the limb shortening that occurs when the femur and tibia are brought together.
- The selection of an appropriate knee incision is of paramount importance to enhance exposure and also to minimize the risk of local skin necrosis, when a knee has multiple scars. Avoid incisions less than 7 cm from previous scars and adhere to the principles outlined in Chapter 33.

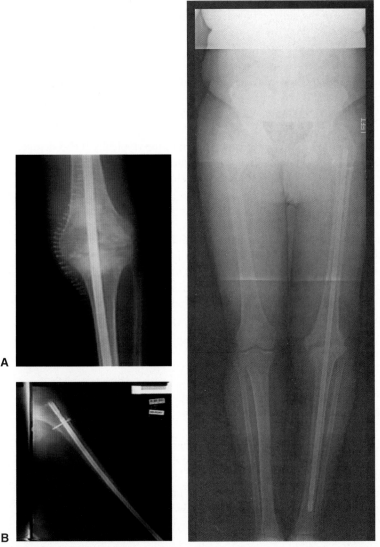

A

B

FIGURE 34-8

(A) Postoperative x-ray of knee. **(B)** Postoperative x-ray of proximal nail with interlocking screw. **(C)** At 1 year postoperatively, the limb is pain free, and there are no clinical signs of persistent infection, but there appears to have been some local bone resorption.

C

Positioning

- Lateral positioning of the patient resembles a hip replacement procedure.
- Position the C-arm over the patient.
- Make sure that there is ample access available for antegrade nail insertion. Insufficient proximal sterile field and exposure at the level of the trochanter increases risk for contamination during the procedure.

Procedure: Bone Preparation

- Localizing the greater trochanter in large patients or those with poorly defined anatomy can be challenging. Consider using fluoroscopy with a percutaneous guide pin to assist in this effort.
- An excessively medial femoral neck starting point may increase the risk of femoral head or neck fracture or postoperative osteonecrosis. Be sure to start the nail in the greater trochanter or piriformis fossa (this may vary according to features of the nail and specific technical aspects that vary with systems).
- An anterior knee incision will facilitate passage of the guidewire and nail from the distal femur into the proximal tibia, as well as allow appropriate preparation of the bone surfaces.
- Remove the collateral ligament and capsular attachments from the distal femur through the knee incision to aid in alignment during wire and nail passage.
- A pair of matched convex and concave reamers may be useful in preparation of the bone ends to enhance bone apposition.
- Poor bone quality in the distal femur may allow the guidewire to penetrate the cortex prior to passage from the distal femur; pass with care and under fluoroscopic visualization.
- The femur is reamed 2 mm larger than the planned nail diameter to accommodate the femoral bow.
- The tibia is reamed to the diameter of the nail to allow rigid fixation.

Procedure: Implant Placement

- Without proper visualization and alignment across the knee joint, the nail may fracture the distal femur or proximal tibia when passed at this level.
- Correct rotation of the lower extremity should be secured prior to passing the nail into the tibial diaphysis.
- Limb rotation should approximate the rotation of the contralateral limb (typically 0 to 5 degrees of external rotation). This is verified before inserting the distal interlocking screw, if the decision is made to use one. It is performed with the "perfect circles" freehand technique.

Proximal Interlocking Technique

- During the insertion and advancement of the nail, make sure that the insertion/targeting guide does not loosen and that the soft tissue protector/drill sleeve is directed to the interlocking holes in the nail. After seating the nail, it is impossible to confirm that the targeting guide has not loosened. If it has loosened, the proximal interlocking screw may miss the hole and be inserted anterior or posterior to the nail. It may appear that the screw is appropriately positioned in the interlocking hole on the anteroposterior fluoroscopic view, but it is imperative to confirm its position with oblique and lateral fluoroscopic views before closing the wounds and applying the dressings.

Final Assessment

- Make a final assessment of limb rotation and arthrodesis-site bone approximation. Although conical reamers may enhance bone contact, use liberal amounts of bone graft to fill the metaphyseal regions where there is no bone apposition.
- Make sure that rotational alignment of the patient's limb is proper before completing interlocking screw placement. Correct rotation of the lower extremity is critical. It may be helpful to compare to the contralateral limb before draping.
- Wound closure may be more difficult after the arthrodesis as the tibia tends to translate anteriorly relative to the femur during intramedullary arthrodesis. Use a saw to trim prominent bone off the femur and tibia (usually anterior on the tibia and medial/lateral on the femur) to facilitate closure.

ALTERNATIVE TECHNIQUE: DOUBLE PLATING

Double plating is more effective than unilateral plating or external fixation techniques. The patient is positioned supine on the operating table. The patient's previous midline anterior vertical incision is used for access to the knee or an alternative incision as you would for a knee revision. Maintain full-thickness skin flaps and minimize undermining of the subcutaneous tissues. Perform a medial parapatellar arthrotomy, or if there is no patella, incise along the medial border of the extensor mechanism. Patellectomy is performed. Viable bone (if present) can be used as bone graft. Use tibial and femoral cutting guides from the knee arthroplasty instrumentation sets to cut the femur and tibia. Cut the femur at approximately 5 degrees of valgus with an intramedullary guide. Cut the tibia perpendicular to its axis in the coronal planes, in slight flexion (back slope), and in the sagittal plane (which will provide slight knee flexion). Alternatively, male and female conical reamers can be used, as described in the technique for intramedullary fusion. Trim enough bone to provide good apposition between the femur and the tibia. Avoid excessive bone trimming to avoid additional limb shortening.

Hold the arthrodesis in proper axial and rotational alignment with the bone surfaces compressed together. Contour a large fragment plate to fit anteromedially. To prevent the plate from being too prominent, small troughs can be made in the metaphyseal flare of the femur to allow the plate to sit well. Next, contour another large fragment plate to sit anterolaterally. Place the plate at approximately 90 degrees to the first plate. Overbend the plates slightly to provide compression across the arthrodesis site. Place multiple screws through the femur and tibia using a dynamic compression technique. Try to obtain fixation with at least four bicortical screws proximal and distal to the arthrodesis site through each plate (Fig. 34-9A–C). Bone graft the arthrodesis site with autogenous bone using the sources mentioned for intramedullary arthrodesis. Close the wound in a layered fashion. Handle and close the skin with care.

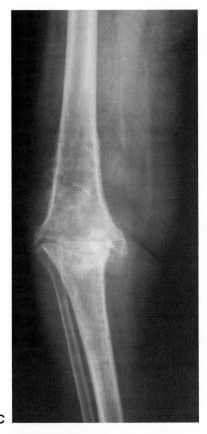
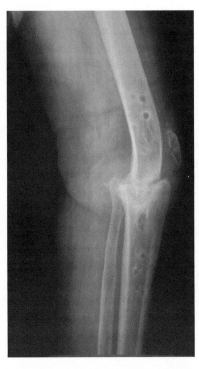
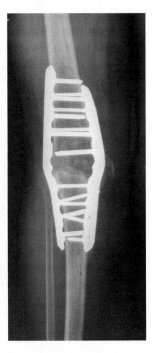

A–C

FIGURES 34-9

(A,B) Anteroposterior and lateral x-rays after unsuccessful arthrodesis using biplanar external fixator. **(C)** The knee was successfully fused with a dual-plating technique.

POSTOPERATIVE MANAGEMENT

Upon completion of intramedullary knee arthrodesis, weight bearing as tolerated should be allowed (4). When the patient has excessive bone loss, limited weight bearing may be necessary to prevent fracture; however, ample bone grafting should be used in these cases. Stabilizing the knee with cast or bracing techniques is not necessary unless rod (or plate) fixation is compromised. An appropriately sized shoe lift should be fitted by a certified orthotist.

COMPLICATIONS

Skin- or wound-related problems may occur, particularly because these knees have often undergone multiple surgeries through the same atrophic scars, as well as a result of the bunching up of the soft tissues that occurs when the limb is shortened during the fusion. Wound problems should be treated meticulously with care that ranges from local debridement to flap coverage depending on the extent of the problem (5). If deep infection occurs, the surgeon attempts to treat the infection surgically with debridement and parenteral antibiotics followed by chronic suppression. Try not to remove the fixation device until the arthrodesis has healed. Long intramedullary nails can be removed through the hip area; plates and screws by exposing the knee. Once the knee has fused, short modular nails, however, cannot be removed unless the fusion is taken down or if a large anterior cortical window is made. This makes the use of short modular fusion nails less desirable in our hands for fusing chronically infected knees. Nonunion or delayed union can occur, particularly when multiple previous revisions had been performed and if there is considerable metaphyseal bone loss. It is more common with external fixators. When nonunion or delayed union occurs, dynamizing the nail can be helpful if a long nail had been used and if distal interlocking screws are present. Additionally, autogenous bone grafting, or allografting with bone-forming stimulants can be considered when a nail or plates have been used. Pin site infections are common with external fixators and one of the reasons we prefer not to use them. Limb shortening of between 2 and 6 cm is not uncommon after knee arthrodesis performed for infection after TKA. The extent of shortening depends on whether the preceding procedure was a primary or revision arthroplasty and how much bone had been removed during prior knee revisions or during debridement to deal with the infection. Finally, the absence of knee motion after arthrodesis imposes some very practical drawbacks; nonetheless, as a salvage operation, successful fusion is a desirable outcome compared to the alternatives such as resection arthroplasty or above-knee amputation.

RESULTS

Historically, nonintramedullary techniques (such as plating and external fixation) for knee arthrodesis as a salvage for infection after TKA has had successful fusion rates between 70% and 80%. In contrast, intramedullary techniques have success rates above 90% (1,2,4,6,7). One recent study found that infection was eradicated in 94% of difficult and compromised patients. Successful fusion was achieved in 96% of patients treated with intramedullary nailing compared to 67% treated with external fixation, although surgical time and blood loss was higher in the intramedullary nailing group. Supplemental bone graft was used during index fusion in 34%. Forty-one percent of patients had complications, including pin-site infections (21%), delayed unions (10%), fractures through pin sites (8%), and deep infections (5%) (1).

REFERENCES

1. Mabry TM, Jacofsky DJ, Haidukewych GJ, et al. The Chitranjan Ranawat Award. Comparison of intramedullary nailing and external fixation knee arthrodesis for the infected knee replacement. *Clin Orthop* 2007;464:11–15.
2. Incavo SJ, Lilly JW, Bartlett CS, Churchill DL. Arthrodesis of the knee: experience with intramedullary nailing. *J Arthrop* 2000;15:9871–9876.
3. Bargiotas K, Wohhlrab D, Sewecke JJ, et al. Arthrodesis of the knee with a long intramedullary nail following the failure of a total knee arthroplasty as the result of infection: surgical technique. *J Bone Joint Surg Am* 2007;89 (Suppl 2):103–110.
4. Donley BG, Matthews LS, Kaufer H. Arthrodesis of the knee with an intramedullary nail. *J Bone Joint Surg Am* 1991;73:907–913.
5. Morrey BF, Shives TC. The Knee: Arthrodesis. In: Morrey BF, ed. *Reconstructive Surgery of the Joints*, 2nd ed. New York: Churchill Livingstone; 1996.
6. Waldman BJ, Mont MA, Payman KR, et al. Infected total knee arthroplasty treated with arthrodesis using a modular nail. *Clin Orthop* 1999;367:230–237.
7. Stiehl JB, Hanel DP. Knee arthrodesis using combined intramedullary rod and plate fixation. *Clin Orthop* 1993;294:238.

Index

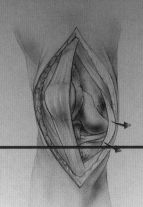

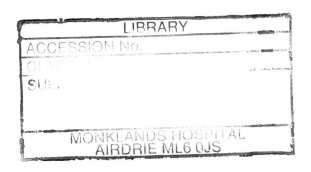